Musculoskeletal Ultrasound with MRI Correlations

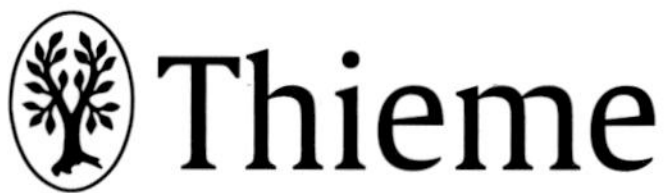

Thieme

Musculoskeletal Ultrasound with MRI Correlations

Vikram S. Dogra, MD
Professor of Radiology
Director of Ultrasound
Associate Chair for Education and Research
Department of Imaging Sciences
University of Rochester Medical Center
Rochester, New York

Diana Gaitini, MD
Associate Clinical Professor
Director, Ultrasound Unit
Department of Medical Imaging
Rambam Medical Center and Faculty of Medicine
Technion, Israel Institute of Technology
Haifa, Israel

Associate Editor

Johnny U. V. Monu, MD
Professor
Department of Imaging Sciences
University of Rochester Medical Center
Rochester, New York

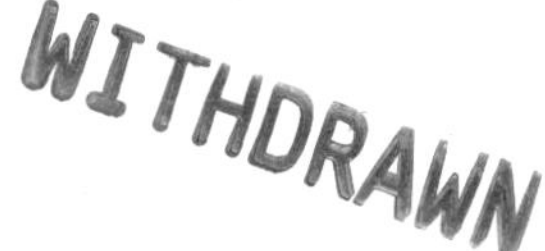

Thieme
New York • Stuttgart

Thieme Medical Publishers, Inc.
333 Seventh Avenue
New York, NY 10001

Editorial Director: Michael Wachinger
Executive Editor: Timothy Y. Hiscock
Managing Editor: J. Owen Zurhellen IV
Editorial Assistant: Emma Lassiter
International Production Director: Andreas Schabert
Production Editor: Martha L. Wetherill, MPS Content Services
Vice President, International Marketing and Sales: Cornelia Schulze
Chief Financial Officer: James Mitos
President: Brian D. Scanlan
Compositor: MPS Content Services, A Macmillan Company
Printer: Everbest

Library of Congress Cataloging-in-Publication Data
Musculoskeletal ultrasound with MRI correlations / [edited by] Vikram S. Dogra, Diana Gaitini.
p. ; cm.
Includes bibliographical references.
ISBN 978-1-60406-244-1
1. Musculoskeletal system—Ultrasonic imaging. 2. Musculoskeletal system—Magnetic resonance imaging.
3. Musculoskeletal system—Diseases—Diagnosis. I. Dogra, Vikram S. II. Gaitini, Diana.
[DNLM: 1. Musculoskeletal Diseases—ultrasonography—Atlases. 2. Magnetic Resonance Imaging—Atlases.
3. Musculoskeletal System—ultrasonography—Atlases. WE 17 M9855 2010]
RC925.7.M89 2010
616.7'07548—dc22

2010002163

Important note: Medical knowledge is ever-changing. As new research and clinical experience broaden our knowledge, changes in treatment and drug therapy may be required. The authors and editors of the material herein have consulted sources believed to be reliable in their efforts to provide information that is complete and in accord with the standards accepted at the time of publication. However, in view of the possibility of human error by the authors, editors, or publisher of the work herein or changes in medical knowledge, neither the authors, editors, nor publisher, nor any other party who has been involved in the preparation of this work, warrants that the information contained herein is in every respect accurate or complete, and they are not responsible for any errors or omissions or for the results obtained from use of such information. Readers are encouraged to confirm the information contained herein with other sources. For example, readers are advised to check the product information sheet included in the package of each drug they plan to administer to be certain that the information contained in this publication is accurate and that changes have not been made in the recommended dose or in the contraindications for administration. This recommendation is of particular importance in connection with new or infrequently used drugs.

Printed in China

5 4 3 2 1

ISBN 978-1-60406-244-1

This book is dedicated to all my teachers.

—VSD

This book is dedicated to my beloved family, for their support and encouragement, and to my wise teachers, for introducing me to the world of medical imaging.

—DG

Contents

Preface .... **ix**

Acknowledgments .... **xi**

Contributors .... **xiii**

1 Imaging of the Shoulder 1
Diana Gaitini, Daniela Militianu, Alicia Nachtigal, and Vikram S. Dogra

2 Imaging of the Elbow 22
Gerd Gruber and Werner Konermann
Translated by Axel W. E. Wismueller and Vikram S. Dogra

3 Imaging of the Wrist 46
Ximena Wortsman and Patricio Azocar

4 Imaging of the Hand 71
Ian Yu-Yan Tsou, Seng Choe Tham, and Gervais K. L. Wansaicheong

5 Imaging of the Knee 92
Ian Beggs

6 Imaging of the Foot and Ankle 106
Gervais K. L. Wansaicheong, Ian Yu-Yan Tsou, and Seng Choe Tham

7 Imaging of the Hip 117
Ahmet Tuncay Turgut, Elif Ergun, Pınar Koşar, and Vikram S. Dogra

8 Bone Imaging 132
Diana Gaitini, Daniela Militianu, Alicia Nachtigal, and Vikram S. Dogra

9 Skin Imaging 147
Ximena Wortsman and Jacobo Wortsman

10 Peripheral Nerve Imaging 171
Siegfried Peer and Werner Judmaier

11 Ultrasound for Rheumatoid Arthritis 194
Robert R. Lopez-Ben

12 Imaging of Muscle, Soft Tissue, and Foreign Bodies 207
Michael A. Bruno, Ashok Kumar Nath, A. U. Sethu, and Khamis Al Muzahmi

13 Ultrasound-Guided Procedures 220
Cesare Romagnoli, Tobias De Zordo, Andrea S. Klauser, and Rethy Chhem

Index **245**

Preface

Imaging is an indispensable tool in the diagnosis and treatment of musculoskeletal disorders. Despite advances in magnetic resonance imaging (MRI) and computed tomographic (CT) imaging, ultrasound remains a useful imaging tool that boasts the advantage of real-time dynamic imaging, lack of radiation, and cost effectiveness. Musculoskeletal (MSK) ultrasound provides a multiplanar real-time high resolution imaging method for anatomy and pathology investigation. Ultrasound is a widely available and low-cost modality that in well-trained hands becomes an invaluable diagnostic tool. Although MRI is widely used in the Western world to diagnose MSK disorders, increasing healthcare costs are leading to a shift in utilizing ultrasound for MSK disorders, especially in the United States.

This book, *Musculoskeletal Ultrasound with MRI Correlations*, is presented in an atlas format. High-quality exemplary ultrasound images with MRI (and occasionally CT) correlation have been included to aid in the understanding of the different pathologies. The book is composed of 13 chapters. The chapters cover clinical indications; technical guidelines; normal anatomy; and degenerative, inflammatory, traumatic, tumoral, and miscellaneous pathologies. Pearls and pitfalls are included at the end of each chapter. The book details a practical, point-by-point checklist of how to perform MSK ultrasound.

We intended to present a well-organized and easy-to-read book, with key facts highlighted separately and in a bulleted style to facilitate learning. We hope and expect that this book will be a valuable addition to the technical know-how of MSK ultrasound as well as a pleasant reading at every level, during and after the training period in medical imaging. The information will be beneficial for sonographers, radiologists, orthopedic specialists, emergency medicine physicians, rheumatologists, and in-training physicians. Our goal was to provide a useful resource in their day-to-day practice.

We have assembled a group of leading MSK experts to contribute. This brings a global perspective to this book. Their valuable knowledge and experience in this field as well as their dedication and hard work allowed this project to materialize. We are very grateful to them.

Vikram S. Dogra, MD
Diana Gaitini, MD

Acknowledgments

It has been our privilege to be the editors of this book. We wish to thank our contributors for their outstanding work and cooperation without which this book would not have been possible. We also thank Timothy Hiscock, J. Owen Zurhellen, and Emma Lassiter of Thieme's editorial department. We would like to express our gratitude to Patricia Miller for her hard work and dedication in providing the secretarial assistance for the preparation of this book. We would also like to acknowledge Margaret Kowaluk, Katie Tower, and Sarah Peangatelli for their graphic support.

Contributors

Patricio Azocar, MD
Radiology Department
Hospital del Trabajador
Santiago, Chile

Ian Beggs, MB ChB, FRCR
Royal Infirmary of Edinburgh
Edinburgh, United Kingdom

Michael A. Bruno, MS, MD
Associate Professor of Radiology and Medicine
Department of Radiology
The Penn State Milton S. Hershey Medical Center
Hershey, Pennsylvania

Rethy Chhem, PhD
Adjunct Professor
Department of Radiology
Medical University of Vienna
Vienna, Austria

Tobias De Zordo, MD
Radiology Research Fellow
Department of Diagnostic Radiology and Nuclear Medicine
London Health Science Centre–University Hospital
London, Ontario
Department of Diagnostic Radiology
Medical University Innsbruck
Innsbruck, Austria

Vikram S. Dogra, MD
Professor of Radiology
Director of Ultrasound
Associate Chair for Education and Research
Department of Imaging Sciences
University of Rochester Medical Center
Rochester, New York

Elif Ergun, MD
Instructor in Radiology
Department of Radiology
Ankara Training and Research Hospital
Ankara, Turkey

Diana Gaitini, MD
Associate Clinical Professor
Director, Ultrasound Unit
Department of Medical Imaging
Rambam Medical Center and Faculty of Medicine
Technion, Israel Institute of Technology
Haifa, Israel

Gerd Gruber, Dr Med
Privat Docent
Atos-Klinik
Heidelberg, Germany

Werner Judmaier, MD
Institute of MR Imaging and Spectroscopy
Innsbruck University Hospital
Innsbruck, Austria

Andrea S. Klauser, MD
Associate Professor of Radiology
Department of Radiology
Medical University Innsbruck
Innsbruck, Austria

Werner Konermann, Dr Med
Chefarzt
Rotes Kreuz Krankenhaus Kassel
Gemeinnützige GmbH
Klinik für Orthopädie, Unfallchirurgie und Rehabilitative Medizin
Kassel, Germany

Pınar Koşar, MD
Instructor in Radiology
Department of Radiology
Ankara Training and Research Hospital
Ankara, Turkey

Robert R. Lopez-Ben, MD
Associate Professor
Department of Radiology
University of Alabama at Birmingham School of Medicine
Birmingham, Alabama

Daniela Militianu, MD
Director of the Musculoskeletal Unit
Deputy Director
Department of Medical Imaging
Rambam Health Care Campus
Haifa, Israel

Johnny U. V. Monu, MD
Professor
Department of Imaging Sciences
University of Rochester Medical Center
Rochester, New York

Khamis Al Muzahmi, MD
Senior Consultant
Department of Radiology
Khoula Hospital
Muscat, Sultanate of Oman

Alicia Nachtigal, MD
Director
Department of Medical imaging
Hillel Yaffe Medical Center
Hadera, Israel

Ashok Kumar Nath, MD
Senior Specialist
Department of Radiology
Khoula Hospital
Muscat, Sultanate of Oman

Siegfried Peer, MD
Professor of Radiology
Department of Radiology
Innsbruck University Hospital
Innsbruck, Austria

Cesare Romagnoli, MD
Department of Radiology
University of Western Ontario
London, Ontario
Canada

A. U. Sethu, MD
Senior Consultant
Department of Orthopedics
Khoula Hospital
Muscat, Sultanate of Oman

Seng Choe Tham, MD
Department of Diagnostic Radiology
Tan Tock Seng Hospital
Singapore

Ian Yu-Yan Tsou, MD, FRCR (UK)
Department of Radiology
Mount Elizabeth Hospital and Medical Centre
Singapore

Ahmet Tuncay Turgut, MD
Associate Professor of Radiology
Department of Radiology
Ankara Training and Research Hospital
Ankara, Turkey

Gervais K. L. Wansaicheong, MBBS
Department of Diagnostic Radiology
Tan Tock Seng Hospital
Singapore

Axel W. E. Wismueller, MD, PhD
Department of Radiology
University of Rochester
Rochester, New York

Jacobo Wortsman, MD
Department of Medicine
Southern Illinois University School of Medicine
Springfield, Illinois

Ximena Wortsman, MD
Radiology Department
Clinica Servet
Santiago, Chile

1 Imaging of the Shoulder

Diana Gaitini, Daniela Militianu, Alicia Nachtigal, and Vikram S. Dogra

Shoulder pain is a common complaint in patients over 40 years old and following trauma or infection, at any age. The underlying pathology is variable, from rotator cuff strain to full thickness rotator cuff tear, tendinosis, calcific tendonitis, acromioclavicular arthritis, and cervical radiculopathy. Similar symptoms and physical findings for different pathologic entities make the differential diagnosis a clinical challenge. Diagnosis and therapy, therefore, is increasingly dependent on medical imaging. Plain radiographs and arthrography have been the primary radiologic examinations used to distinguish among the different conditions. A cross-sectional imaging battery, including magnetic resonance imaging (MRI), spiral computerized tomography (CT), and ultrasound, has been incorporated in the routine clinical practice during the last two decades. The decision on which imaging test is the one to start with is in the hands of the clinician, who is not always aware of the advantages and limitations of each test. Our aim in this chapter is to illustrate the appearance of the normal shoulder and different pathologies on multiplanar modalities, emphasizing ultrasound advantages, such as availability and cost-effectiveness that makes it the modality of choice to start with in most patients.

Technical Guidelines and Normal Anatomy

Transducer and Equipment Capabilities

A shoulder examination is performed with a high-resolution linear array transducer. A 5 to 12 MHz and even higher frequency broad bandwidth is optimal; a lower 4 to 8 MHz frequency is useful in heavier patients. New software and hardware technologies such as tissue harmonic, compound, and extended field-of-view (FOV) imaging are essential for a technically successful shoulder examination; in fact, they have become standard techniques for musculoskeletal ultrasonography.

Patient Position

Patients are examined while seated on a revolving stool, which allows easy positioning during scanning. The examiner is seated on a wheeled chair in front of the patient.

Examination Protocol and Normal Anatomy

Shoulder sonography includes scanning the long tendon of the biceps brachialis, the rotator cuff tendon, which includes the subscapularis, infraspinatus, teres minor, and supraspinatus tendons, the glenohumeral joint, the spinoglenoid notch, and the acromioclavicular joint. The examination is completed with a series of dynamic maneuvers to assess rotator cuff impingement and glenohumeral joint fluid.

Transverse Image of the Bicipital Groove and Long Head of the Bicipital Tendon

The patient is seated facing the operator; his or her hands are placed palms up on the thighs. The operator places the transducer at the humeral head (**Fig. 1.1A**). In an axial scan, the bicipital groove appears as a concavity in the surface of the humeral head, detected as a hyperechoic line between the greater and lesser tuberosities. The groove is an anatomic landmark to differentiate between the subscapularis tendon, which is placed medially to it, from the laterally placed supraspinatus tendon. Within the groove, the long head of the biceps tendon is seen as a hyperechoic oval structure (**Fig. 1.1B**). Care should be taken to avoid probe stirring that might make the tendon appear hypoechoic due to anisotropy of normal tendons (**Fig. 1.1C**).

Longitudinal Image of the Bicipital Groove and Long Head of the Bicipital Tendon

The whole long biceps tendon is visualized from the humeral head extending as far down as the musculotendinous junction in the humeral shaft (**Fig. 1.2A**). The tendon reveals a fine fibril pattern (**Fig. 1.2B**).

Transverse Image of the Subscapularis Tendon

The patient is asked to externally rotate his or her arm with abduction of the forearm; the transducer is turned to a transverse position and moved medially from the bicipital groove (**Fig. 1.3A**). The subscapularis tendon is visualized as a band of medium-level echoes (**Fig. 1.3B**). The subdeltoid bursa, placed over the tendon, is seen as a thin convex echogenic line. Passive internal and external rotation helps in assessing integrity of the tendon.

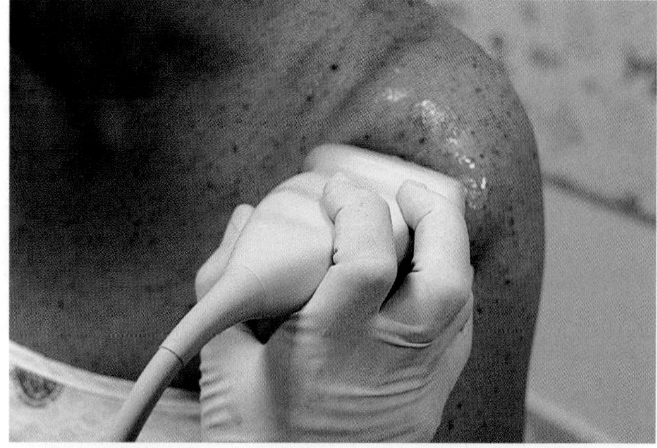

A

Fig. 1.1 Normal long head of the biceps tendon on transverse ultrasound view. **(A)** The probe positioning is over the anterior shoulder on the humeral head. **(B)** A transverse image of the long head of the biceps (*arrows*) that can be seen as a rounded hyperechogenic structure within the bicipital groove (*arrowhead*). **(C)** Tendon anisotropy. There is artifactual low echogenicity of normal biceps tendon (*arrowheads*), while tilting the transducer because of tendon anisotropy.

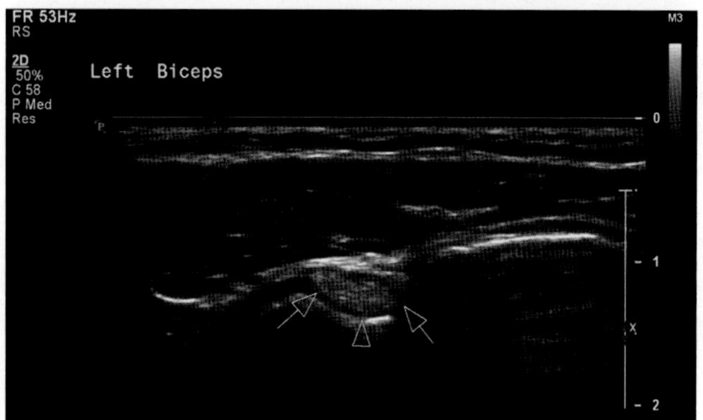

B

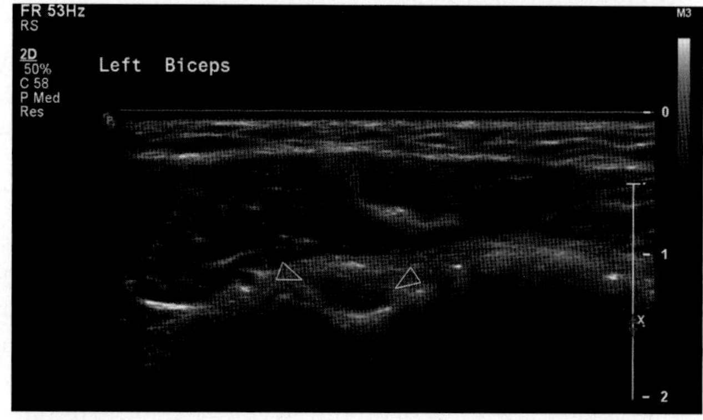

C

Longitudinal Image of the Subscapularis Tendon

The transducer is turned 90 degrees to scan perpendicularly to the tendon axis (**Fig. 1.4A**). The tendon is seen as several groups of fascicles in transverse orientation (**Fig. 1.4B**).

Transverse Image of the Infraspinatus and Teres Minor Tendons

The patient is rotated to be examined from the back, his or her hand is resting on the thigh or is elevated to the opposite

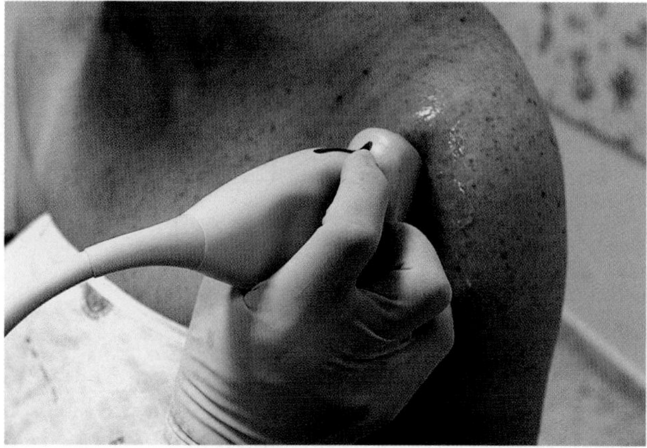

A

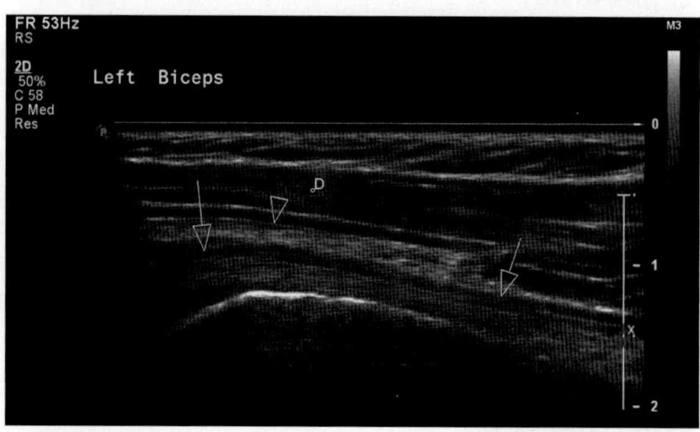

B

Fig. 1.2 Normal long head of the biceps tendon on longitudinal ultrasound view. **(A)** The probe is positioned over the anterior shoulder on the humeral head. **(B)** The tendon is seen as a fine fibril structure laterally (*arrows*). The collapsed subacromial-subdeltoid bursa (*arrowhead*) can be seen between the tendon and the overlying deltoid muscle (D).

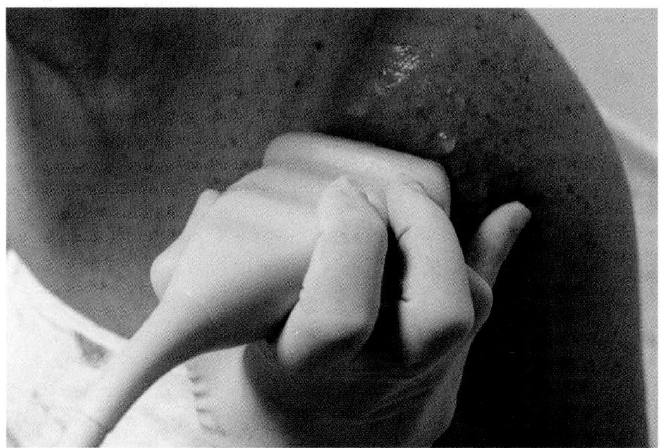

A B

Fig. 1.3 Normal subscapularis tendon on transverse ultrasound view. **(A)** The probe is positioned medial to the bicipital groove for an axial scan. Note the abduction of the patient's forearm. **(B)** The tendon has a convex superficial margin (*arrows*) and is outlined by the subacromial subdeltoid bursa (*arrowhead*), deep to the subdeltoid fat.

shoulder (**Fig. 1.5A**). The infraspinatus tendon appears as a beak-shaped soft tissue structure attaching to the greater tuberosity (**Fig. 1.5B**). Passive external and internal rotation is useful to examine the infraspinatus tendon. By moving the transducer distal on the humerus, the teres minor may be visualized as a trapezoidal structure, differentiated from the infraspinatus by its oblique internal echoes. This small tendon may be not scanned routinely.

Transverse Image of the Glenohumeral Joint

The transducer is moved slightly laterally to the infraspinatus tendon (**Fig. 1.6A**). The articular cartilage of the humeral head is seen as a thin hypoechogenic layer adjacent to the high-level echoes originating from the bony surface. A portion of the posterior glenoid labrum is seen as a hyperechoic triangular structure (**Fig. 1.6B**).

Transverse Image of the Spinoglenoid Notch

The transducer is moved medially to the glenohumeral joint (**Fig. 1.7A**). A slightly concave bone surface is seen, which contains the suprascapular artery, and beside it, the suprascapular nerve (**Fig. 1.7B**). The artery may be detected as a pulsating structure on grayscale ultrasound, better detected on color Doppler.

Transverse Image of the Supraspinatus Tendon

The patient is again seated facing the operator, his or her arm adducted and externally rotated, placing the hand on

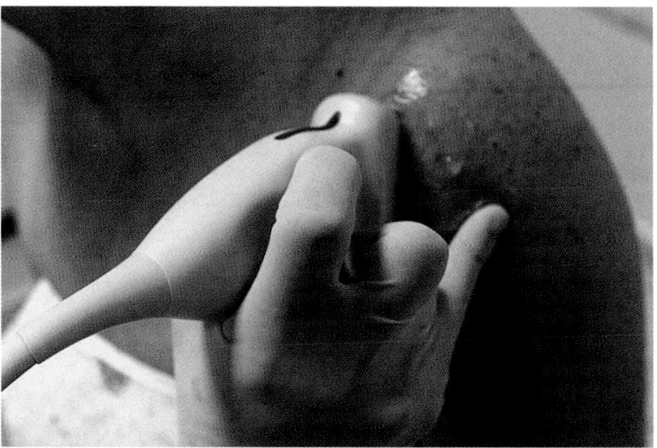

A

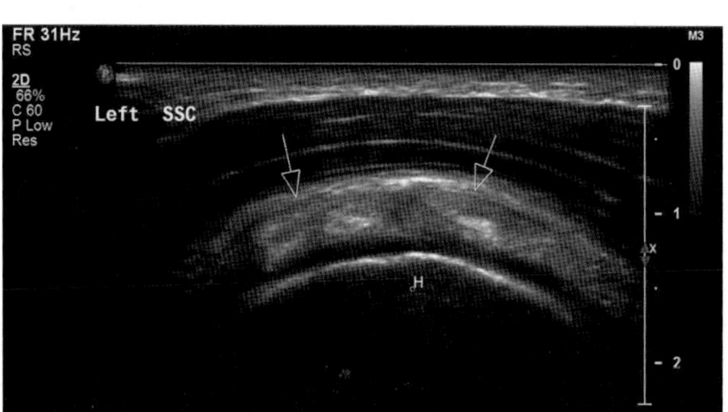

B

Fig. 1.4 Normal subscapularis tendon on longitudinal ultrasound view. **(A)** The probe is positioned medial to the bicipital groove for a sagittal scan. **(B)** The tendon is seen as a convex cuff of fibers (*arrows*) over the underlying hypoechogenic cartilage and the echogenic line of the humeral head (H).

A

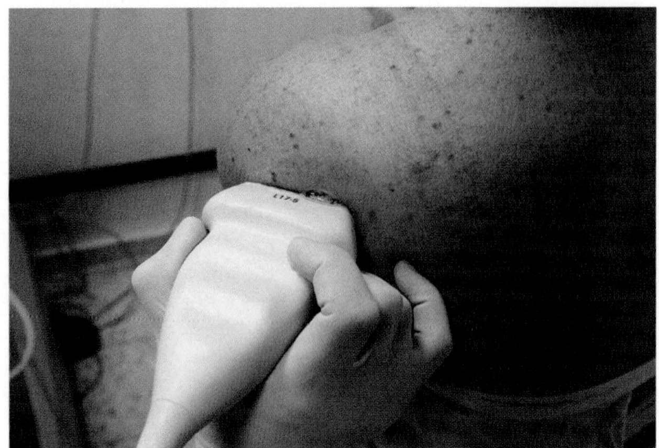

B

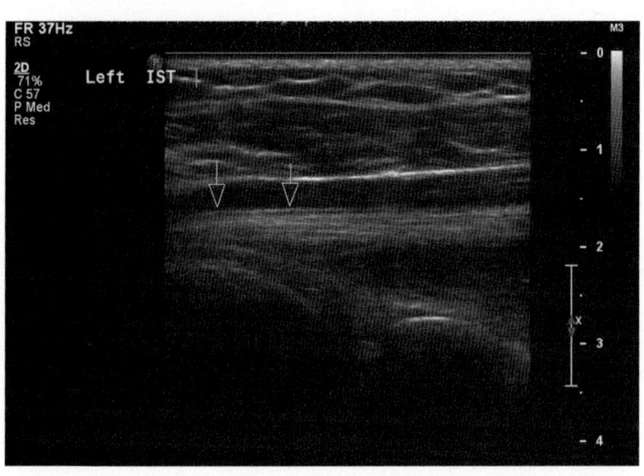

Fig. 1.5 Normal infraspinatus tendon. **(A)** The patient is examined from the back with his or her hand on the opposite shoulder. The probe position is over the posterolateral shoulder. **(B)** A beak-shaped fibril echogenic band (*arrows*) can be seen attached to the greater tuberosity.

A

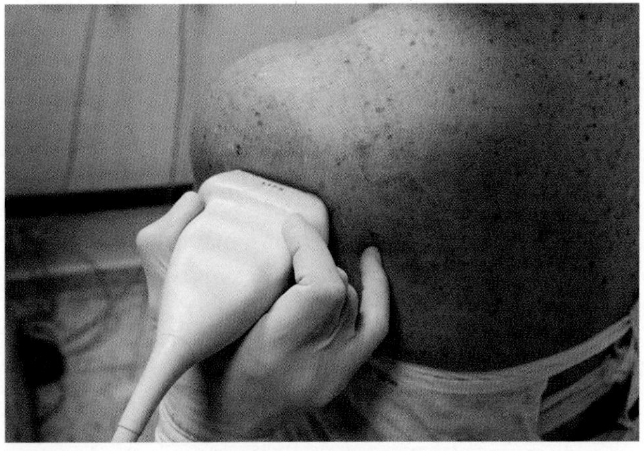

B

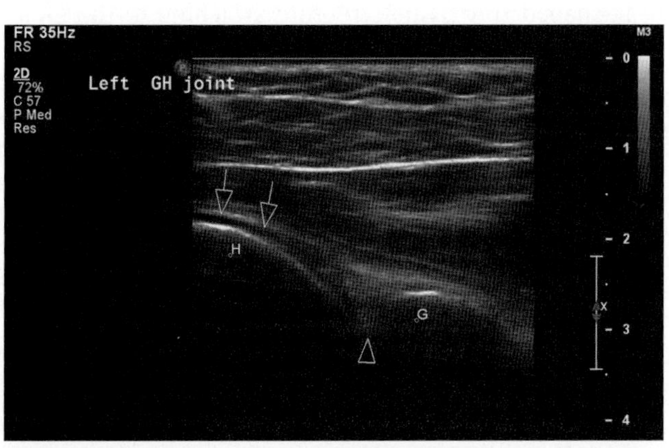

Fig. 1.6 Normal glenohumeral joint. **(A)** The probe is positioned slightly lateral to the infraspinatus tendon. **(B)** A normal rounded hyperechoic contour of the posterior humeral head (H) is seen with hypoechogenic adjacent hyaline cartilage (*arrows*) opposite to the glenoid ridge (G). The normal posterior glenoid labrum is seen as a triangular hyperechoic structure in the depth of the joint (*arrowhead*).

A

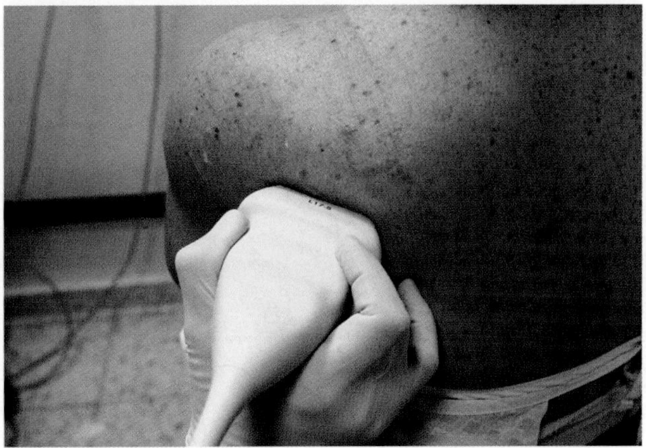

B

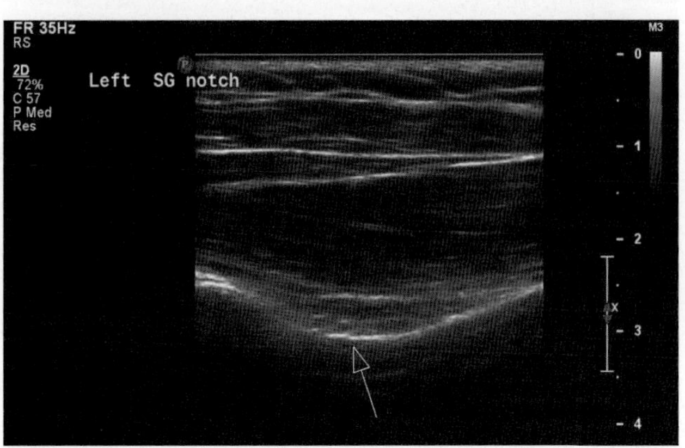

Fig. 1.7 Normal spinoglenoid notch. **(A)** The probe is positioned medial to the joint. **(B)** A slightly concave bone surface (*arrow*) is seen medial to the glenohumeral joint.

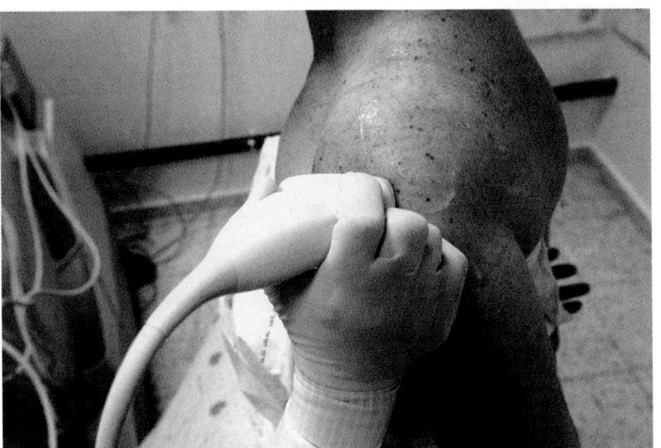

Fig. 1.8 Normal supraspinatus tendon on transverse ultrasound view. **(A)** The probe is positioned lateral and posterior to the bicipital groove. Note the patient's arm is adducted and externally rotated, the hand placed backward on the waist on the opposite side. **(B)** The tendon is seen as a band of echogenic fibers, above the hypoechogenic hyaline cartilage on the humeral head (*arrowheads*) and deep to the thin hypoechogenic layer of the subdeltoid bursa and the echogenic subdeltoid fat (*arrows*).

the back or in the rear pocket with the palm against the body and the elbow directed posteriorly. The transducer is moved laterally from the bicipital groove, in a transverse position (**Fig. 1.8A**). The supraspinatus tendon is seen as a band of medium-level echoes (**Fig. 1.8B**). The convex echogenic line of the subdeltoid bursa is seen above the tendon. The hypoechoic layer of the articular cartilage and the bony layer of the humeral head and greater tuberosity are seen below it. The "critical zone" of the supraspinatus tendon is an area of relative avascularity, more susceptible to injury, and thus, essential to be visualized. It is located in the anterior part of the tendon, one centimeter posterolateral to the biceps tendon. The subacromial subdeltoid bursa is seen above the tendon as a very thin hypoechoic layer surrounded by hyperechoic peribursal fat. The bursa is no more than 2 mm thick including a thin internal layer of fluid.

Longitudinal Image of the Supraspinatus Tendon

The transducer is turned 90 degrees to scan perpendicularly to the tendon axis (**Fig. 1.9A**). The tendon appears as a beak-shaped structure of medium-level echogenicity extending below the acromion to its attachment along the greater tuberosity (**Fig. 1.9B**).

Dynamic Maneuvers for Assessment of Rotator Cuff Impingement

The patient places his or her hand again over the thigh, palm up. The transducer is placed transversally over the acromion, the rotator cuff tendon seen below and lateral to the acromion. The patient is asked to raise his or her arm while in internal rotation, pointing the elbow up (**Fig. 1.10A**).

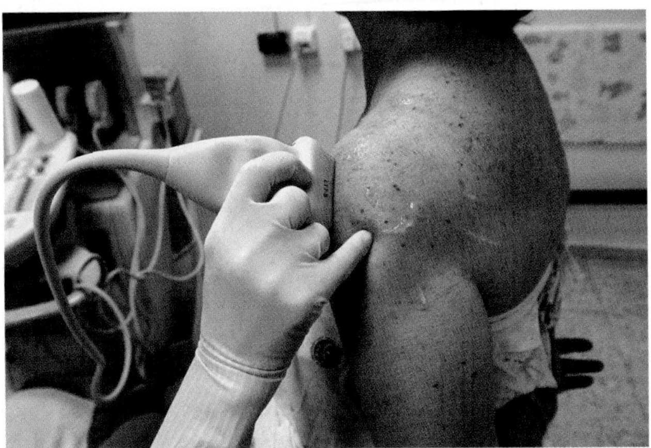

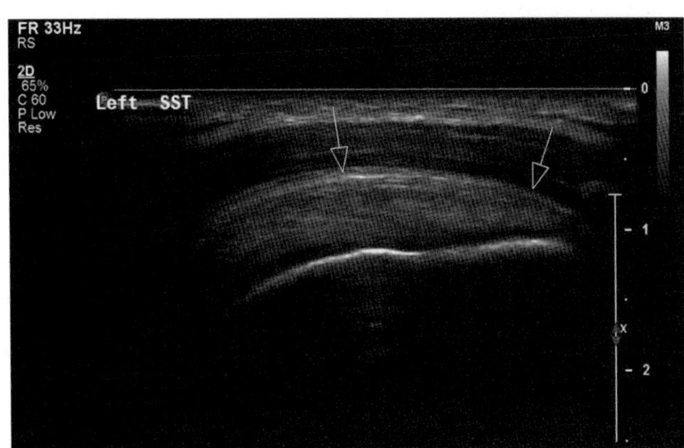

Fig. 1.9 Normal supraspinatus tendon on longitudinal ultrasound view. **(A)** The probe is positioned perpendicular to the tendon. **(B)** The "parrot-beak" appearance of the tendon (*arrow*) is seen in this view.

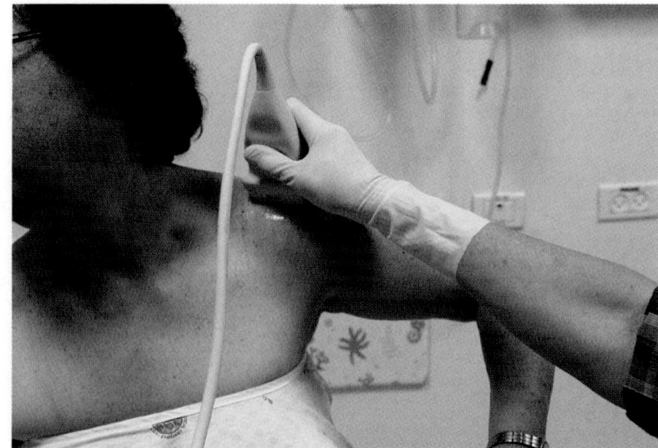

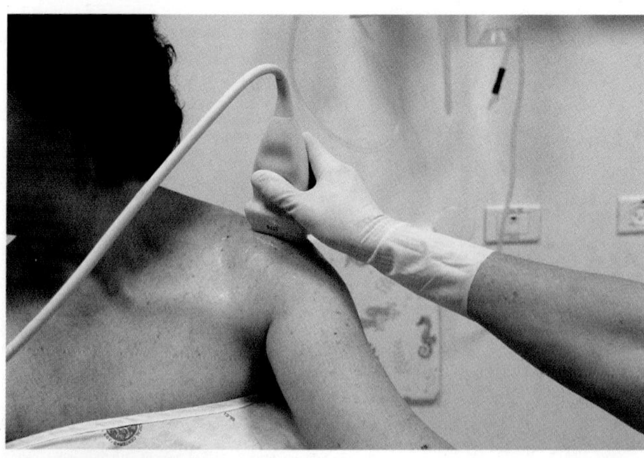

Fig. 1.10 Normal rotator cuff tendon on dynamic maneuvers. **(A)** The patient's elbow is raised. **(B)** The patient's arm is moved forward. **(C)** Left plot: the supraspinatus tendon (*arrow*) is seen under the acromion (A). Right plot: the tendon is hidden under the acromion (A) during a dynamic maneuver.

Afterward, the patient is asked to extend the arm with the palm facing backward and to move it forward (**Fig. 1.10B**). During these dynamic maneuvers, the tendon slides below the acromion being hidden by the bone acoustic shadow (**Fig. 1.10C**).

Transverse Image of the Acromioclavicular Joint

The patient turns his or her hand palm up on the thigh; the transducer is placed over the shoulder on a coronal plane (**Fig. 1.11A**). The bone echogenic lines of the clavicular dis-

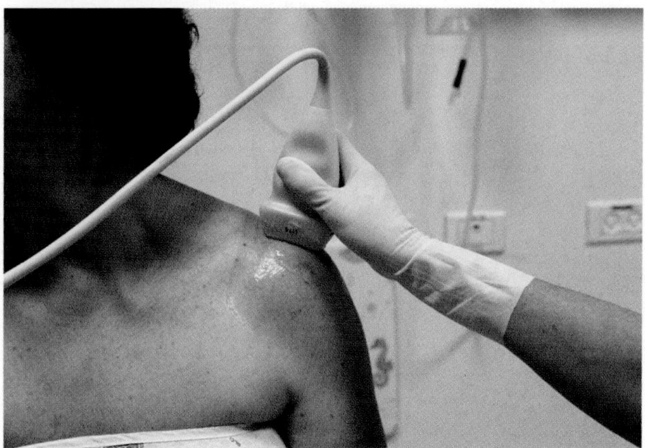

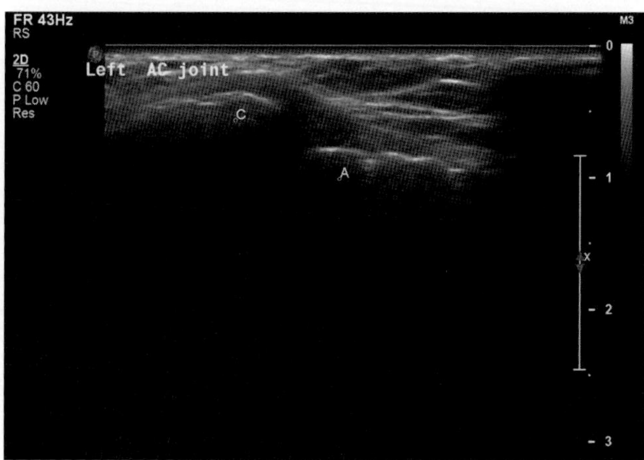

Fig. 1.11 Normal acromioclavicular joint. **(A)** The probe is positioned in a coronal plane over the shoulder. **(B)** On coronal view, the acromioclavicular ligament is seen as a hypoechogenic structure bridging the bone echogenic lines of the clavicle (C) and the acromion (A).

tal end and the acromion are seen bridged by a hypoechoic convex structure that represents the acromioclavicular ligament (**Fig. 1.11B**).

Pathologies

Rotator Cuff Tear

Full-Thickness Tear

A full-thickness tear leads to a total (large full-thickness tear) (**Figs. 1.12, 1.13**) or a focal (small full-thickness tear) (**Figs. 1.14, 1.15**) nonvisualization of the rotator cuff. The majority of focal full-thickness tears are located in the critical zone at the anterior part of the tendon (**Fig. 1.15**). The cuff is compressible by the transducer and the defect may be accentuated by extension and internal rotation of the arm. Full-thickness tears may be filled with synovial fluid or hyperechoic granulation tissue, hypertrophied synovium, or hemorrhage. Passive arm movement is helpful to confirm the absence of cuff tendon. Tears must be confirmed on two perpendicular planes.

Partial-Thickness Tear

A partial-thickness tear is a localized absence in the cuff involving either the articular (**Fig. 1.16**) or the bursal surface, the first being more common. It is seen as a hypoechoic or mixed hypo- and hyperechoic focal discontinuity, sharply demarcated from the surrounding normal cuff. An additional appearance is a large dominant linear echogenic focus within the cuff substance, with or without narrowing of cuff thickness. A partial tear must be confirmed on two orthogonal planes. An 82% positive predictive value and a 98% negative predictive value have been reported for the sonographic demonstration of rotator cuff tears.

A

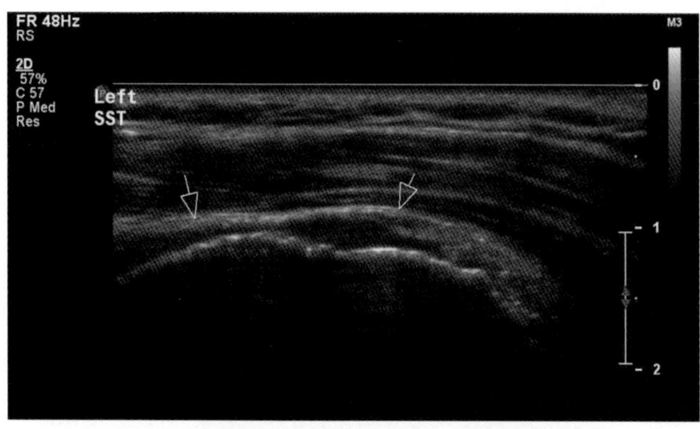

B

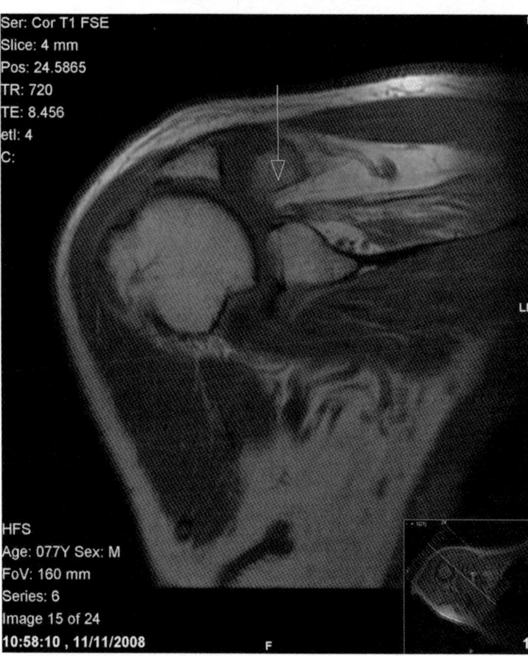

C

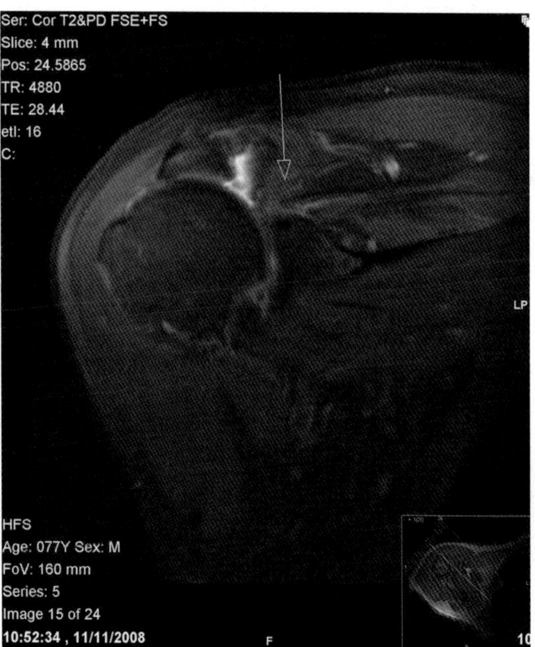

Fig. 1.12 Supraspinatus tendon large full-thickness tear. **(A)** Transverse ultrasound view. The tendon is not seen and a thin layer of fluid fills the gap between the subdeltoid bursa (*arrows*) and the humeral head. **(B)** Coronal T1-weighted fast spin echo (FSE) and **(C)** coronal proton density (PD) FSE fat-suppressed (FS) magnetic resonance images demonstrate a complete tear and retraction of the supraspinatus tendon (*arrow*). Supraspinatus fat replacement due to muscle atrophy and upper subluxation of the humeral head are secondary findings.

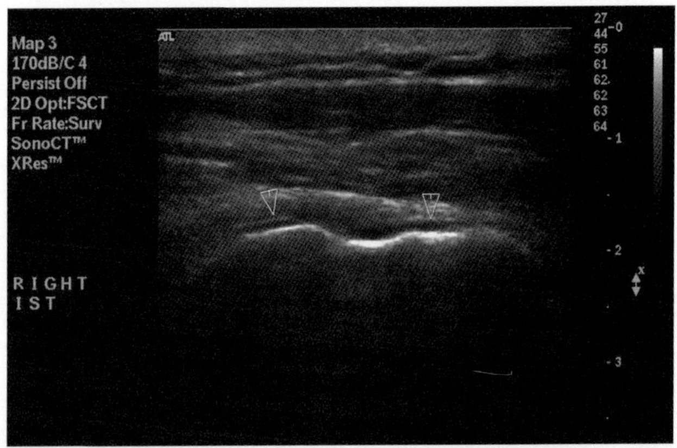

Fig. 1.13 Full-thickness tear of the infraspinatus tendon. **(A)** The articular cartilage is well seen on ultrasound due to absence of the tendon above the humeral head (*arrowheads*). **(B)** Coronal T1-weighted fast spin echo (FSE) and **(C)** coronal proton density (PD) FSE fat-suppressed (FS) magnetic resonance images show a complete distal tear (*arrow*), proximal retraction of the tendon, and muscle atrophy with fat infiltration.

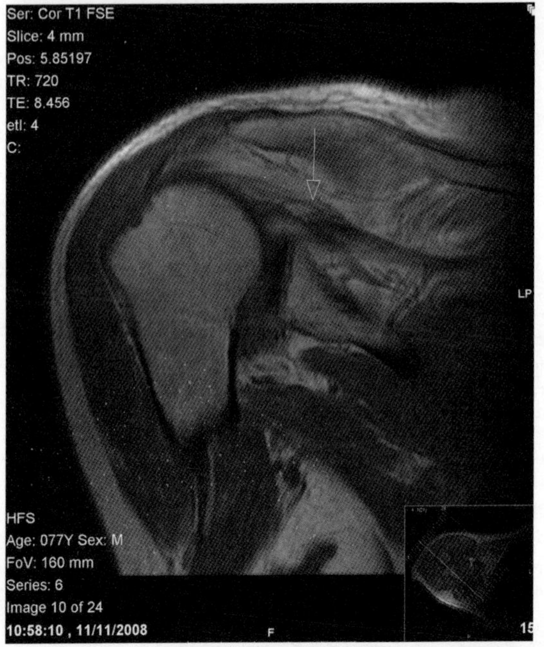

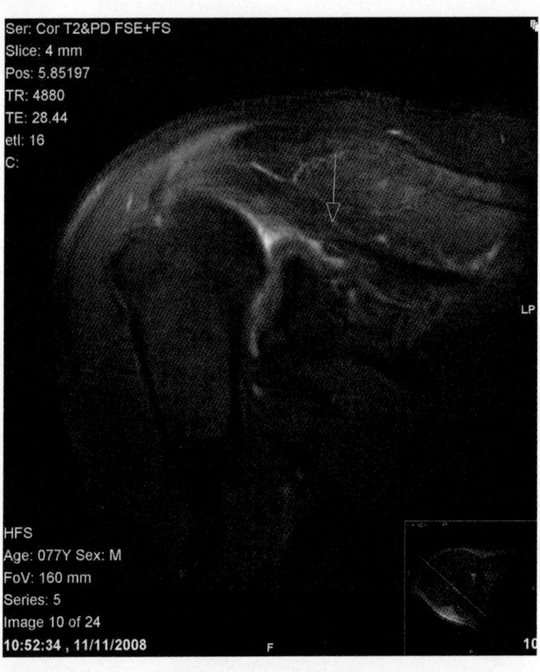

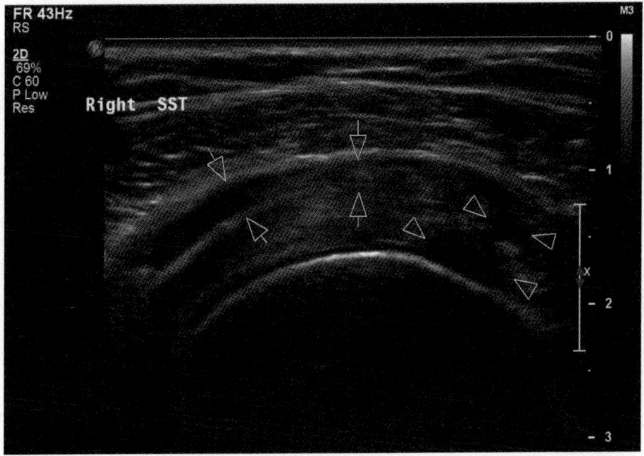

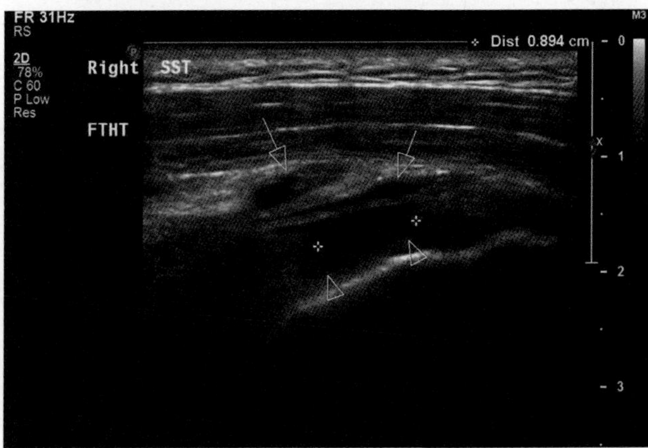

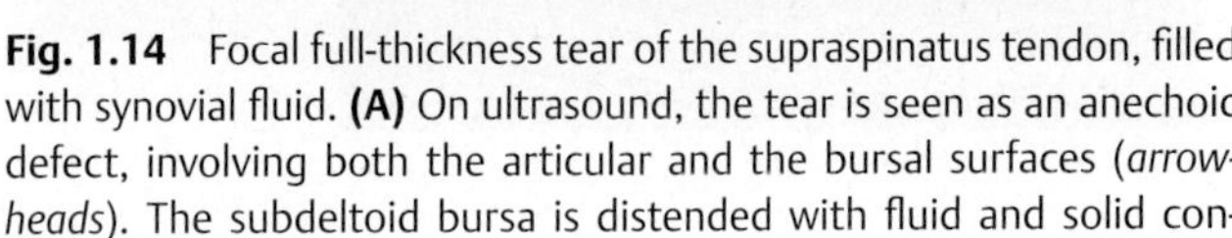

Fig. 1.14 Focal full-thickness tear of the supraspinatus tendon, filled with synovial fluid. **(A)** On ultrasound, the tear is seen as an anechoic defect, involving both the articular and the bursal surfaces (*arrowheads*). The subdeltoid bursa is distended with fluid and solid contents probably due to hemorrhage (*arrows*). **(B)** In another example, a 9-mm-length tear filled with fluid (*arrows*) in the echogenic tendon and a small amount of fluid in the subdeltoid bursa (*arrows*) are seen. (*Continued*)

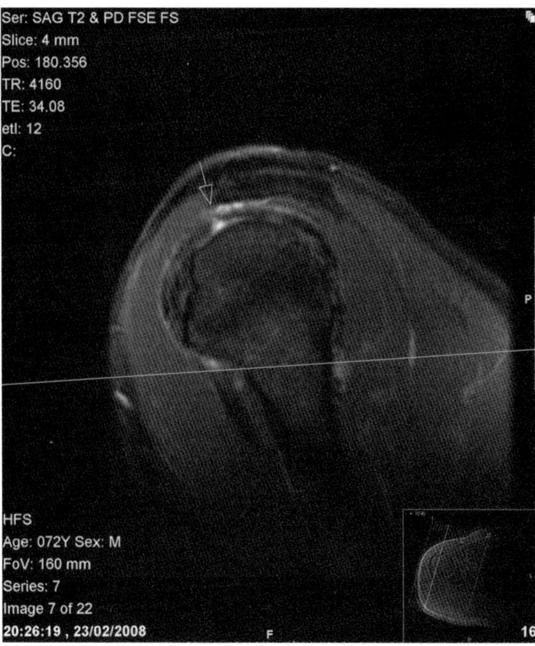

C

Fig. 1.14 (*Continued*) **(C)** Sagittal proton density (PD) fast spin echo (FSE) fat-suppressed (FS) magnetic resonance image shows a focal high intensity signal representing a tear in the supraspinatus tendon (*arrow*) within the normal low signal intensity tendon.

Intrasubstance Tear

An intrasubstance tear is a focal hypoechoic zone within the cuff, not extending to the bursal or articular surfaces (**Fig. 1.17**). Van Holsbeeck and Introcaso do not consider these intrasubstance defects as real tears.

Minor Criteria for Rotator Cuff Tear

- Subacromial bursal effusion: It is the most reliable secondary finding. Bursal fluid may be the only abnormality in small tears (**Fig. 1.18**).
- Concave subacromial bursal contour: In a full-thickness tear, the subacromial bursa is generally thickened up to 5 mm in width, has a concave downward contour, and is directly adjacent to the humeral head surface (**Fig. 1.19**).
- Humeral head elevation: Elevation of the humeral head toward the acromion may be seen (**Fig. 1.12**) corresponding to plain film findings. Detection is easier when comparing with the normal side.
- Joint effusion: Presence of fluid in the glenohumeral joint increases the suspicion of a full-thickness tear (**Fig. 1.20**).

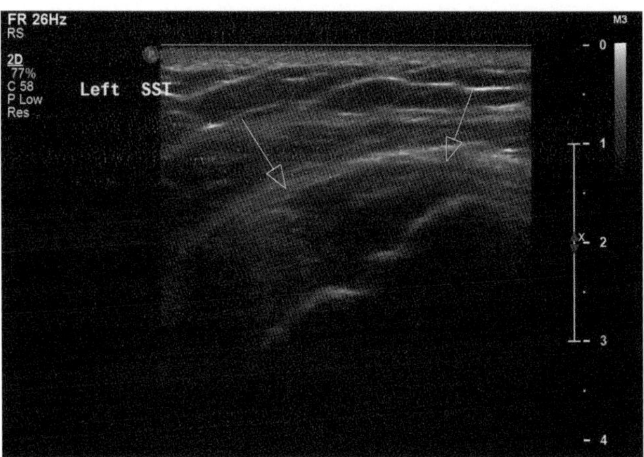

A

Fig. 1.15 Focal full-thickness tear of the supraspinatus tendon at the "critical zone." **(A)** A sonolucent defect extending from the articular to the bursal surface is seen at the anterior part of the tendon (*arrow*), which is considered to be relatively avascular—therefore more vulnerable. **(B)** Coronal proton density (PD) fast spin echo (FSE) fat-suppressed (FS) magnetic resonance image shows high intensity signal (*arrow*) at a complete tear site.

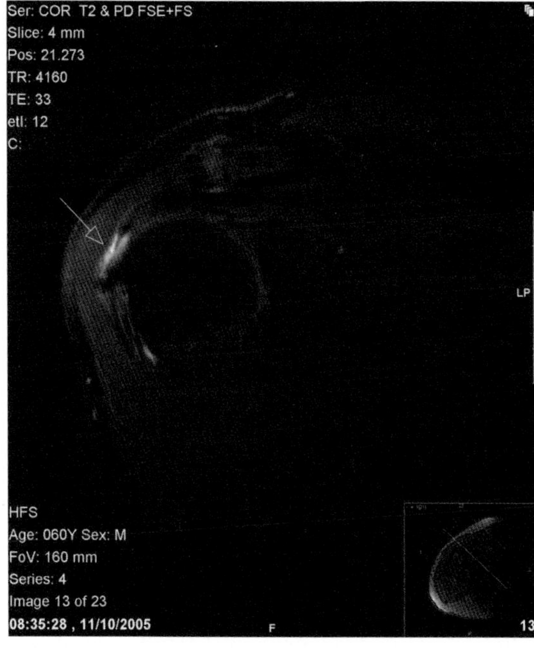

B

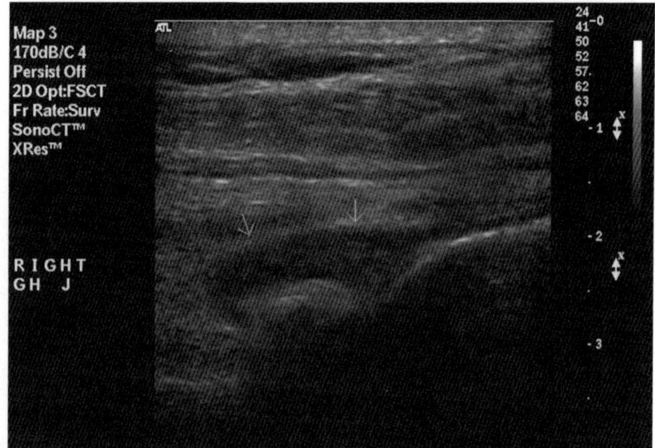

A

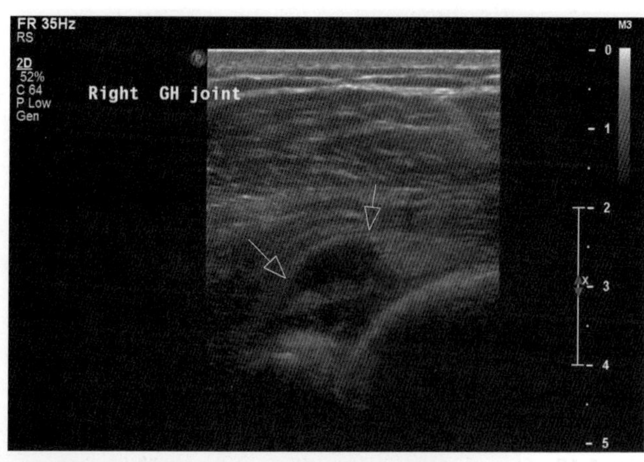

B

C

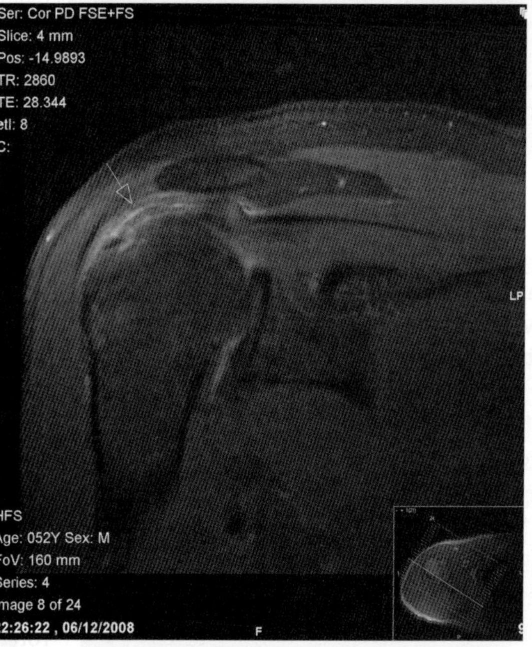

D

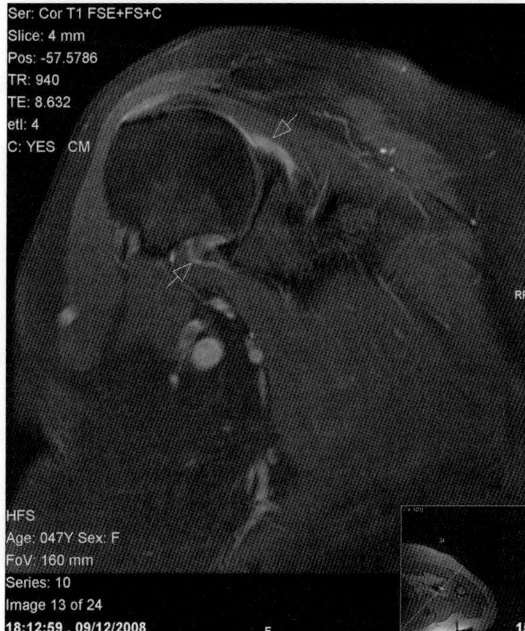

E

Fig. 1.20 Glenohumeral joint effusion. **(A,B)** Anechoic **(A)** and low echogenic **(B)** fluid is seen at the glenohumeral joint (*arrows*) in two cases, secondary to complete tear of the rotator cuff. **(C)** Axial proton density (PD) fast spin echo (FSE) fat-suppressed (FS) magnetic resonance image (MRI) shows high intensity fluid (*arrows*) in the glenohumeral joint. **(D)** Coronal PD FSE FS MRI shows a complete tear of the supraspinatus tendon (*arrow*) with tendon proximal retraction. **(E)** Coronal T1 FSE FS MRI scan after gadolinium injection shows synovial enhancement in the joint (*arrows*) representing synovitis.

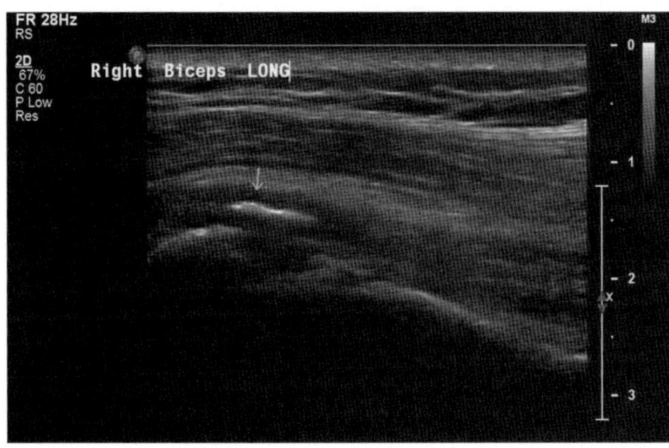

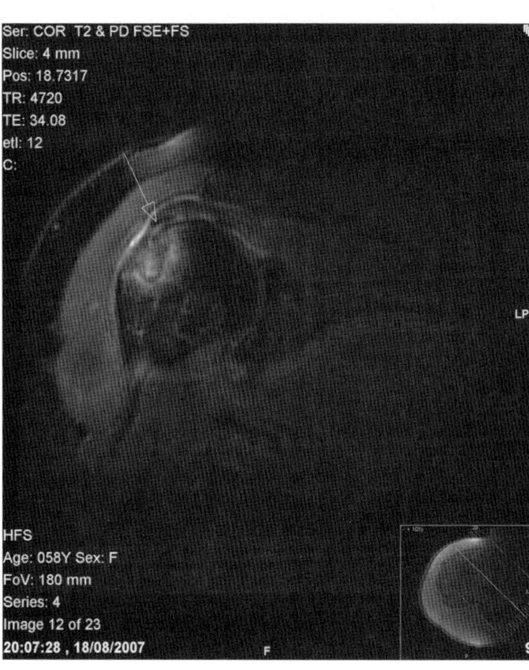

Fig. 1.21 Greater tuberosity fracture. **(A)** Discontinuity in the normally smooth bony surface and avulsion fracture. The osteochondral fragment is seen as a hyperechogenic focus (*arrow*) adjacent to the biceps tendon at the proximal part of the bicipital groove. **(B)** Coronal proton density (PD) fast spin echo (FSE) fat-suppressed (FS) magnetic resonance image shows a fracture line surrounded by intramedullary contusion and mild compression of the greater tuberosity (*arrow*).

normal nutrient pathway. Arthropathy may be seen on ultrasound as an irregularity of a bony surface and a loss of hypoechoic articular cartilage.

Pitfalls

An inadequate position of the transducer is the most common cause of inaccuracies. Failure to orient the transducer parallel to the fibers of the tendon may result in artifactual decreased echogenicity due to anisotropy (**Fig. 1.1C**). Scanning the supraspinatus with the transducer placed laterally may mimic a tear. Obesity and large bursal effusions decrease penetration and limit the accuracy of the exam.

Conclusions

Rotator cuff ultrasound is an accurate test when performed with modern equipment and correct examination technique. Although published results vary widely, 100% sensitivity, 85% specificity, and overall 96% accuracy compared

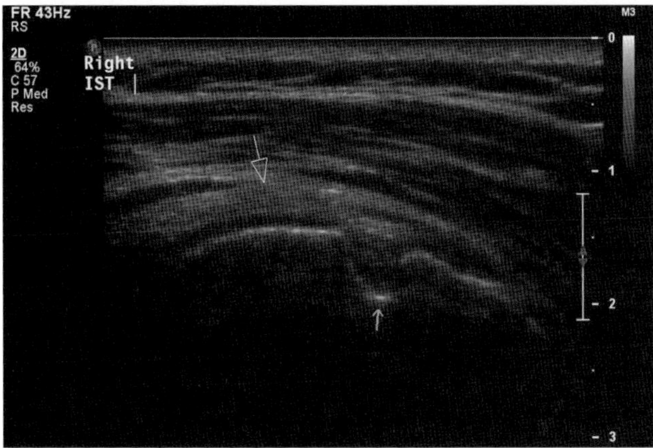

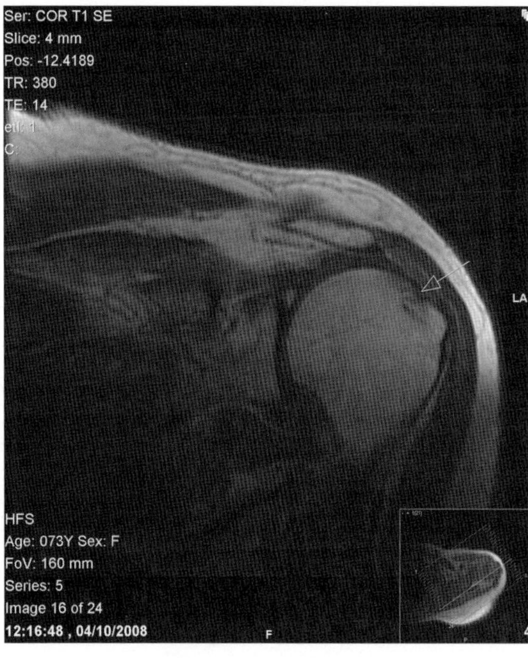

Fig. 1.22 Compression fracture of the humeral head. **(A)** Hill–Sachs fracture. A triangular notch at the posterior area of the humeral head (*small arrow*), below the supraspinatus tendon (*arrow*) is seen. The defect is filled by synovial fluid. **(B)** Hill–Sachs fracture (*arrow*) seen on coronal T1-weighted spin echo (SE) magnetic resonance image (MRI). (*Continued*)

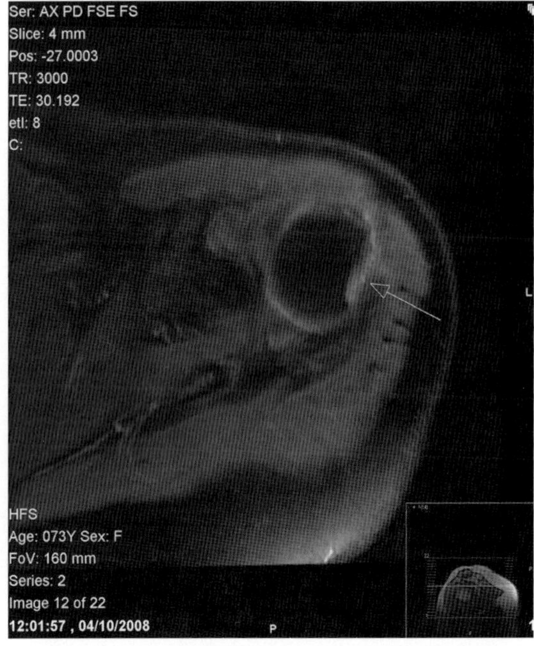

C

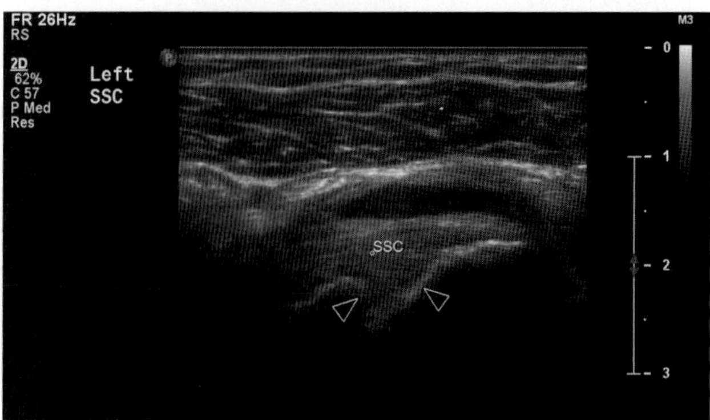

D

Fig. 1.22 (*Continued*) **(C)** The defect in the humeral head (*arrow*) is seen also on axial proton density (PD) fast spin echo (FSE) fat-suppressed (FS) MRI. **(D)** McLaughlin fracture (*arrowheads*) at the anterior humeral head below the subscapularis tendon. Fluid is seen in the subacromial bursa.

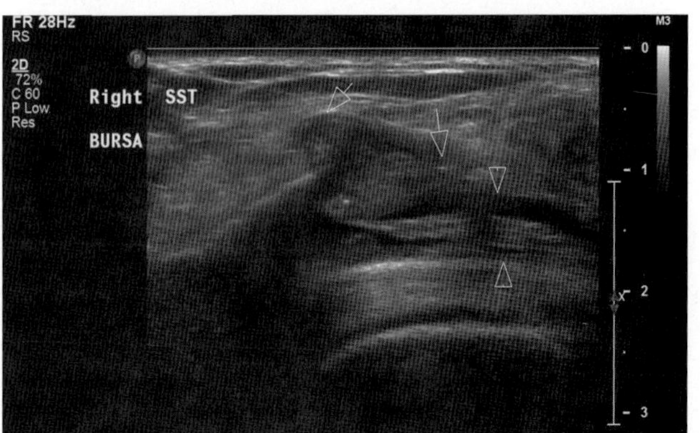

A

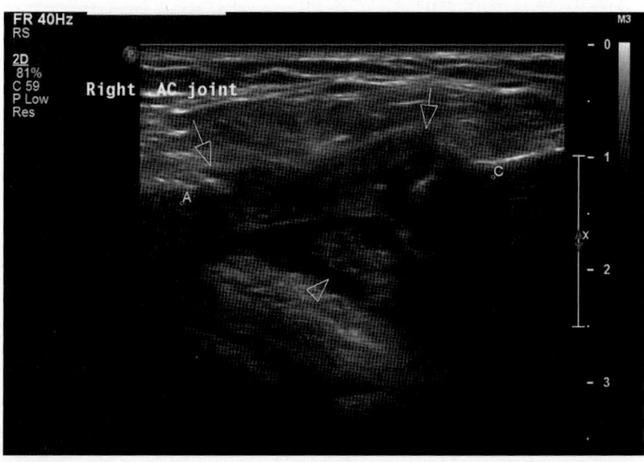

B

C

Fig. 1.23 Postacromioplasty hematoma. **(A)** A low echogenic hematoma (*arrows*) is seen at the bed of the resected acromion. The hematoma is connected with the subdeltoid subacromial bursa (*arrowheads*), which contains fluid and echogenic material compatible with clots. **(B)** A widened acromio- (A) clavicular (C) joint (*arrows*) by a hematoma at the bottom (*arrowhead*) is shown. **(C)** Inflammatory changes at the acromioclavicular joint depicted as hyperemia on power Doppler (*arrows*).

with arthroscopy and surgery were reported by Teefey et al. It is most useful in patients over 50 years old, those expected to have larger lesions, and in the postoperative patient. In a younger patient with persistent symptoms, a negative sonography should be followed by additional imaging tests.

Impingement Syndrome

Subacromial impingement during forward flexion and abduction of the glenohumeral joint may be secondary to muscle weakness due to trauma, inflammation, or tears of the rotator cuff leading to failure of depression of the humeral head. The supraspinatus and the subacromial bursa are compressed against the coracoacromial arch. On dynamic maneuvers, impingement is diagnosed as bunching up of the supraspinatus or distention of the subdeltoid bursa, pressured against the acromion (**Fig. 1.24**). Impingement causes trauma, inflammation, and tendinopathy, predisposing to further tearing which worsens the severity of impingement.

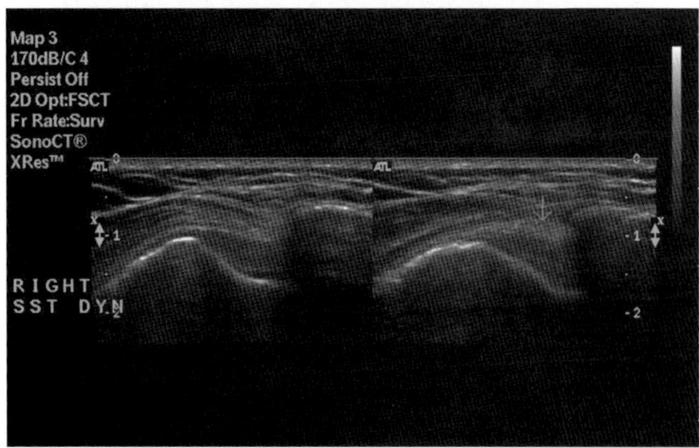

Fig. 1.24 Impingement syndrome. The supraspinatus tendon and the subacromial bursa (*arrow*) are compressed against the coracoacromial arch on dynamic maneuvers. A side-by-side comparison is provided: on the left plot, at rest, and on the right plot, during dynamic maneuvers.

Calcifying Tendonitis

Calcifying tendonitis is most commonly an idiopathic primary condition, although it may also be secondary to calcinosis due to end-stage renal failure, tumors, vitamin D intoxication, and collagen disease. The supraspinatus and the long head of the biceps are the most commonly involved tendons. A calcium deposition in the rotator cuff is detected as a hyperechoic focus in the tendon substance. A well-defined posterior shadow may be seen in the hard stage (**Figs. 1.25A,B**). A faint or lack of shadowing is seen in the soft form known as a "slurry" calcification, which is proven to be liquid in most cases (**Fig. 1.25C**). Calcium excites an inflammatory reaction leading to tendon edema and secondary impingement. Calcium may rupture into the subacromial bursa, causing severe exacerbation of symptoms.

Calcifying Bursitis

A calcium deposit within the bursa leads to the development of calcifying bursitis. On ultrasound, a thickened bursa filled with echogenic debris is seen (**Fig. 1.26**). Ultrasound-guided calcium aspiration from the calcified tendon or bursa de-

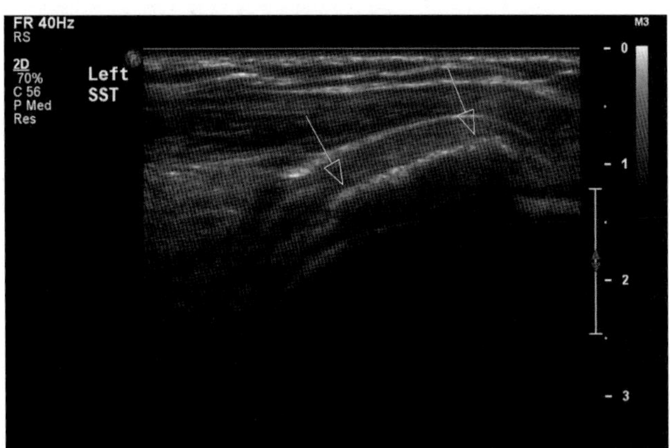

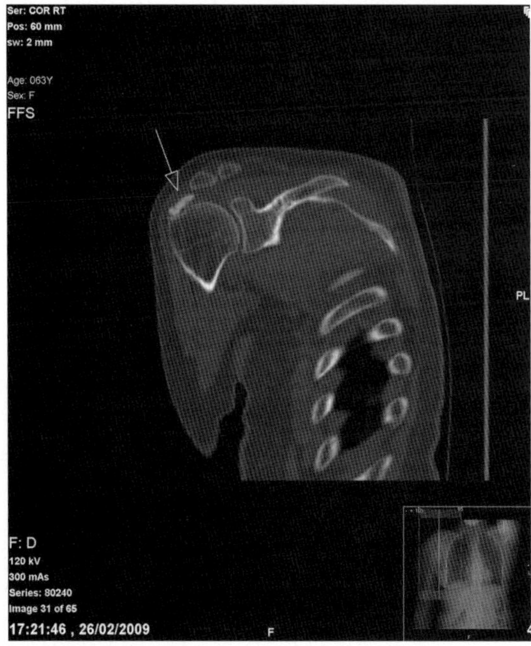

Fig. 1.25 Calcifying tendinosis of the supraspinatus tendon. **(A)** On ultrasound, a large hyperechoic focus is detected in the tendon (*arrows*) with a wide posterior acoustic shadow, obscuring the humeral head, compatible with a large heavy calcification. **(B)** Reformatted coronal computed tomography shows a highly dense linear calcification (*arrow*) along the supraspinatus tendon. (*Continued*)

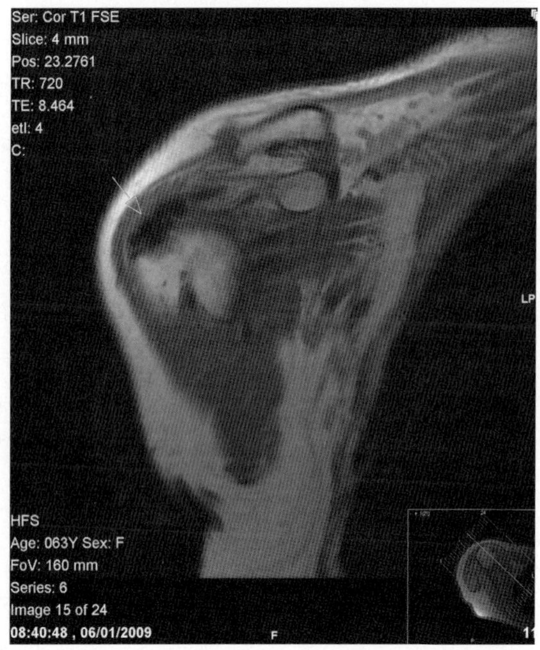

C

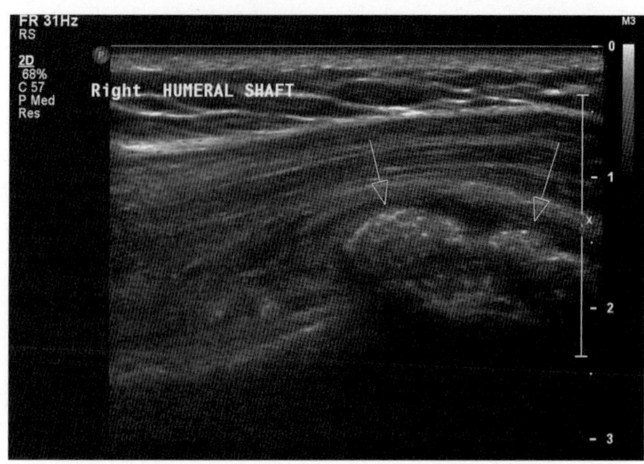

D

Fig. 1.25 (*Continued*) **(C)** Coronal T1 fast spin echo (FSE) magnetic resonance image shows low intensity signal along the tendon calcification. **(D)** A wide hyperechogenic focus (*arrows*) is seen in this case, lacking posterior shadowing, compatible with a soft form of calcifying tendonitis.

Fig. 1.26 Calcifying subdeltoid bursitis. **(A)** Ultrasound shows a thickened and hyperechoic bursa (*cursors*) over the subscapularis tendon. **(B)** Linear calcification (*arrow*) in the subdeltoid bursa seen on axial proton density (PD) fast spin echo (FSE) fat-suppressed (FS) magnetic resonance image (MRI). **(C)** Soft form of calcification is seen in the subscapularis bursa. **(D)** Soft calcifications seen in the anterior recess of the subdeltoid bursa (*arrows*). (*Continued*)

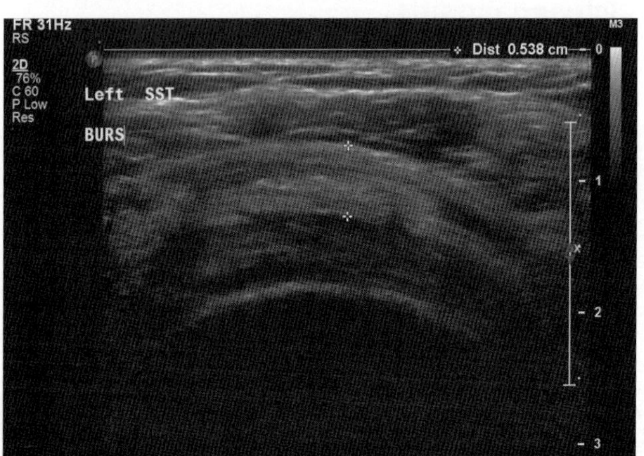

A

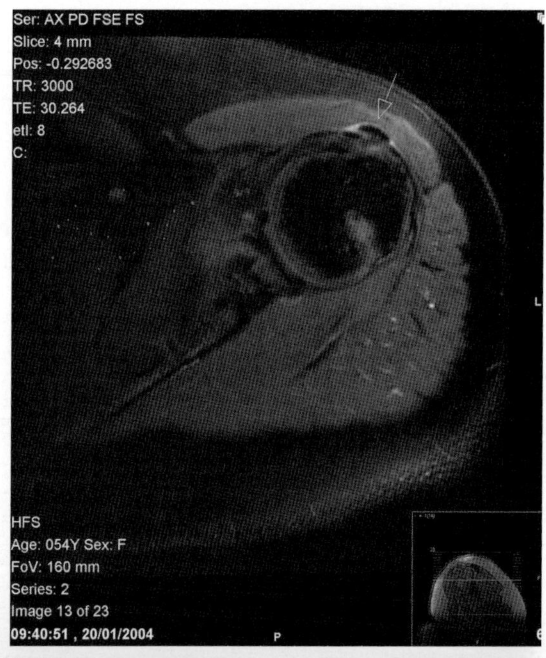

B

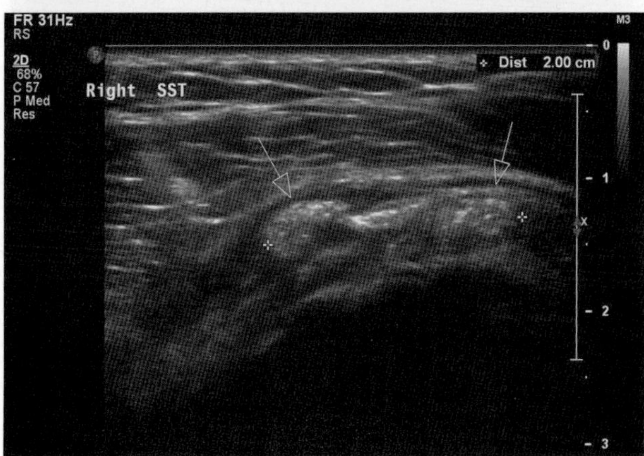

C

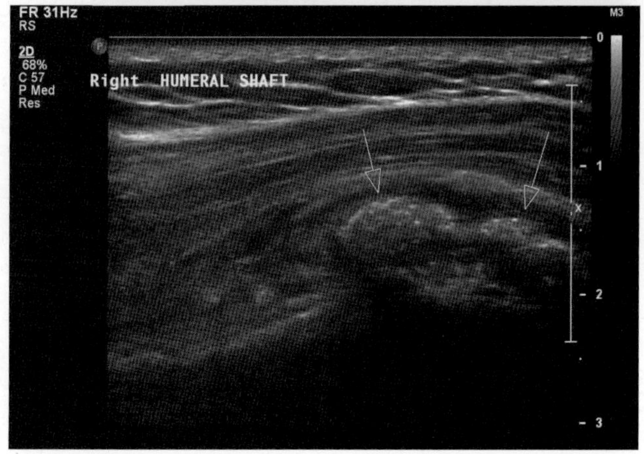

D

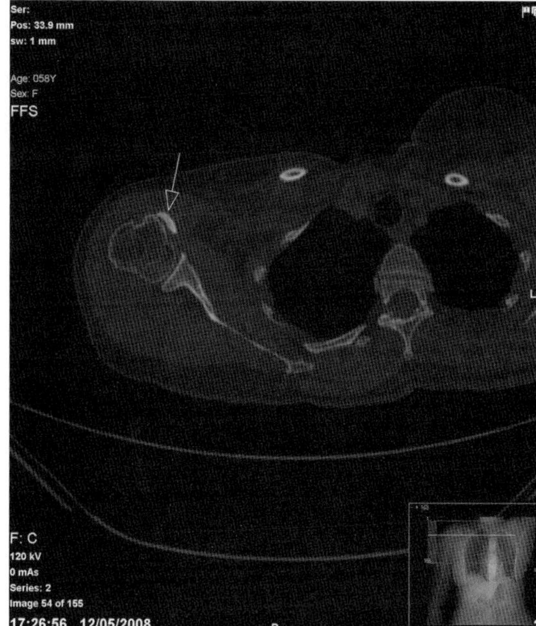

E

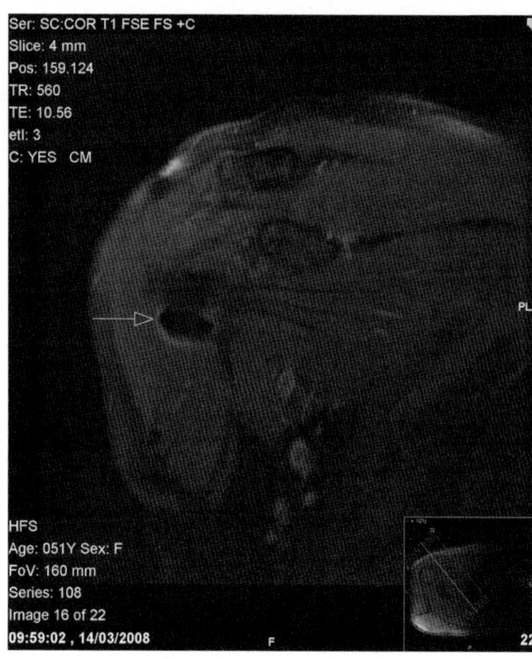

F

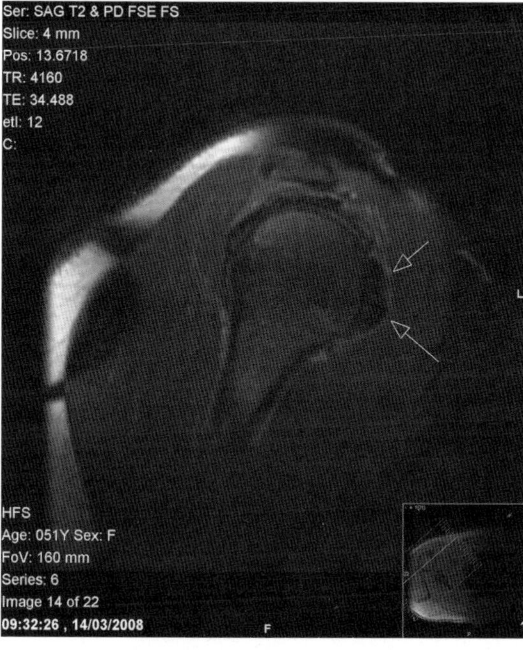

G

Fig. 1.26 (*Continued*) Calcifying subdeltoid bursitis. **(E)** Calcification seen as a high linear density in the subscapularis bursa (*arrow*) on computed tomography. **(F)** Coronal T1 FSE FS MRI with gadolinium shows a big calcified focus and mild enhancement in the subscapular bursa (*arrow*) representing mild bursitis. **(G)** Calcifications are seen as a low intensity signal on a sagittal PD FSE FS MRI into the subscapular bursa (*arrows*).

creases pressure and produces localized bleeding, aiding in the resorption of the remaining calcified material. Milwaukee shoulder, a rare arthropathy that mainly affects elderly women, is characterized by hydroxyapatite crystal deposits intra- or periarticular, calcific bursitis, significant rotator cuff disease and shoulder arthritis leading to the rapid destruction of the rotator cuff and the glenohumeral joint. The inciting process remains unidentified.

Bursal and Joint Effusion

The subacromial–subdeltoid bursa is the largest bursa in the body. Effusion in the subacromial–subdeltoid bursa is highly specific of rotator cuff tear. Fluid in the bursa may be communicating with a joint effusion (**Figs. 1.27** and **1.28**) or noncommunicating. A noncommunicating bursitis may be posttraumatic from a direct blow, causing hemorrhagic

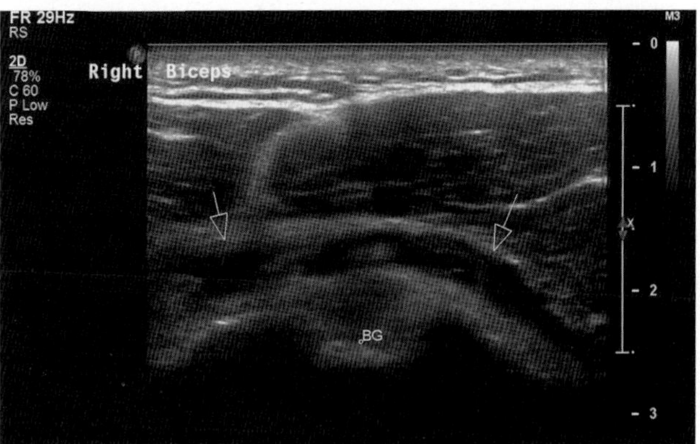

A

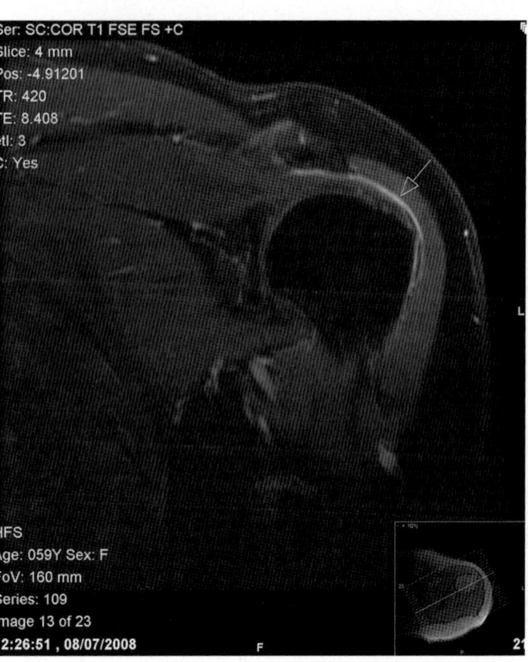

B

Fig. 1.27 Subacromial subdeltoid bursal fluid. **(A)** Synovial fluid is detected in the subacromial subdeltoid bursa (*arrows*) superficial to the subscapularis tendon and the bicipital groove (BG). Note the hypoechogenicity of the bicipital tendon due to anisotropy. Bursal fluid was associated with a full thickness tear of the rotator cuff. **(B)** Coronal T1-weighted fast spin echo (FSE) fat-suppressed (FS) magnetic resonance image with gadolinium shows subacromial subdeltoid bursitis seen as enhancement of the synovium in the bursae (*arrow*).

A

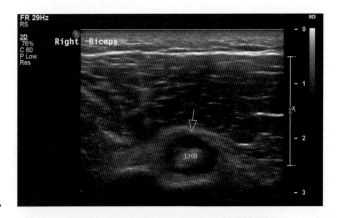

Fig. 1.28 Fluid in biceps sheath. **(A)** Axial ultrasound view shows synovial fluid (*arrow*) surrounding the long head of the biceps (LHB). **(B)** Fluid is seen as high intensity signal (*arrow*) on an axial proton density (PD) fast spin echo (FSE) fat-suppressed (FS) magnetic resonance image (MRI). **(C)** Axial T1-weighted FSE FS MRI with gadolinium shows enhancement (*arrow*) in the bicipital grove surrounding the low intensity biceps tendon, which is compatible with biceps tenosynovitis.

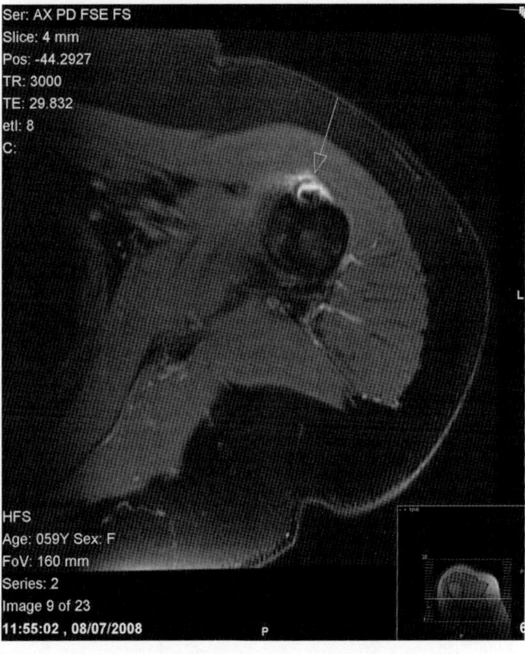

B

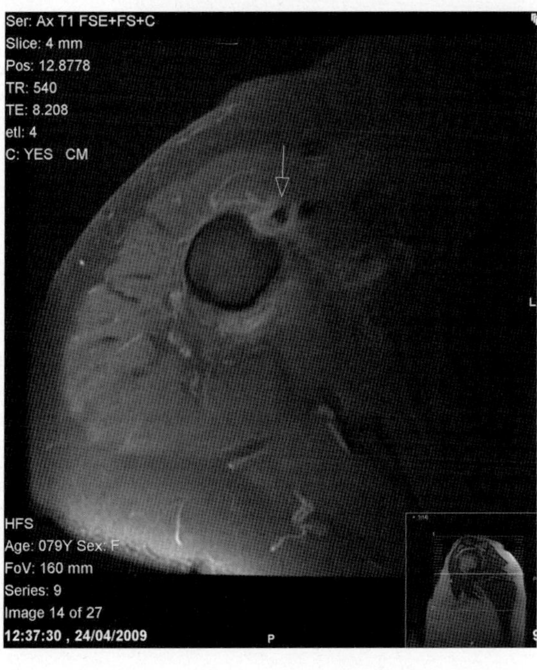

C

bursitis, or secondary to a chronic irritation in impingement syndrome, associated with synovial thickening and fluid (**Fig. 1.28**). Bursitis may also be secondary to inflammatory arthropathy, polymyalgia rheumatica, amyloidosis, and calcium deposition. The sonographic observation of fluid in the subacromial–subdeltoid bursa, either isolated or combined with a joint effusion, should prompt a careful evaluation of the supraspinatus tendon for tear.

Biceps Tendon Tenosynovitis, Tear, and Dislocation

Tenosynovitis of the long head of the biceps is seen as fluid in the sheath surrounding the tendon; synovial enhancement after gadolinium injection is seen on MRI (**Fig. 1.28**). Biceps tendonitis may be associated with rotator cuff tear, shoulder osteoarthritis, and bursitis secondary to rheumatoid arthritis. The diagnosis of biceps tendon-sheath fluid prompts a detailed evaluation of the shoulder. Total tear of the long biceps tendon at the musculotendinous junction appears as a total disruption of the tendon with a hematoma filling in the gap (**Fig. 1.29**). The long head of the biceps tendon always dislocates medially, either superficial or deep to the subscapularis tendon (**Fig. 1.30**). A congenital narrow or shallow bicipital groove, less than 3 mm in depth, with a flat medial wall are predisposing factors to dislocation of the long head of the biceps tendon. Dislocations are associated in most cases with a full-thickness tear of the supraspinatus tendon, but they can also occur as a consequence of lifting or carrying a heavy load. Bilateral congenital dislocations have also been described. When intermittent, the displacement may be detected dynamically by externally rotating the arm while scanning the bicipital groove in a transverse view.

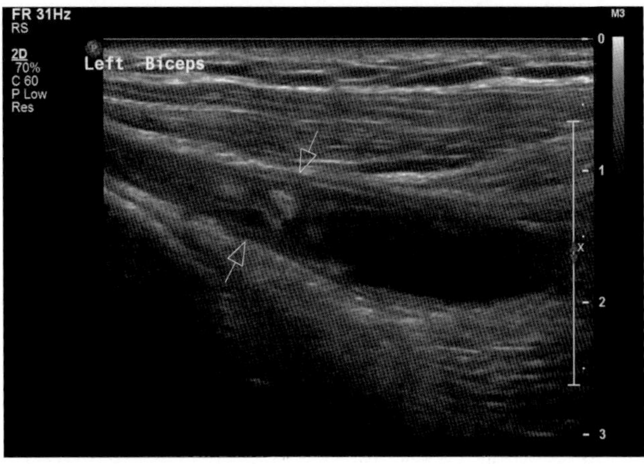

Fig. 1.29 Complete tear of biceps tendon. This is a full-thickness tear after acute trauma. Ultrasound shows discontinuity of tendon fibers (*arrows*) and a large fluid collection distending the sheath distal to the rupture.

Artifacts

Near-field artifacts, narrow superficial image field, and tendon anisotropy are sources of confusion in a shoulder examination. Tendon echogenicity depends on the transducer angle relative to the tendon. Hypoechogenicity is an artifact caused by the anisotropic structure of tendons (**Fig. 1.1C**). A high-resolution multifrequency linear array transducer with a center frequency of 12 MHz decreases near-field artifacts and is state-of-the art imaging. Marked improvements in

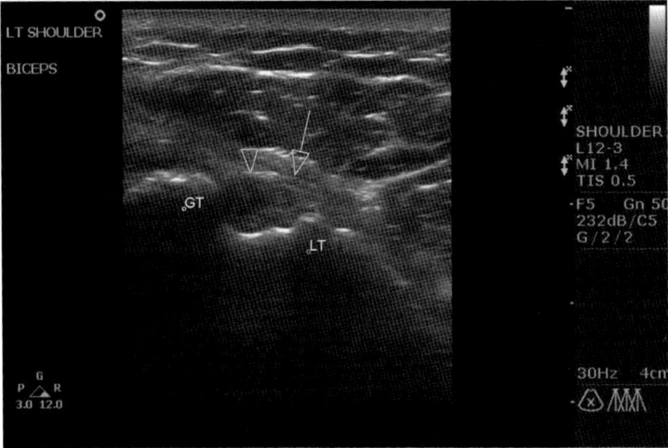

A

Fig. 1.30 Dislocation of long head of biceps tendon. **(A)** Ultrasound view shows the biceps tendon (*arrow*) subluxed over the lesser tuberosity (LT). Fluid is seen in the tendon sheath (*arrowhead*). GT, greater tuberosity. **(B)** Axial proton density (PD) fast spin echo (FSE) fat-suppressed (FS) magnetic resonance image shows medially dislocated tendon (*arrow*) and empty bicipital grove (*arrowhead*).

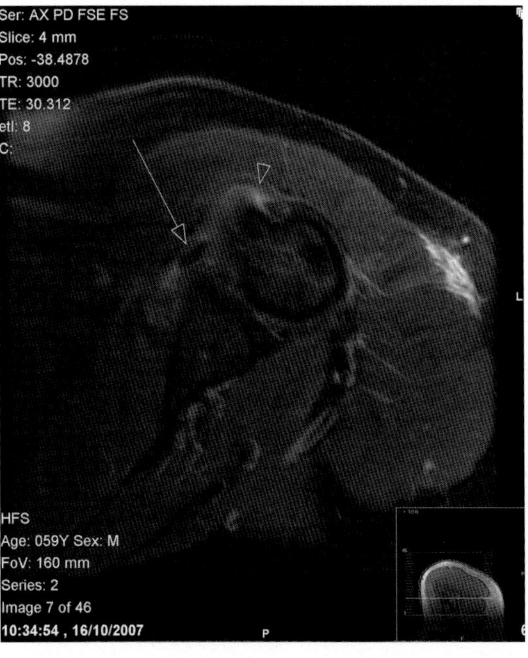

B

near-field resolution, compound imaging, large field of view, and panoramic imaging greatly reduce imaging artifacts and improve image quality.

Comparison between Ultrasound, MRI, CT, and Arthrography

Ultrasound, magnetic resonance imaging, computed tomography, and arthrography are compared (**Table 1.1**) in relation to their role in diagnosing shoulder pathology. The use of ultrasound as the initial imaging modality is the safest, most sensitive and cost-effective approach for the investigation of shoulder pathology.

Proposed Algorithm for Shoulder Imaging Investigation

Plain radiography
Ultrasound—first imaging examination for soft tissue pathologies
MRI—for technically difficult ultrasound (very obese, immobile patients), suspected lesions of labrum or joint capsule, and proximal subacromial impingement not seen on ultrasound
CT—for suspected bone pathology such as fractures not detected on plain radiography and spurs
Arthrography—mostly combined with CT imaging, for optimal imaging of the joint space

Pearls and Pitfalls

- High-resolution multifrequency transducers, with advanced imaging capabilities such as real-time compound, tissue harmonic, color, power flow, and extended field of view have improved the diagnostic quality, in particular tissue contrast and spatial resolution, of ultrasound images of the musculoskeletal system.
- Dynamic examination for the diagnosis of impingement, tendon instability or dislocation, joint subluxation, nerve entrapment among other conditions, and side-to-side comparison are unique features of ultrasound.
- Sonographic "palpation" is a valuable technique in localizing the region of interest. Occult fractures may be demonstrated by a step-off bone deformity or angulation.
- Be aware of the anisotropic characteristics of tendons. Reflectivity, attenuation, and backscatter of the ultrasound signal depend on the orientation of the ultrasound beam relative to the tendon structure.
- Be aware of "mirror" artifact in very reflective large structures such as extremity bones, which may make structures on the opposite side of a cortical bone appear as real anatomic structures.
- Despite the technological advances in ultrasound equipment, a good knowledge of anatomy and pathology of the musculoskeletal system, as well as experience in performing ultrasound examinations are essential for a precise diagnosis and treatment planning.
- Interventional ultrasound is rapidly achieving an important role for the definitive diagnosis and treatment of many musculoskeletal disorders.

Table 1.1 Comparison between Different Imaging Modalities for Shoulder Diagnoses

Feature	Ultrasound	Magnetic Resonance Imaging	Computed Tomography	Arthrography
Cost	Low	High	Moderate	Moderate
Patient compliance	High	Low (claustrophobia, long immobilization)	Moderate	Low
Operator dependence	High	Moderate	Moderate	High
Sensitivity for large full tears	High	High	Low	High
Sensitivity for small full and partial tears	High	Moderate	None	Moderate
Sensitivity for calcium deposit	High	Low	High	Low
Invasiveness	Absent Arthrosonography: saline injection	MRI arthrography: Gd intraarticular injection	CM intravenous injection	CM intraarticular injection
Dynamic exam, bilateral exam	Yes	No	No	No
Availability	High	Low	Moderate	Moderate
Radiation	None	None	Yes	Yes

Abbreviations: CM, contrast media (ionic); Gd, gadolinium.

Suggested Readings

Bianchi S, Martinoli C. Ultrasound of the Musculoskeletal System. Springer-Verlag Berlin Heidelberg 2007.

Bouffard JA, Lee SM, Dhanju J. Ultrasonography of the shoulder. Semin Ultrasound CT MR. 2000;21(3):164–191

Menias CO, Middleton WD, Teefey SA. An overview of ultrasonography of the shoulder. Ultrasound Q 2000;16(4):171–183

Teefey SA, Middleton WD, Yamaguchi K. Shoulder sonography. State of the art. Radiol Clin North Am 1999;37(4):767–785, ix

van Holsbeeck MT, Introcaso JH. Musculoskeletal Ultrasound. St. Louis, MO: Mosby, Inc. 2001

Winter TC III, Teefey SA, Middleton WD. Musculoskeletal ultrasound: an update. Radiol Clin North Am 2001;39(3):465–483

2 Imaging of the Elbow

Gerd Gruber and Werner Konermann
Translated by Axel W. E. Wismueller and Vikram S. Dogra

The standard examination of the elbow joint includes the ventral and dorsal elbow joint regions. The ventral sectional planes are positioned with extended elbow, the dorsal ones with flexed elbow. For the dorsal sectional planes, using a standoff pad is recommended, as this facilitates the coupling of the transducer over the olecranon process. In the dorsal region, the elbow joint is examined in two almost perpendicular planes (transverse and longitudinal), and in the ventral region the elbow joint is examined in one transverse and two longitudinal planes.

Both typical and rare pathologic findings and indications for an ultrasound examination of the elbow joint are listed in **Table 2.1**.

■ Technique for Examination of the Elbow

Ventral Region: Transverse View (Humeroradial)

The ventral transverse views are obtained with the elbow joint in an extended and supinated position with the patient sitting. In patients with a significant reduction of shoulder joint motion, these views can be obtained in a supine position.

To obtain transverse views, the transducer is positioned in the distal third of the humeral shaft and then moved in a distal direction over the elbow joint. The trochlea and the capitulum humeri can be seen with their hyalin cartilage coating as a curly brace. The brachialis and brachioradialis muscles are visualized anterior to hyalin cartilage (**Fig. 2.1**).

Differential Diagnosis

See **Figs. 2.2, 2.3, 2.4, 2.5, 2.6** for various pathologies found with a transverse view of the ventral region of the elbow.

Ventral Region: Longitudinal View (Humeroradial)

Longitudinal views of the ventral region are obtained with the elbow in an extended position. The transducer is positioned parallel to the longitudinal axes of the humeral and

Table 2.1 Typical and Rare Pathologic Findings and Indications

Classification	Diseases
Bony changes	Cubital osteoarthritis Avascular osteonecroses and osteochondroses Free joint bodies Fracture: Fracture of coronoid process Radial head fracture
Changes of bursae and joint cavity	Intraarticular volume increase (synovialis, joint effusion) Bursitis olecrani
Changes of tendons and ligaments	Distal biceps tendon rupture Triceps tendon calcification
Combined changes and other findings	Cubital osteoarthritis (with synovitis, joint effusion) Cubital arthritis Gouty tophus Rheumatoid node Lymphadenitis Fracture Tumor

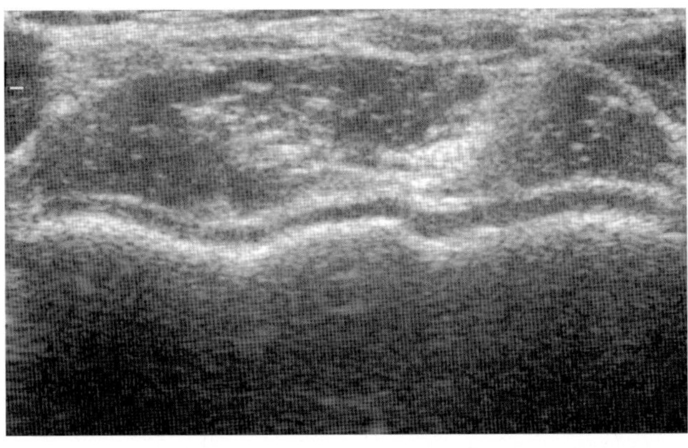

A

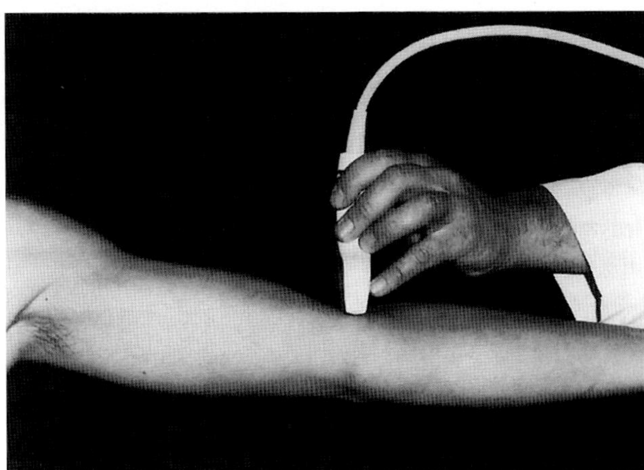

B

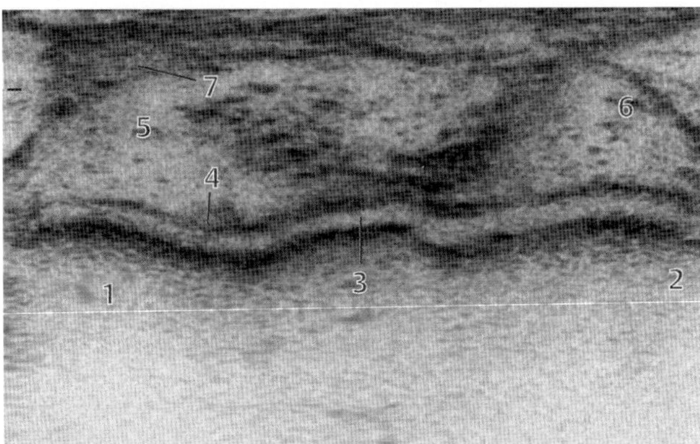

C

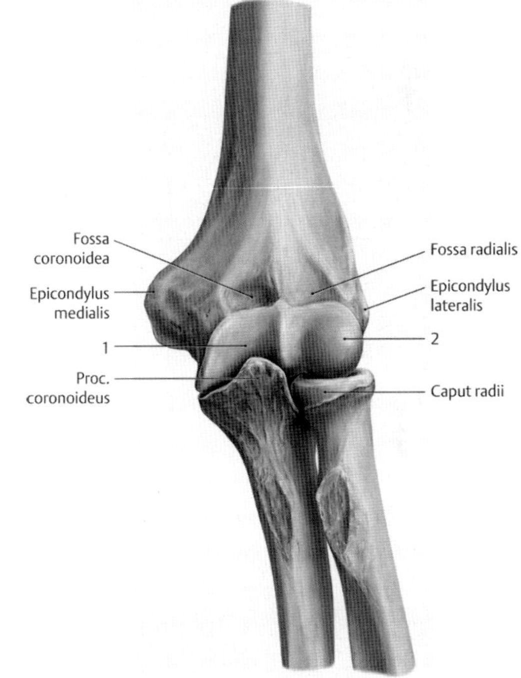

D

Fig. 2.1 **(A)** Transverse view in the distal third of the humeral shaft. **(B)** Transducer position. **(C)** Anatomic structures visualized by ultrasound, annotated in (D). **(D)** Anatomic position of the structures visualized in (C): 1, Trochlea humeri; 2, capitulum humeri; 3, hyalin cartilage; 4, joint capsule; 5, M. brachialis; 6, M. brachioradialis; 7, A. brachialis.

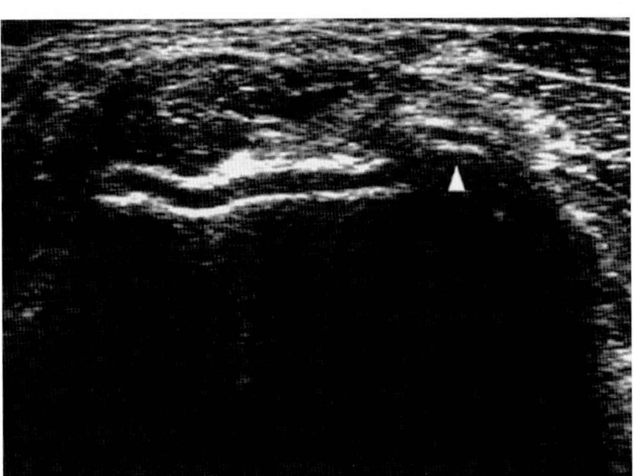

Fig. 2.2 Free joint body (*arrowhead*) (see Fig. 2.36C).

radial shafts. In this sectional view, the distal humeral shaft, the radial fossa, the capitulum humeri, the radial head, and the proximal radial shaft can be seen. The brachioradialis is seen anterior to the capitulum of the humerus and head of the radius. Starting at the radial head, the supinator muscle can be seen in longitudinal view anterior to the radial shaft (**Fig. 2.7**).

Differential Diagnosis

See **Figs. 2.8, 2.9. 2.10, 2.11, 2.12** for various pathologies found with a longitudinal view of the ventral region of the elbow.

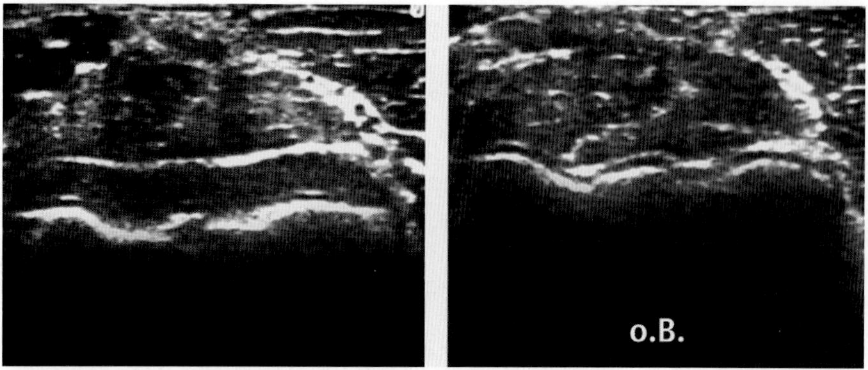

Fig. 2.3 Radial head fracture (see Fig. 2.39A).

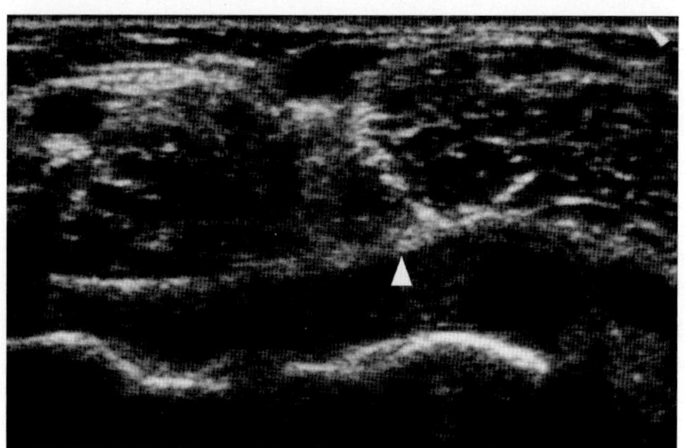

Fig. 2.4 Cubital arthritis (*arrowhead*) (see Fig. 2.44B).

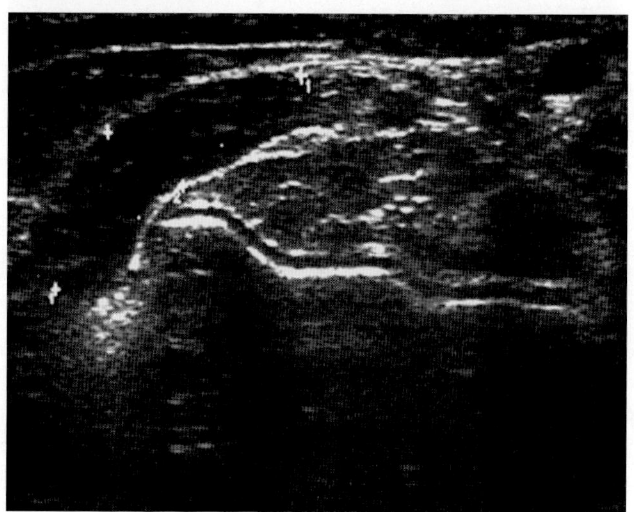

Fig. 2.5 Lymphadenitis (see Fig. 2.49A).

A

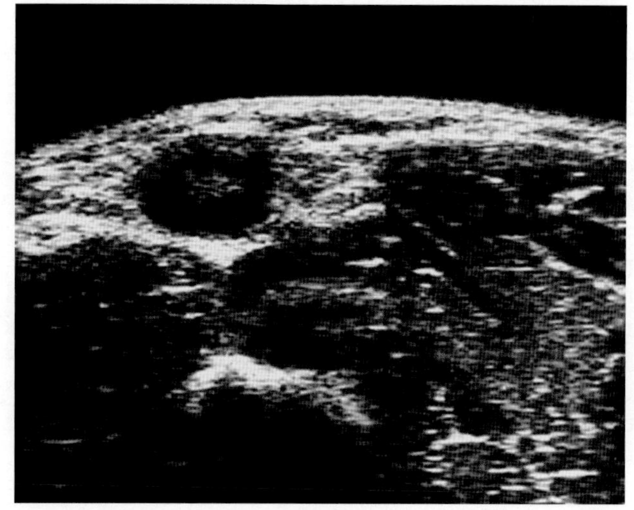

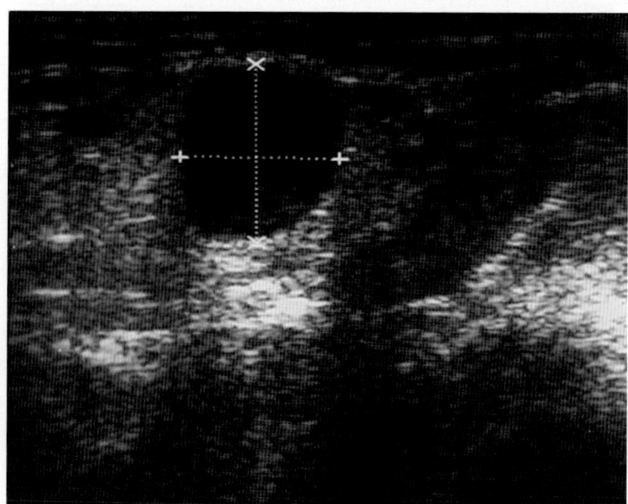

B

Fig. 2.6 **(A,B)** Tumor (see Figs. 2.50B,D).

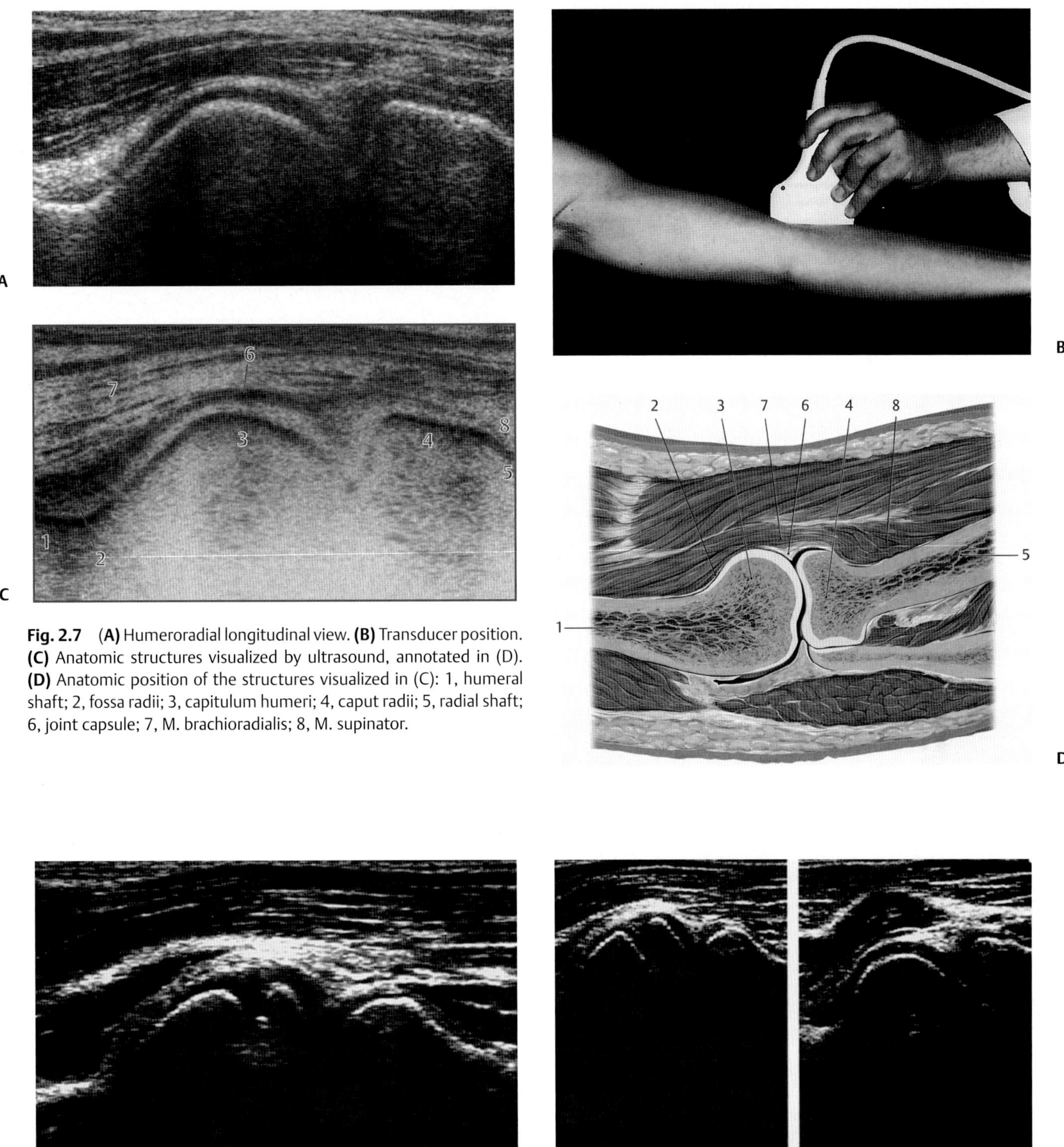

Fig. 2.7 **(A)** Humeroradial longitudinal view. **(B)** Transducer position. **(C)** Anatomic structures visualized by ultrasound, annotated in (D). **(D)** Anatomic position of the structures visualized in (C): 1, humeral shaft; 2, fossa radii; 3, capitulum humeri; 4, caput radii; 5, radial shaft; 6, joint capsule; 7, M. brachioradialis; 8, M. supinator.

Fig. 2.8 **(A,B)** Osteochondrosis dissecans (see Figs. 2.35A,B).

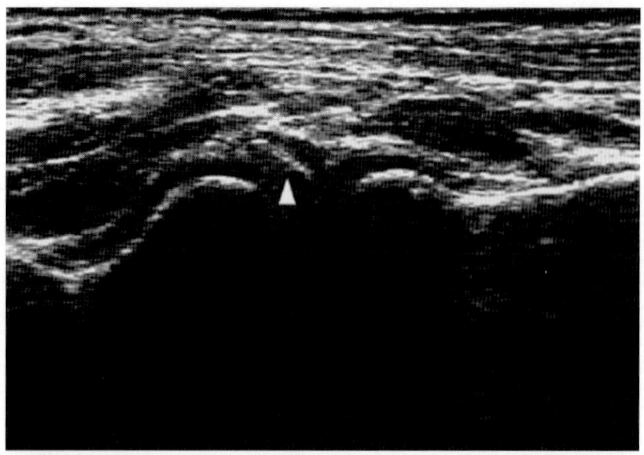

Fig. 2.9 Free joint body (*arrowhead*) (see Fig. 2.36A).

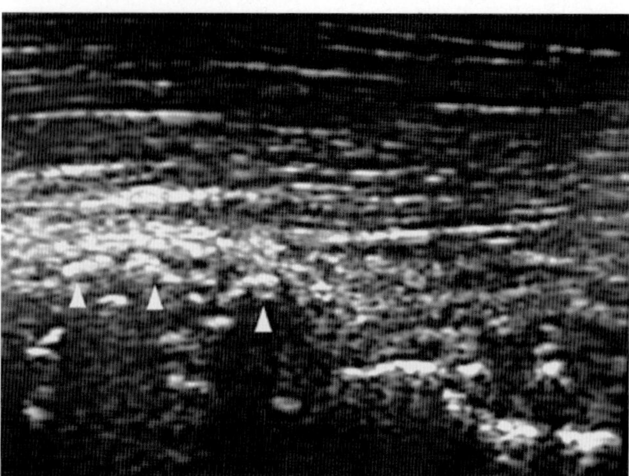

A

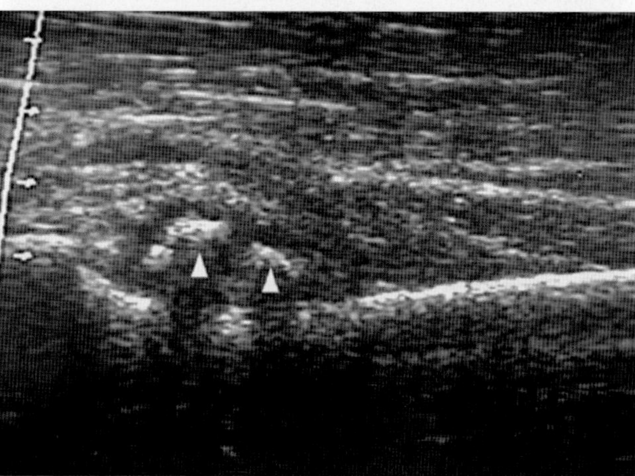

B

Fig. 2.10 **(A,B)** Chondromatosis (*arrowheads*) (see Figs. 2.37A,B).

Ventral Region: Humeroulnar Longitudinal Section

Starting from the humeroradial longitudinal view, the transducer is moved in longitudinal axes to visualize the humerus and ulna. In this longitudinal view, the distal humeral shaft, the coronoid fossa, the humeral trochlea, the coronoid process, the proximal ulna, as well as the brachial muscle and the forearm flexors are visualized (**Fig. 2.13**). The humeral shaft is positioned parallel to the upper border of the screen.

Under normal conditions, the coronoid fossa appears echogenic. The positioning of the proximal ulna is frequently alleviated by a moderate flexion of the elbow joint. If extension is impaired, use of a convex transducer is recommended.

Differential Diagnosis

See **Figs. 2.14, 2.15, 2.16, 2.17** for various pathologies found with a humeroulnar longitudinal view of the elbow.

A

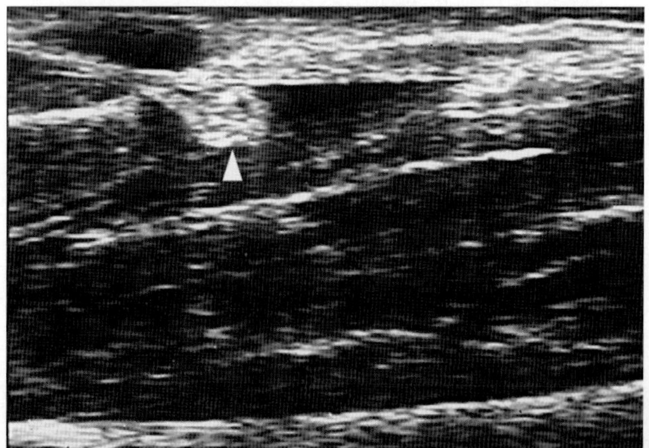

B

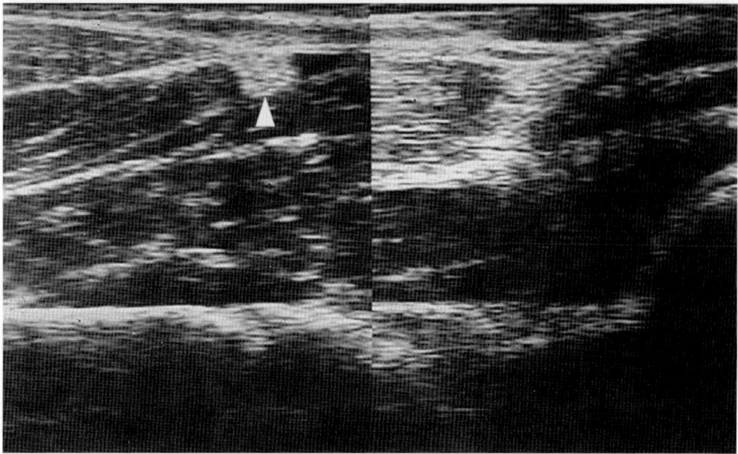

Fig. 2.11 **(A,B)** Distal biceps tendon rupture (*arrowhead*) (see Figs. 2.42A,B).

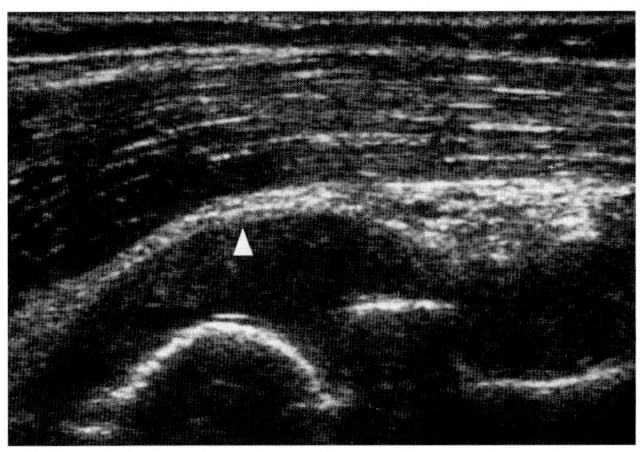

Fig. 2.12 Cubital arthritis (*arrowhead*) (see Fig. 2.44A).

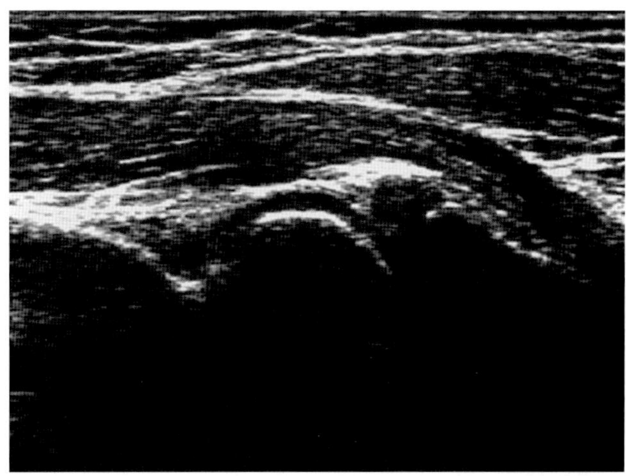

Fig. 2.14 Free joint body (see Fig. 2.36B).

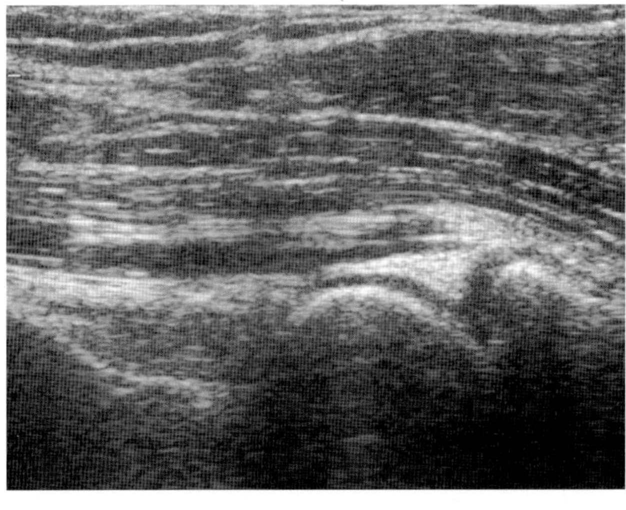

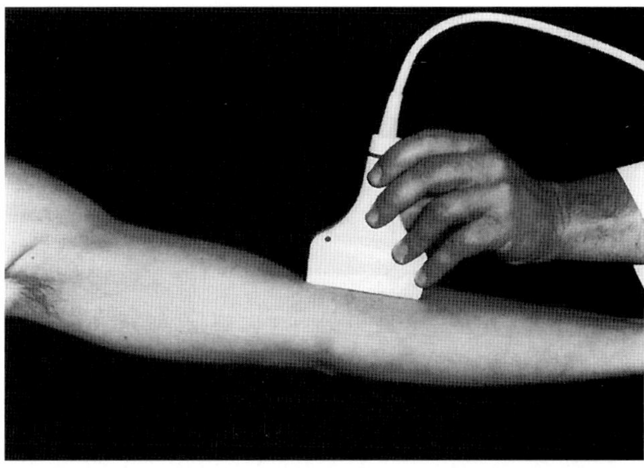

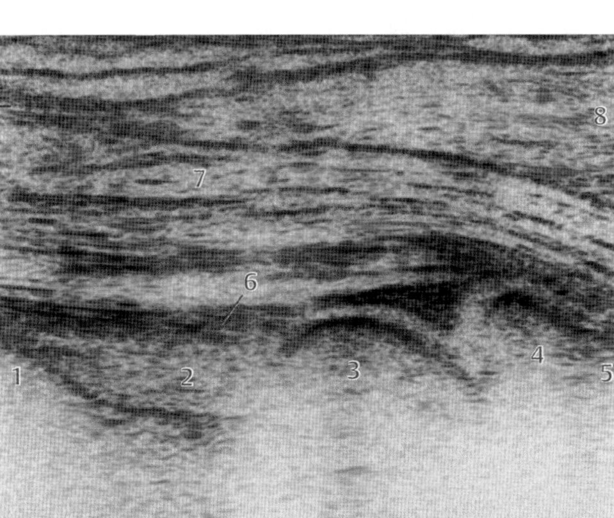

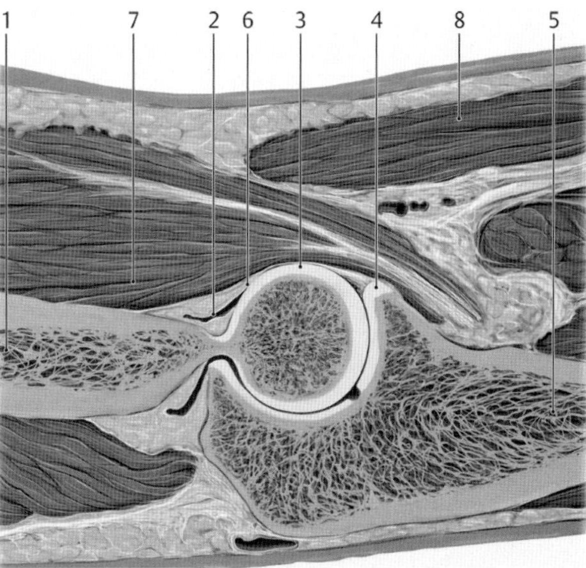

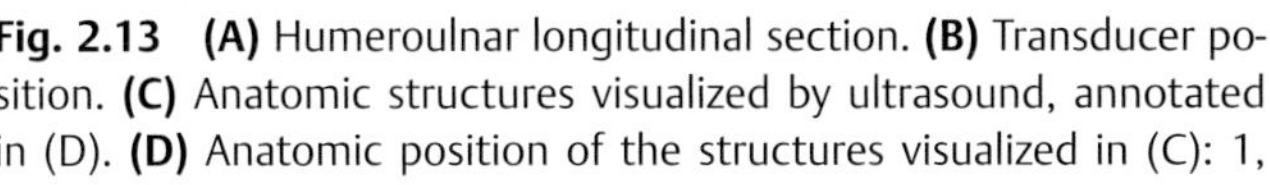

Fig. 2.13 **(A)** Humeroulnar longitudinal section. **(B)** Transducer position. **(C)** Anatomic structures visualized by ultrasound, annotated in (D). **(D)** Anatomic position of the structures visualized in (C): 1, humeral shaft; 2, fossa coronoidea; 3, trochlea humeri; 4, processus coronoideus; 5, ulnar shaft; 6, joint capsule; 7, M. brachialis; 8, forearm flexors.

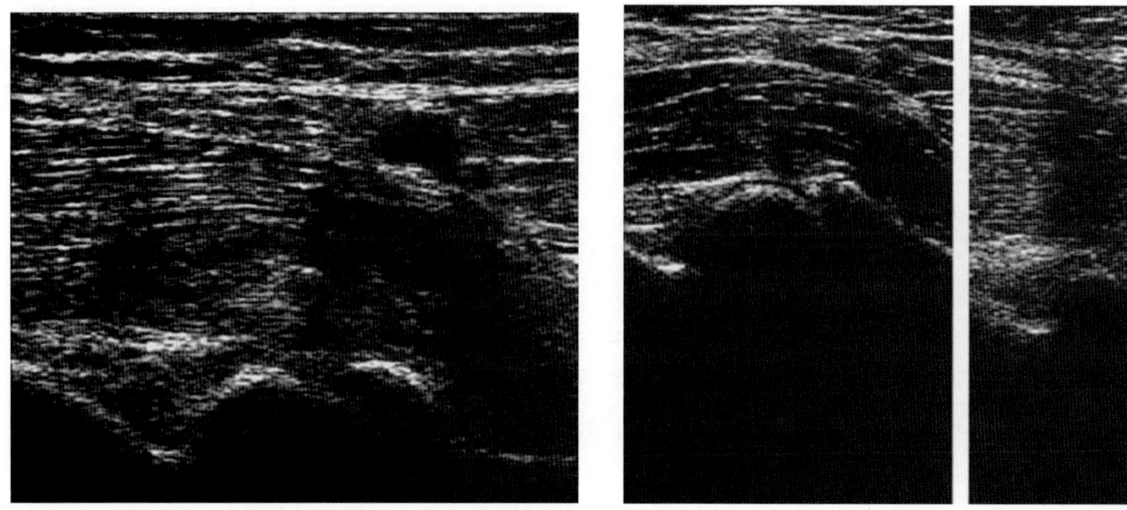

Fig. 2.15 **(A,B)** Fracture of the coronoid process (see Figs. 2.38A,B).

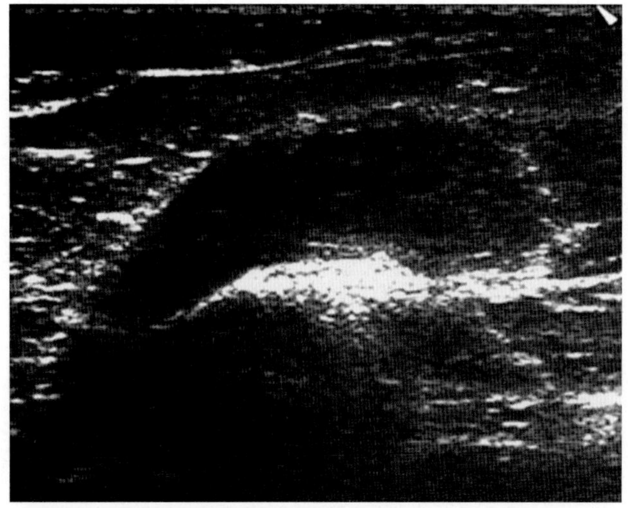

Fig. 2.16 Lymphadenitis (see Figs. 2.49B).

Dorsal Region: Transversal Section

The dorsal longitudinal and transverse views are obtained in a sitting position with the elbow flexed. If the patient is unable to sit, then the transducer is moved distally from the distal third so views can be obtained in supine position. The olecranon fossa forms a typical "u" shape. It is filled with fatty tissue, which appears moderately more echogenic than the triceps muscle that is running above and is imaged in a transverse view. An imaginary tangent line touching the condyles runs parallel to the upper screen edge (**Fig. 2.18**).

Differential Diagnosis

See **Figs. 2.19, 2.20, 2.21, 2.22, 2.23, 2.24** for various pathologies found with dorsal longitudinal and transverse views of the elbow.

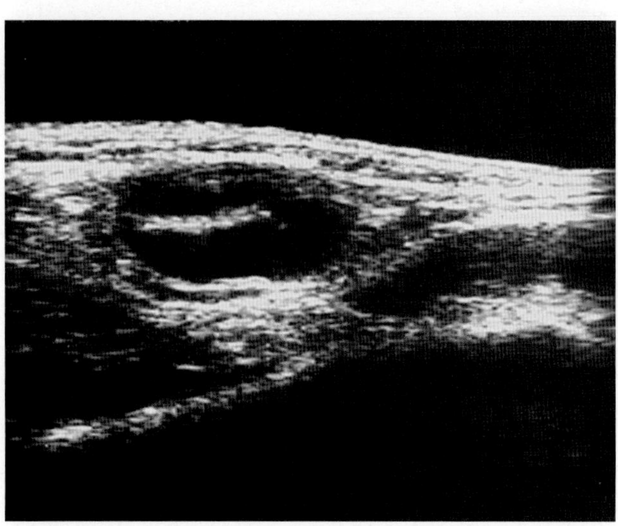

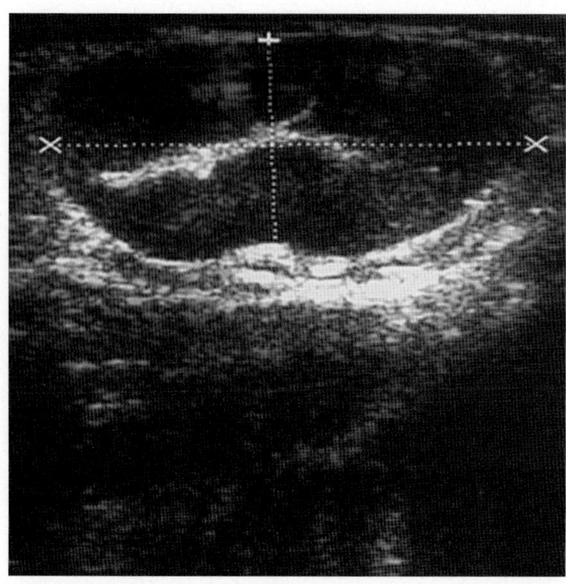

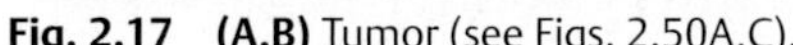

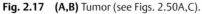

Fig. 2.17 **(A,B)** Tumor (see Figs. 2.50A,C).

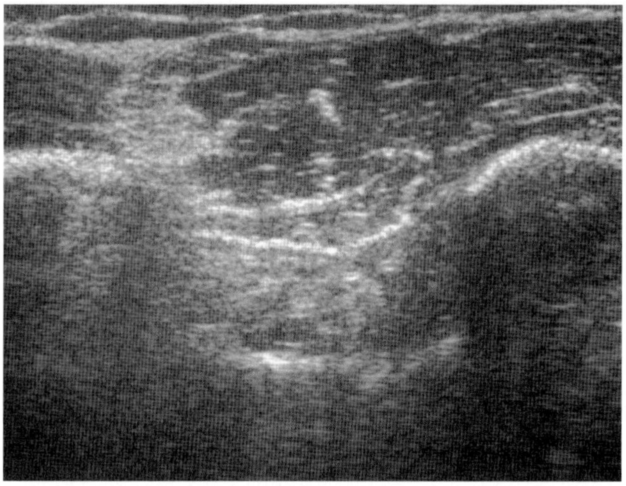

Fig. 2.18 **(A)** Transversal section, dorsal region. **(B)** Transducer position. **(C)** Anatomic structures visualized by ultrasound, annotated in (D). **(D)** Anatomic position of the structures visualized in (C): 1, condylus humeri ulnaris; 2, fossa olecrani; 3, condylus humeri radialis; 4, joint capsule; 5, M. triceps brachii.

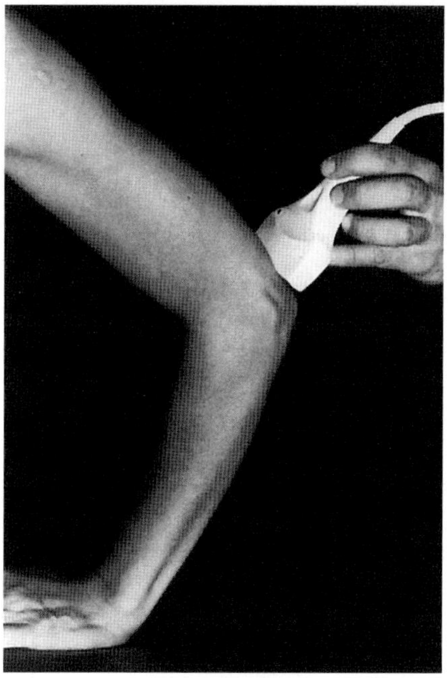

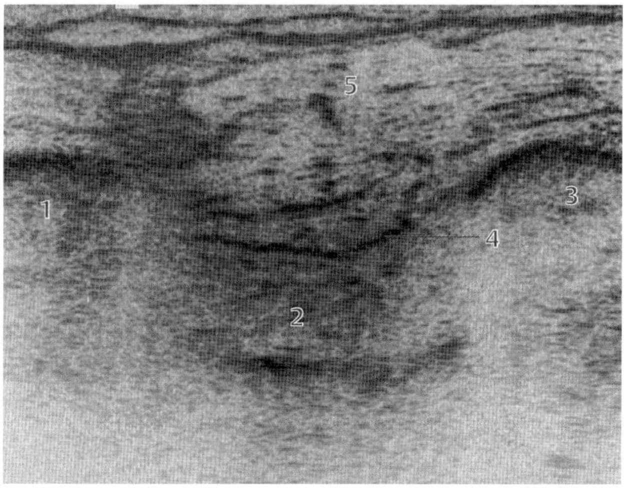

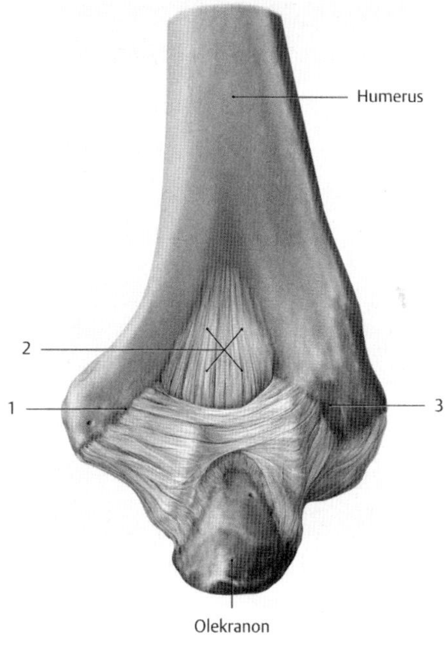

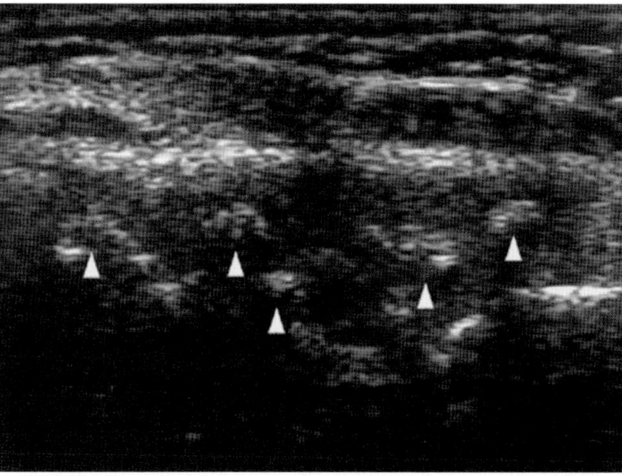

Fig. 2.19 Chondromatosis (*arrowheads*) (see Fig. 2.37D).

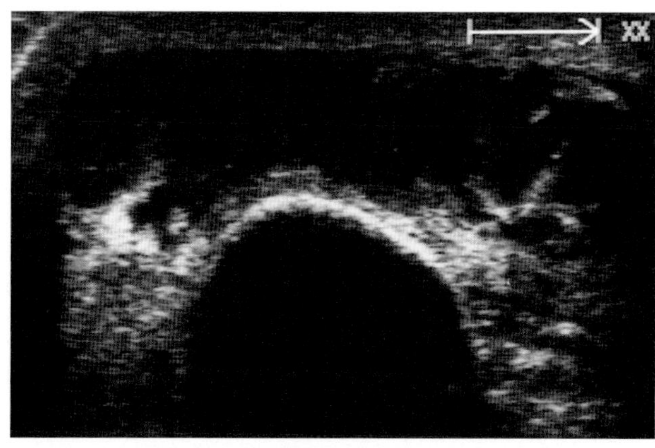

Fig. 2.20 Bursitis olecrani (see Fig. 2.40B).

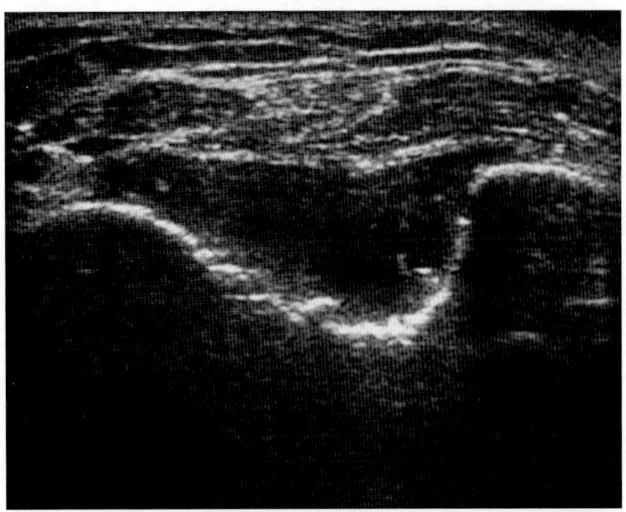

A

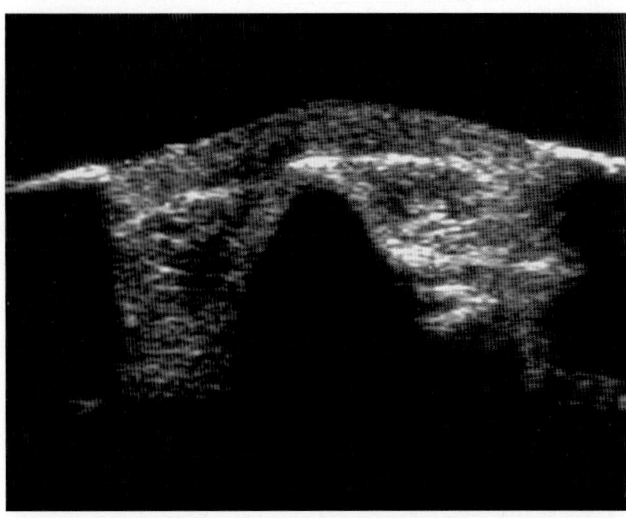

B

C

Fig. 2.21 **(A,B,C)** Cubital arthritis (see Figs. 2.44D, 2.45B, 2.46B).

Dorsal Region: Longitudinal Section

The transducer is positioned parallel to the longitudinal axes of the humeral shaft over the distal humerus and the olecranon with flexed elbow. Here, the distal humeral shaft, the olecranon fossa appears as a cavity between the trochlea and the humeral shaft. The olecranon can be seen as well. The triceps muscle is anterior to the olecranon process. The distal triceps tendon appears as a beak-shaped hyperechoic structure in continuity with the hypoechoic bellies of the triceps muscle that inserts ~1 cm distal to the apex of the

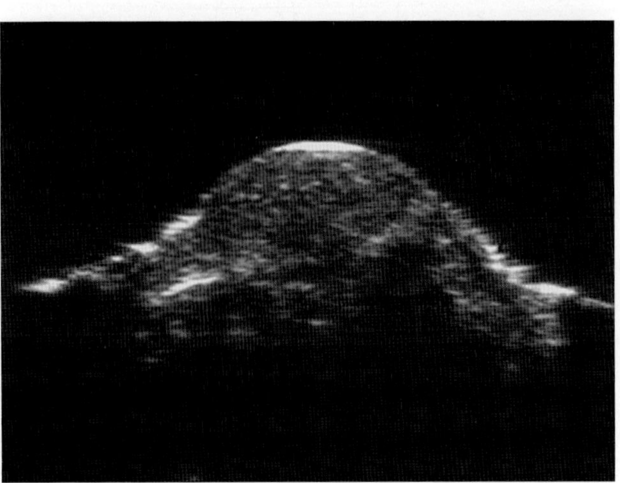

Fig. 2.22 Gouty tophus (see Fig. 2.47B).

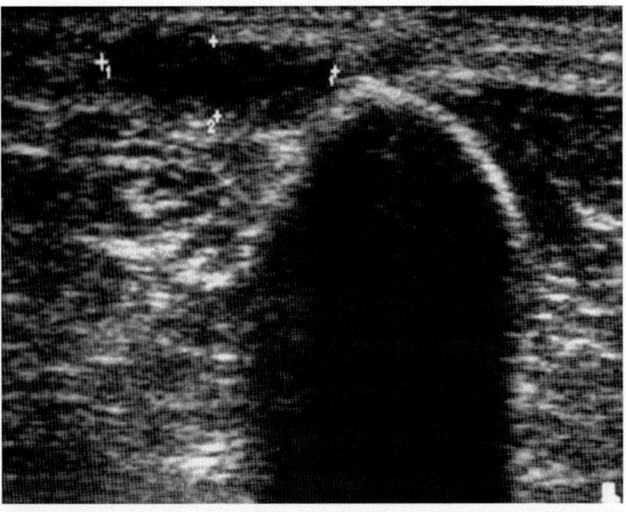

Fig. 2.23 Rheumatoid node (see Fig. 2.48B).

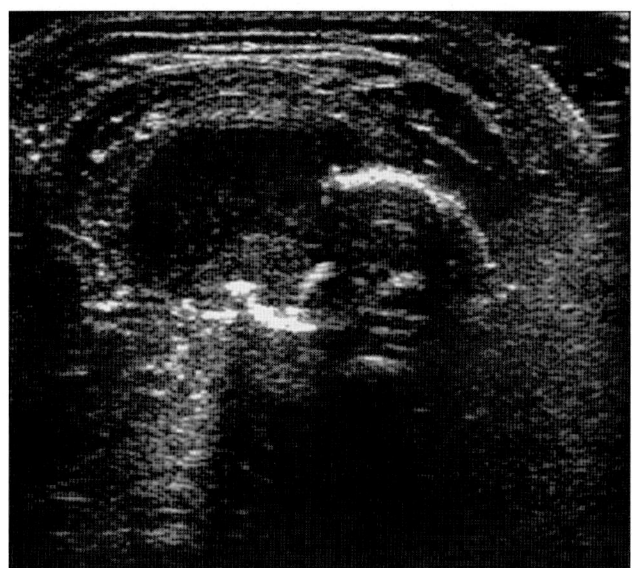

Fig. 2.24 Tumor (see Fig. 2.51B).

olecranon. The humeral shaft is positioned parallel to the upper border of the screen. Under normal conditions, the olecranon fossa appears echogenic (**Fig. 2.25**).

Differential Diagnosis

See **Figs. 2.26, 2.27, 2.28, 2.29, 2.30, 2.31, 2.32, 2.33, 2.34** for various pathologies found with dorsal longitudinal views of the elbow.

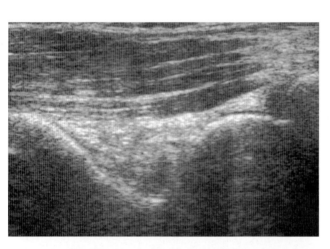

A

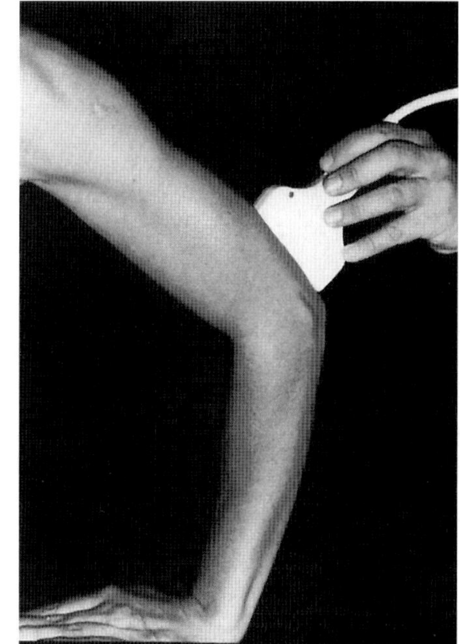

B

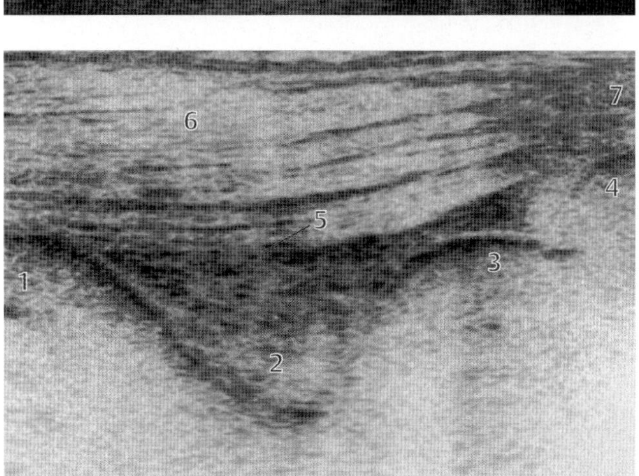

C

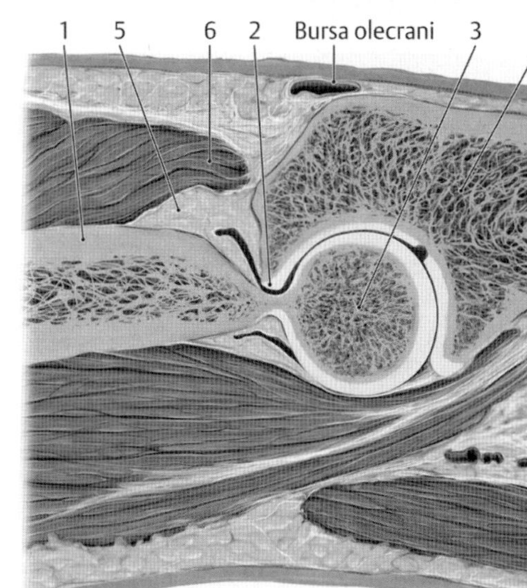

D

Fig. 2.25 **(A)** Longitudinal section, dorsal region. **(B)** Transducer position. **(C)** Anatomic structures visualized by ultrasound, annotated in (D). **(D)** Anatomic position of the structures visualized in (C): 1, humeral shaft; 2, fossa olecrani; 3, trochlea humeri; 4, olecranon; 5, joint capsule; 6, M. triceps brachii; 7, triceps tendon.

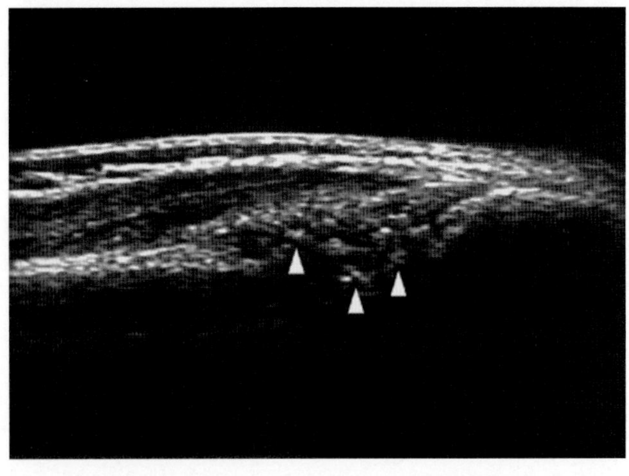

Fig. 2.26 Chondromatosis (*arrowheads*) (see Fig. 2.37C).

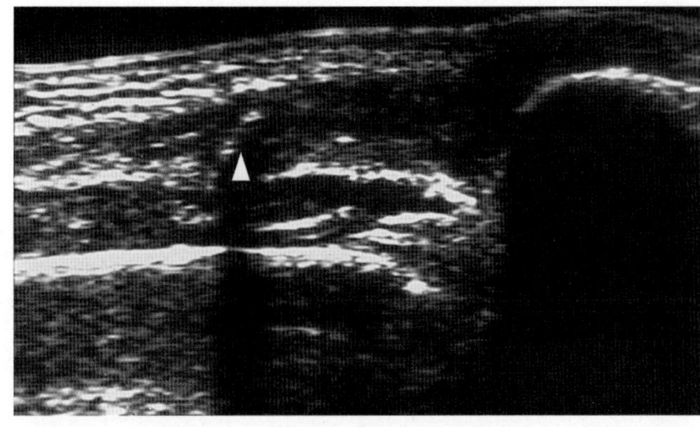

Fig. 2.28 Triceps tendon calcification (*arrowhead*) (see Fig. 2.43A).

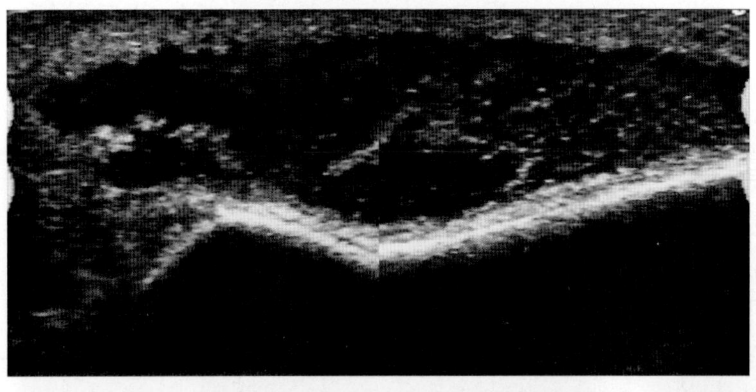

A

Fig. 2.27 **(A,B,C)** Bursitis olecrani (see Fig. 2.40A,C and Fig. 2.41).

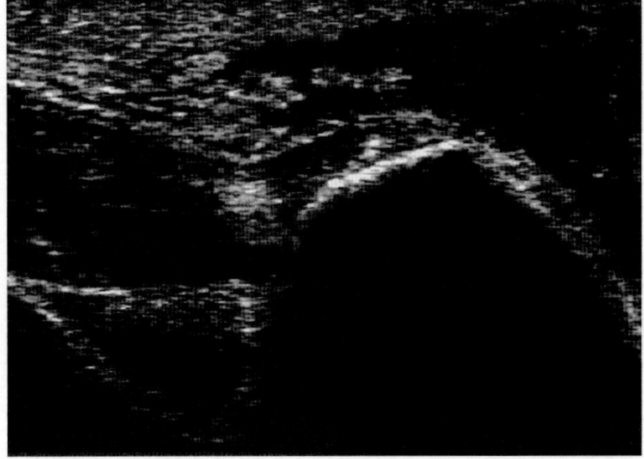

B

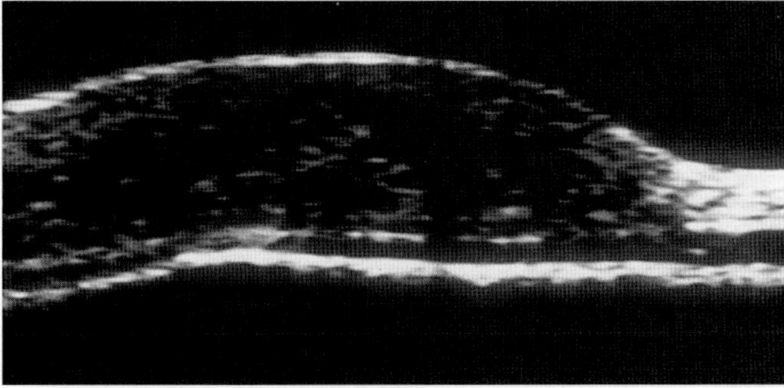

C

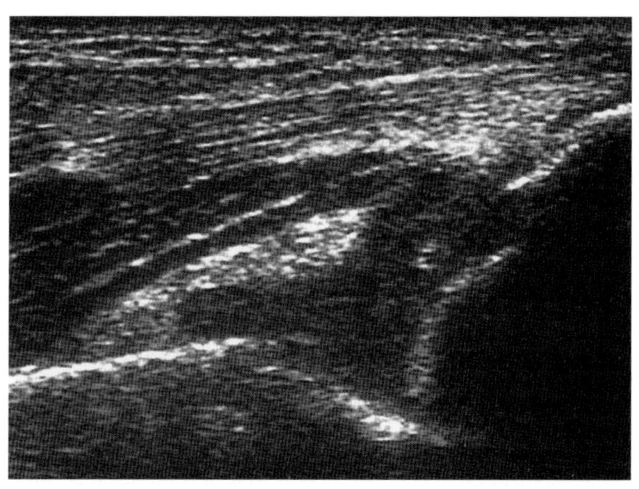

A

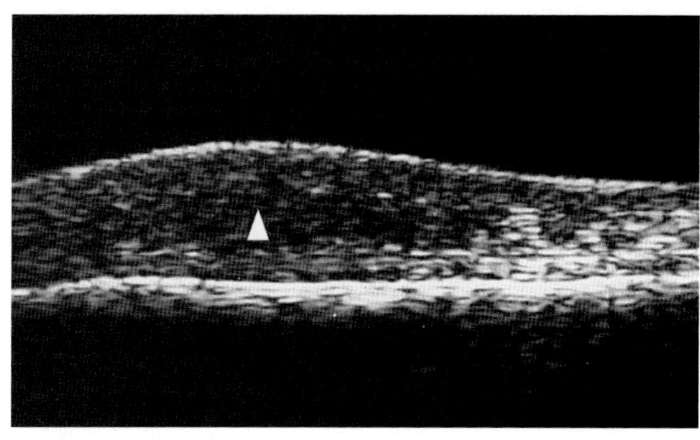

Fig. 2.31 Soft tissue changes in rheumatoid arthritis (*arrowhead*) (see Fig. 2.45A).

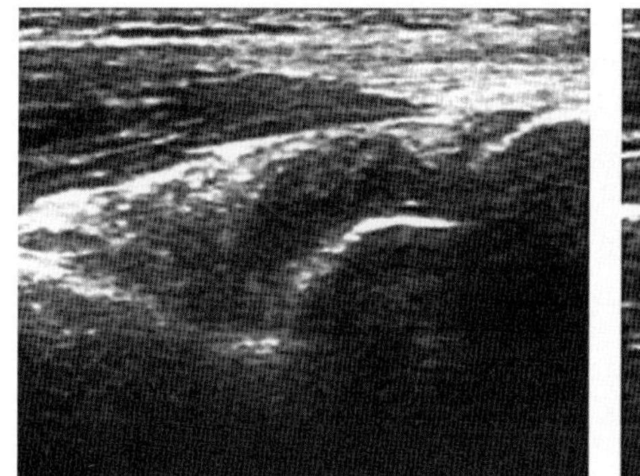

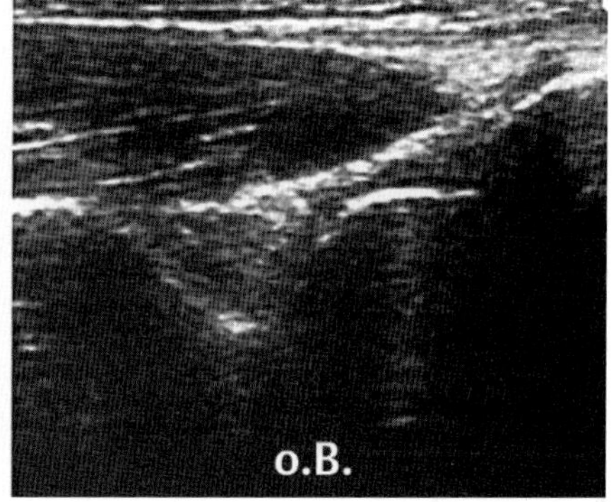

B

Fig. 2.29 **(A,B)** Radial head fracture (see Figs. 2.39B,C).

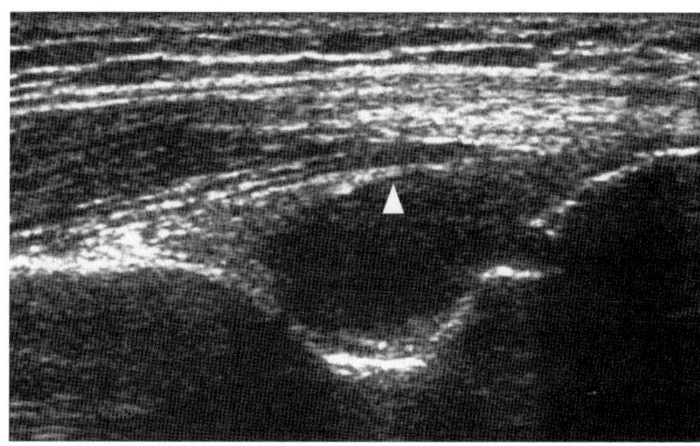

A

Fig. 2.30 **(A,B)** Cubital arthritis (see Fig. 2.44C and Fig. 2.46A).

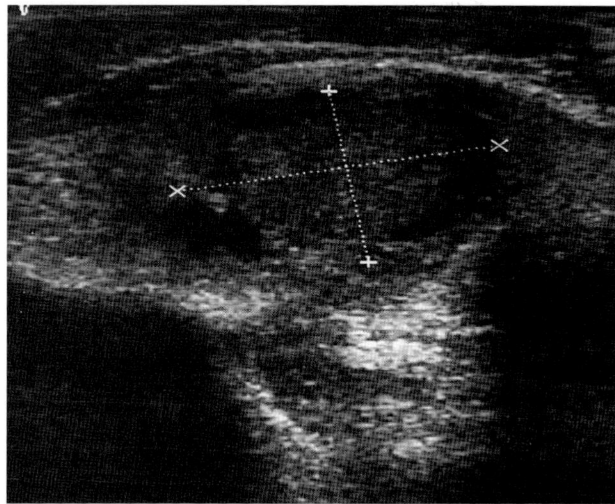

B

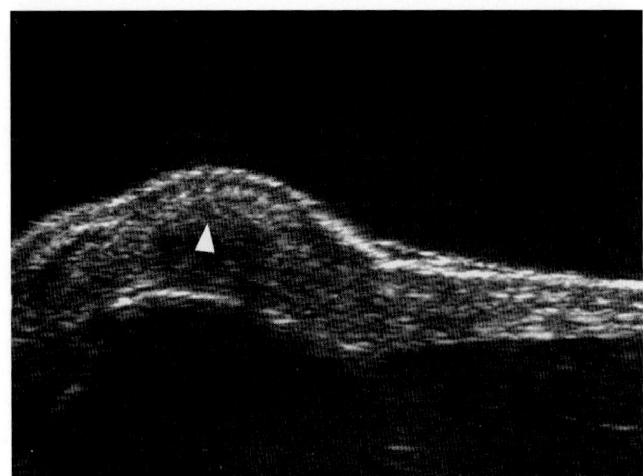

Fig. 2.32 Gouty tophus (*arrowhead*) (see Fig. 2.47A).

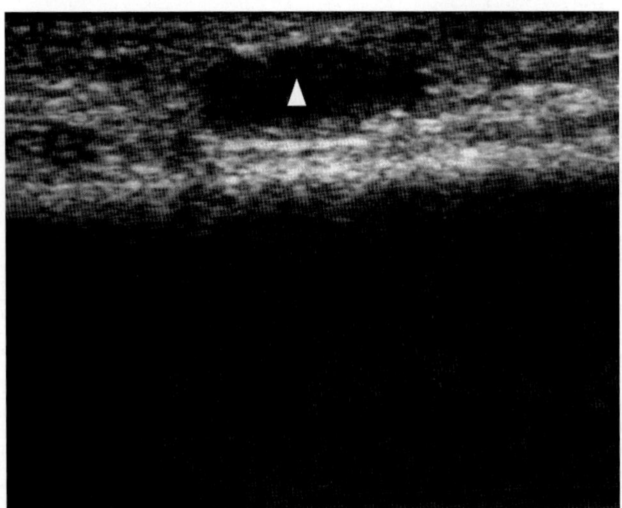

Fig. 2.33 Rheumatoid node (*arrowhead*) (see Fig. 2.48A).

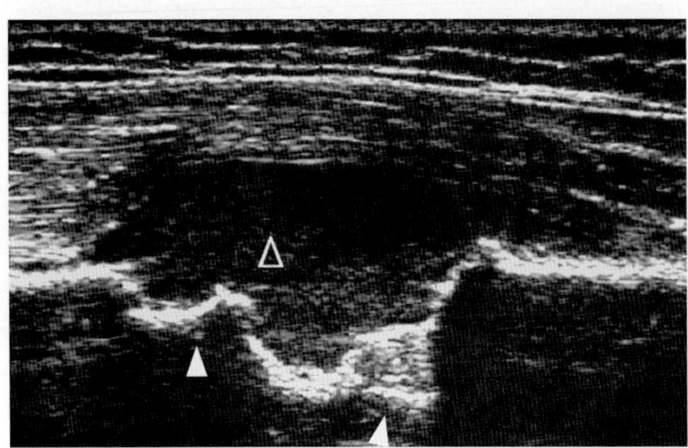

Fig. 2.34 Tumor (see Fig. 2.51A).

Pathologic Findings

Avascular Osteonecroses and Osteochondroses

Clinical Appearance

The etiopathogeneses of the avascular cartilage-bone necroses has not yet been fully elucidated. In the elbow joint, the most frequent localization is the capitulum humeri (Panner disease) and the second most frequent localization is the trochlea humeri (Hageman disease). Apart from the knee joint, the second most frequent localization of the osteochondrosis dissecans is the elbow joint. The main localizations are the convex joint surfaces. Osteochondrosis dissecans affects males twice as often as females and usually develops between 10 to 50 years of age. If the osteochondrotic fragment breaks loose, it can be seen as a loose body in the joint (joint mouse). This can be found predominantly in the olecranon fossa and the coronoid fossa.

Ultrasound

Using ultrasound the bony changes as well as the potential joint capsule distention are evaluated (**Fig. 2.35**).

Free Joint Body

Clinical Appearance

In order of frequency, free joint bodies can be observed in chondromatosis, osteochondrosis dissecans, osteoarthritis, and intraarticular fracture. They can lead to joint blockings.

Ultrasound

Free joint bodies can be found at different positions in the joint space. The most frequent localizations are the olecranon fossa and the coronoid fossa (**Fig. 2.36**).

Chondromatosis

Clinical Appearance

Chondromatosis is a rare disease that most frequently affects the elbow joint. Based on a metaplastic change of the plica synovialis, sometimes more than 100 chondromas are formed in the joint cavity.

Ultrasound

Initially, the chondromas are cartilaginous (sonographically low echogenicity without acoustic shadowing) and increasingly ossify over time (sonographically with high echogenicity and acoustic shadowing). They move freely in the joint space and typically lead to recurrent joint blockings (**Fig. 2.37**).

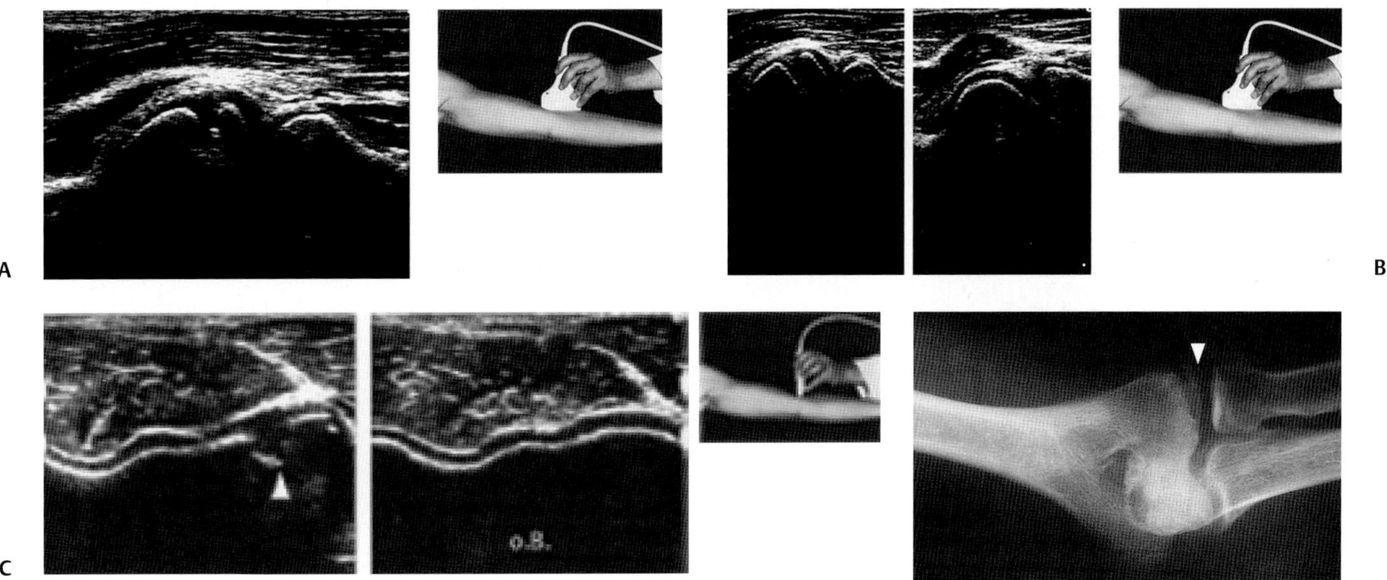

Fig. 2.35 A 14-year-old patient, left elbow joint. **(A)** Ventral humeroradial longitudinal section, left side. The capitulum humeri reveals an interruption of its contour with a base reflex (*arrow*). The cartilage coating cannot be evaluated properly. An intraarticular volume increase can be definitely excluded. **(B)** Ventral humeroradial longitudinal section, right and left side. The contralateral side (right image) shows a normal ultrasound scan. **(C)** Ventral transversal section normal, right and left side. **(D)** X-ray in anteroposterior projection. The x-ray image clarifies the findings. Osteochondrosis dissecans of the capitulum humeri can be seen (*arrowhead*).

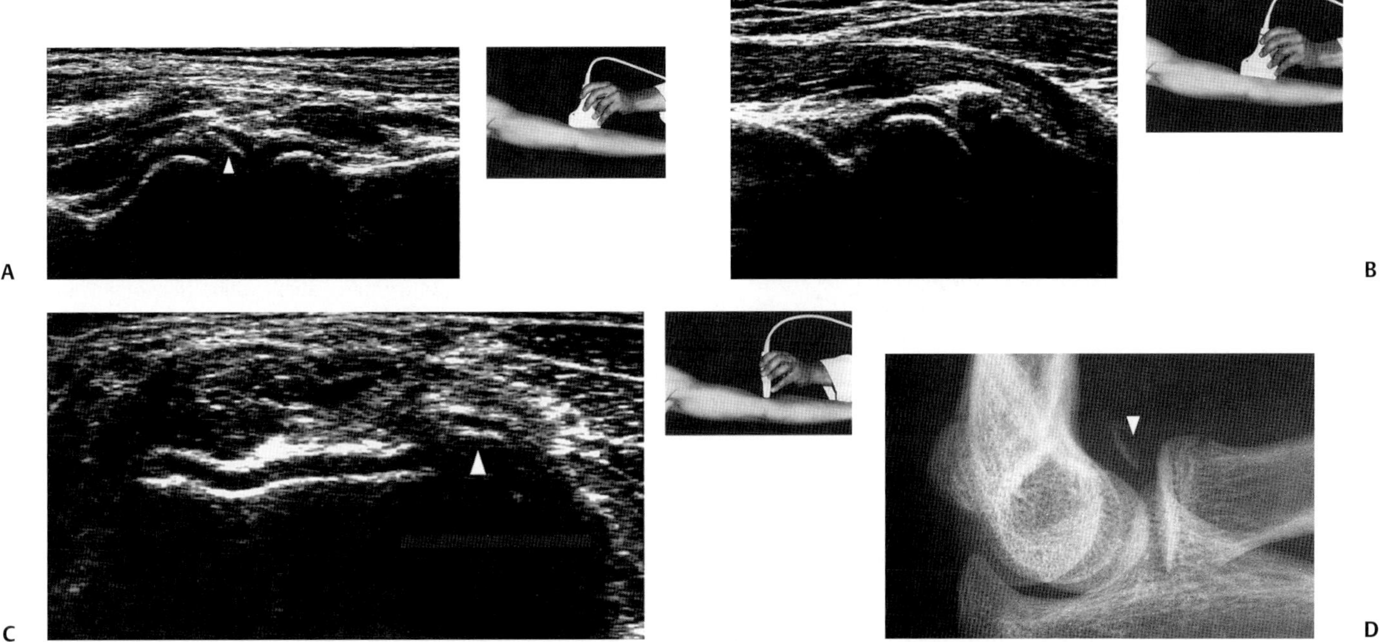

Fig. 2.36 A 12-year-old female patient, right elbow joint. **(A)** Ventral humeroradial longitudinal section, right side. The adherent joint body is seen as an echogenic longitudinal structure with acoustic shadowing in the region of the capitulum humeri (*arrowhead*). **(B)** Ventral humeroulnar longitudinal section, right side. In the humeroulnar longitudinal section, normal findings are observed. **(C)** Ventral transversal section, right side. **(D)** X-ray in lateral projection. The x-ray image clarifies the findings (*arrowhead*).

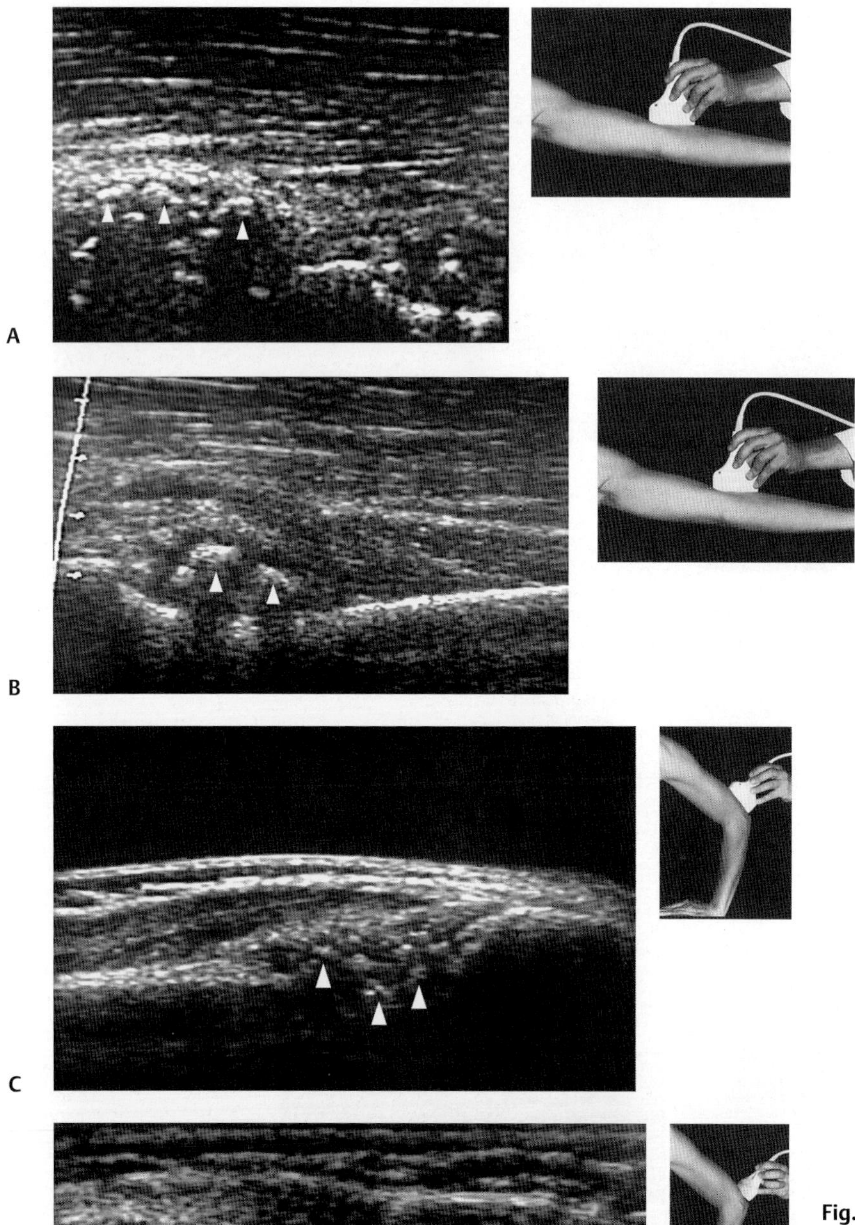

Fig. 2.37 A 34-year-old patient, right elbow joint. **(A)** Ventral humeroradial longitudinal section, right side. Multiple chondromas can be observed partly as structures with low echogenicity, partly as structures with high echogenicity and acoustic shadowing (*arrowheads*). Thus, the capitulum humeri can no longer be visualized. **(B)** Ventral humeroradial longitudinal section, right side. **(C)** Dorsal longitudinal section, right side. In the olecranon fossa, multiple chondromas can be seen as well. Consequently, the base of the olecranon fossa is sonographically not observable. **(D)** Dorsal transversal section, right side.

Fracture of the Coronoid Process

Ultrasound

To evaluate a fracture, an x-ray is the primary imaging choice. By ultrasound examination, one can observe an osseous discontinuity and an eventual axis deviation in each plane, as well as a fracture-induced hematoma that usually appears as a structure with low echogenicity (**Fig. 2.38**).

Radial Head Fracture

Clinical Appearance

Although the dislocated radial head fracture with clear history, clinical findings, and x-ray-based confirmation does not create significant problems, one may sometimes observe cases where no clear signs of fracture can be found despite a typical history and clinical findings. In radial head fracture, the intraarticular fracture localization leads to intraarticular hemorrhage.

Ultrasound

Based on the pain-induced protective posture with flexion in the elbow joint, the dorsal region can be examined by ultrasound without any problems. In the presence of an intraarticular hemorrhage, a convex-shaped elevation of the joint capsule can be observed in ultrasound. In addition, the radial head as well as the radial neck can eventually be examined ventrally using a convexly bended transducer. In some cases, one can find a discontinuity. A sonographically guided puncture with aspiration of the intraarticular hemorrhage can be done to relieve the pressure in the joint (**Fig. 2.39**).

A

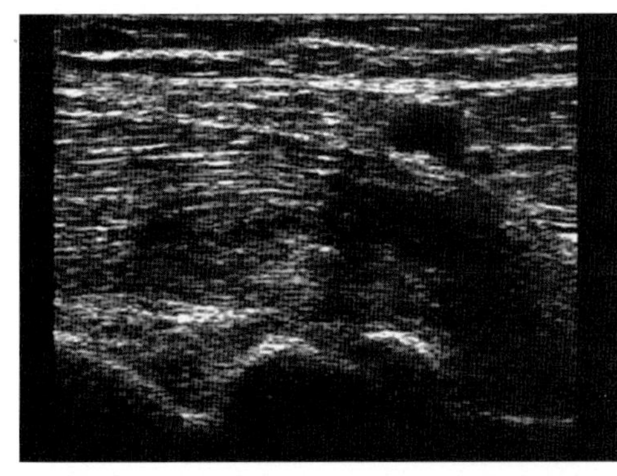

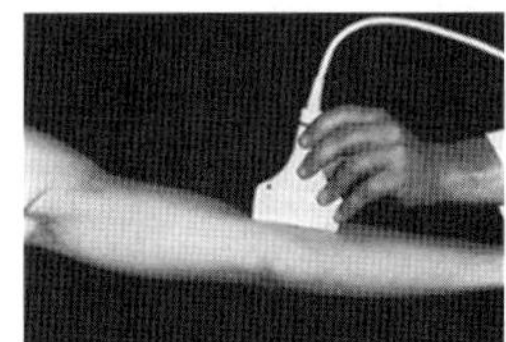

B

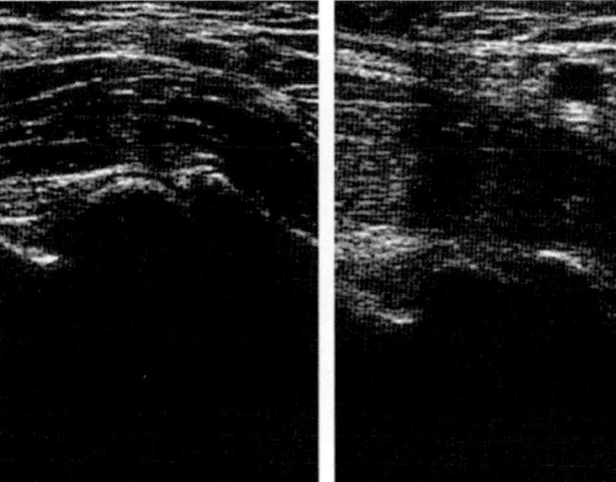

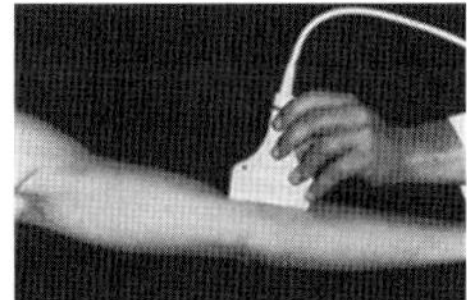

Fig. 2.38 A 52-year-old patient, right elbow joint. **(A)** Ventral humeroulnar longitudinal section, right side. If the coronoid process is fractured, it does not appear as a narrow-angled echogenic reflex as under normal conditions, but as a broad echogenic reflex (*arrow*). In addition, one can observe a discrete distension of the joint capsule based on interarticular hemorrhage. **(B)** Ventral humeroulnar longitudinal section, right and left side.

A

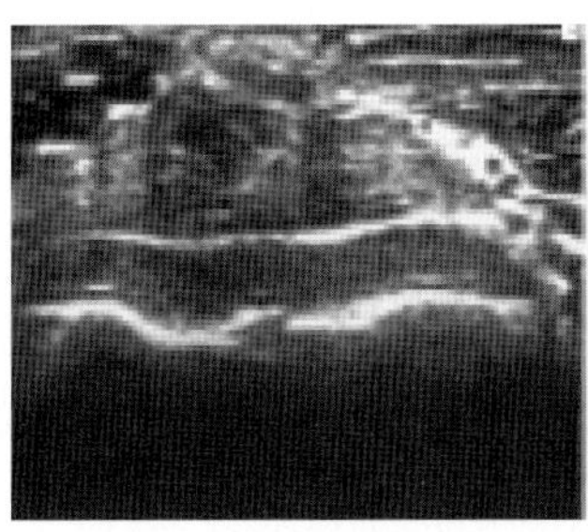

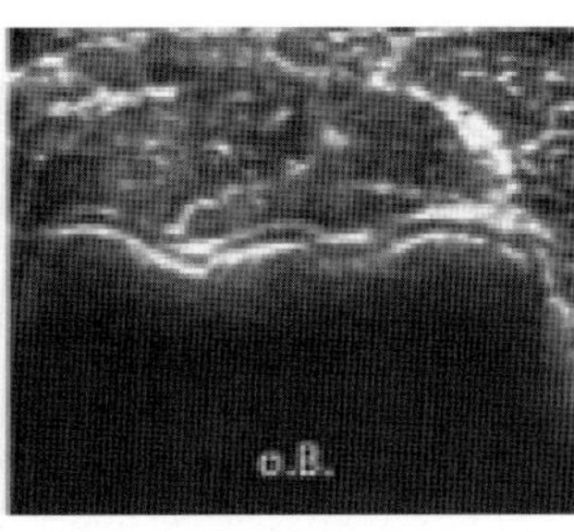

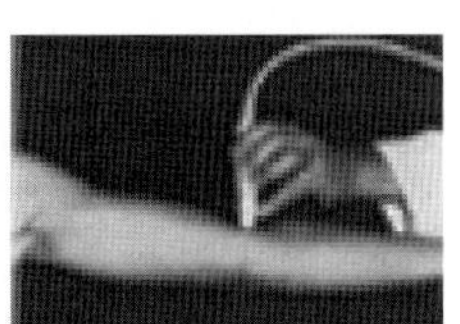

Fig. 2.39 A 32-year-old patient, left elbow joint. **(A)** Ventral transversal section comparing right and left sides. In both section planes a distension of the capsule can be observed as a result of intraarticular hemorrhage in the sense of an intraarticular volume increase with low echogenicity. (*Continued*)

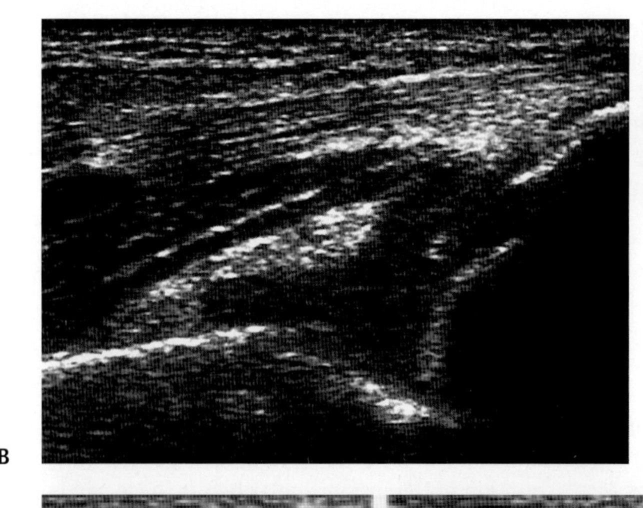

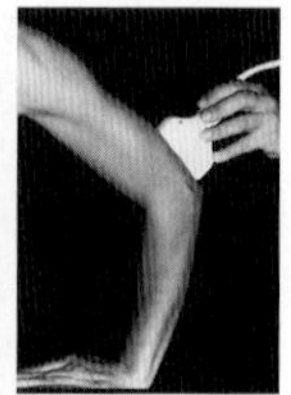

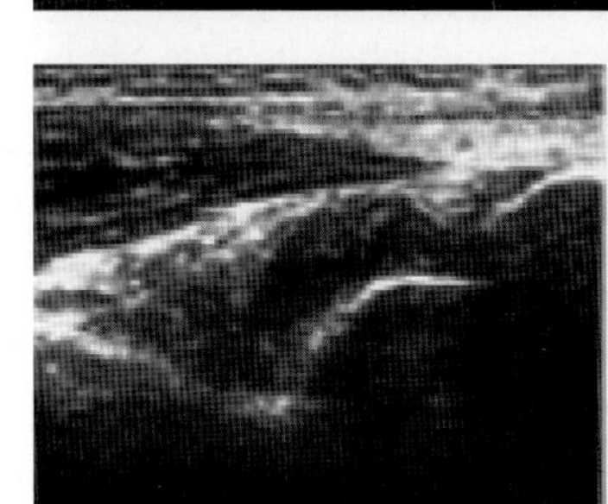

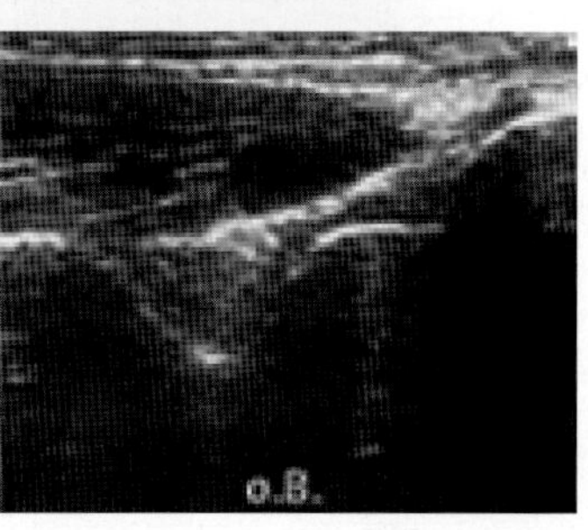

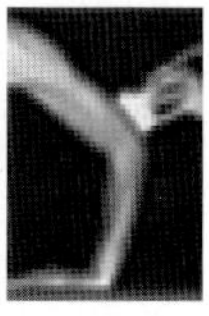

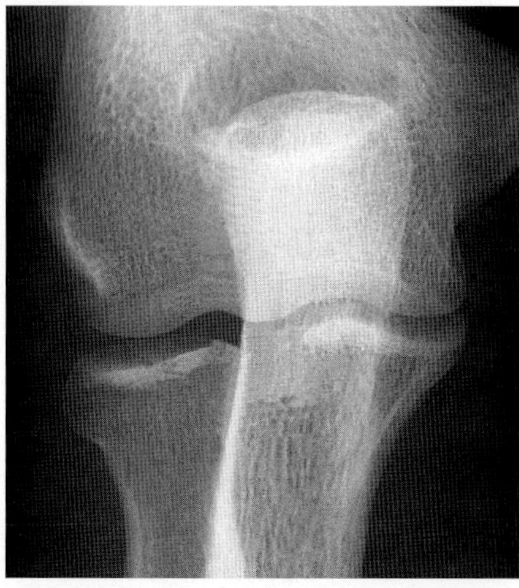

Fig. 2.39 (*Continued*) **(B)** Dorsal longitudinal section, left side. **(C)** Dorsal longitudinal sections comparing right and left sides. **(D)** X-ray in anteroposterior (AP) projection. The x-ray does not clearly reveal a discontinuity.

Olecranon Bursitis

Clinical Appearance

The olecranon bursitis is located between the subcutaneous tissue and the olecranon; it cannot be observed sonographically under normal conditions. The olecranon bursitis is a localized fluctuating swelling dorsal to the olecranon. It has to be distinguished from a rheumatic note and a gouty tophus.

Ultrasound

In general, the ultrasound examination of an olecranon bursitis is performed with the elbow extended (**Figs. 2.40, 2.41**).

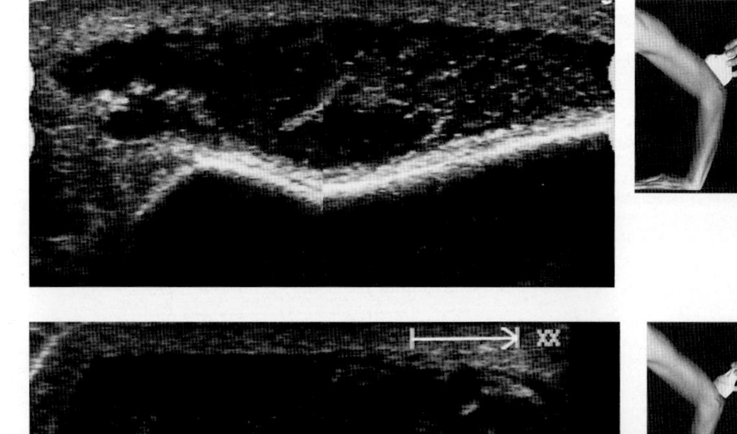

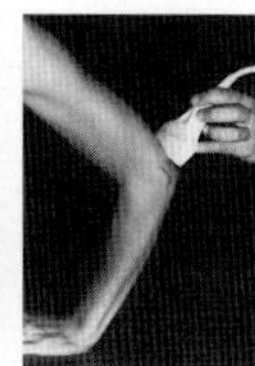

Fig. 2.40 A 26-year-old patient, left elbow joint. **(A)** Dorsal longitudinal section in extended position, left side. In this case the septic olecranon bursitis can be observed as a widespread mass lesion with predominantly low echogenicity and echogenic internal structures. **(B)** Dorsal transversal section, left side. (*Continued*)

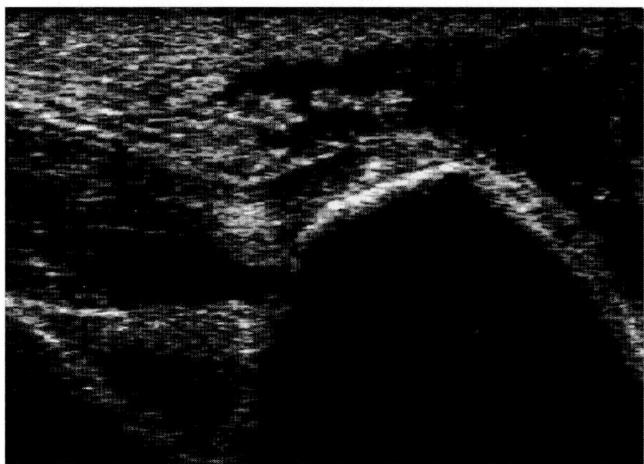
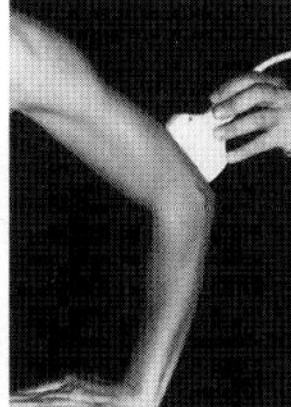

C

Fig. 2.40 (*Continued*) **(C)** Dorsal longitudinal section in flexed position, left side. The triceps tendon and the intraarticular space appear normal in the dorsal region.

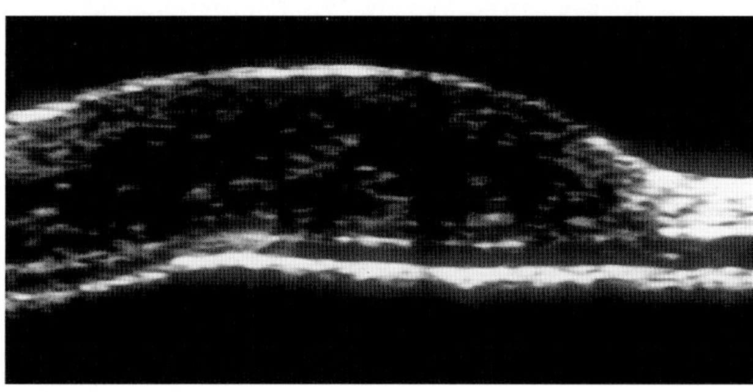
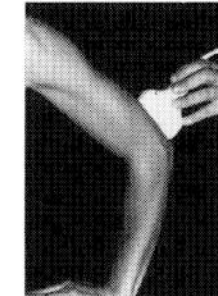

Fig. 2.41 A 70-year-old patient, left proximal forearm. Dorsal longitudinal section left side. In the immediate dorsal vicinity of the cortical surface of the ulna, a structure with predominantly low echogenicity is visualized. It is a septic olecranon bursitis.

Distal Biceps Tendon Rupture

Clinical Appearance

A distal biceps tendon rupture occurs very rarely when compared with the proximal rupture of the long biceps tendon. In most cases, it is caused by trauma and is most often observed in athletes.

Ultrasound

Ultrasound should be performed at the insertion region of the tendon at the tuberositas radii. The transducer is moved proximally from this position along the biceps muscle in a longitudinal direction (**Fig. 2.42**).

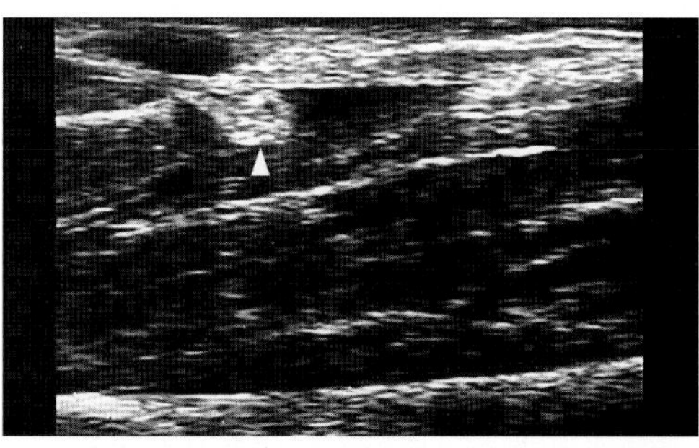
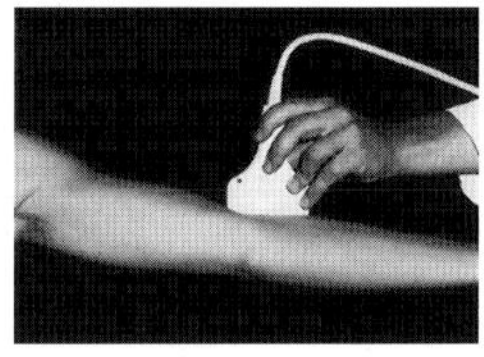

A

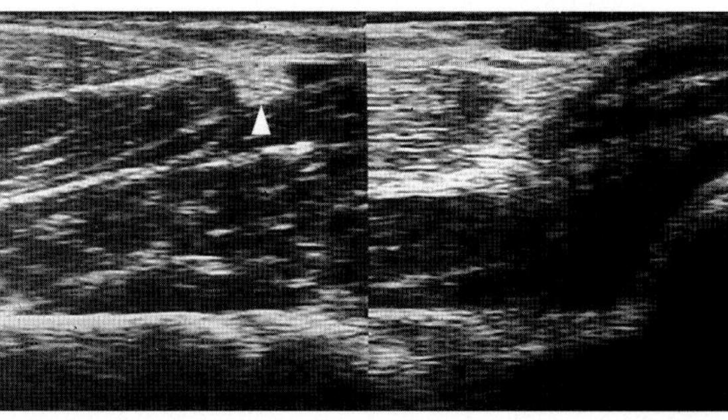
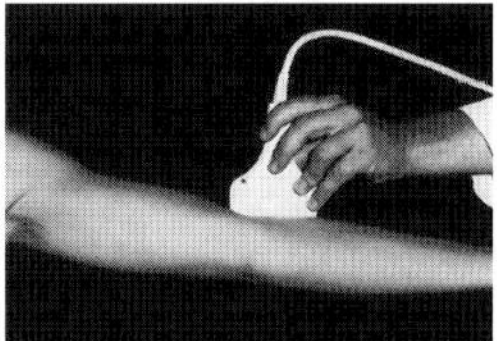

B

Fig. 2.42 A 33-year-old patient, right elbow joint. **(A)** Ventral humeroradial longitudinal section, right side. The rupture zone can be seen as a triangular-shaped region with low echogenicity at the distal, volar upper arm (*arrowhead*). The proximal ending of the distal biceps tendon can be seen as an echogenic region. **(B)** Ventral humeroradial longitudinal section, right side. The composed image shows the localization in relation to the capitulum humeri (*arrowhead*).

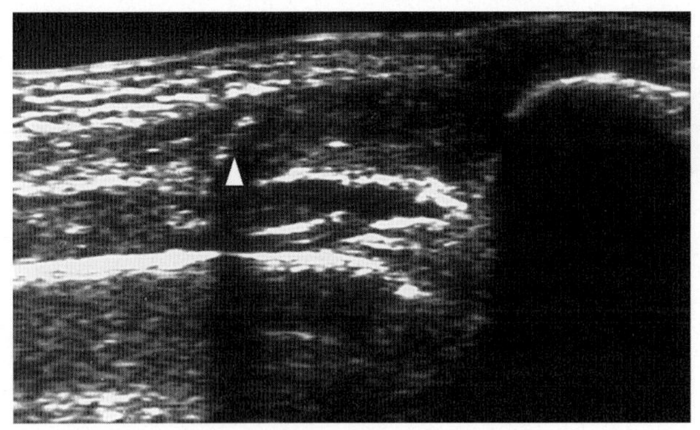
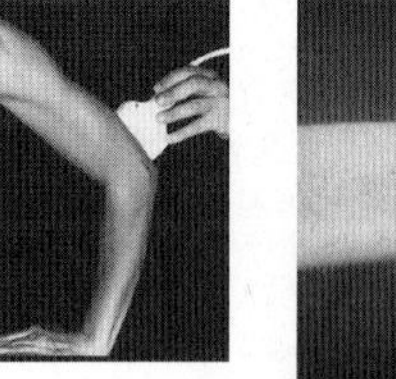
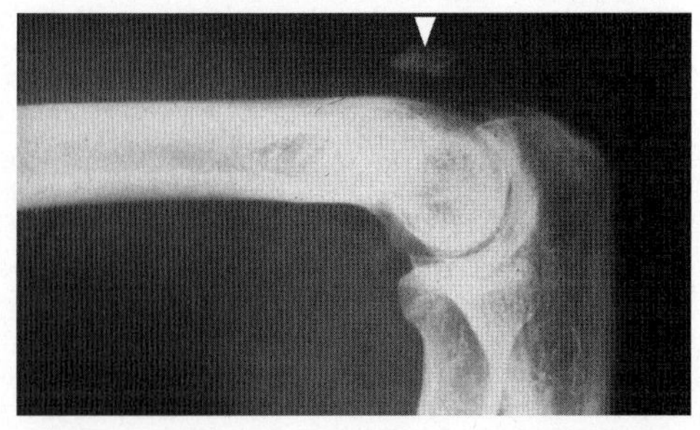

Fig. 2.43 A 41-year-old patient, left elbow joint. **(A)** Dorsal longitudinal section, left side. Along the triceps tendon the calcification presents as an echogenic reflex with acoustic shadowing (*arrowhead*). **(B)** X-ray in lateral projection. The x-ray confirms the findings (*arrowhead*).

Calcification of the Triceps Tendon

Clinical Appearance

Calcification affecting muscles or tendons can be observed as degenerative, posttraumatic, as well as postinfectious changes.

Ultrasound

Calcification cannot reliably be distinguished from ossifying myositis; both conditions appear with an echogenic reflex with acoustic shadowing (**Fig. 2.43**).

Cubital Arthritis

Clinical Appearance

In the context of a manifestation of rheumatic disease in the elbow joint, bony structures, the joint cavity, as well as the periarticular soft tissue can be involved.

Ultrasound

In healthy individuals, the contents of the olecranon fossa and the coronoid fossa appear more echogenic than the muscles located above these structures. In contrast, in the presence of a rheumatoid arthritis, one can observe the contents of the fossae with low or even missing echo signal, eventually associated with a distension of the joint capsule. Cartilaginous and bony destructions can be visualized sonographically (**Figs. 2.44, 2.45, 2.46**).

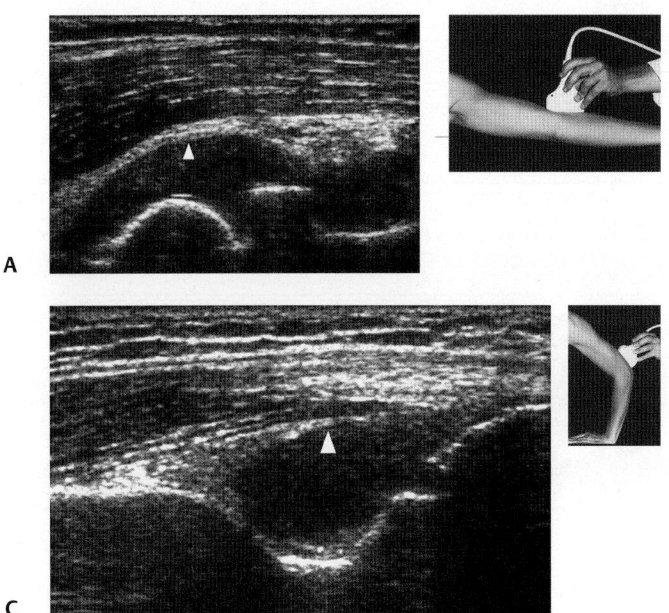
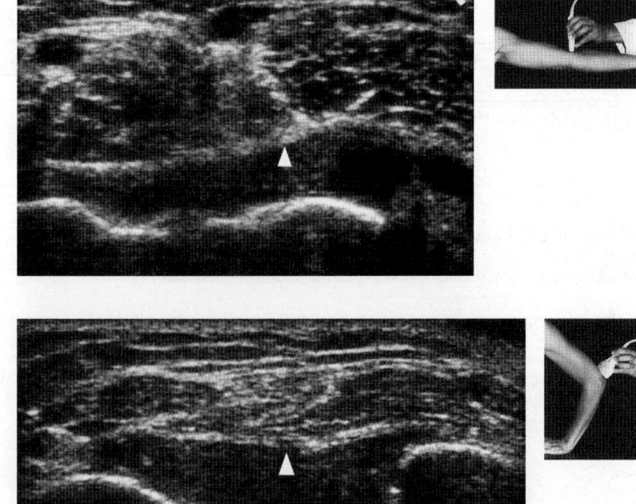

Fig. 2.44 A 59-year-old female patient, right elbow joint. **(A)** Ventral humeroradial longitudinal section, right side. In the visualized sections, one can observe a significant distension of the capsule associated with an intraarticular increase in volume (*arrowhead*). Bony changes cannot be detected sonographically. The findings indicate the presence of rheumatoid arthritis. **(B)** Ventral transversal section, right side. **(C)** Dorsal longitudinal section, right side. **(D)** Dorsal transversal section, right side.

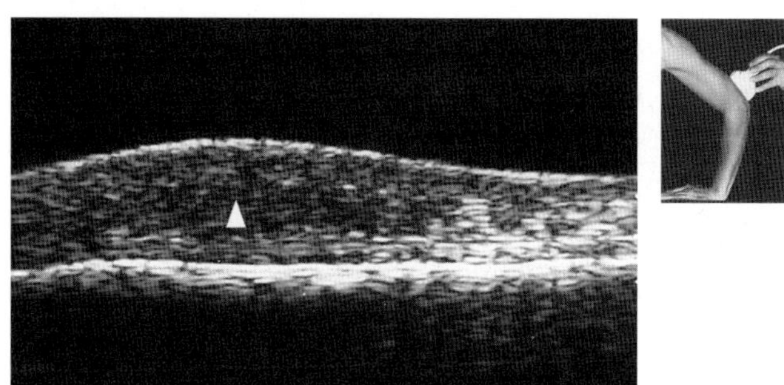
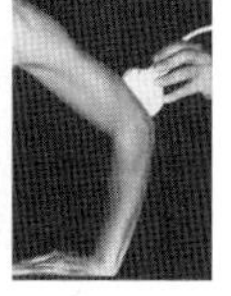
A

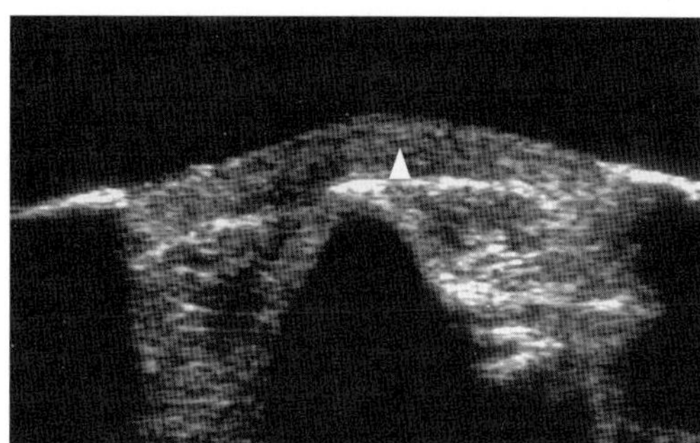

B

Fig. 2.45 A 50-year-old patient, right proximal dorsal ulna. **(A)** Dorsal longitudinal section, right side. In both sectional planes, a homogeneous soft tissue formation with high echogenicity can be observed dorsoradial to the cortical surface of the ulna (*arrowhead*). The findings represent a soft tissue change associated with rheumatoid arthritis. **(B)** Dorsal transversal section, right side.

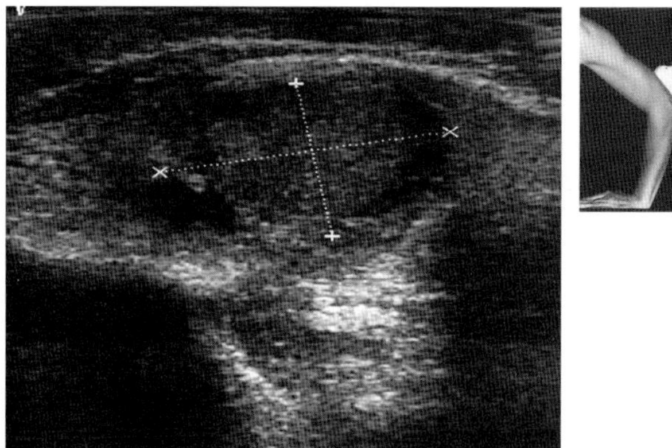
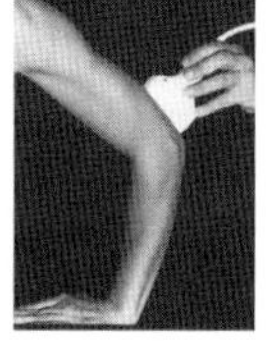
A

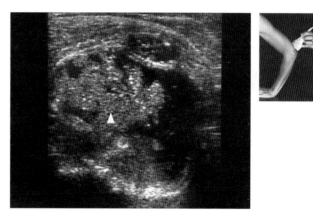

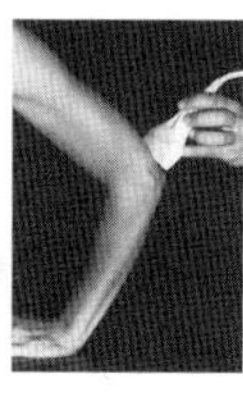
B

Fig. 2.46 A 63-year-old female patient, left elbow joint. **(A)** Dorsal longitudinal section, left side. A soft tissue formation, predominantly echogenic with hypoechoic margins appears dorsal to the olecranon fossa in both sectional planes. **(B)** In the transversal section, left side, the surface exhibits villous appearance (*arrowhead*). The triceps muscle is displaced in dorsal direction. The findings represent a soft tissue change in rheumatoid arthritis.

Gouty Tophus

Clinical Appearance

In chronic hyperuremia, depositions of urate crystals can be observed in the joint cartilage and in the joint capsule as well as in the subcutaneous tissue.

Ultrasound

The gouty tophus appears sonographically echogenic without acoustic shadowing, and it is usually more echogenic than a rheumatic node (**Fig. 2.47**).

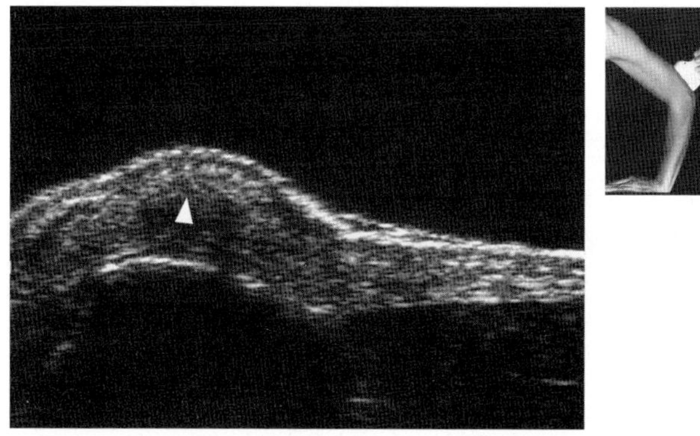
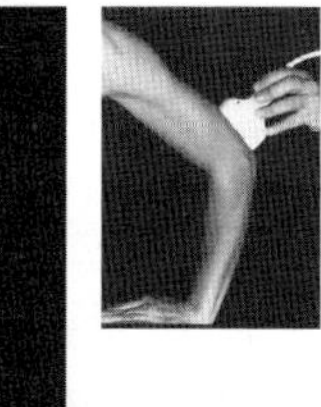
A

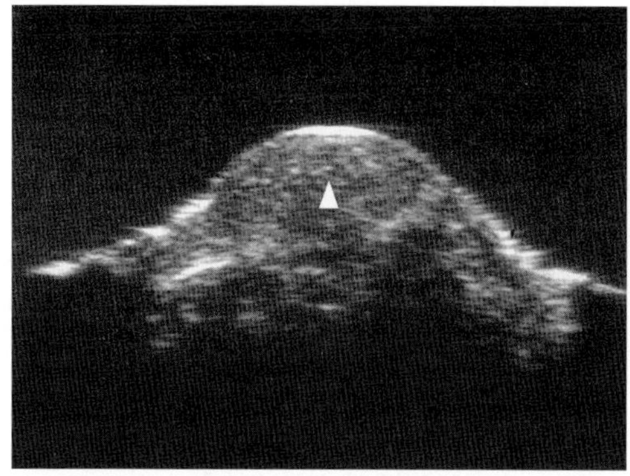
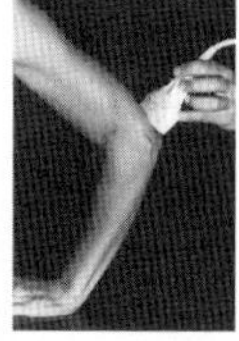
B

Fig. 2.47 A 54-year-old patient, right elbow joint. **(A)** Dorsal longitudinal section, right side. In both sectional planes, a predominantly echogenic formation appears dorsal to the olecranon (*arrowhead*). **(B)** Dorsal transversal section, right side.

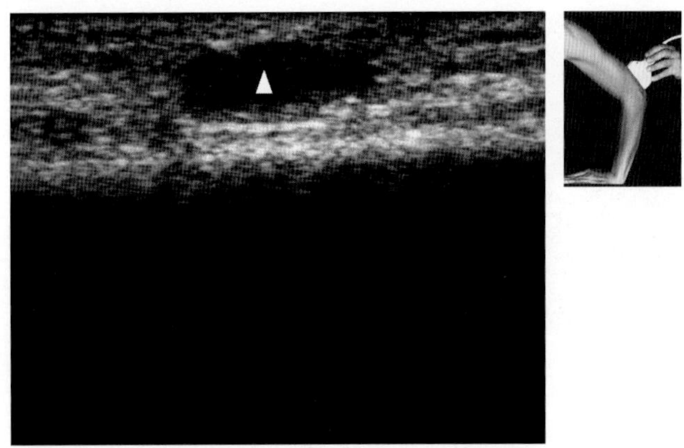

A

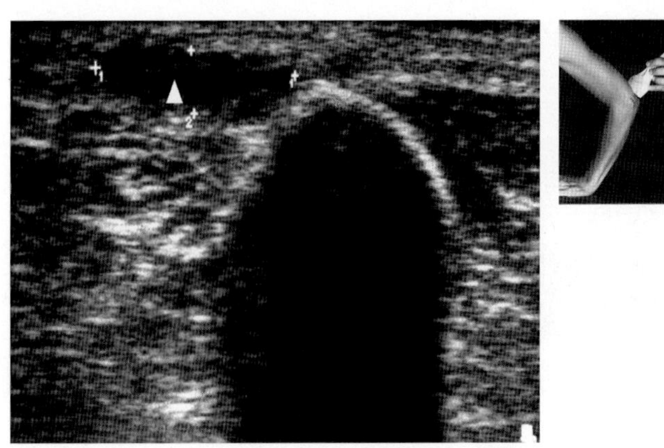

B

Fig. 2.48 A 50-year-old female patient, left proximal forearm. **(A)** Dorsal longitudinal section, left side. A hypoechogenic ovoid structure in the subcutaneous tissue is a reactive lymph node in rheumatoid arthritis (arrowhead). Calipers outline the lesion in **(B)** dorsal transversal section, left side.

Rheumatic Node

Clinical Appearance and Ultrasound

Rheumatic nodes can typically be found close to the joint at the dorsal aspect of the proximal ulna. They usually appear hypoechogenic and have an oval shape (**Fig. 2.48**).

Lymphadenitis

Clinical Appearance and Ultrasound

Severe inflammations result in regional lymphangitis and, based on the exudative inflammation, in involvement of the regional lymph nodes presenting with the histologic appearance of lymphadenitis (**Fig. 2.49**).

Tumor

Clinical Appearance

In the elbow region, benign and malignant soft tissue and bone tumors as well as metastases can be observed.

Ultrasound

Frequently, such changes are diagnosed in the context of a multiregional ultrasound examination. This underlines the necessity of a multiregional ultrasound work-up. In benign and malignant soft tissue and bone tumors as well as metastases, bone surface and soft tissue changes can be detected sonographically. However, a detailed histopathologic specification cannot be based on ultrasound. Besides the obligatory biplanar x-ray diagnostics, further imaging studies and a histopathologic tissue examination are required for further diagnostic work-up (**Figs. 2.50, 2.51**).

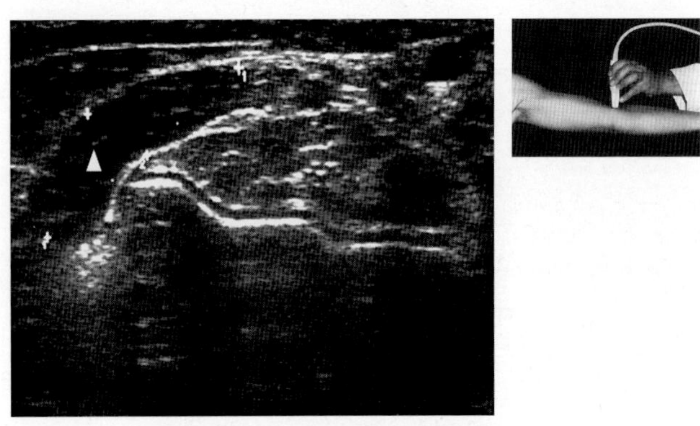

A

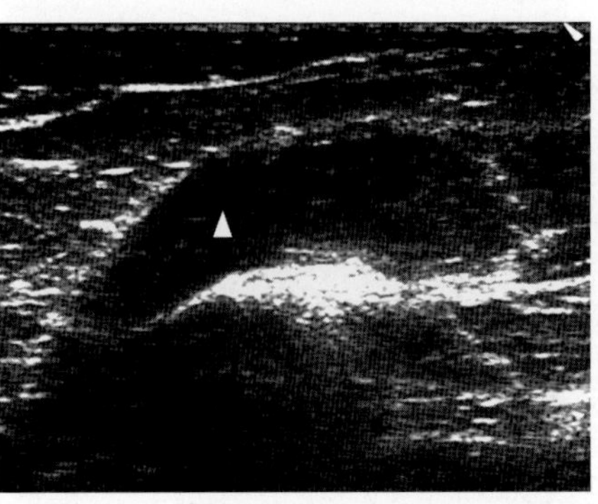

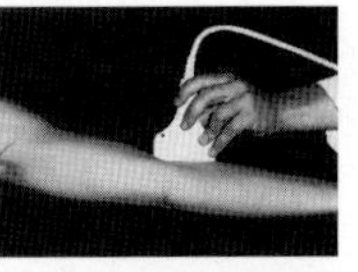

B

Fig. 2.49 A 25-year-old female patient, left elbow joint. **(A)** Ventral transversal section, left side. In both sectional planes, a hypoechoic structure with echogenic margin appears volar/ulnar to the trochlea. Intraarticular volume increase cannot be observed sonographically. Histologic analysis revealed a nonspecific lymph node alteration. **(B)** Ventral longitudinal section over the lymph node, left side.

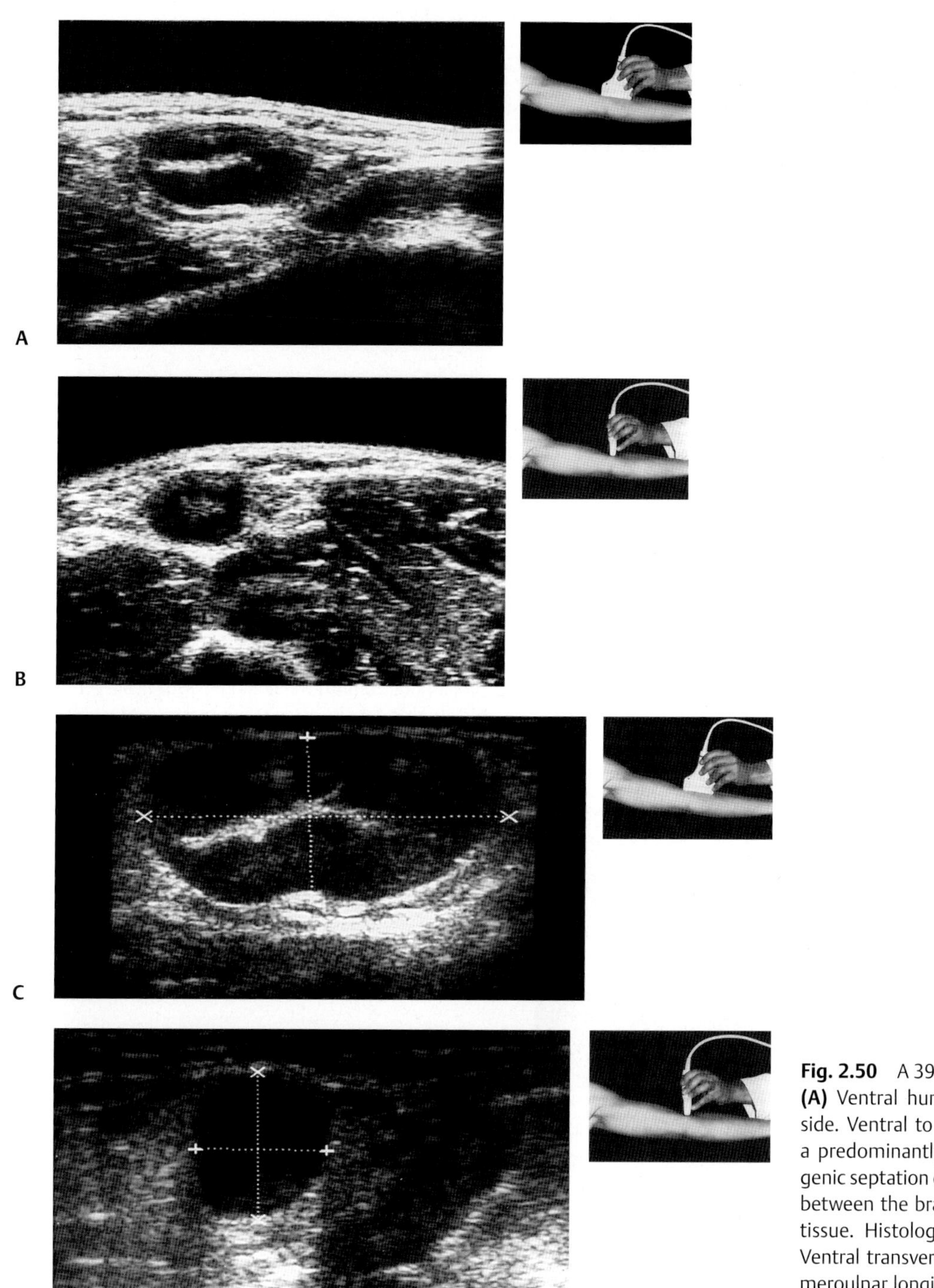

Fig. 2.50 A 39-year-old patient, right distal humerus. **(A)** Ventral humeroulnar longitudinal section, right side. Ventral to the cortical surface of the humerus, a predominantly hypoechoic mass lesion with echogenic septation can be observed in both section planes between the brachialis muscle and the subcutaneous tissue. Histologic analysis revealed a ganglion. **(B)** Ventral transversal section, right side. **(C)** Ventral humeroulnar longitudinal section, right side. **(D)** Ventral transversal section, right side.

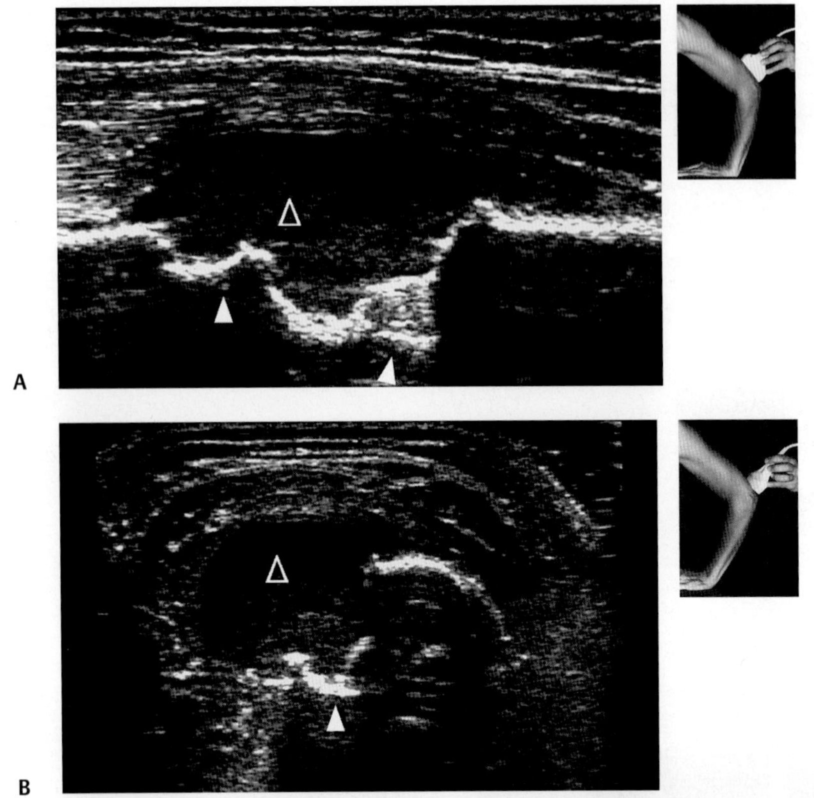

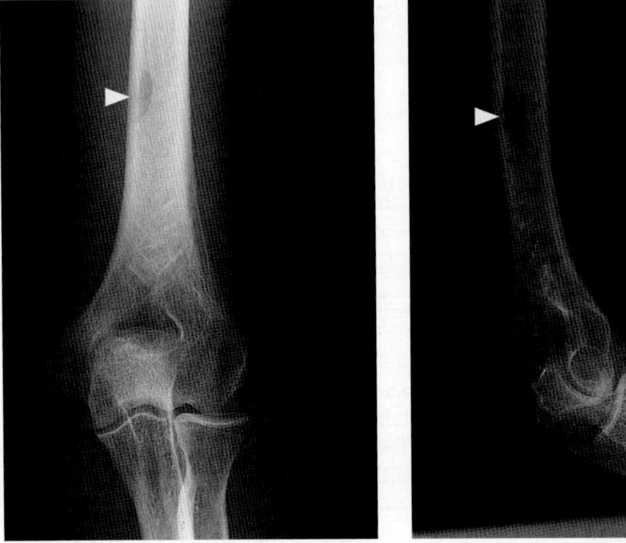

Fig. 2.51 A 60-year-old patient, right distal humerus. **(A)** Dorsal longitudinal section, right side. The destroyed distal cortical surface of the humerus appears sonographically interrupted and located below the level of the adjacent cortical bone in both sectional planes (*arrowheads*). The predominantly hypoechogenic localized tumor soft tissue component displaces the triceps muscle dorsally (*open arrowhead*). **(B)** Dorsal transversal section, right side. **(C,D)** The x-ray images in two projections confirm the findings (*arrowheads*). The histologic analysis revealed a metastasis of a bronchial carcinoma.

Pearls and Pitfalls

- The main advantage of elbow ultrasound is its ease of performance, ready availability, and dynamic capability.
- Ultrasound can assess the presence of capsular and synovial processes and differentiate them from other soft tissue tumors.
- The elbow is second only to the knee in incidence for the development of intraarticular loose bodies. Loose bodies may be chondral, osseous, or osteochondral in origin.
- Olecranon bursitis is the most common site of superficial bursitis and is easily confirmed by ultrasound.
- The most common tendon ruptures of the elbow involve the biceps and triceps tendons.
- The deposition of calcium hydroxyapatite within periarticular soft tissues, predominantly tendons, is commonly referred to as calcific tendinopathy.
- Coronoid fractures usually occur in association with elbow dislocations.
- Occult fractures can be diagnosed with ultrasound.

Suggested Readings

Finlay K, Ferri M, Friedman L. Ultrasound of the elbow. Skeletal Radiol 2004;33(2):63–79

Kijowski R, De Smet AA. The role of ultrasound in the evaluation of sports medicine injuries of the upper extremity. Clin Sports Med 2006;25(3):569–590, viii

Martinoli C, Bianchi S, Giovagnorio F, Pugliese F. Ultrasound of the elbow. Skeletal Radiol 2001;30(11):605–614

3 Imaging of the Wrist

Ximena Wortsman and Patricio Azocar

The newest ultrasound systems capture high-definition images of tissues and lesions in real time. For the wrist, which is easily accessible, the studies can be performed at rest or during dynamic testing as they are performed rapidly, without exposing the patient or the imager to ionizing radiation.

When properly performed, ultrasound in addition to anatomic details provides functional data such as blood flow. Thus, ultrasound can be used for diagnostic purposes, for monitoring the results of treatments, or to guide percutaneous procedures. Pathology of the wrist includes both injuries and systemic diseases involving the wrist's complex anatomy of bones, a network of soft tissues, and thin skin layers. Hence, ultrasound is the ideal imaging modality.

Clinical Indications

- Inflammatory and degenerative diseases—De Quervain disease, distal intersection syndrome, tenosynovitis, inflammatory arthritis (rheumatoid arthritis [RA], crystal-related arthritis)
- Traumatic lesions of extensor and flexor tendons, nerves, vessels, and occult fractures of the carpal bones
- Entrapment neuropathies—tunnel syndromes (carpal and Guyon)
- Space-occupying lesions—dorsal or ventral ganglia, neurogenic tumors, lipomatous tumors, presence of accessory muscles

Technical Guidelines

For an ultrasound of the wrist, the patient rests the wrist in his or her lap and is seated in front of the examiner. Alternatively, the patient may be seated at an examination table with both hands resting on the table. The screening on ultrasound examination includes transverse and longitudinal views of the local structures at rest or after dynamic testing positions. In addition, oblique approaches or a heel-toe maneuver (to increase the pressure on one side of the probe) can be helpful to remove anisotropy artifacts. For the examination of the volar aspect of the wrist, the hand is positioned palm up with mild extension and radial or ulnar deviation; for examination of the dorsal aspect of the wrist, the hands are moved into a palm down position. Maneuvers of gentle flexion and/or extension of the digits can help identify the different tendons. These flexo-extension maneuvers are performed along a longitudinal sonographic axis; this dynamic study shows the normal and gentle movement of the tendons and can be helpful in the detection of tendon entrapments or for the identification of the median nerve inside the carpal tunnel that does not show any movement.

Normal Anatomy

The wrist can be subdivided into four segments: the volar, dorsal, medial, and lateral aspects (**Figs. 3.1** and **3.2**).

The *volar aspect* comprises a roof made by the flexor retinaculum, which is a fibrous band best identified on transverse view as a hyperechoic band. Deeper in this aspect is the carpal tunnel that contains the superficial and deep hand flexor tendons (flexor digitorum superficialis and profundus of the second to fifth finger) and their surrounding single synovial sheath, as well as the flexor pollicis longus tendon surrounded by its sheath. On ultrasound, all these tendinous structures show a hyperechoic fibrillar pattern. Above the

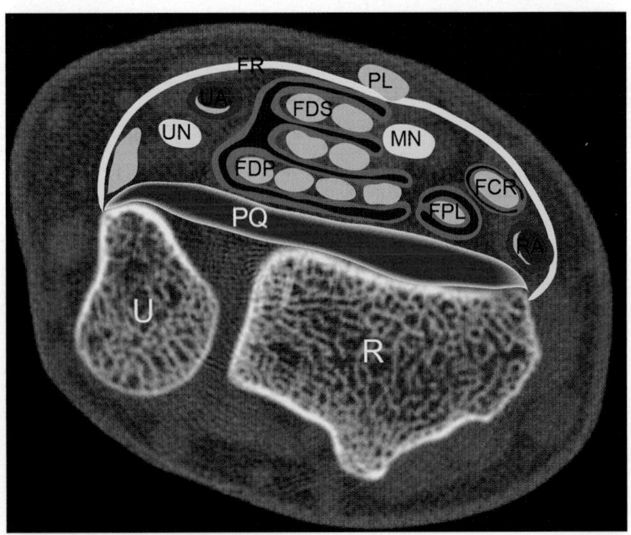

Fig. 3.1 Volar aspect of the wrist, axial ultrasound view. FR, flexor retinaculum; FDS, flexor digitorum superficialis tendons; FDP, flexor digitorum profundus tendons; MN, median nerve; UN, ulnar nerve; FCR, flexor carpi radialis tendon; FPL, flexor pollicis longus tendon; RA, radial artery; UA, ulnar artery; PQ, pronator quadratus muscle; R, radius; U, ulna; PL, palmaris longus tendon; R, radius; U, ulna.

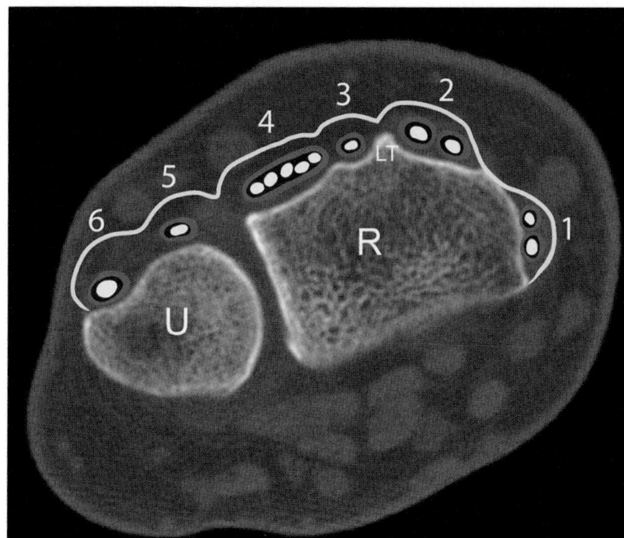

Fig. 3.2 Dorsal aspect of the wrist, axial ultrasound view. Extensor tendons compartments of the wrist (1 through 6, from lateral to medial): (1) abductor pollicis longus and extensor pollicis brevis tendons; (2) extensor carpi radialis longus and brevis tendons; (3) extensor pollicis longus tendon; (4) common extensor tendons (extensor digitorum longus and extensor indicis proprius); (5) extensor digiti minimi tendon; (6) extensor carpi ulnaris tendon. R, radius; U, ulna; LT, Lister tubercle

flexor tendons and below the flexor retinaculum is the median nerve. The median nerve, a hyperechoic structure that contains small hypoechoic dots representing the neuronal fascicles; these are best shown on transverse ultrasound view. The bone margins of the tunnel, going from lateral to medial and proximal to distal are the scaphoid tubercle and pisiform bone and more distally, the ridge of the trapezium and the hook of the hamate; all these bone margins are hyperechoic. Outside the carpal tunnel are the tendons for the flexor carpi radialis, flexor carpi ulnaris and the palmaris longus. The palmaris longus tendon may be absent in up to 16% of the population as a normal variant. It may also vary in shape presenting different types of muscular and tendinous components as anatomic variants.

The Guyon canal is a triangular space lateral to the pisiform bone and medial to the hamate that contains the ulnar nerve and ulnar artery. The ulnar nerve is smaller than the median nerve but has similar echostructure. More commonly, the ulnar artery is located lateral to the nerve and shows flow signals on color Doppler. Proximal to the carpal tunnel and deeper to the flexor tendons is the pronator quadratus muscle, a square-shaped muscle that lies above the distal ends of the radius and ulna.

The dorsal aspect has a transverse hyperechoic fibrous band, the extensor retinaculum, that holds the six extensor tendon compartments. The first compartment contains the tendons for the abductor pollicis longus and extensor pollicis brevis, each having its own synovial sheath. The second compartment contains the tendons for the extensor radialis longus and brevis, sharing a common synovial sheath. The Lister tubercle is a bony prominence that serves as a landmark separating the second from the third extensor compartments. The third compartment contains only one structure, the tendon for the extensor pollicis longus with its synovial sheath. The fourth extensor compartment contains the common extensor tendons (common extensor digitorum longus tendons and extensor indicis proprius tendon) that share a common synovial sheath. The fifth extensor compartment contains the tendon for the extensor digiti minimi. Last, the sixth extensor compartment contains the tendon for the extensor carpi ulnaris; both fifth and six compartments have separate synovial sheaths.

The lateral aspect houses the radial artery and the tendon for the extensor carpi radialis; and the medial aspect contains the tendon for the extensor carpi ulnaris and the triangular fibrocartilage complex (TFCC), which is located deep to the extensor carpi ulnaris tendon, between the distal segment of the ulna and the triquetrum. The TFCC comprises a meniscus homologue, the triangular fibrocartilage, an articular disk, the ulnar collateral ligament, the dorsal and volar radioulnar ligaments, and the extensor carpi ulnaris tendon and sheath. TFCC separates the carpal bones from the radius and ulna and serves as a major stabilizer of the radioulnar joint as well as a cushion for ulnar axial loads. On ultrasound, TFCC appears as a triangular hypoechoic and slightly heterogeneous structure in the medial aspect of the wrist. Because the components of TFCC cannot be defined clearly by sonography, when a lesion is suspected it is suggested that magnetic resonance imaging (MRI) be obtained for confirmation.

■ Pathologies

Inflammatory

Tenosynovitis

Inflammation of the tendons and/or their synovial sheaths is one of the most common disorders of the wrist. The main causes are repetitive motion at work, pregnancy, inflammatory arthropathies, and diabetes. Sonographically, there is enlargement of the tendons and their synovial sheath; more chronic cases may be associated with peritendinous anechoic cysts or small hypoechoic nodules in the synovial sheath. Color Doppler ultrasound may detect increased vascularity in the synovial sheath or intratendinous (in more advanced stages) (**Fig. 3.3**).

De Quervain Tenosynovitis

De Quervain tenosynovitis is a common tenosynovitis of the wrist and affects the first extensor compartment, composed

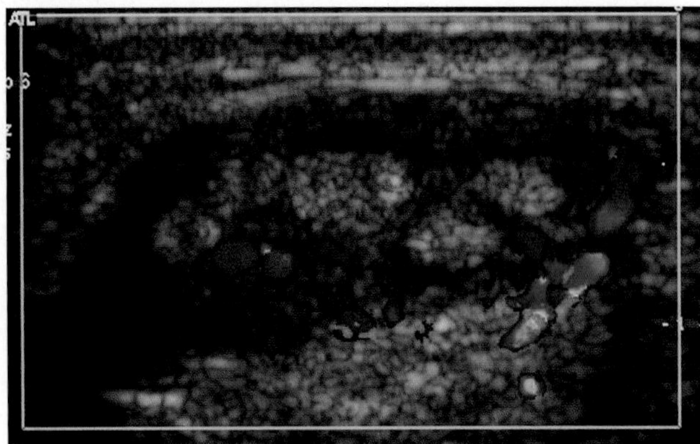

Fig. 3.3 Tenosynovitis. Color Doppler ultrasound transverse view: the common extensor tendons compartment is swollen, and the synovial sheath thickened with enhanced color Doppler ultrasound signals.

of the tendons for the abductor pollicis longus and the extensor pollicis brevis muscles. Symptoms include chronic pain, tenderness or swelling in the thumb side of the wrist as well as limitation of movement. Sonographic thickening of the first extensor compartment is seen on ultrasound, which also helps in severe cases when it is necessary to rule out the presence of accessory tendons, or septa in the synovial sheaths (**Figs. 3.4, 3.5, 3.6, 3.7**). In the postsurgical follow-up of patients with De Quervain tenosynovitis, an ultrasound examination can rule out the development of neuromas of the terminal branches of the radial nerve (**Fig. 3.8**).

Distal Intersection Syndrome

Distal intersection syndrome, also called crossover syndrome, is a tenosynovitis at the intersection between the second (extensor carpi radialis longus and brevis) and third

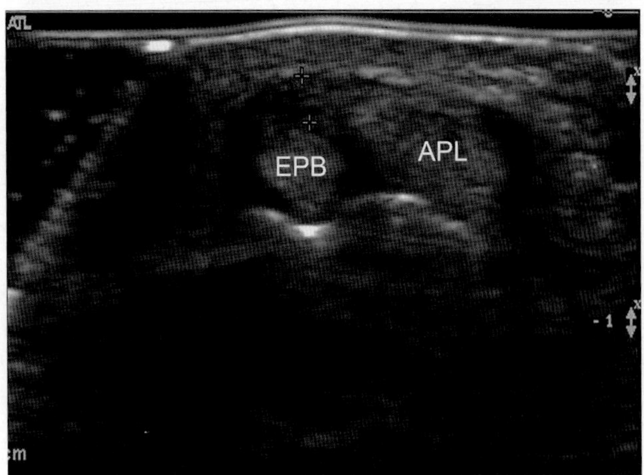

Fig. 3.4 De Quervain tenosynovitis. Transverse ultrasound view shows an abnormal swollen first extensor compartment and its synovial sheath (*between markers*). APL, abductor pollicis longus; EPB, extensor pollicis brevis.

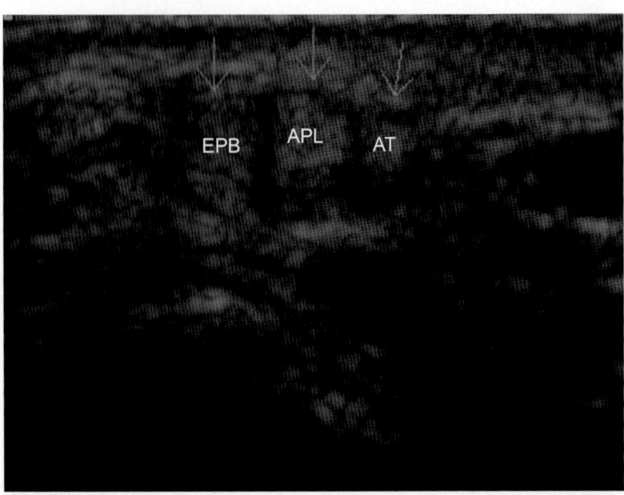

Fig. 3.5 De Quervain tenosynovitis variant, with accessory tendon. Transverse ultrasound view demonstrates enlargement of the tendons in the first extensor compartment including an accessory tendon (AT; *arrows*). APL, abductor pollicis longus; EPB, extensor pollicis brevis.

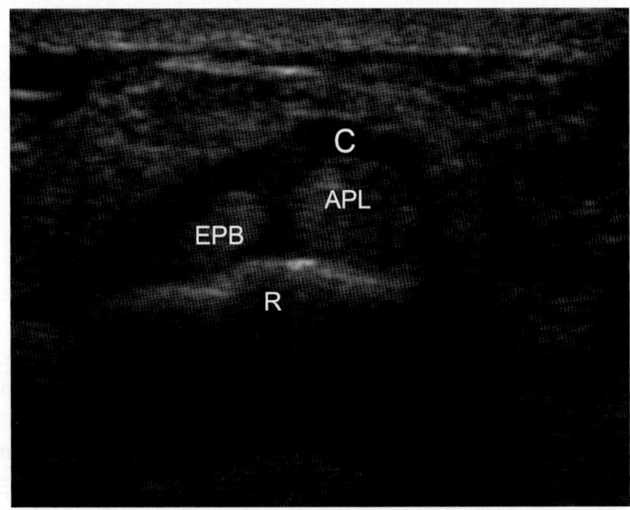

Fig. 3.6 De Quervain tenosynovitis variant, with ganglia. Transverse ultrasound view: swelling of structures as in Figs. 3.4 and 3.5, and a small ganglia cyst (C) attached to the abductor pollicis longus tendon. APL, abductor pollicis longus; EPB, extensor pollicis brevis; R, Radius.

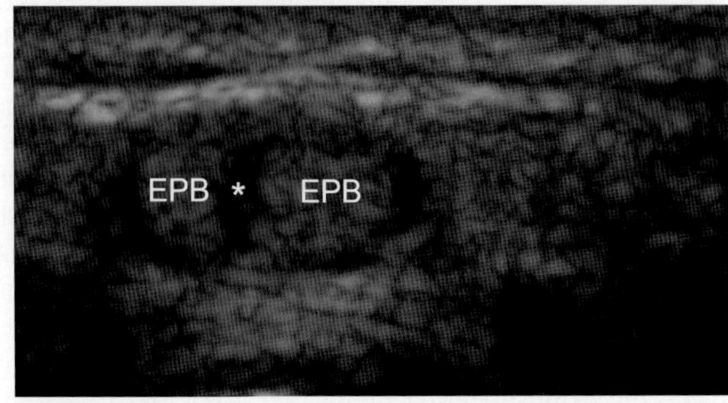

Fig. 3.7 De Quervain tenosynovitis, with a septa variant. Transverse ultrasound view shows a septa (*) dividing the swollen extensor pollicis brevis tendon (EPB) in two separate fascicles.

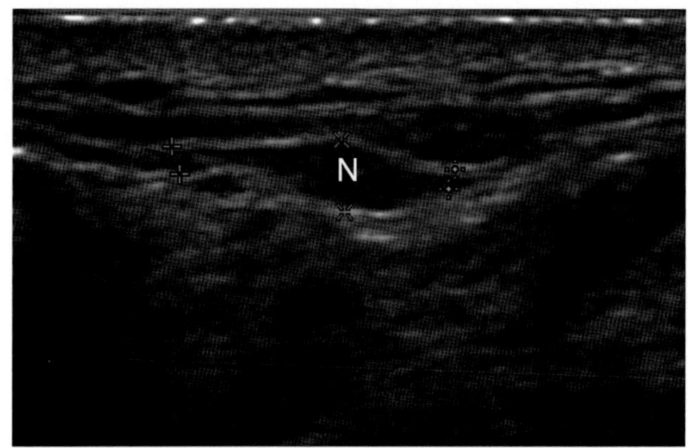

Fig. 3.8 Postoperative complication of De Quervain tenosynovitis. Longitudinal ultrasound view demonstrates a neuroma (N) of a distal branch of the radial nerve. A hypoechoic fusiform structure with connecting neurogenic tracts to the mass (*between markers*) is identified.

(extensor pollicis longus) compartments. It is caused by repetitive prono-supination or flexo-extension movements and commonly presents with pain and tenderness proximal to the Lister tubercle in the distal forearm. The most affected tendon is the extensor pollicis longus that develops tendon swelling and thickening of the sheath that may be associated with synovial sheath fluid (**Fig. 3.9**). There is also another less common crossing syndrome that represents a *proximal* intersection syndrome; this affects the distal forearm at the level of the musculotendinous junction of the first extensor compartment with the second extensor compartment tendons (radialis longus and brevis tendons). This syndrome is seen in patients with repetitive prono-supination movements and overload.

Pronator Quadratus Syndrome

The pronator quadratus syndrome, as its name indicates, affects the pronator quadratus muscle, a square-shaped muscle, located in the anterior aspect of the distal forearm, overlying the interosseus membrane. This muscle is supplied by the anterior interosseus artery and may become inflamed during maintained forced dorsiflexion of the wrist as for example, when carrying a heavy tray for a prolonged period. The muscle becomes enlarged and hyperechoic and an early diagnosis is necessary to avoid development of a full-fledged compartment syndrome (**Figs. 3.10** and **3.11**).

Carpometacarpal Boss

Carpometacarpal boss, also known as carpal boss, is a bony protuberance that develops at the base of the second and/or

A

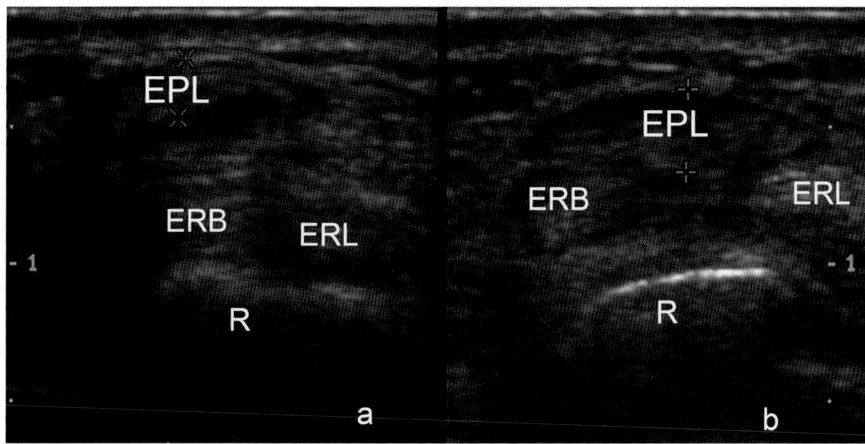

B

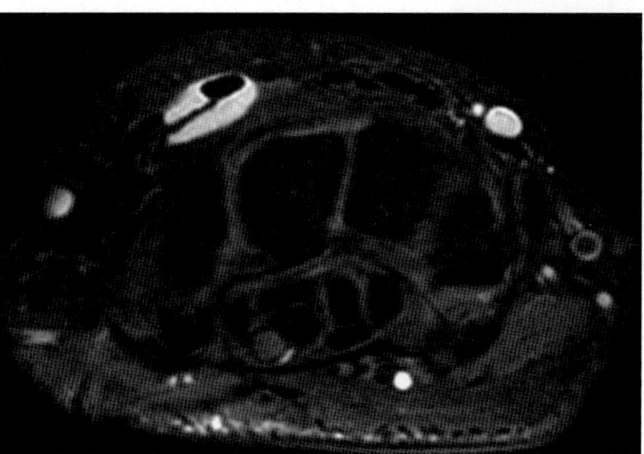

Fig. 3.9 **(A)** Distal intersection syndrome. Transverse comparative ultrasound views show swelling of the extensor pollicis longus tendon (EPL; *between calipers*) at the crossing with the second extensor compartment tendons (extensor carpi radialis longus [ERL] and brevis [ERB] tendons) in the proximal (a) and distal (b) segments of the wrist. R, radius. **(B)** Patient with tenosynovitis of the EPL. Axial fat-suppressed fast spin echo (FSE) T2-weighted magnetic resonance image showing fluid around the second dorsal compartment compatible with tenosynovitis.

A

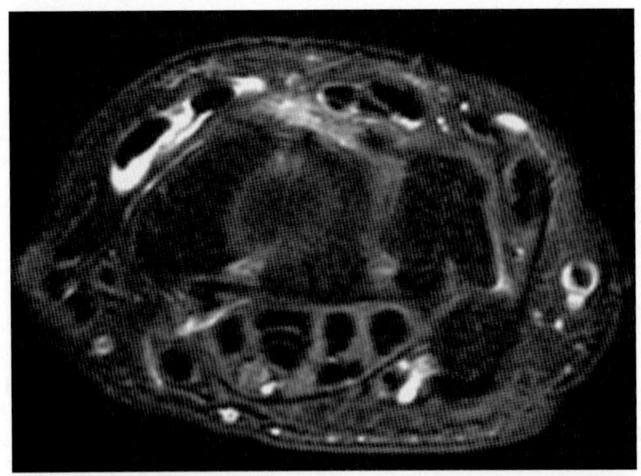

B

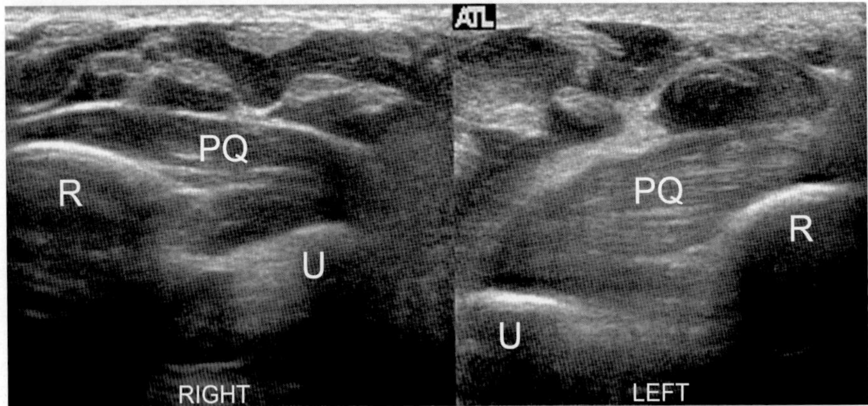

Fig. 3.10 **(A)** Normal pronator quadratus muscle. Axial proton density (PD) magnetic resonance image showing pronator quadratus muscle in the distal forearm attaching to the radius and ulna. **(B)** Pronator quadratus muscle syndrome. Transverse comparative views show swelling and hyperechogenicity of the pronator quadratus muscle (PQ) in the affected side (LEFT). The normal side is marked RIGHT. R, radius; U, ulna.

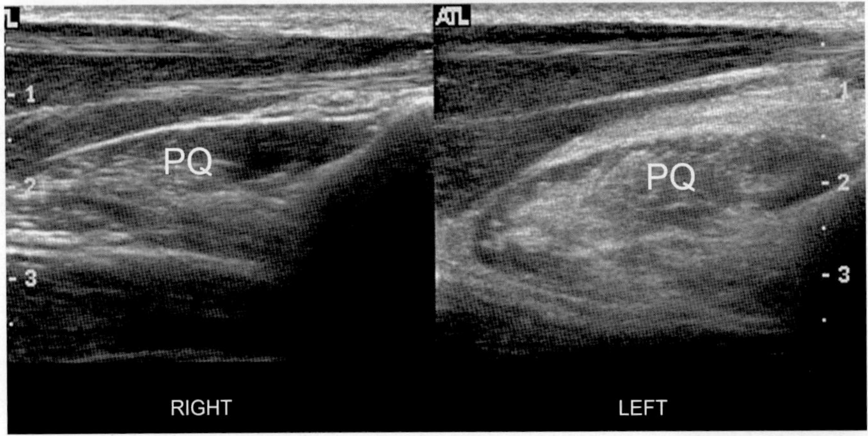

Fig. 3.11 Pronator quadratus muscle syndrome. Longitudinal comparative ultrasound views demonstrate enlargement and hyperechogenicity of the pronator quadratus muscle (PQ) in the affected side (LEFT). In contrast, the normal side (RIGHT) presents a normal hypoechoic muscular pattern in the same muscle.

third carpometacarpal joint close to the capitate and trapezoid bones. It may represent a degenerate osteophyte and/or an os styloideum (an accessory ossification center). Clinically, patients may report pain and limitation of movement in the affected hand, likely due to an overlying ganglion cyst, or an extensor tendon that may be slipping over the bony protuberance. On ultrasound, it is possible to detect the hyperechoic bony abnormality and/or the anechoic round or oval shaped ganglion cyst, and a dynamic study can detect the slipping tendon movement (**Figs. 3.12, 3.13, 3.14**).

Extensor Carpi Ulnaris Tenosynovitis

The extensor carpi ulnaris (ECU) inserts into the midportion of the fifth metacarpal. Tenosynovitis of the ECU can be caused by the persistent ulnar deviation of RA and may be associated with a ganglion cyst. On ultrasound, there is enlargement of the tendon and its synovial sheath (**Figs. 3.15** and **3.16**); in RA patients, synovial pannus is an important cause for thickening of the synovial sheath.

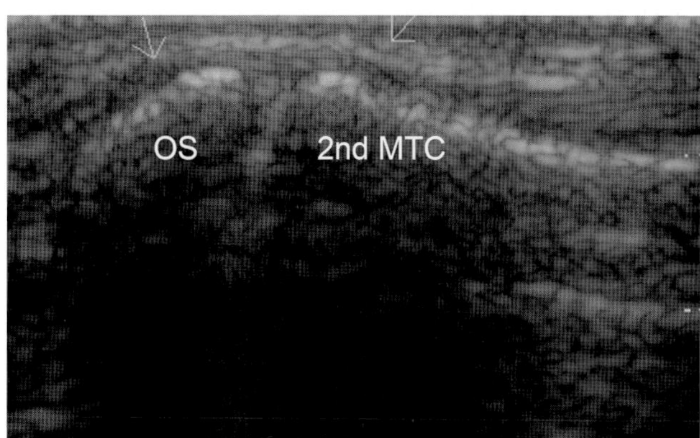

Fig. 3.12 Carpal boss. Longitudinal ultrasound view shows a hyperechoic fragment corresponding with an accessory bone (os styloideum; OS), in the dorsal aspect of the wrist close to the base of the second metacarpal bone (2nd MTC).

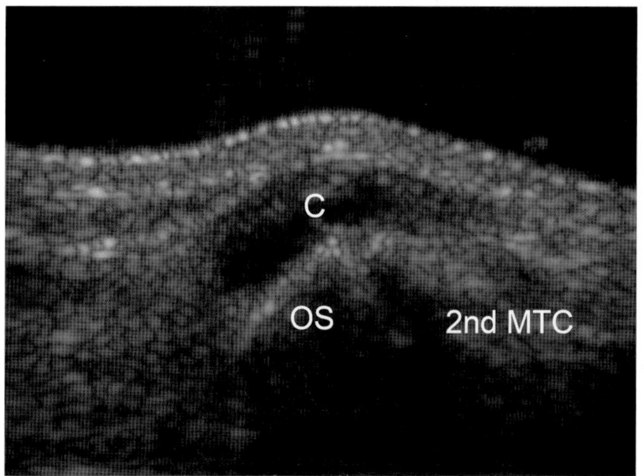

Fig. 3.13 Carpal boss and ganglia cyst. Longitudinal ultrasound view presents a round anechoic cyst (C) above the dorsum of the os styloideum (OS) at the base of the second metacarpal bone (2nd MTC).

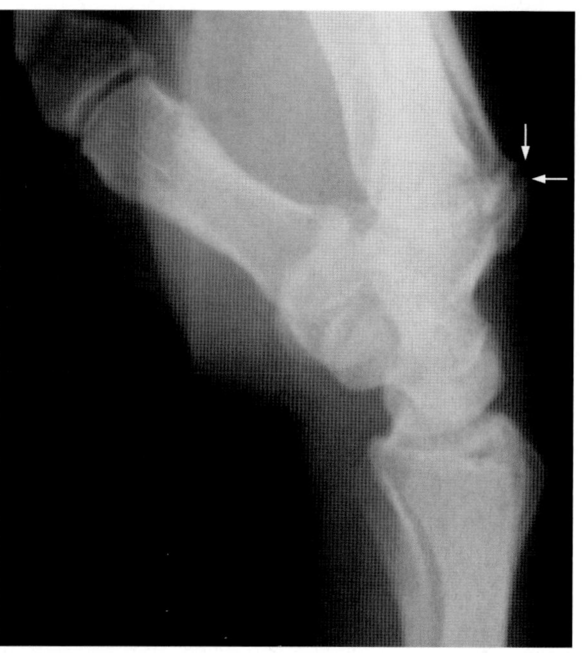

Fig. 3.14 Carpal boss. X-ray projection (lateral view) shows bony prominences with degenerative osteophytes (*arrows*).

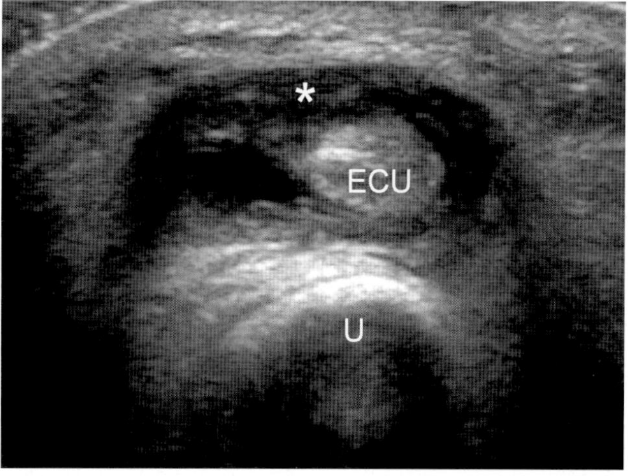

Fig. 3.15 Extensor carpi ulnaris tendon (ECU) tenosynovitis. Transverse ultrasound view demonstrates swelling of the tendon as well as thickening and fluid in the synovial sheath (*). U, ulna.

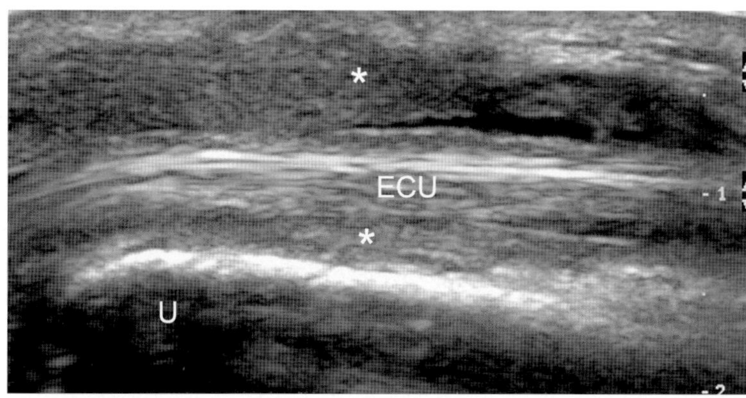

Fig. 3.16 Extensor carpi ulnaris tendon (ECU) tenosynovitis in longitudinal ultrasound view demonstrates an important thickening of the synovial sheath (*). U, ulna.

Flexor Carpi Ulnaris Tendinitis

Flexor carpi ulnaris (FCU) tendinitis is a common problem in players of racquet sports, due to the chronic repetitive trauma associated with forced wrist flexion or ulnar deviation. Symptoms are pain along the tendon or in its distal insertion around the pisiform; the FCU tendon does not have synovial sheath covering. Pain in FCU tendinitis may also arise from arthrosis of the pisotriquetral joint or instability of the pisiform. Because calcific tendinitis of the FCU has been reported in relation to trauma, its primary mechanism may be local hypoxia from mechanical causes or vascular abnormalities.

Flexor Carpi Radialis Tendinitis

Flexor carpi radialis (FCR) tendinitis is seen less frequently than FCU tendinitis and is also associated with repetitive trauma. The flexor carpi radialis tendon passes through a separate compartment of the transverse ligament apart from the rest of the flexor tendons and overlies the scaphoid tubercle and trapezial crest. Adhesions in the tunnel or constriction of the distal tendon secondary to trauma or arthrosis may trigger the typical pain. The close relationship between the FCR and the median nerve may occasionally generate secondary irritation of the nerve.

Inflammatory Arthropathies

Ultrasound is a sensitive imaging technique for the evaluation of joint fluid, synovitis, erosions, cartilage destruction, or calcifications. Rheumatoid arthritis and crystal disease are common causes of inflammatory diseases affecting the wrist.

Rheumatoid Arthritis

Rheumatoid arthritis is characterized by proliferative and hypervascularized synovitis, bone erosion, cartilage damage, joint destruction, and long-term disability. Proliferative synovitis (i.e., rheumatoid pannus) is the earliest pathologic abnormality in RA and may be associated with small amounts of fluid in the joint. Doppler color imaging shows synovial thickening and high signals in the synovial sheath that together suggest proliferative, hypervascularized pannus tissue that can be quantified and subsequently monitored (**Figs. 3.17** and **3.18**). Furthermore, use of microbubbles sonographic contrast agents may enhance detection of synovial vascularization, a marker of disease activity. The data generated can be applied to a scoring system developed by EULAR (European League Against Rheumatism) used to assess and standardize RA and its complications. Tenosynovitis is a common finding in RA. It is usually bilateral and affects mainly the tendons for the flexor digitorum, extensor digitorum longus, and extensor carpi ulnaris. Bone erosions are detected on ultrasound as intraarticular discontinuities of the bone surface visible on two planes perpendicular to each other. Most commonly, bone erosions affect the capitate, triquetrum and lunate in the carpal region, and the ulnar styloid process (**Fig. 3.18b**).

Crystal-Related Arthritis

Crystal-related arthritis is a group of disorders characterized by deposition of microcrystals in the joints resulting in acute or chronic arthritis or periarthritis. Disease-producing crystal deposits are mostly monosodium urates, causing gout, and calcium pyrophosphate dihydrate (CPPD) causing pseudogout.

Gout

Gout is the most common crystal-induced arthritis and is characterized by pain, edema, and inflammation affecting the metatarsophalangeal joint of the great toe, ankle, wrist, and knee. Uric acid crystals precipitate predominantly on the surface of the articular cartilage. Ultrasound of the affected joints shows a hyperechoic and slightly irregular band over the hypoechoic articular cartilage, corresponding to the uric acid deposits, producing the image known as "double contour" (**Fig. 3.19**). The hyperechoic heterogeneous material surrounding the joints is tophaceous material and is described as "wet sugar clumps." These clumps frequently form at the pressure points (**Fig. 3.20**). Bone erosions, seen as breaks in the hyperechoic outline of the bony cortex in two perpendicular planes can also be seen. Although small joint effusions may be detected, they are not specific to gout.

In pseudogout, the deposits of the crystals tend to locate in the center of the hyaline and fibrous cartilage, instead of on the surface of cartilage as seen in gout.

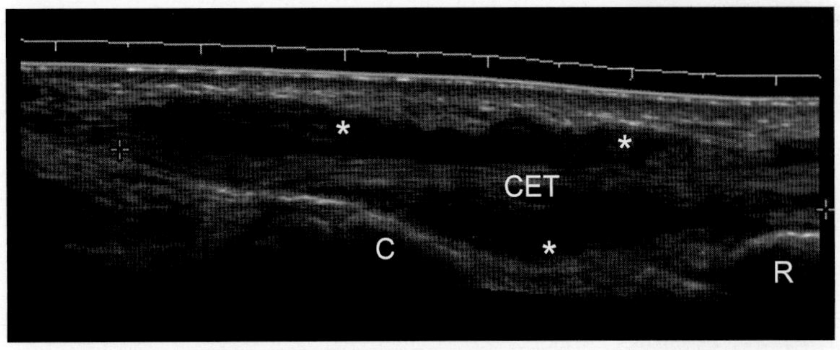

Fig. 3.17 Rheumatoid arthritis tenosynovitis. Panoramic longitudinal ultrasound view shows swelling of the fourth extensor compartment (CET) with marked pannus (*). R, radius; C, capitate.

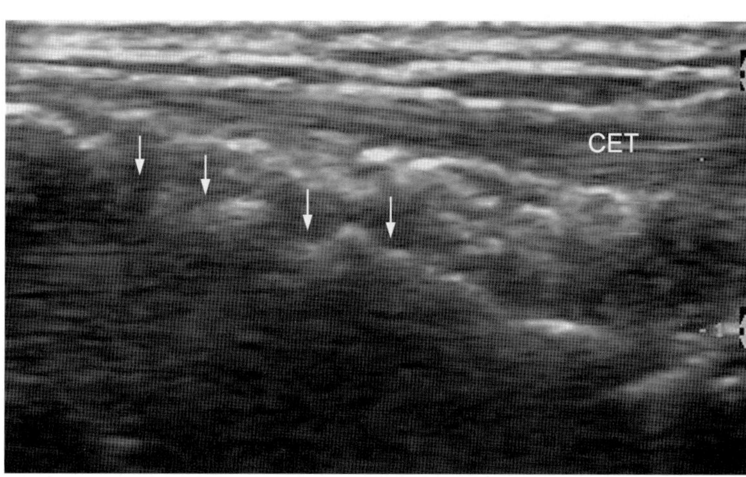

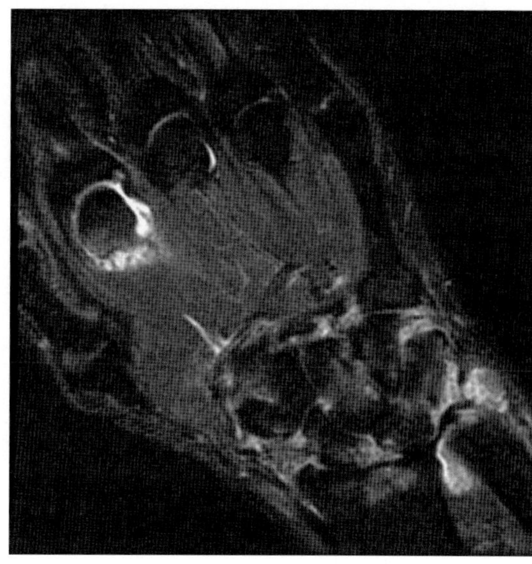

Fig. 3.18 **(A)** Bone erosions in rheumatoid arthritis. Longitudinal ultrasound view shows disruptions of continuity in the cortical bone margin (*arrows*). CET, common extensor tendons of the 4th compartment in the dorsum of the wrist. **(B)** Inflammatory and erosive changes in a patient with active rheumatoid arthritis. Coronal short T1 inversion recovery (STIR) magnetic resonance image (MRI) of the wrist shows erosions in the proximal scaphoid and capitate. There is fluid signal seen around the distal radioulnar joint and at the second metacarpophalangeal (MCP) joint. Observe the complete loss of joint space at the radiocarpal joint and the area of subarticular high signal compatible with an evolving subchondral cyst. Patient has active rheumatoid arthritis in the wrist and the second MCP joint.

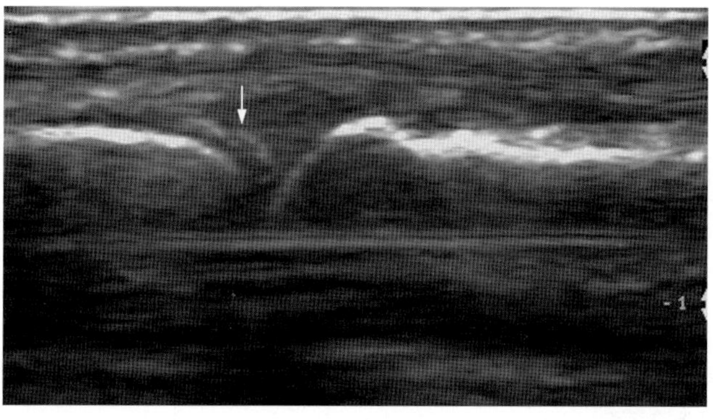

Fig. 3.19 Uric acid deposits in the wrist. Longitudinal ultrasound scan shows hyperechoic linear deposits of uric acid on the surface of hyaline cartilage, which corresponds with the "double contour sign" (*arrow*).

Traumatic

Rupture of the Extensor or Flexor Tendons

Tendons are susceptible to lacerations, burns, or blunt trauma. At the wrist, injuries of the extensor tendons are more common than flexor tendons because the protecting dorsal tissue cover is thinner. Flexor tendons are damaged mainly by direct cuts that can also injure nerves and vessels close to the flexor sheath. Other causes of flexor tendon injuries are intense pulling or stretching frequently associated with sports such as football, wrestling, rugby, or rock climbing.

Traumatic lesions of the tendons are divided into inflammation and partial or total (full thickness) tears.

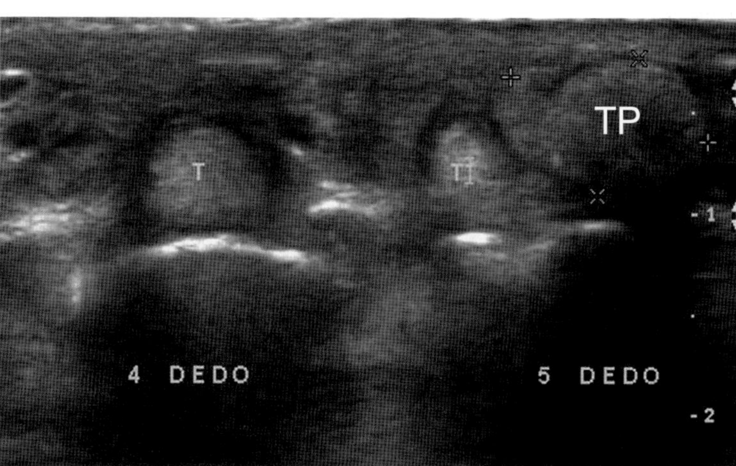

Fig. 3.20 Gouty tophi. Transverse ultrasound view shows a tophi nodule (TP, *between markers*) that is attached and compressing the flexor tendon of the fifth finger. The tophi (TP) is seen as a hyperechoic nodule with a "wet sugar clump" appearance.

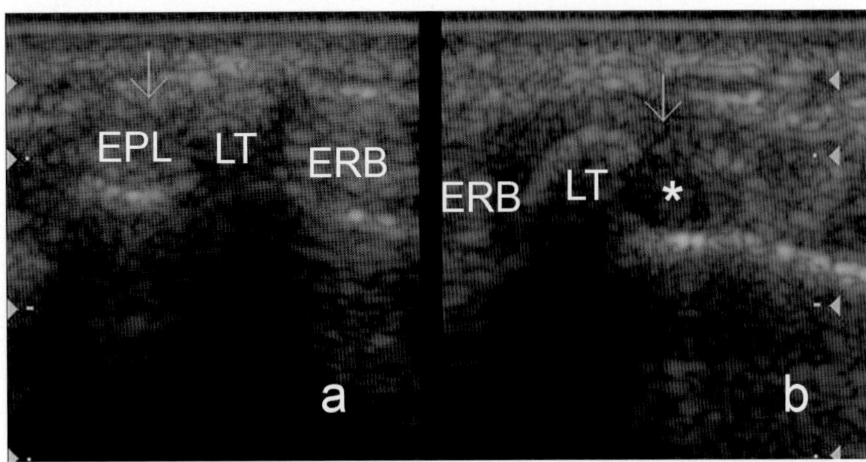

Fig. 3.21 Tendon rupture in the extensor pollicis longus (EPL). Comparative transverse ultrasound images. (a) normal side; (b) affected side showing absence (*) of the EPL tendon. LT, Lister tubercle; ERB, extensor radialis brevis tendon.

On ultrasound, the area of rupture is seen as discontinuity of the fibrillar pattern in the tendon. The ends of the tendon may be seen and retraction of the tendon ends toward the hand or the forearm can be demonstrated (**Figs. 3.21** and **3.22**).

The tendon of the extensor pollicis longus runs in proximity to the Lister tubercle and it may be ruptured by fractures of the tubercle and/or by articular inflammation as in RA. Clinically, tendon rupture presents with instability of the phalangeal joint of the thumb; when rupture of the extensor pollicis brevis is also present, the deformity can extend to the metacarpophalangeal joint of the thumb.

Damage from multiple lacerations may be difficult to define because it can include more than one extensor compartment. Ultrasound can help in the follow-up of tenodesis performed after repair or tendon transfer; and most importantly, it can rule out recurrent tears.

A

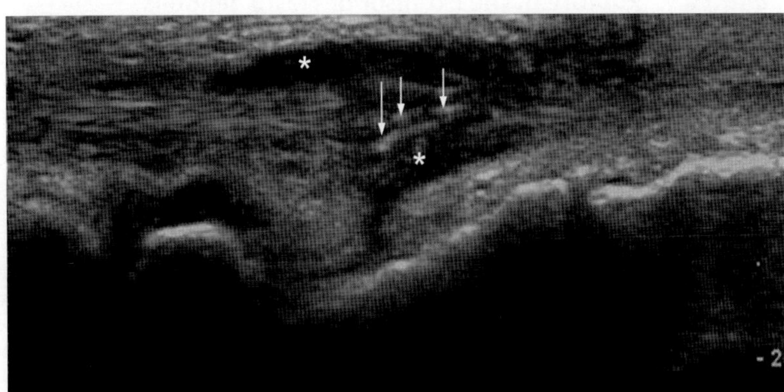

B

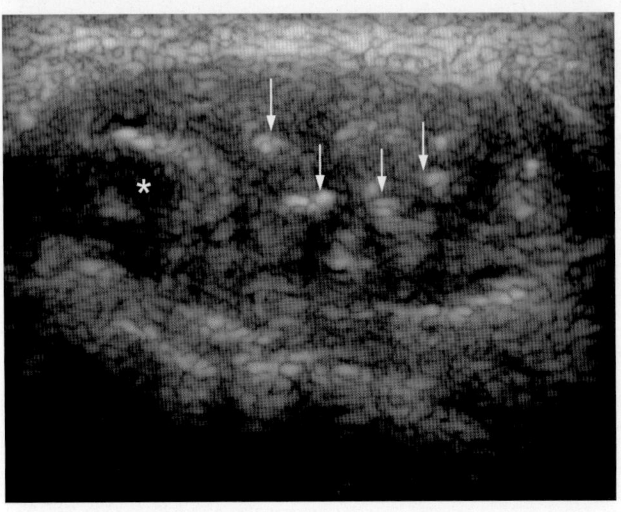

Fig. 3.22 Surgical repair of a rupture of the common extensor tendons (fourth extensor compartment) at 7 days postsurgery. **(A)** Longitudinal ultrasound view shows fluid (*) in the tendinous sheath; hyperechoic dots (*arrows*) inside the tendons correspond to suture material (*arrows*). **(B)** Follow-up ultrasound after surgical repair of the common extensor tendons compartment. Transverse view of the same case as **(A)** shows enlargement and hypoechogenicity of the tendons. The hyperechoic dots (*arrows*) correspond to suture material. No evidence of rerupture was found.

Recurrent Dislocation of the Tendon of the Extensor Carpi Ulnaris

The tendon of the ECU passes through a groove in the distal end of the ulna and is covered by an annular ligament. Subluxation of the tendon can be recurrent and is characterized by a painful snap over the ulnodorsal aspect of the wrist, mainly during forearm rotation; it is seen more commonly after injury or insufficiency of the extensor retinaculum, styloid process fractures, or RA. With the wrist under ulnar deviation, supination will produce subluxation of the tendon out of the groove, often with an audible snap. Pronation will relocate the ECU tendon onto the sulcus.

Hidden Bone Fractures

The scaphoid and the distal radius are the most commonly fractured bones at the wrist, whereas scaphoid fractures are the most frequent of the occult fractures. In a setting of wrist pain and negative x-ray an occult fracture should be suspected. Ultrasound can be used to assess for cortical discontinuities and irregularities in the hyperechoic cortical margin or to detect loose hyperechoic fragments adjacent to the bone. Computed tomography is generally performed following ultrasound to obtain better definition of the trabecular architecture and confirm an occult fracture (**Figs. 3.23** and **3.24**).

Scaphoid Fracture

A scaphoid fracture is the most common fracture of the intrinsic carpal bones. The fracture is usually caused by a fall with the outstretched hand in dorsiflexion and radial deviation. In 70% of cases the fracture occurs at the waist of the bone, 20% are reported in the proximal scaphoid pole, and the remaining 10% in the distal pole. In the scaphoid, the arterial supply for the proximal pole enters at the waist and the blood supply to the proximal pole can be disrupted by a fracture at the waist thus predisposing the proximal fracture moiety to avascular necrosis. Fracture of the waist of the scaphoid may also be associated with lesions to the scapholunate ligament. Fractures at the distal pole of the scaphoid may occur in conjunction with injury to the radial collateral ligament. On ultrasound, these fractures are characterized by interruption of the hyperechoic bony margin of the scaphoid with or without disruption of the fibrillar pattern of the scapholunate ligament (**Figs. 3.25, 3.26, 3.27, 3.28, 3.29**).

Fractures of the Triquetrum

These are the second most common fractures in the carpal bones. They are produced by axial loading of the ulnar deviated outstretched hand or by direct blow to the dorsum of the hand. This type of fracture occurs more commonly as an avulsion of a dorsal fragment, also called a chip fracture at the insertion of the radioulnar ligament. Ultrasound may detect the hyperechoic bony fragment (**Fig. 3.30**).

Fractures of the Hamate

The hamate is commonly fractured at the base of the hook, generally by a direct blow on a dorsiflexed ulnar deviated hand. Fracture of the hook of the hamate may be seen in players of sports with racquets, bats, or golf clubs. Affected patients complain of pain over the hypothenar eminence.

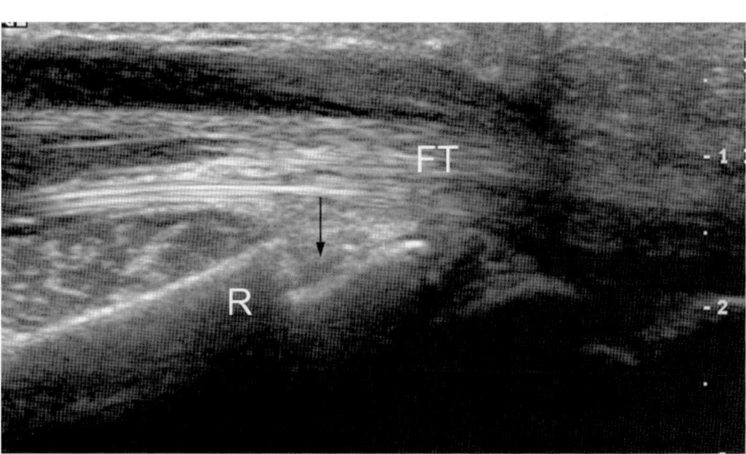

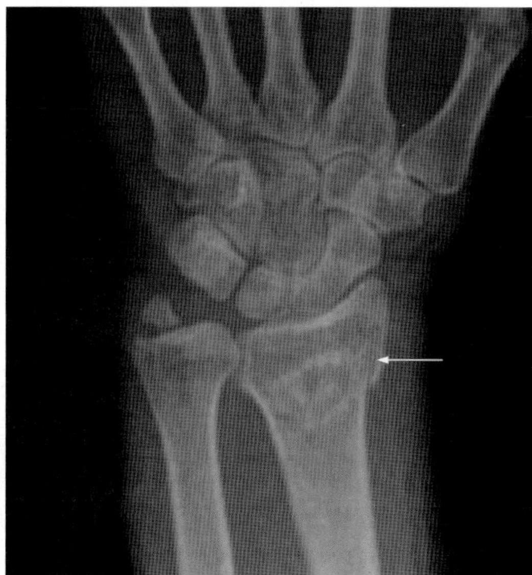

Fig. 3.23 Fracture of the radius at the distal end. **(A)** Longitudinal ultrasound scan performed in the volar aspect of the wrist shows interruption in the hyperechoic pattern of the radius cortex (*arrow*) corresponding with the fracture site. FT, flexor tendons; R, radius. **(B)** Fracture of the radius at the distal end. X-ray projection (anteroposterior) of the same case as **(A)** shows an impacted fracture of the radius (*arrow*) with concomitant fracture of the ulna styloid.

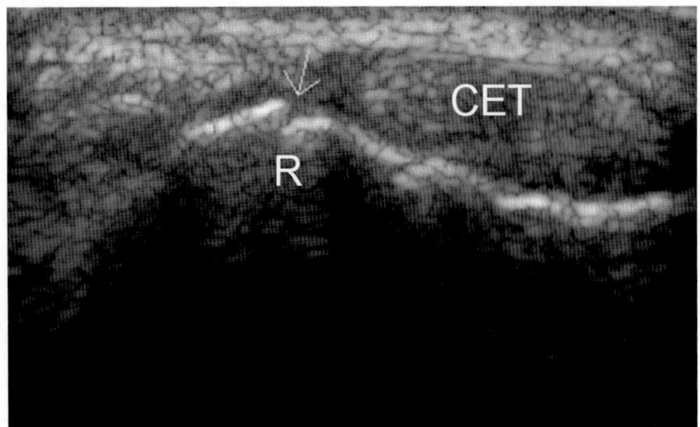

A

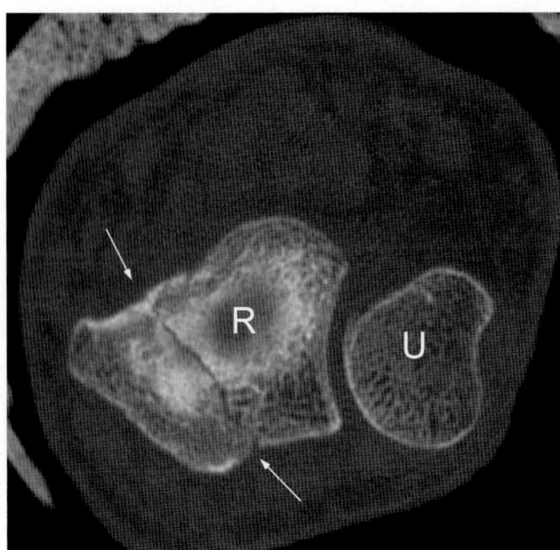

B

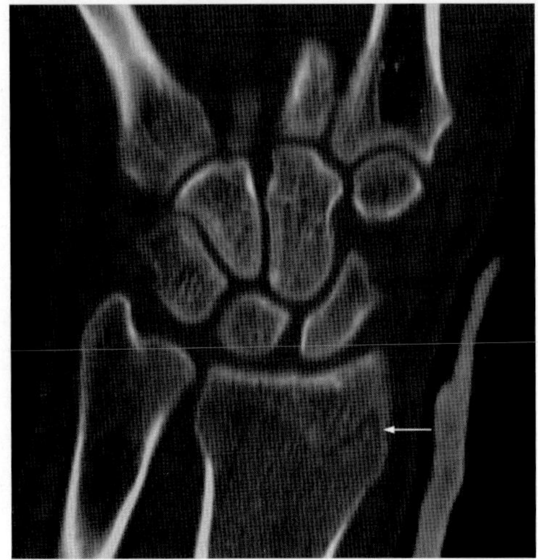

C

Fig. 3.24 Fracture of the radius at the distal end without displacement. **(A)** Transverse ultrasound view shows a discontinuity of the radial cortex (*arrow*) in a patient with normal x-rays. R, radius; CET, common extensor tendons. **(B)** Axial computed tomography (CT) scan of the same case as **(A)** demonstrates the fracture of the distal end of the radius to the articular zone (*arrows*). U, ulna. **(C)** Coronal CT reconstruction of the same case as **(A)** and **(B)** shows a linear hypodense fracture (*arrow*) in the distal end of the radius.

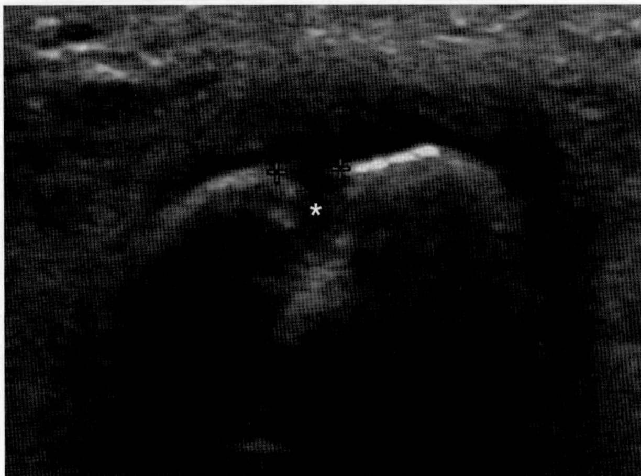

Fig. 3.25 Fracture of the pisiform bone. Transverse ultrasound view performed in the volar aspect of the wrist shows an interruption of the cortical outline of the pisiform (* *between markers*).

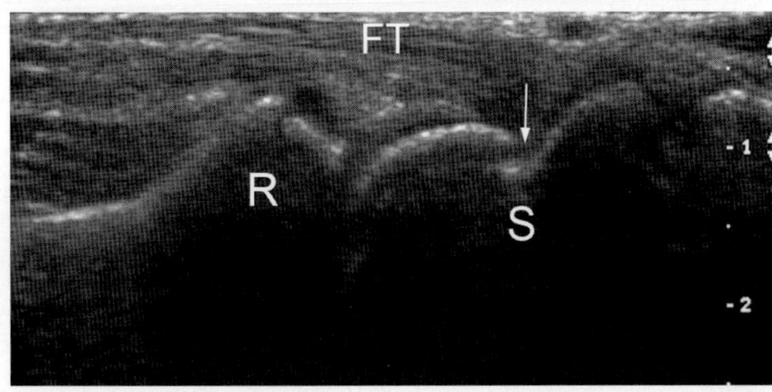

Fig. 3.26 Fracture of the waist of the scaphoid bone. Longitudinal ultrasound view shows an interruption (*arrow*) of the cortical outline in the scaphoid bone (S). R, radius; FT, flexor tendons.

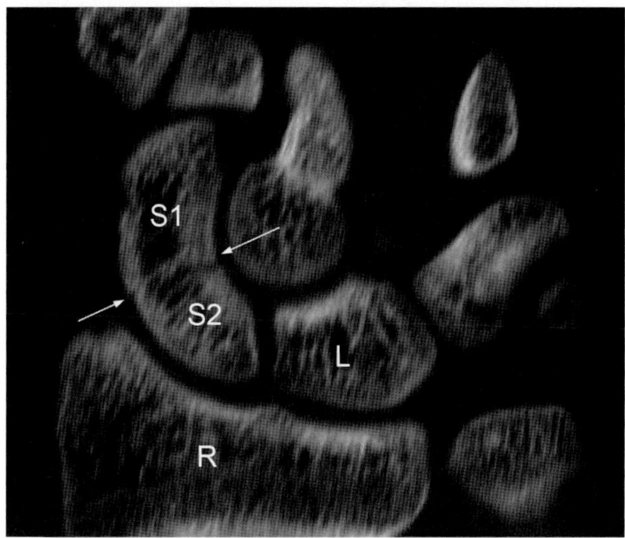

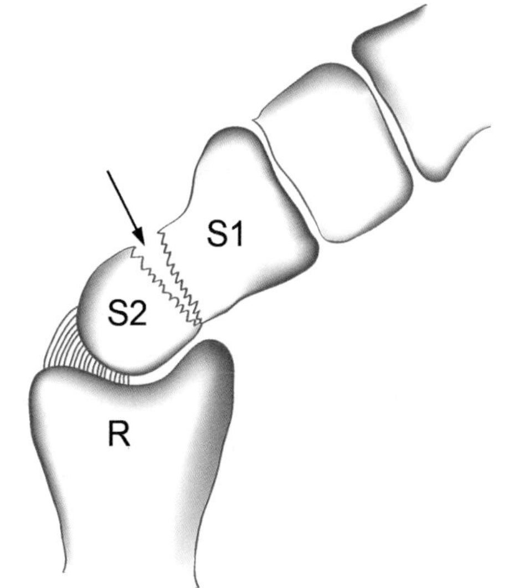

Fig. 3.27 Fracture of the scaphoid bone. **(A)** Coronal computed tomography (CT) reconstruction confirmed the fracture (*arrows*) in the same case as Fig. 3.24. The fracture separated the scaphoid bone into two fragments (S1 and S2). L, lunate; R, radius. **(B)** Digital drawing shows the gap of the fracture seen in the waist of the scaphoid bone that separated the bone in two fragments (S1 and S2). R, radius.

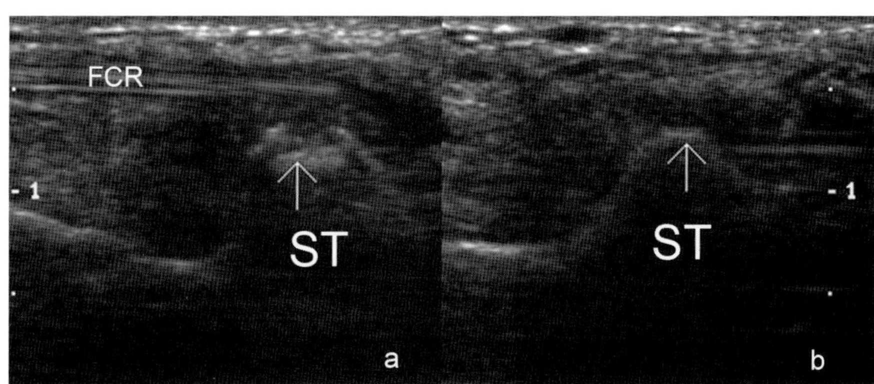

Fig. 3.28 Fracture of the tubercle of the scaphoid bone. Comparative longitudinal ultrasound images of the volar aspect of the wrists. The affected side (a) shows fragmentation of the tubercle of the scaphoid (ST); (b) corresponds to the normal side. FCR, flexor carpi radialis tendon.

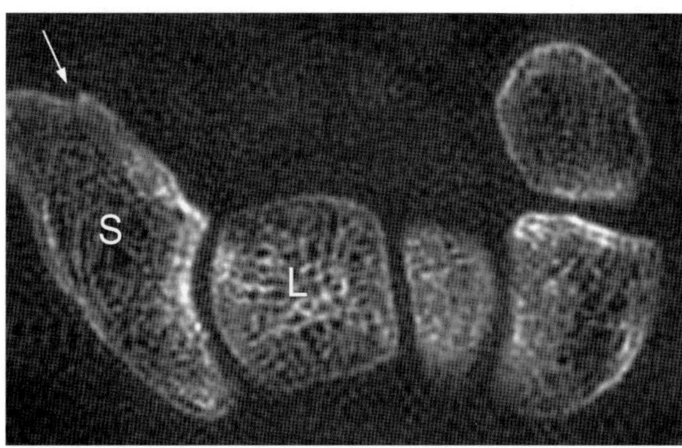

Fig. 3.29 Fracture of the scaphoid. Axial computed tomography (CT) scan of the same patient as in Fig. 3.27 demonstrates the fracture (*arrow*). S, scaphoid; L, lunate.

On sonography, there is discontinuity of the hyperechoic cortex margin at the level of the base of the hook that may be associated with injury to a deep branch of the ulnar nerve.

Fractures of the Capitate

The capitate is the largest carpal bone, but its fractures are generally part of complex injuries. Capitate fractures may occur with scaphoid waist fractures in the so-called scaphocapitate syndrome. The mechanism is a direct blow to the wrist or forced dorsiflexion. Blood supply to the capitate enters the bone at the waist. Similarly, fractures in the waist of the capitate may result in avascular necrosis of the proximal fracture moiety. On ultrasound, there may be discontinuity of the hyperechoic bony margin of the capitate.

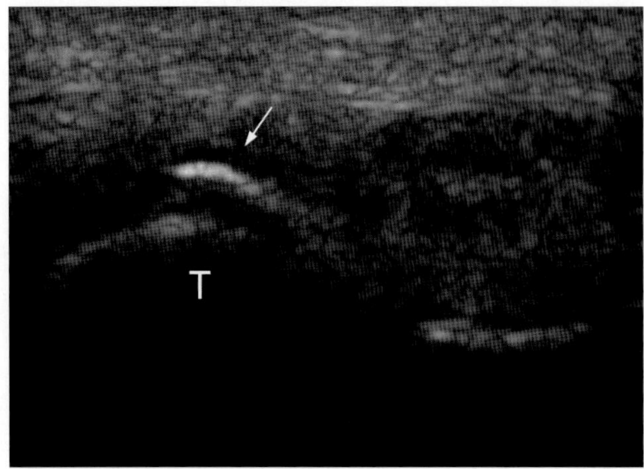

A

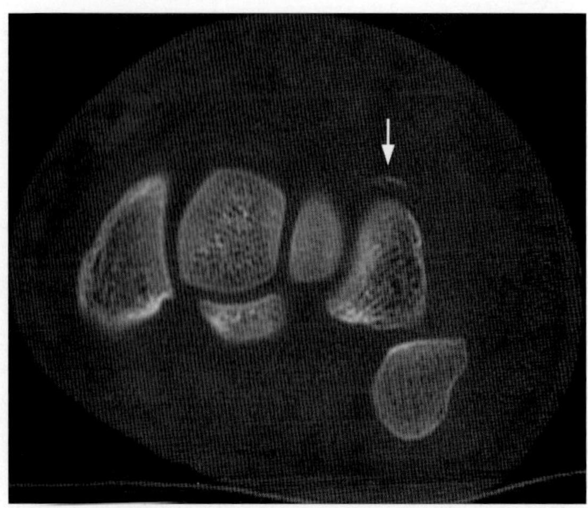

B

C

Fig. 3.30 Fracture of the dorsum of the triquetrum bone (T). **(A)** Longitudinal ultrasound scan shows an hyperechoic fragment (*arrow*) corresponding with the avulsion fragment, by the tearing of the radiotriquetral ligament. **(B)** Avulsion fracture of the dorsum of the triquetrum. Axial computed tomography (CT) scan of the same patient as in **(A)**, demonstrates the avulsion fragment (*arrow*). **(C)** Digital drawing of an avulsion fracture of the triquetrum (arrow). T, triquetrum; RTL, radiotriquetral ligament; R, radius; L, lunate.

Arterial Lesions

Most arterial lesions of the wrist may manifest as pseudoaneurysm, thrombosis, and arteriovenous fistulas. The two main arterial vessels in the wrist are the radial and ulnar arteries and the main cause of lesions in these vessels is direct trauma.

Arterial Thrombosis

The affected vessel may be enlarged and filled with a hypoechoic thrombus with absence of signals on color Doppler. Sometimes a compensatory collateral vessel may be seen in the vicinity (**Fig. 3.31**).

Pseudoaneurysm

Pseudoaneurysms are caused by a partial laceration of the arterial wall that results in a cystic-like structure connected to the arterial lumen and producing turbulent blood flow. The cystic mass is seen attached to the artery, often filled with hypoechoic thrombotic material. Color Doppler shows turbulent flow inside the pseudoaneurysm and its communication with the main artery (**Fig. 3.32**). At the earliest stages, and when the lesion is still small, it may be possible to perform ultrasound-guided compression of the pseudoaneurysm.

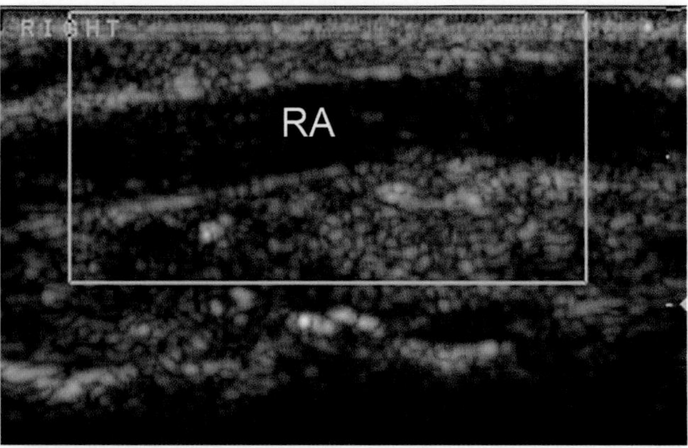

Fig. 3.31 Thrombosis of the radial artery after a direct trauma to the wrist. Color Doppler ultrasound longitudinal view shows absence of blood flow in the lumen of the radial artery (RA).

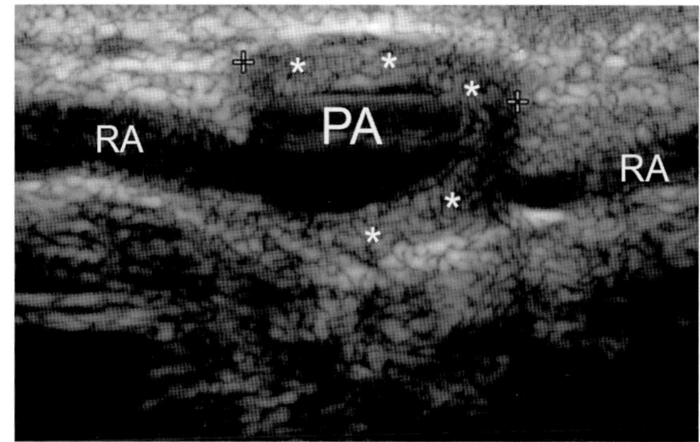

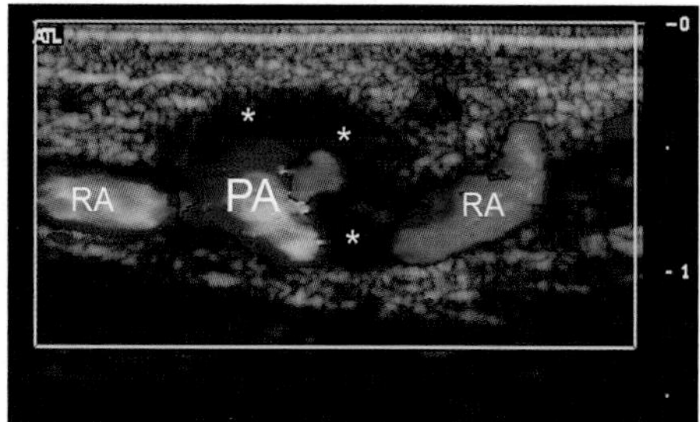

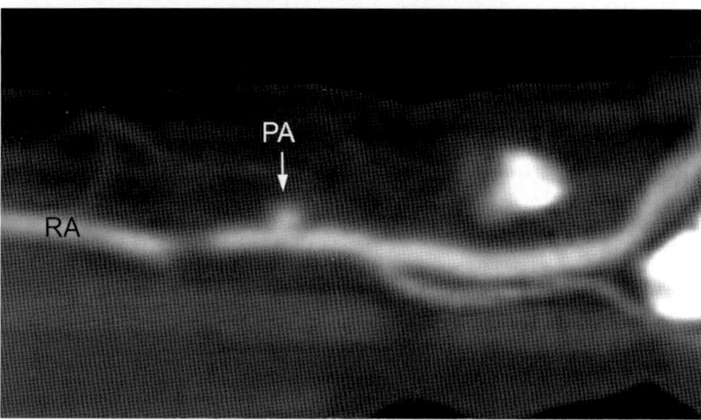

Fig. 3.32 Pseudoaneurysm of the radial artery (RA) following a direct injury with an electric drill. **(A)** Longitudinal view shows saccular enlargement corresponding with a pseudoaneurysm (PA, *between markers*) of the radial artery (RA); there is also hypoechoic thrombotic material (*) attached to the arterial walls. **(B)** Color Doppler ultrasound in longitudinal axis of the same case as in **(A)** shows turbulent blood flow inside the pseudoaneurysm (PA) and the lumen is partially thrombosed (*). **(C)** AngioCT (computed tomography) reconstruction in longitudinal axis in the same case as **(A)** and **(B)** shows the presence of a pseudoaneurysm (PA) in the distal radial artery (RA).

Arteriovenous Fistulas

Arteriovenous fistulas are anomalous connections between arterial and venous vessels, commonly the result of direct trauma such as penetrating wounds. Color Doppler shows turbulent and pulsed flow inside the venous side of the fistula and extremely turbulent flow inside the communication. The arterial side of the fistula shows low resistance flow.

Radial Artery Lesions

The radial artery arises from the bifurcation of the brachial artery and runs distally on the anterior part of the forearm, close to the flexor carpi radialis and abductor pollicis longus; it serves as a landmark to separate the anterior and posterior compartments of the forearm. The artery winds laterally around the wrist, crossing the deep aspect of the tendons of the abductor pollicis longus and extensor pollicis brevis (first extensor compartment) and extensor pollicis longus (third extensor compartment), passes through the anatomic snuff box and ends between the heads of the first dorsal interosseus muscle. Along its course, the radial vein accompanies it. Injuries to the radial artery may result from synovial cyst surgery in the radial aspect of the wrist, or from other invasive procedures **(Fig. 3.33)**.

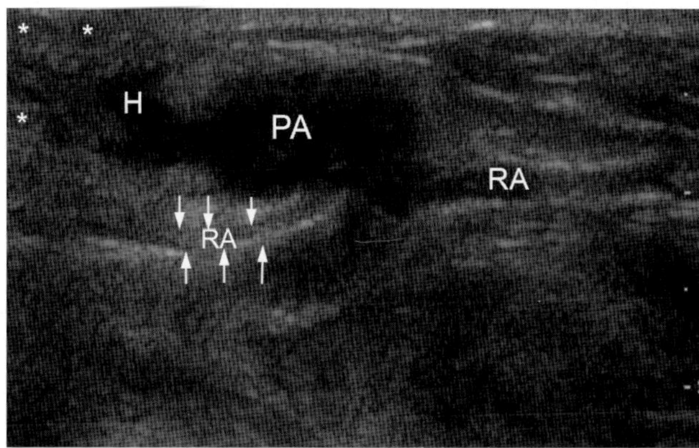

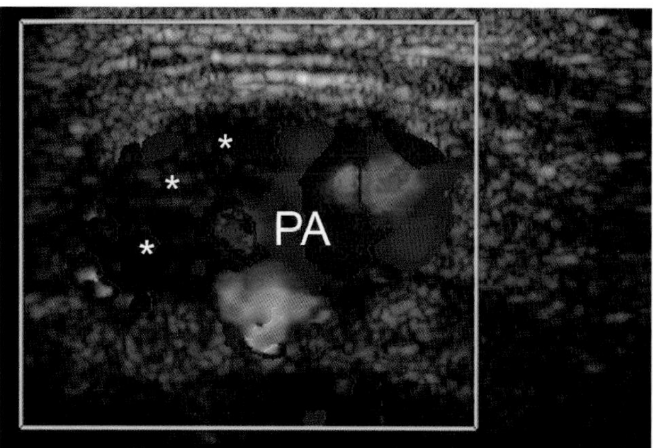

Fig. 3.33 Pseudoaneurysm of the radial artery following knife cut. **(A)** Longitudinal ultrasound view shows saccular enlargement (PA) of the radial artery (RA) surrounded by edema of the subcutaneous tissue (*) and a hematoma (H). Also, distal narrowing of the radial artery (*arrows*) can be seen. **(B)** Pseudoaneurysm of the radial artery (PA). Color Doppler ultrasound of the same patient as in **(A)** shows turbulent flow inside the partially thrombosed pseudoaneurysm.

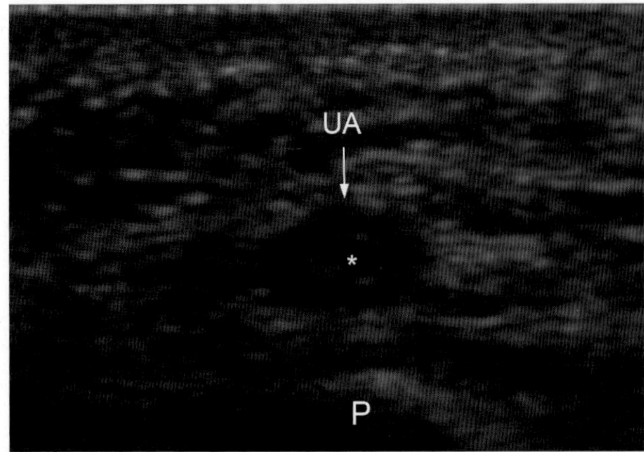

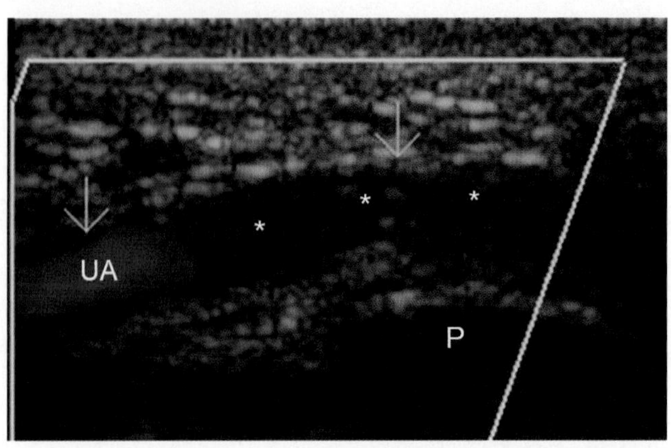

Fig. 3.34 Thrombosis of the ulnar artery in a worker with repetitive use of a hammer (hammer hand syndrome). **(A)** Transverse ultrasound image shows hypoechoic thrombotic material (*) filling the lumen of the ulnar artery (UA). P, pisiform. **(B)** Ulnar artery thrombosis. Color Doppler ultrasound longitudinal view shows thrombotic material (*) filling the lumen of the ulnar artery (UA). P, pisiform.

Ulnar Artery Lesions

The ulnar artery arises from the brachial artery and runs in the medial aspect of the forearm. In the lower half of the forearm, it lies on the flexor digitorum profundus tendon, and then travels between the tendons of the flexor carpi ulnaris and flexor digitorum superficialis. At the wrist the ulnar artery goes through the Guyon tunnel, covered by the volar carpal ligament lying on the transverse carpal ligament. The ulnar artery is surrounded on its medial side by the pisiform bone, and somewhat behind and lateral by the ulnar nerve. Repetitive trauma on the ulnar aspect of the wrist may cause thrombosis of the ulnar artery and/or secondary neurologic symptoms from compression of the ulnar nerve (hypothenar hammer syndrome) **(Fig. 3.34)**.

Venous Thrombosis

Venous thrombosis may occur after a direct injury to the wrist such as during an invasive procedure, or accompanying paraneoplastic or hematologic disorders. Commonly, it affects a subcutaneous vein which becomes non compressible and sometimes painful. On sonography, the lumen is dilated and filled with hypoechoic material corresponding to the thrombus. Color Doppler shows the absence of flow in the affected vessel (**Fig. 3.35**).

Entrapment Neuropathies

Carpal Tunnel Syndrome

Carpal tunnel syndrome (CTS) is generally caused by chronic compression of the median nerve inside the carpal tunnel from the trauma of longstanding and repetitive movements, such as typing, carpentry, or jackhammer operation. Other causes are intrinsic nerve dysfunction caused by edema, inflammation, or tumor; or less commonly by extrinsic compression by tunnel-occupying lesions.

CTS is the most frequent peripheral entrapment neuropathy affecting 3.7% of the general population, but with an increasing prevalence in individuals whose work entails

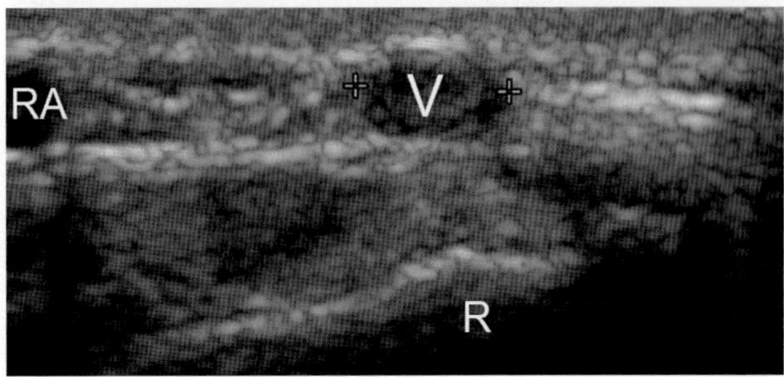

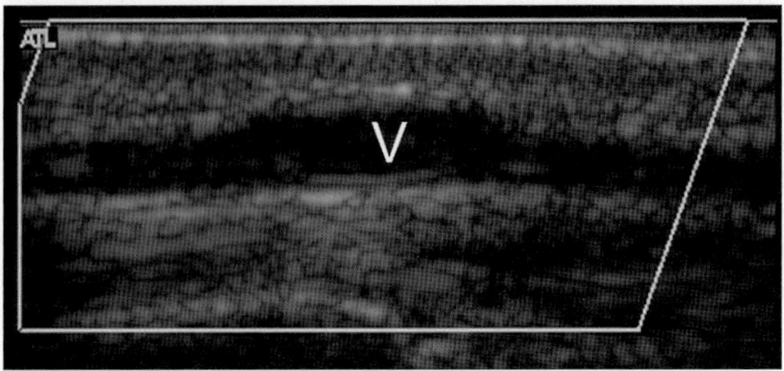

Fig. 3.35 Thrombosis of a subcutaneous vein in the wrist. **(A)** Transverse ultrasound image shows hypoechoic thrombotic material filling the lumen of a subcutaneous vein (V) running close to the radial artery (RA), after direct trauma to the wrist. R, radius. **(B)** Color Doppler ultrasound longitudinal view shows absence of flow signals inside the subcutaneous vein (V) of the wrist in the same case as **(A)**.

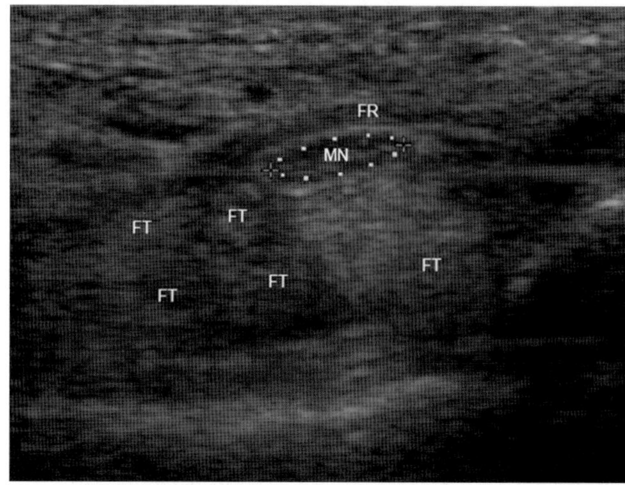

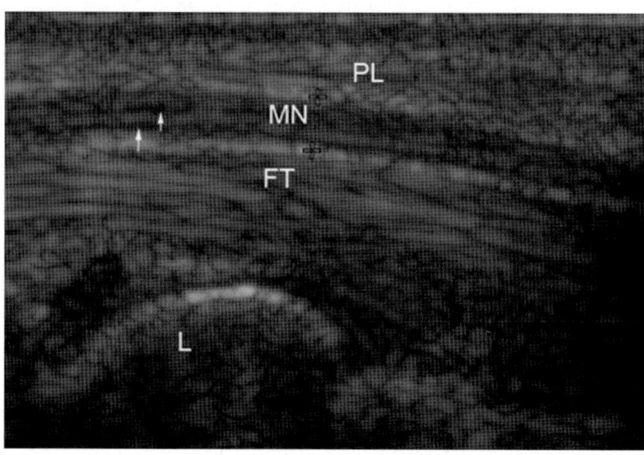

Fig. 3.36 Median nerve (MN) normal anatomy. **(A)** Transverse ultrasound view shows the fascicular pattern with inner hypoechoic dots typical of the neural tissue (*between markers*). Calculation of the nerve area was made by the ellipsoid formula (indirect method). FT, flexor tendons; FR, flexor retinaculum. **(B)** Longitudinal axis shows hypoechoic lines corresponding with the neural fascicles (*arrows*). FT, flexor tendons; PL, palmaris longus tendon; MN, median nerve.

repetitive motion of the wrist, those who are pregnant, or in patients with diabetes or arthritis. The disease affects women more commonly and has a peak incidence between 40 and 60 years of age.

Among the symptoms of CTS are pain, numbness, a tingling sensation of the fingers excluding the little finger, and loss of sensation in the hand and the fingers.

CTS Ultrasound Diagnosis Criteria

The sonographic diagnosis of CTS is based on the abnormalities seen in the median nerve or its surrounding structures (**Figs. 3.36** and **3.37**). They can be classified as follows:

1. Median nerve changes
   - Nerve swelling in the proximal tunnel
   - Nerve flattening in the distal tunnel
   - Nerve thickening as measured on cross-sectional area in the transverse axis greater than 10 mm^2 (transverse diameter x anteroposterior diameter × 3.14/4, by ellipsoid formula, also called indirect method) or greater than 9 mm^2 (continuous boundary trace, also called direct method)
   - Decrease in overall nerve echogenicity with loss of the fascicular pattern
   - Presence of nerve inner hypervascularity

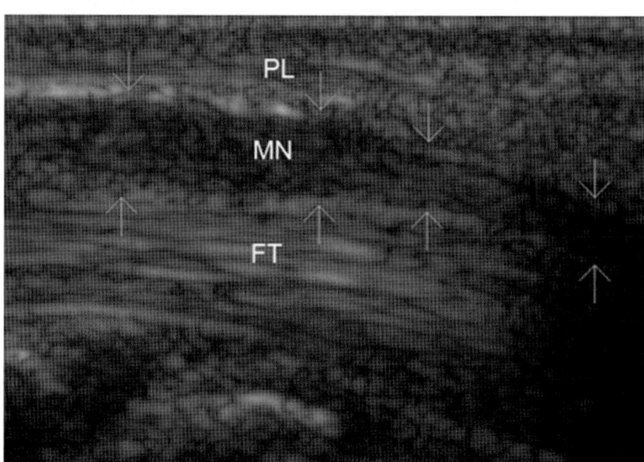

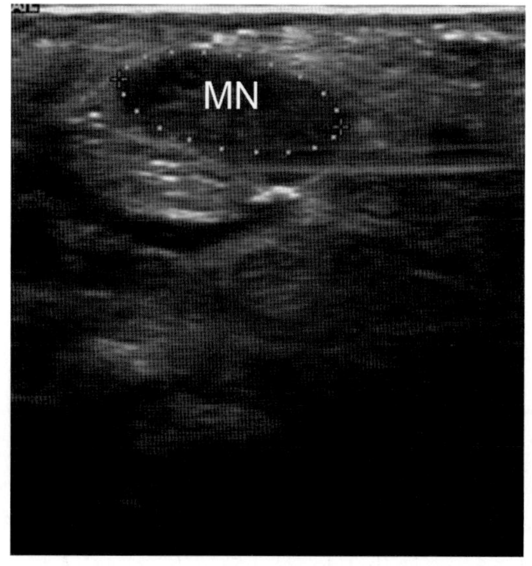

Fig. 3.37 Carpal tunnel syndrome. **(A)** Longitudinal ultrasound view shows swelling and hypoechogenicity of the median nerve (MN and *arrows*). FT, flexor tendons; PL, palmaris longus tendon. **(B)** Transverse ultrasound view shows diffuse swelling of the median nerve (MN) with a nerve area of 32 mm^2 and loss of the fascicular pattern that becomes heterogeneous and hypoechoic. (*Continued*)

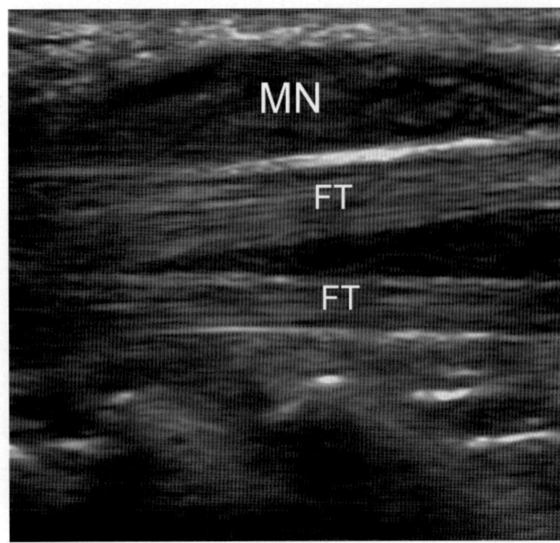

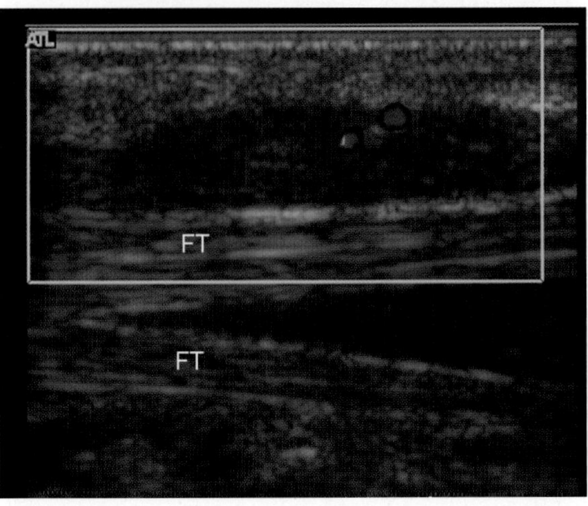

Fig. 3.37 (*Continued*) Carpal tunnel syndrome. **(C)** Longitudinal ultrasound view shows marked swelling and heterogeneous structure of the median nerve (MN). The flexor tendons (FT) present a normal hyperechoic fibrillar appearance. **(D)** Color Doppler ultrasound of the affected side in the same patient as in Fig. 3.36 shows flow signals (in color) seen within the fascicular pattern of the median nerve compatible with neuritis. FT, flexor tendons.

2. Flexor retinaculum changes
   - Bulging of the volar flexor retinaculum, as assessed by distance from the retinaculum to a line joining the tip of the hook of the hamate and the tubercle of the trapezium. A value greater than 4 mm is abnormal.
   - Thickening of flexor retinaculum as compared with the contralateral side
3. Changes in the carpal tunnel content
   - Enlargement of the surrounding structures, most frequently from tenosynovitis
   - Tunnel-occupying lesions, the leading cause is a volar ganglia

Guyon Tunnel Syndrome

The Guyon tunnel contains the ulnar nerve and the ulnar artery. The syndrome, less common than CTS, is due to compression of these structures. The symptoms depend on degree and site of compression of the ulnar nerve. The pisiform level (zone I) is most proximal; at that level the ulnar nerve is represented by the main trunk with its sensory and motor branches; at the hamate level, the deep portion of the tunnel contains a separate motor branch (zone II), more distally, the superficial portion of the tunnel houses a separate sensory branch (zone III). The main causes of compression of the ulnar nerve are ganglia cysts that frequently arise from the hamate-triquetrum or piso-triquetrum joints. These cystic lesions can be connected to the joints through thin and tortuous tracts (**Figs. 3.38** and **3.39**). Less frequent causes of Guyon tunnel syndrome are ulnar artery injuries with thrombosis or pseudoaneurysm, and anatomic variants of muscles such as the accessory abductor digiti minimi that can also compress the nerve. Fractures and benign tumors of the nerve can generate Guyon tunnel syndrome symptoms as well.

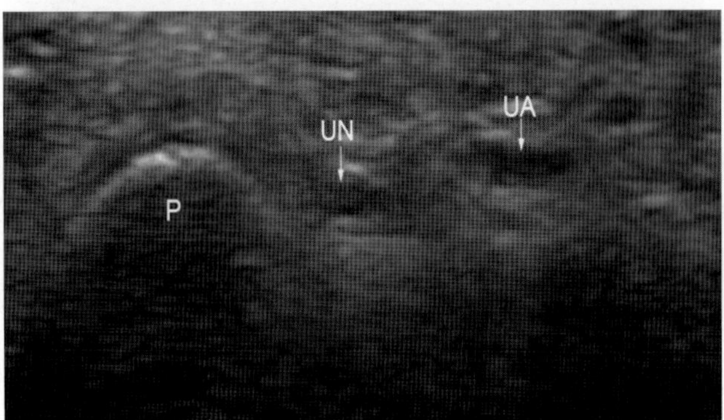

Fig. 3.38 Guyon tunnel normal anatomy. Transverse view shows the ulnar nerve (UN) between the pisiform bone (P) and the ulnar artery (UA).

Miscellaneous

Space-Occupying Lesions

Ganglia

Ganglia are the most common space-occupying lesions in the wrist and one of the most frequent indications for an ultrasound exam; they appear to be caused by trauma or chronic tissue irritation that produces extrusion of the synovial membrane that over time loses its synovial origin. Other causes may be changes in the para-articular connective tissue with secondary myxoid degeneration. The cystic wall is made of collagen and differs histologically from a true

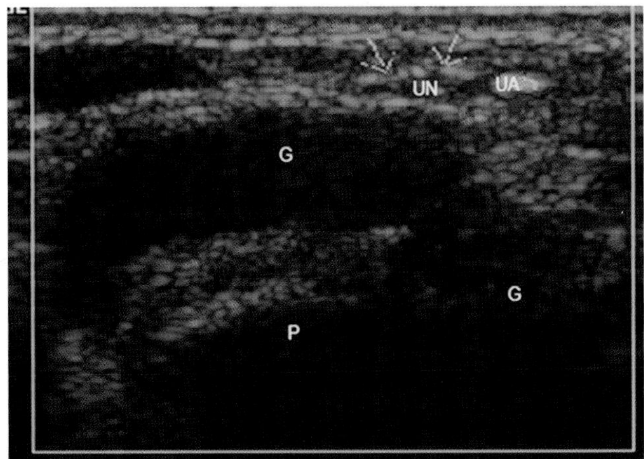

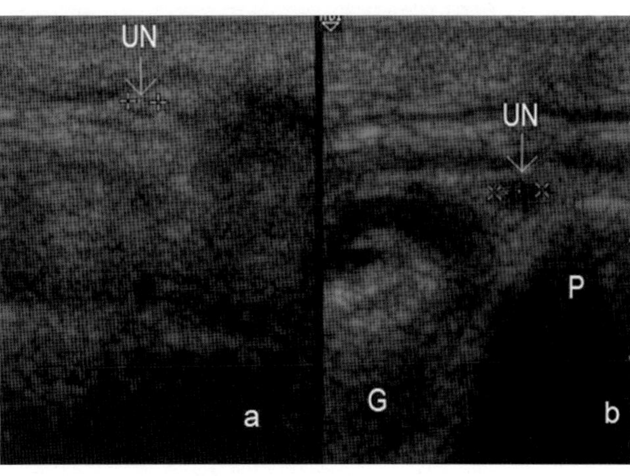

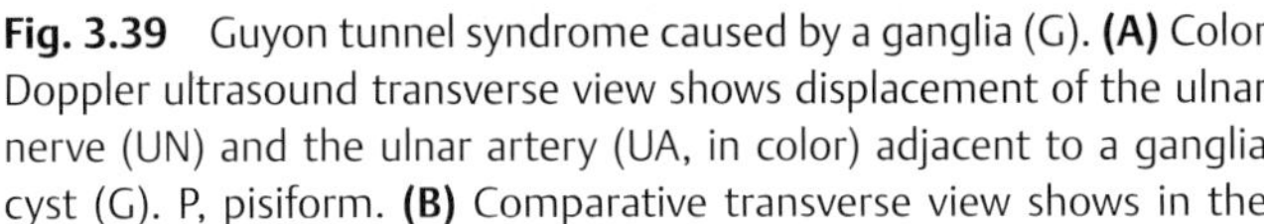

Fig. 3.39 Guyon tunnel syndrome caused by a ganglia (G). **(A)** Color Doppler ultrasound transverse view shows displacement of the ulnar nerve (UN) and the ulnar artery (UA, in color) adjacent to a ganglia cyst (G). P, pisiform. **(B)** Comparative transverse view shows in the affected side (b) thickening of the ulnar nerve (UN, *between markers*) adjacent to a ganglia cyst. The normal side (a) shows a normal diameter of the ulnar nerve. P, pisiform.

synovial cyst because of the lack of synovial lining. The cysts may or may not communicate with the adjacent joint or tendon sheath structures; they contain a gelatinous, mucoid, or thick fluid composed of hyaluronic acid, albumin, globulin, and glucosamine.

Most ganglia are asymptomatic, although associated pain, motion limitation, weakness, and paresthesias have also been described.

The most common locations of ganglia are the dorsal aspect of the wrist overlying the scapholunate ligament followed by the radial volar aspect of the wrist between the flexor carpi radialis and the radial artery **(Fig. 3.40A)**.

On ultrasound, ganglia are seen as anechoic round, oval, or lobulated structures that may be unilocular or septated; in 40% of ganglia there is presence of internal echoes; and 15% of ganglia may show a pattern of mixed echogenicity (anechoic and hypoechoic). Color Doppler ultrasound may show a hypervascular wall in larger cysts (**Figs. 3.40** and **3.41**). Frequently, a thin communication between the cyst and the radiocarpal joint is detectable and the persistence of a valve-like mechanism in that connection may result in varying size of the ganglia over time. Rarely, arterial thrombosis may be seen as a complication of ganglia surgery (**Fig. 3.42**).

Neurogenic Tumors

These are rare tumors of the upper extremity, representing less than 5% of the soft tissue tumors in this location. The most frequent neurogenic tumors are the schwannomas, also called neurilemomas (**Fig. 3.43**); neurofibromas are less common. Most lesions are solitary and present as a painless mass. In patients that present amputation in their limbs, it is not uncommon to detect neuromas in the ending

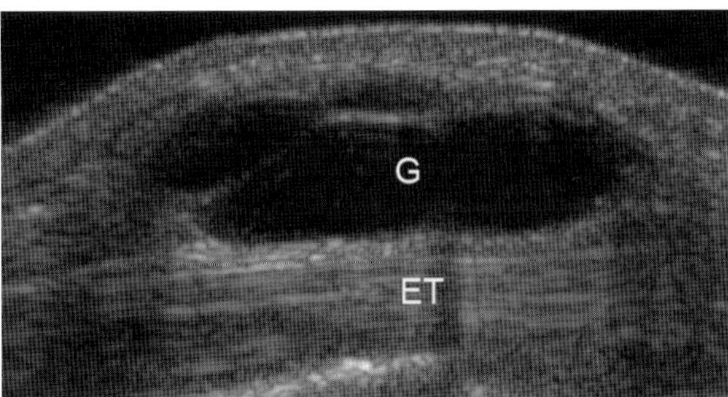

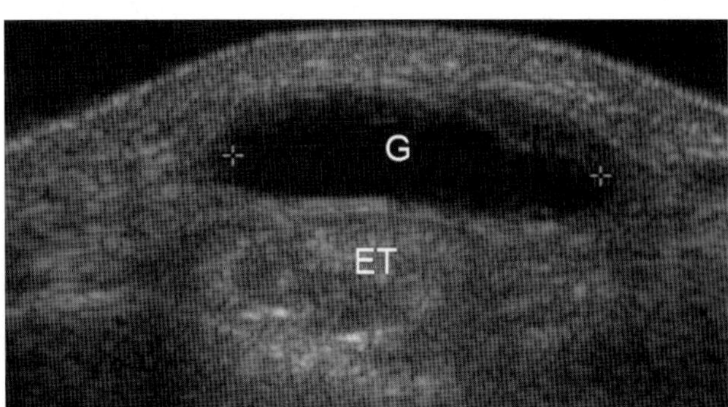

Fig. 3.40 Ganglia in the dorsal aspect of the wrist. **(A)** Longitudinal and **(B)** transverse view ultrasound scans show a lobulated and anechoic cystic structure (G) above the fourth extensor compartment (ET). (*Continued*)

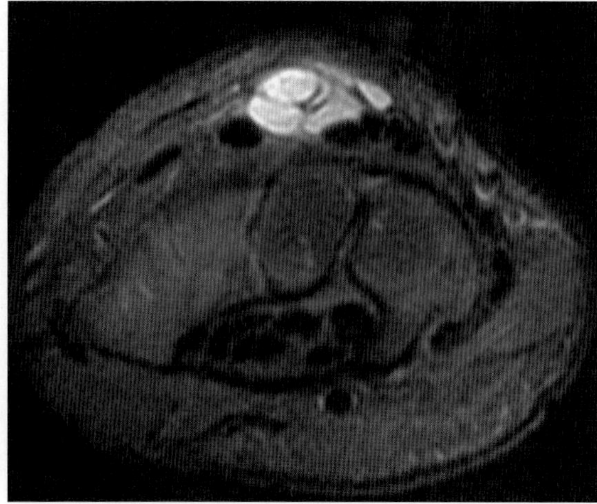

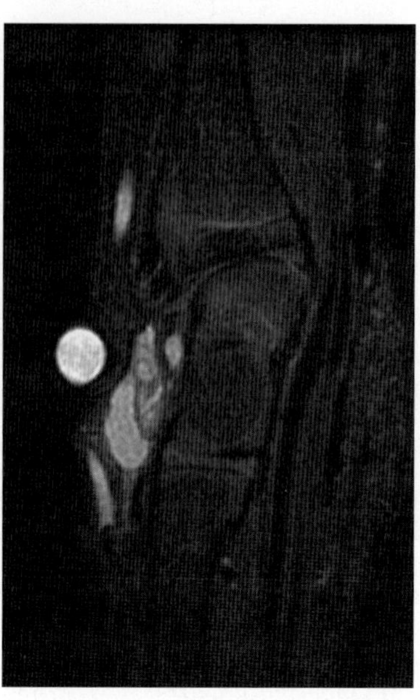

Fig. 3.40 (*Continued*) Ganglia in the dorsal aspect of the wrist. **(C)** Axial and **(D)** sagittal fat-suppressed proton density weighted magnetic resonance images showing multiloculated focus of high signal in the dorsum of the wrist consistent with a dorsal ganglion. (Rounded high signal superficial high signal structure is a marker on the skin)

sites of the nerves that used to be very painful (**Fig. 3.44**). On ultrasound, both types of tumors appear as oval or round hypoechoic nodules attached to a nerve tract. Sonographic differentiation between schwannomas and neurofibromas is difficult, but schwannomas tend to have a more eccentric location in relation to the nerve tract and neurofibromas, a more central location and fusiform shape. Frequently, tubular hypoechoic tracts connecting the nerve and the mass can be defined.

Fig. 3.41 Ganglia attached to the dorsal scapholunate ligament. Transverse ultrasound image shows a small round anechoic cyst (G, *between markers*) above the dorsal scapholunate ligament (SLL). S, scaphoid; L, lunate.

Lipomatous Tumors

Lipomatous tumors present as painless swellings and can affect the carpal or ulnar tunnels causing entrapment of its contents, for example, the median nerve (**Fig. 3.45**). Lipomatous tumors are oval or round in shape, and can be hypo-, iso-, or hyperechoic depending on the type of tissue accompanying the main fatty component; these tumors tend to follow the main axis of the skin layers.

Anatomic Variants

Accessory Muscles

These are commonly detected as incidental findings, or may mimic a tumor by causing symptoms due to compression of surrounding structures. On ultrasound, accessory muscles appear as a hypoechoic mass with distinctive internal muscle echostructure. Sonographic examination should be performed at rest and during contraction because they demonstrate the dynamic properties of muscular tissue.

The accessory abductor digiti minimi is the most common accessory muscle in the wrist and is found in ~24% of normal individuals. It runs inside the Guyon canal in close contact with the artery and nerve. Thus, during contraction or abduction of the little finger the muscle may cause secondary compression of the ulnar nerve, although generally it is an asymptomatic variant. The extensor digitorum brevis manus is found in 1 to 3% of normal individuals, arising from the dorsal aspect of the distal radius, to end distally in the index or middle finger. It appears clinically as a fu-

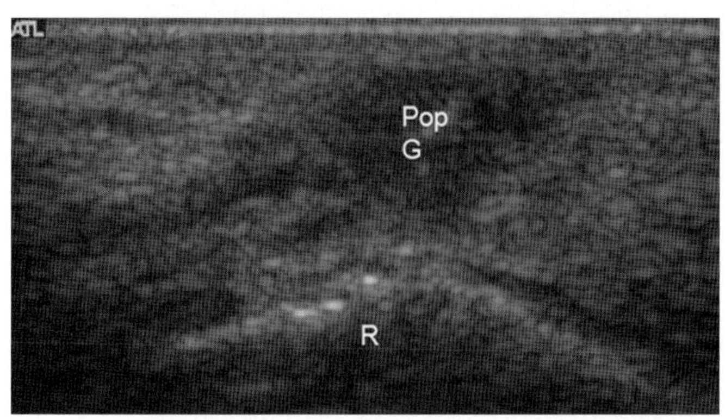

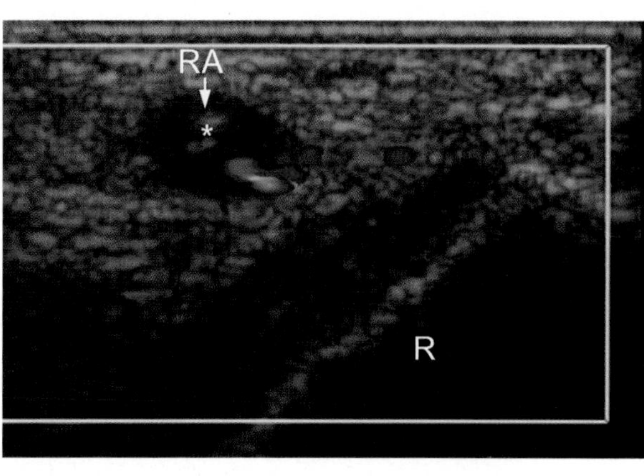

Fig. 3.42 Ganglia postoperative ultrasound follow-up. **(A)** Transverse ultrasound image shows a remnant hypoechoic area (Pop G) in the zone of the ganglia surgery. R, radius. **(B)** Thrombosis of the radial artery, after surgery and in the same patient as in **(A).** Color Doppler ultrasound transverse view shows hypoechoic thrombotic material (*) and scarce marginal flow (colors) inside the radial artery (RA). R, radius.

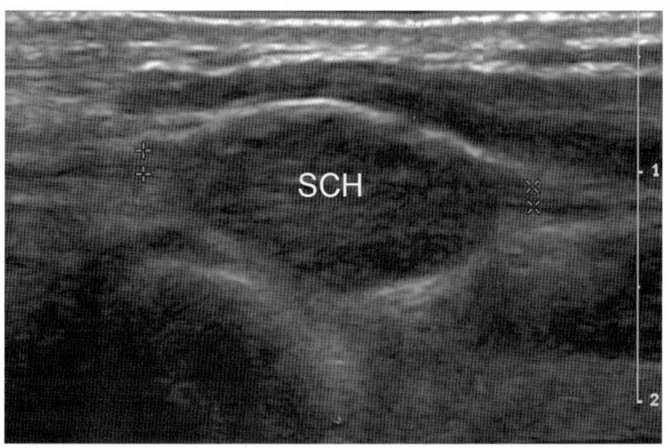

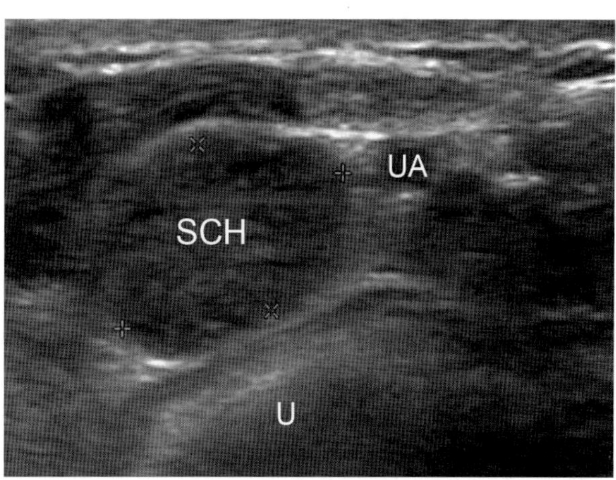

Fig. 3.43 Schwannoma of the ulnar nerve. **(A)** Longitudinal panoramic ultrasound view shows an oval hypoechoic nodule (SCH) attached to the ulnar nerve tract. Neural tracts afferent and efferent to the lesion are shown between markers. **(B)** Transverse ultrasound view shows a round hypoechoic nodule (SCH, between markers) in the same case as in **(A)**. UA, ulnar artery; U, ulna.

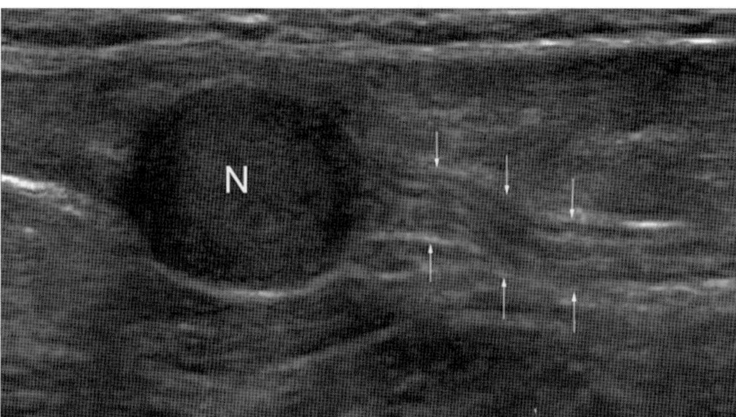

Fig. 3.44 Neuroma of the median nerve postamputation. Longitudinal ultrasound view shows that the median nerve tract (*arrows*) ends in the round hypoechoic nodule that corresponds with the neuroma (N). This nodule is located in the distal forearm close to the beginning of the wrist.

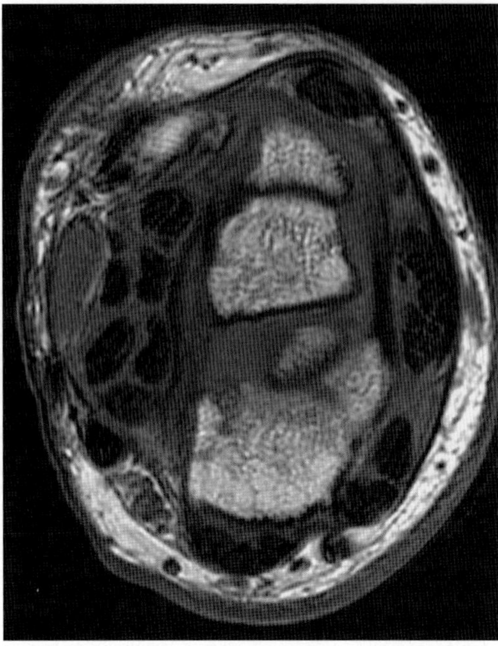

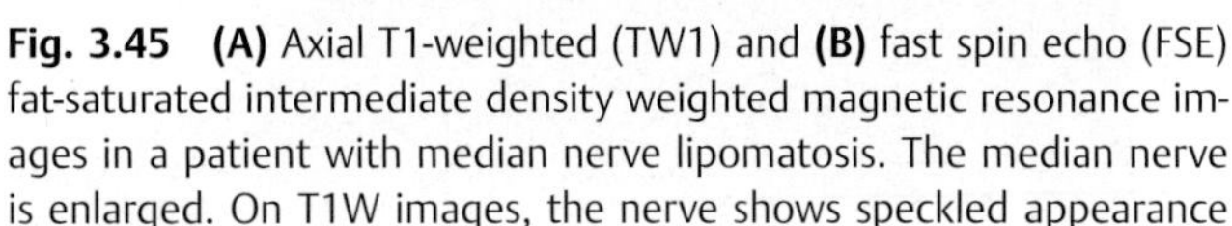

Fig. 3.45 **(A)** Axial T1-weighted (TW1) and **(B)** fast spin echo (FSE) fat-saturated intermediate density weighted magnetic resonance images in a patient with median nerve lipomatosis. The median nerve is enlarged. On T1W images, the nerve shows speckled appearance with interspersed foci of high signal due to presence of fat within the lesion. This speckled pattern is also observed on the intermediate density images. These represent the enlarged nerve sheaths.

siform tumor alongside the extensor tendon of the index finger. Other muscle variants include anomalous bellies of the flexor digitorum muscle and anatomic variations of the palmaris muscle (**Figs. 3.46, 3.47, 3.48, 3.49, 3.50, 3.51**).

Bifid Median Nerve

The bifid median nerve is an anatomic variant produced by the high bifurcation of the nerve and is present in 9% of the normal population. Most of the time this variant is asymptomatic, but it has also been related to carpal tunnel syndrome. The presence of a bifid median nerve is commonly associated with a persistent median artery (**Fig. 3.52**).

Persistent Median Artery

The embryonal median artery provides blood supply to the forearm and hand, and as the radial and ulnar arteries complete their development the median artery atrophies to a small vessel that accompanies the median nerve into the forearm. A persistent median artery (PMA) may extend into the carpal tunnel and join the superficial volar arch, or supply the radial digits with absent arch, or end just as a thrombosed thread. In 2 to 3% of the normal population, the vessel persists prominently and this anatomic variation is commonly bilateral and associated with a bifid median nerve. Because it has a superficial location, it is prone to direct

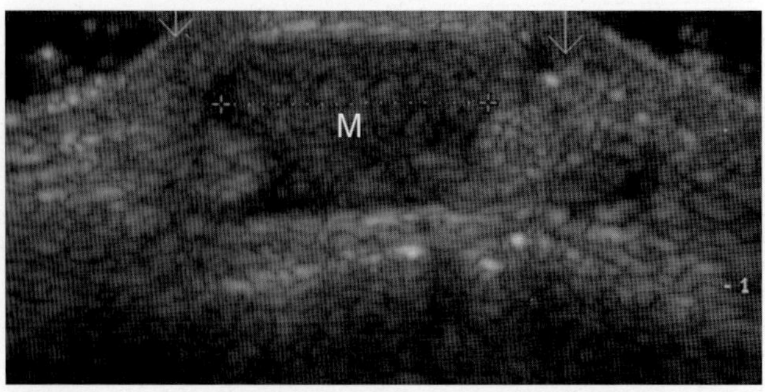

Fig. 3.46 Extensor brevis manus accessory muscle. **(A)** Transverse ultrasound view at rest shows an oval hypoechoic structure in between the extensor tendons of the fourth compartment corresponding to an accessory muscle (M, *between markers*). **(B)** Extensor brevis manus during dynamic maneuver (flexion of the hands). Transverse view of the accessory muscle (M) shows normal contraction pattern in this variant that is seen in the same patient as in **(A)** (*Continued*).

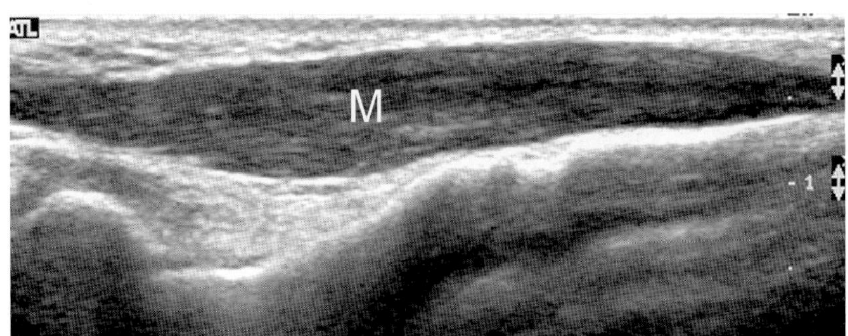

C

Fig. 3.46 (*Continued*) Extensor brevis manus accessory muscle. **(C)** Extensor brevis manus accessory muscle during extension of the hand. Longitudinal ultrasound view shows a hypoechoic fusiform structure corresponding to a thick accessory muscle (M) that crosses the wrist and hand. **(D)** Extensor brevis muscle comparative view. Transverse comparative ultrasound views show in the normal side (a) absence of the accessory muscle and in the affected side (b) presence of the muscular variant (M), attached to the fourth extensor compartment (b).

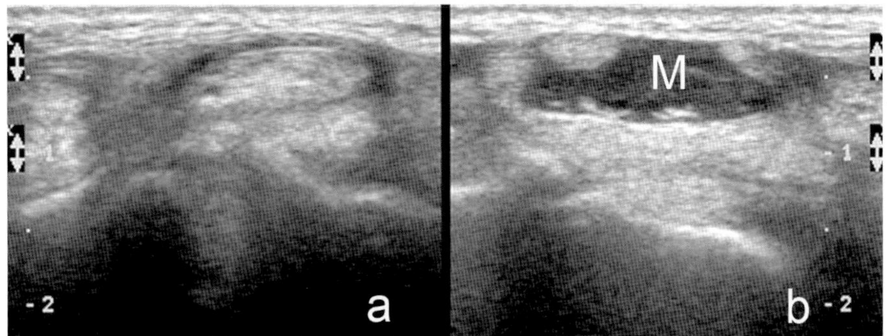

D

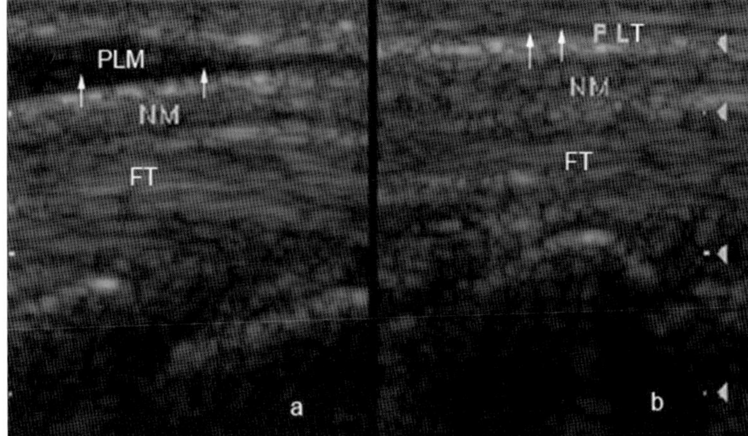

A

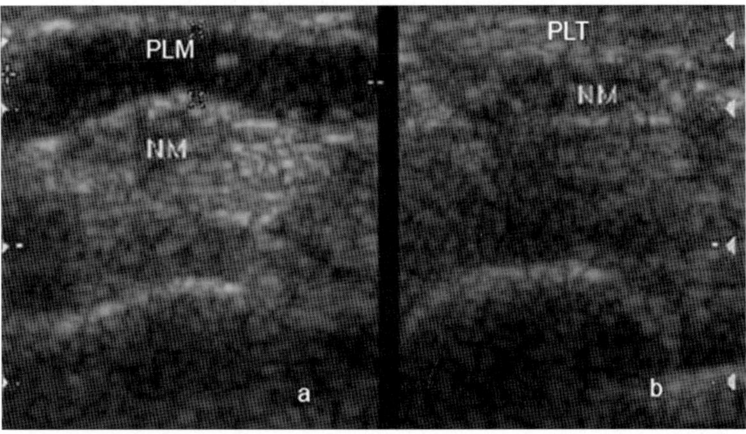

B

Fig. 3.47 Palmaris longus musculotendinous variant. **(A)** Longitudinal comparative ultrasound views show in the affected side (a) a palmaris muscular fascicle (PLM; *arrows*) accompanying the flexor tendons (FT) and median nerve (NM). In contrast, the normal side (b) presents a hyperechoic palmaris longus tendon (PLT; *arrows*) in the same location. **(B)** Palmaris longus musculotendinous variant. Transverse comparative ultrasound images in the same case as in **(A)** shows in the affected side (a) a hypoechoic oval structure above the median nerve (MN) that corresponds with variant of a palmaris longus muscle (PLM). In the normal side (b) there is a palmaris longus tendon (PLT) that is seen as a hyperechoic oval structure in the same location.

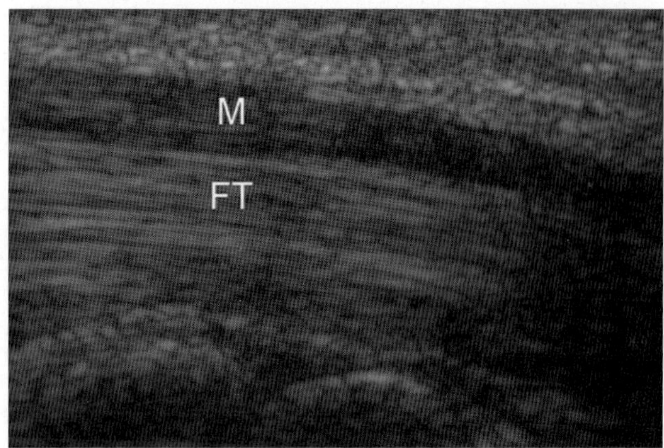

Fig. 3.48 Accessory muscular fascicle accompanying the flexor digitorum superficialis tendon for the second finger. Longitudinal view shows the hypoechoic muscle (M) attached to the hyperechoic flexor tendon (FT).

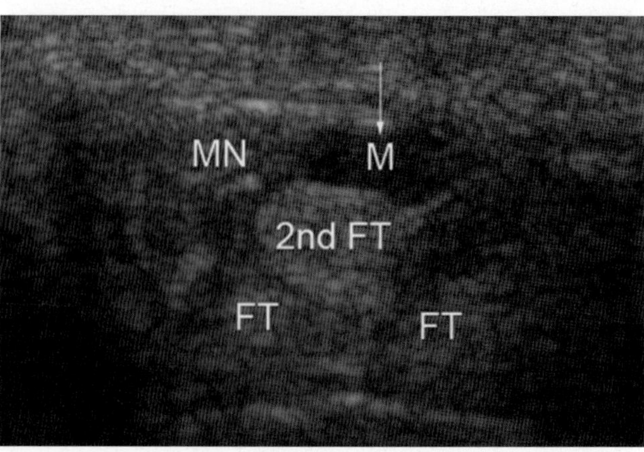

Fig. 3.49 Accessory muscular fascicle accompanying the second flexor digitorum superficialis tendon. Transverse ultrasound view of the same patient of Fig. 3.46 shows the oval hypoechoic structure corresponding with the accessory muscle (M; *arrow*) attached to the flexor tendon for the second finger (2nd FT). MN, median nerve.

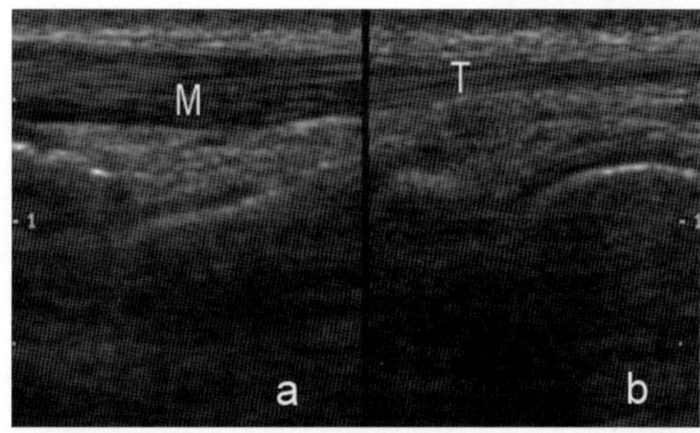

Fig. 3.50 Accessory muscle attached to the second extensor tendon. Longitudinal comparative ultrasound views show in the affected side (a) the presence of a hypoechoic muscle (M). The normal side (b) presents only a hyperechoic fibrillar tendinous structure (T) in the same location.

trauma and may easily become thrombosed. Furthermore, it may be the cause of carpal tunnel syndrome of acute onset (**Figs. 3.53** and **3.54**).

Proposed Algorithm for Wrist Imaging Investigation

1. Plain radiography
2. Ultrasound—first imaging examination for soft tissue pathologies
3. Computed tomography—for suspected bone pathology not detected in plain radiography such as hidden fractures
4. Magnetic resonance imaging—MRI Arthrography for suspected triangular fibrocartilage lesions

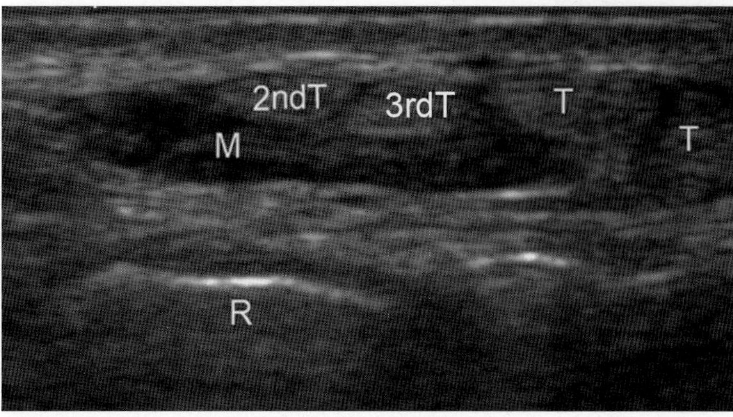

Fig. 3.51 Accessory muscle attached to the second and third extensor tendons in the fourth compartment. Transverse ultrasound view shows an oval hypoechoic structure corresponding to the accessory muscle (M), below the second and third extensor tendons (2nd and 3rd T). T, tendons; R, radius.

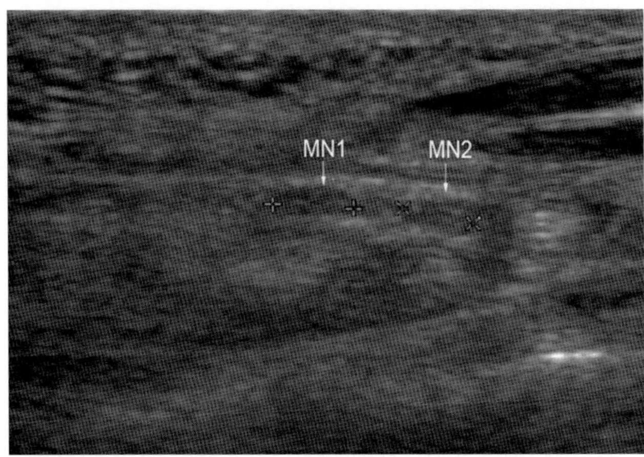

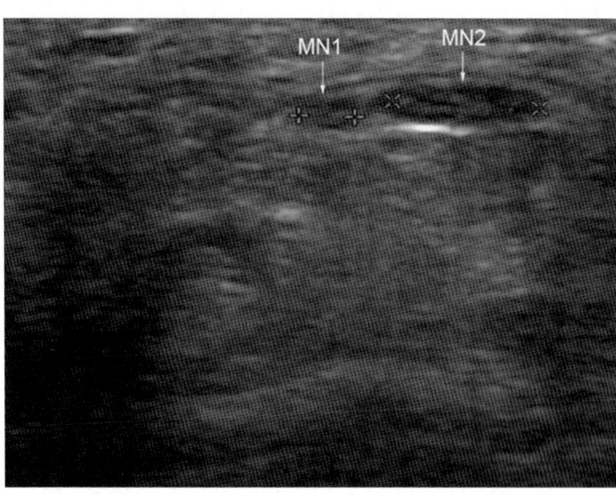

Fig. 3.52 Bifid median nerve. **(A)** Transverse ultrasound image of the carpal tunnel shows two neural tracts of same diameter (MN1 and MN2; *between markers*) instead of one median nerve. **(B)** Transverse ultrasound image shows in the carpal tunnel two neural tracts of different diameters. There is a dominant branch (MN2) and an accessory branch (MN1).

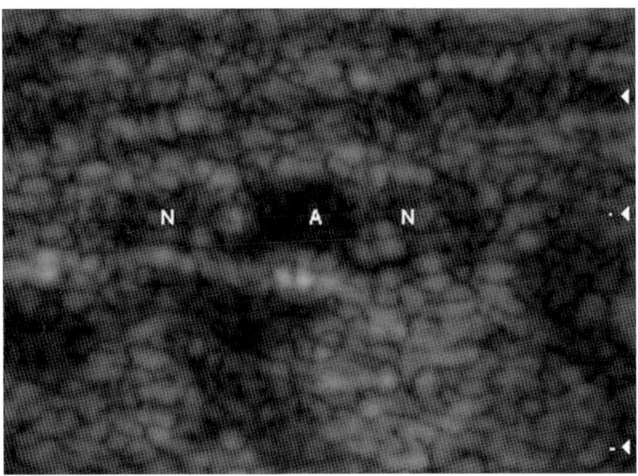

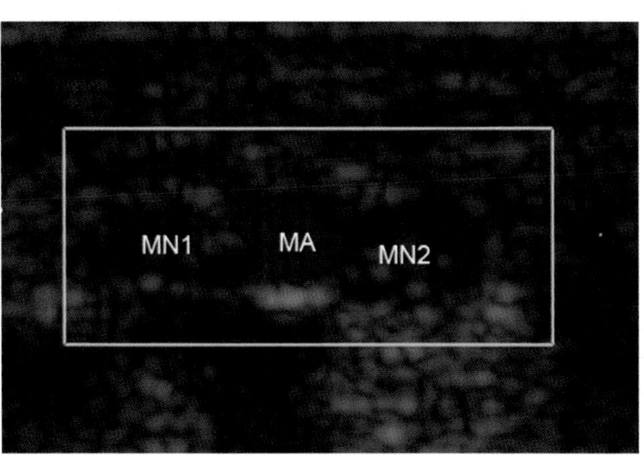

Fig. 3.53 Persistent median artery. **(A)** Transverse view shows an anechoic round structure that corresponds with a median artery (A) seated between two branches of a bifid median nerve (N). **(B)** Color Doppler ultrasound shows blood flow signals inside the persistent median artery (MA) located in between the two branches of a bifid median nerve (MN1 and MN2).

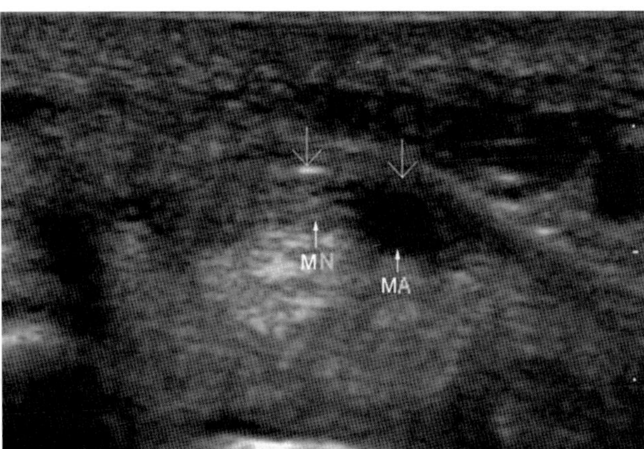

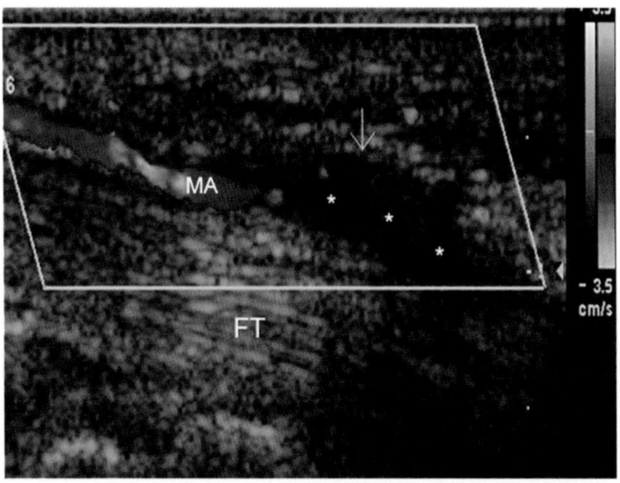

Fig. 3.54 Thrombosis of a persistent median artery. **(A)** Transverse ultrasound view shows a dilatation of a persistent median artery (MA; *arrows*) beside the median nerve (MN) in the carpal tunnel. **(B)** Color Doppler longitudinal ultrasound view of the same case as in Fig. 3.53 shows presence of hypoechoic material (* and *arrow*) corresponding to a thrombus that fills the lumen of the distal portion of the median artery (MA). FT, flexor tendons.

Pearls and Pitfalls

- Systematic sonographic examination of the dorsal aspect of the wrist is best started with a transverse view to identify sequentially the extensor compartments from I to VI. This may be followed with a longitudinal view testing the sequence in reverse order.
- To study the ventral aspect, start with a transverse view; this allows easy separation of the median nerve from the flexor tendons. A subsequent longitudinal axis view will make it possible to identify the tendons by their fibrillar pattern and the median nerve by its fascicular pattern.
- Generally, the extensor tendons of compartment II (extensor carpi radialis longus and brevis) are larger than the extensor tendons of compartment I (abductor longus and extensor brevis of the thumb). When compartment I extensor tendons are larger than the extensor tendons of compartment II, an inflammatory process should be suspected.
- When a bifid median nerve is detected; it is suggested to look for the persistent median artery in the middle of the two branches. With color Doppler ultrasound, it is possible to detect the low blood flow inside the artery. Sometimes, this artery can be seen as a fibrous remnant without flow.
- In the ultrasound examination of synovial cysts, it is important to look for the connecting tract to the joint space. This is important data needed to prevent recurrence after surgery.

Suggested Readings

Bianchi S, Martinoli S. Wrist. In: Bianchi S, Martinoli C, eds. Ultrasound of the Musculoskeletal System. 1st ed. Heidelberg: Springer; 2007:425–494

Boutry N, Morel M, Flipo RM, Demondion X, Cotten A. Early rheumatoid arthritis: a review of MRI and sonographic findings. AJR Am J Roentgenol 2007;189(6):1502–1509

Gassner EM, Schocke M, Peer S, Schwabegger A, Jaschke W, Bodner G. Persistent median artery in the carpal tunnel: color Doppler ultrasonographic findings. J Ultrasound Med 2002;21(4):455–461

Lee D. Wrist. In: Chhem R, Cardinal E, eds. Guidelines and gamuts in musculoskeletal ultrasound. 1st ed. Hoboken, NJ: Wiley-Liss; 1998:107–124

Pinilla I, Martín-Hervás C, Sordo G, Santiago S. The usefulness of ultrasonography in the diagnosis of carpal tunnel syndrome. J Hand Surg Eur Vol 2008;33(4):435–439

Propeck T, Quinn TJ, Jacobson JA, Paulino AF, Habra G, Darian VB. Sonography and MR imaging of bifid median nerve with anatomic and histologic correlation. AJR Am J Roentgenol 2000;175(6):1721–1725

Thiele RG, Schlesinger N. Diagnosis of gout by ultrasound. Rheumatology (Oxford) 2007;46:1116–1121

Van Holsbeeck M, Introcaso J. Sonography of the elbow, wrist and hand. In: Van Holsbeeck M, Introcaso J, eds. Musculoskeletal Ultrasound. 2nd ed. St. Louis: Mosby; 2001: 531-554

4 Imaging of the Hand

Ian Yu-Yan Tsou, Seng Choe Tham, and Gervais K. L. Wansaicheong

Imaging of the hand and fingers with ultrasound has always been challenging. Although the hand and fingers are amenable to ultrasound imaging, the difficulty has been with the small sizes of the anatomic structures under study, as well as the very superficial position of these structures, which places them in the extreme near field of the ultrasound transducer.

However, the development of hand and microsurgery as a subdiscipline of orthopaedic surgery has led to increased demand for imaging of the hand and fingers. Often, the surgeon will have a specific question after the clinical examination, and ultrasound can be directed toward answering this question quickly and easily. As long as the limitations of ultrasound are recognized by both the performing radiologist and the referring clinician, ultrasound will continue to play a large role in hand and wrist imaging.

Clinical Indications

The role of ultrasound in hand and finger imaging is progressively growing. Although much of the current imaging is still based on radiography in terms of traumatic injury and rheumatology, there has been definite recognition of the importance of visualization of the soft tissues, as well as imaging during dynamic movement, both of which are well demonstrated with ultrasound.

Acute hand and finger injuries would still require radiographs as the initial imaging modality, primarily to identify fractures or radiopaque foreign bodies. However, persistent posttraumatic pain or other symptoms in the absence of fracture or bony injury requires further evaluation. Ligament and tendon injuries make up a significant proportion of cases of dysfunction, which are not directly visible on radiographs other than as bony dislocation or subluxation.

Penetrating injuries by foreign bodies are also a frequently encountered indication for ultrasound imaging. It is not uncommon for retained foreign bodies to be nonopaque on radiographs, usually of organic material such as wooden splinters, plant thorn, insect stings, etc. In addition, the foreign bodies may be in multiple small fragments, each of which needs to be identified and removed, to reduce the risk of infection and inciting an inflammatory response. Ultrasound is able to detect such millimeter-sized foreign bodies, providing the hand surgeon with a road map for removal.

Lumps and bumps on the hand have always been a common indication for ultrasound imaging, with the main intention to identify if it is solid or cystic. Ancillary findings would include the relationship or attachment to the surrounding structures, compressibility, vascularity, and location.

The more diffuse swelling in the hand and fingers is usually due to soft tissue edema. The role that ultrasound is able to contribute is to assess if the edema is related to any particular anatomic structure or underlying injury. Joint effusions and fluid collections can also track within the fascial planes and present as swelling. Inflammatory or rheumatologic conditions may also present as joint swelling.

Erosive arthropathy has also become more often imaged with ultrasound, both by radiologists and rheumatologists. Bony erosions demonstrated on radiographs are a late manifestation of disease, and the direct visualization of soft tissue inflammatory pannus with increased vascularity allows earlier detection and diagnosis.

Biopsy, aspiration, or injection of the hand and fingers is easily done by the clinician, knowing the normal anatomy, and with the target area in a superficial location. Ultrasound-guided procedures are occasionally useful in situations where there is an unexpected "dry tap" of a cyst or collection; ultrasound would then be used to both assess if there is sufficient fluid for aspiration, or if the lesion is solid or a diffuse area of soft tissue edema.

Technical Guidelines

With the exception of ultrasound of the skin, the hand and fingers provide the next most superficial body part or organ to be imaged. This by itself demands that high frequency (10 mHz or more) be used to provide adequate resolution. Newer transducers that are commercially available have frequencies up to 17 MHz.

The shape or configuration of the transducer probe is also another matter for consideration. A linear array is a definite requirement, and the two most common forms are the larger (6 to 8 cm width) probes (**Fig. 4.1A**), or the smaller (2 to 3 cm) "hockey-stick" probe (**Fig. 4.1B**). The hockey-stick probe is named as such due to its angled head in relation to the handle of the probe. The larger probes allow greater appreciation at any one point due to the larger field-of-view, which is useful in demonstration of the length of a tendon. The hockey-stick probes are easier to manipulate given their

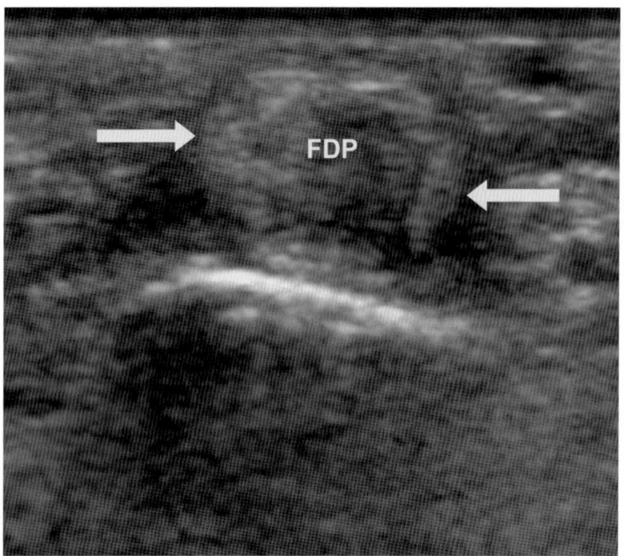

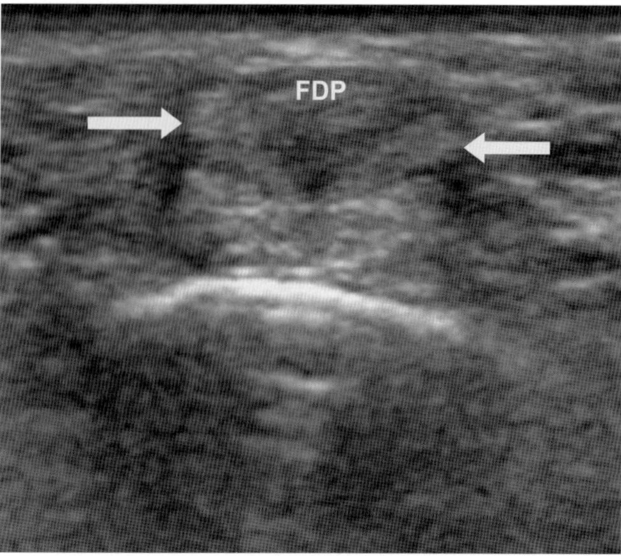

Fig. 4.3 (*Continued*) Within the finger, the FDS tendon divides into two (*white arrows*) and passes around the FDP tendon to end up deep to the FDP before attaching to the middle phalanx **(C,D).**

with each passing around the associated profundus tendon on either side, to wind up deeper than the profundus tendon and attaching on to the base of the middle phalanx. This relationship can be shown on transverse images of the flexor tendons, scanning from proximal to distal (**Fig. 4.3C,D**).

In the longitudinal plane, the flexor tendons show a fibrillar echogenic appearance, with the FDP inserting onto the distal phalanx (**Fig. 4.4**). The flexor tendon sheath around each tendon begins in the palm at the level of the metacarpal neck, and follows the tendon distally. Even with the double layer or synovium, it is extremely thin in the normal state and closely apposed to the flexor tendon.

The flexor tendon of each finger passes through the fibro-osseous tunnel, which is formed by the annular and cruciate pulleys, and the palmar cortical surface of the phalanges and palmar plates. The pulleys are condensations of the tendon sheath, and are attached to the adjacent phalanges (**Fig. 4.5**). There are five annular pulleys designated A1 to A5 and three

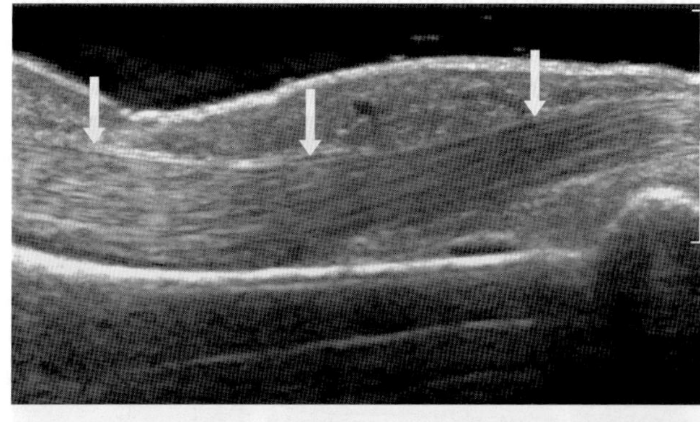

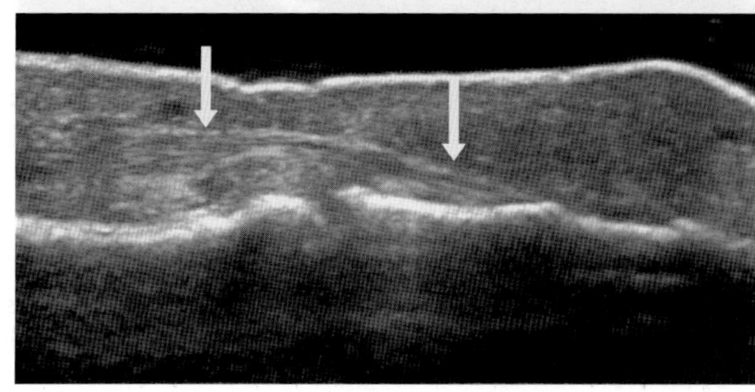

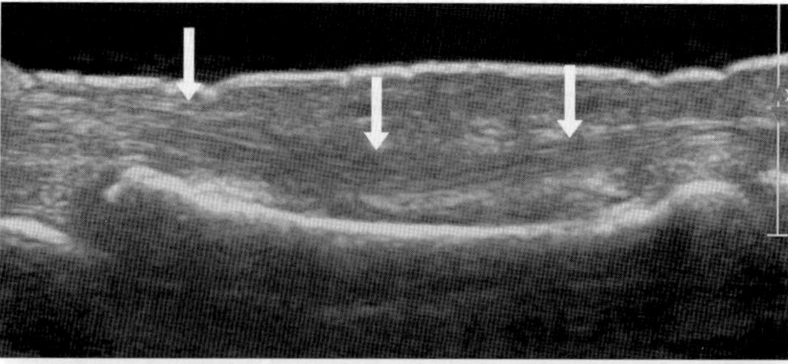

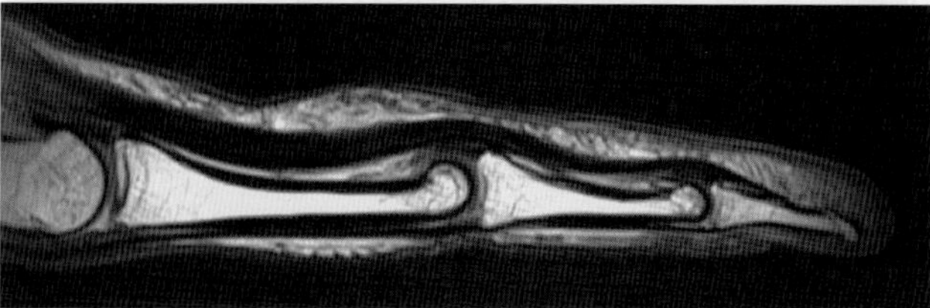

Fig. 4.4 Longitudinal ultrasound **(A–C)** images and corresponding magnetic resonance **(D)** image of the normal flexor tendon in the finger (*white arrows*).

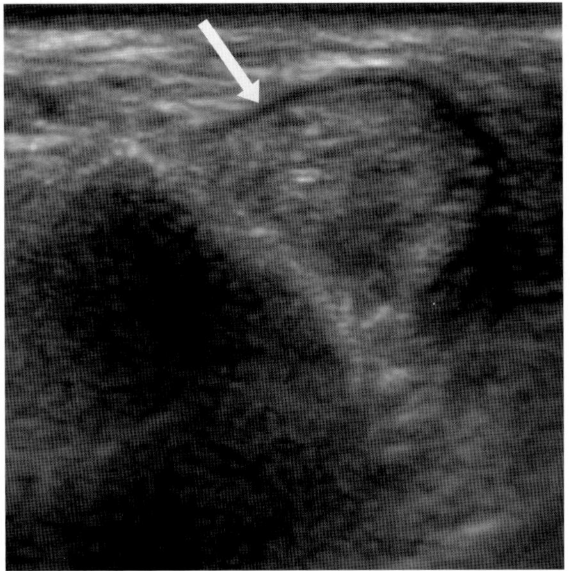

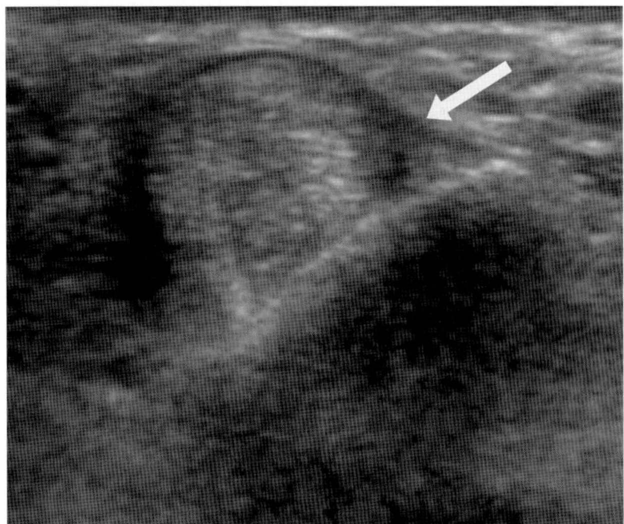

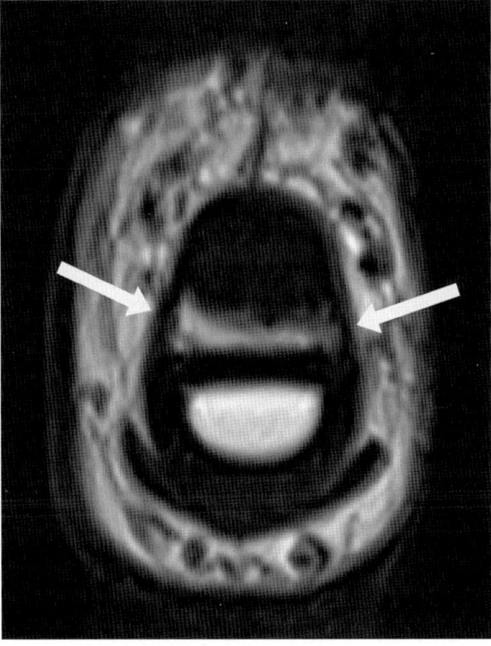

Fig. 4.5 Transverse ultrasound images showing the radial **(A)** and ulnar **(B)** aspects of the A2 pulley of the middle finger, with corresponding magnetic resonance **(C)** image (*white arrows*). Due to the oblique orientation of the pulleys, it is difficult to image both the radial and ulnar arms on the same ultrasound image.

cruciate pulleys designated C1 to C3, from proximal to distal. The pulleys serve to restrain the flexor tendon, holding it against the phalanges, to prevent bow-stringing on flexion of the finger.

The A1, A3, and A5 pulleys are sited at the metacarpophalangeal (MCP), proximal interphalangeal (PIP), and distal interphalangeal (DIP) joints, respectively. The A2 and A4 pulleys are at the level of the midshafts of the proximal and middle phalanges, respectively. The A2 and A4 pulleys are biomechanically the most important, while pathology at the level of the A1 pulley is a common cause of trigger finger.

The course of the flexor tendons are also divided into five zones, which are based on anatomic considerations for tendon injury and repair. The zones are numbered from 1 to 5, from distal to proximal. Zone 1 consists only of the flexor digitorum profundus tendon, at the point distal to the insertion of the flexor digitorum superficialis tendons on the middle phalanx.

Zone 2 extends from the A1 pulley to the level of the middle phalanx, and tendon injury in this region may predispose to formation of adhesions due to the restricted soft tissue space through which the tendons pass. Zone 3 extends from the distal edge of the carpal tunnel to the A1 pulley, and the lumbrical muscles lie in this zone.

Zone 4 includes the carpal tunnel from its proximal to distal boundaries, and zone 5 is from the tendon origins in the distal forearm and wrist until they pass into the carpal tunnel.

The dorsal extensor tendon to each finger is significantly smaller in size than the corresponding flexor tendon (**Fig. 4.6**). Only the central slip inserts on the base of the middle phalanx, while the two lateral bands pass on either side of the central slip and insert onto the base of the distal phalanx. In the index and little fingers, there are also contributions to the extensor tendon by the extensor indicis proprius and extensor digiti minimi tendons as well.

In the thumb, there are corresponding dorsal and volar tendons that perform extension and flexion. The single long tendon arising above the level of the wrist on the volar side is the flexor pollicis longus (FPL) tendon, which passes within the thenar eminence between the two heads of the flexor pollicis brevis muscle, and inserts into the volar aspect of the base of the distal phalanx (**Fig. 4.7**).

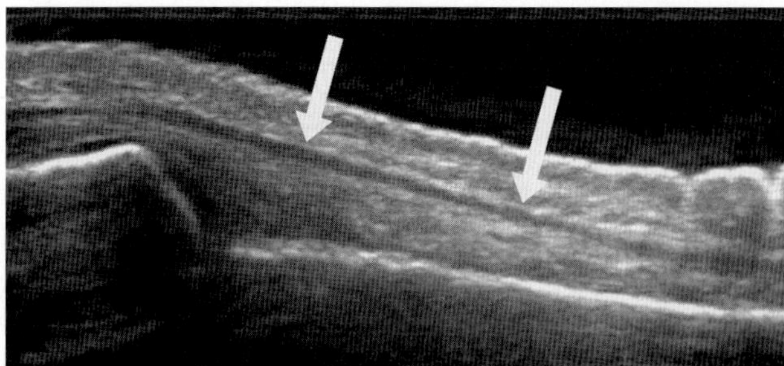

A

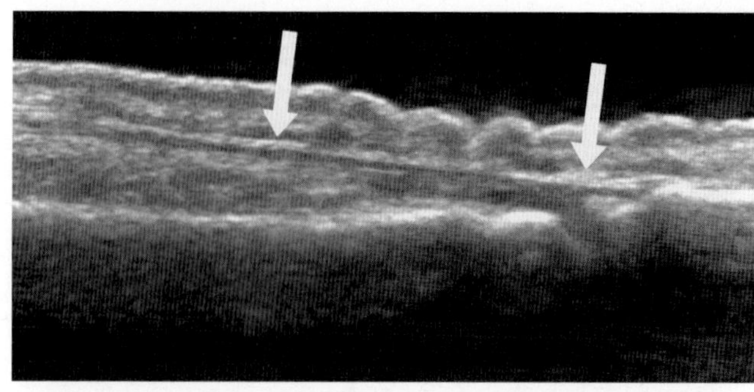

B

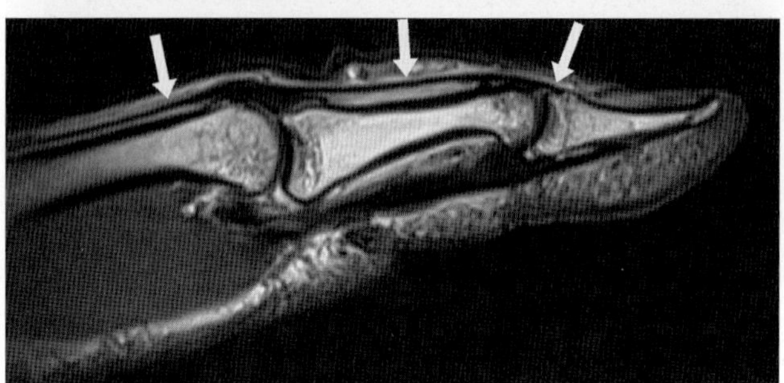

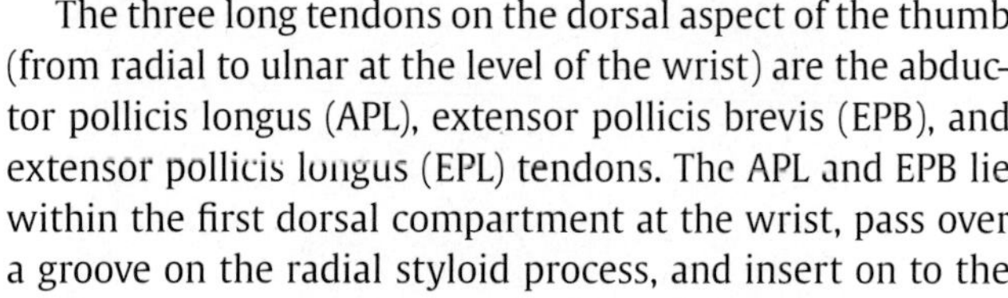

C

Fig. 4.6 Longitudinal ultrasound **(A,B)** images and corresponding magnetic resonance **(C)** image of the normal extensor tendon (*white arrows*) to its distal insertion on the distal phalanx.

The three long tendons on the dorsal aspect of the thumb (from radial to ulnar at the level of the wrist) are the abductor pollicis longus (APL), extensor pollicis brevis (EPB), and extensor pollicis longus (EPL) tendons. The APL and EPB lie within the first dorsal compartment at the wrist, pass over a groove on the radial styloid process, and insert on to the base of the first metacarpal (APL) and base of the proximal phalanx (EPB) (**Fig. 4.8A**). These two tendons form the radial margin of the anatomic snuffbox at the dorsum of the hand.

The extensor pollicis longus tendon lies in the third dorsal compartment of the wrist (**Fig. 4.8B**). As it passes distally, it hooks around the Lister tubercle on the dorsal surface of the distal radius, runs superficial to the extensor carpi radialis longus and extensor carpi radialis brevis tendons in the second dorsal compartment. It provides the ulnar margin for the anatomic snuffbox, and inserts onto the base of the distal phalanx of the thumb.

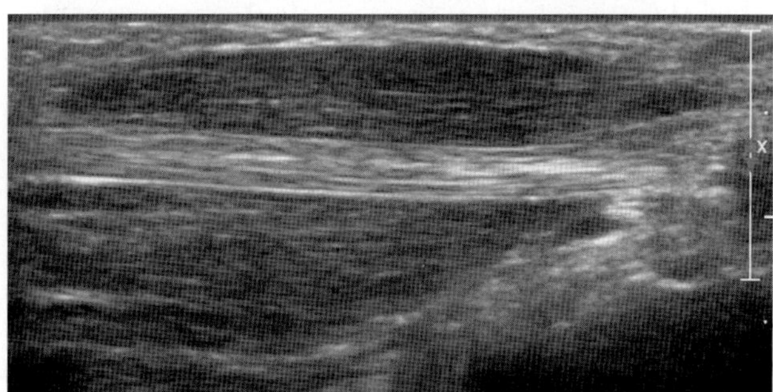

A

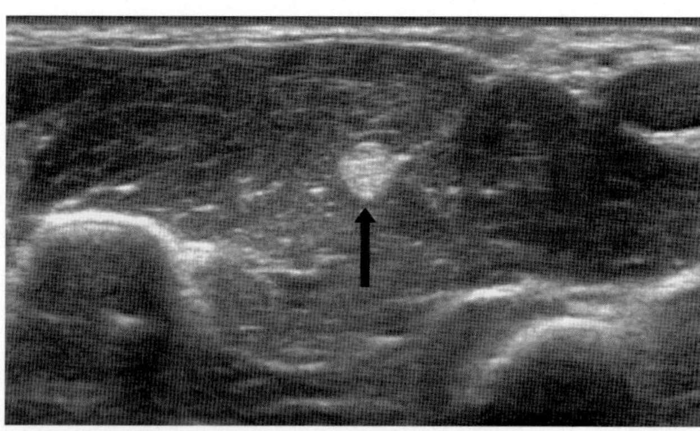

B

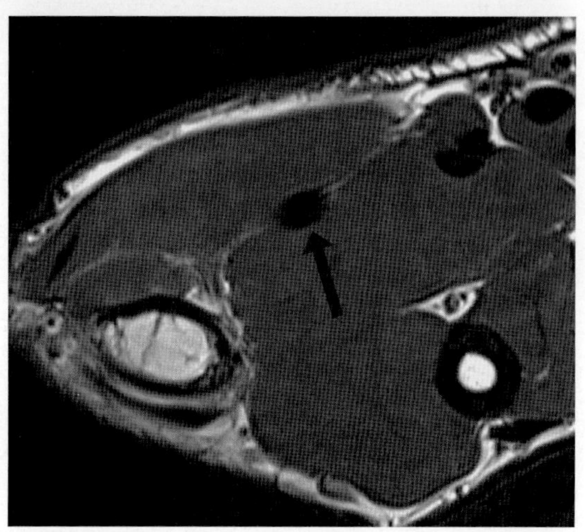

C

Fig. 4.7 Longitudinal **(A)** and transverse **(B)** ultrasound images and magnetic resonance **(C)** image of the flexor pollicis tendon (*black arrow*) in the thenar eminence.

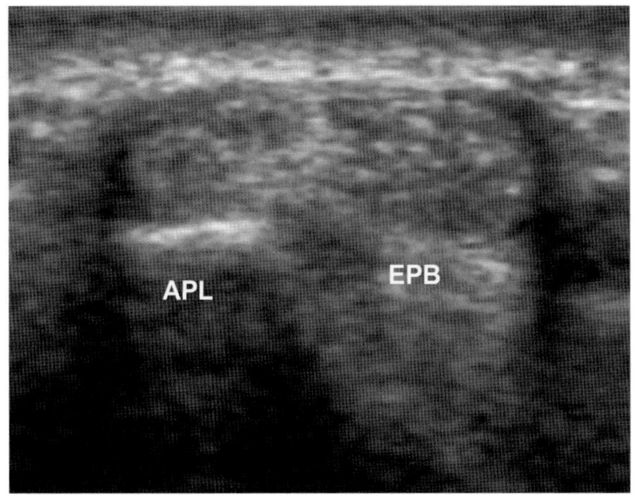

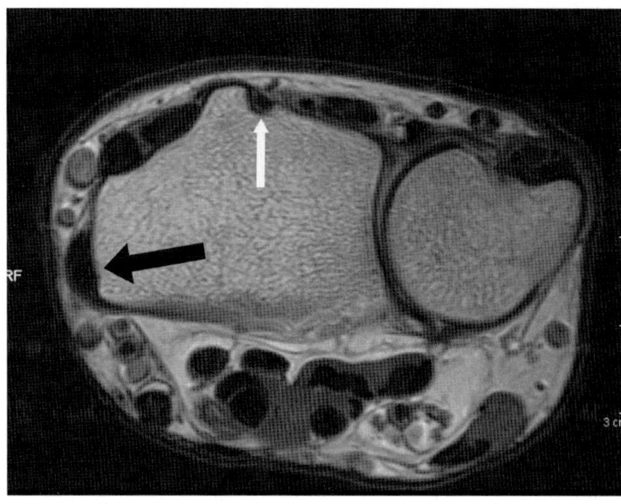

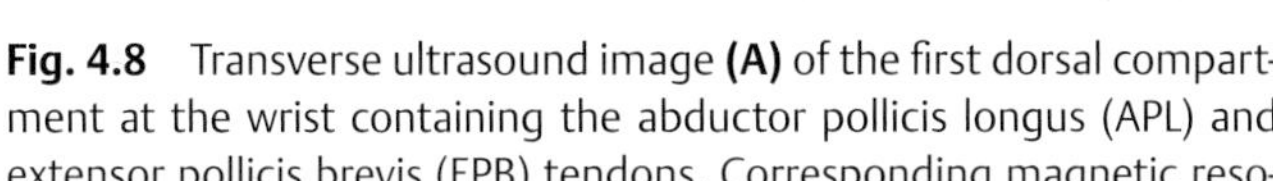

Fig. 4.8 Transverse ultrasound image **(A)** of the first dorsal compartment at the wrist containing the abductor pollicis longus (APL) and extensor pollicis brevis (EPB) tendons. Corresponding magnetic resonance image **(B)** shows these two tendons in the first dorsal compartment (*thick black arrow*) as well as the extensor pollicis longus (EPL) in the third dorsal compartment (*thin white arrow*).

Muscles of the Hand

The small muscles within the hand can be grouped into the thenar muscles acting on the thumb, hypothenar muscles on the little finger, and the lumbricals and interossei muscles within the palm.

Thenar and Hypothenar Muscles

These consist of the abductor pollicis brevis (APB), flexor pollicis brevis (FPB), opponens pollicis (OP) and adductor pollicis (**Fig. 4.9A,C**). The abductor pollicis brevis and flexor pollicis brevis muscles lie superficial on the palmar

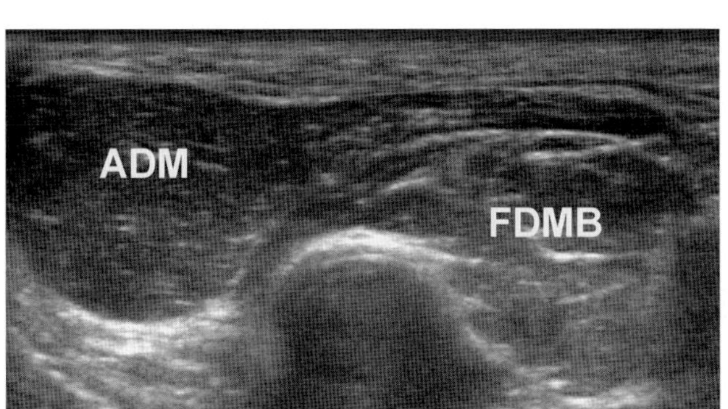

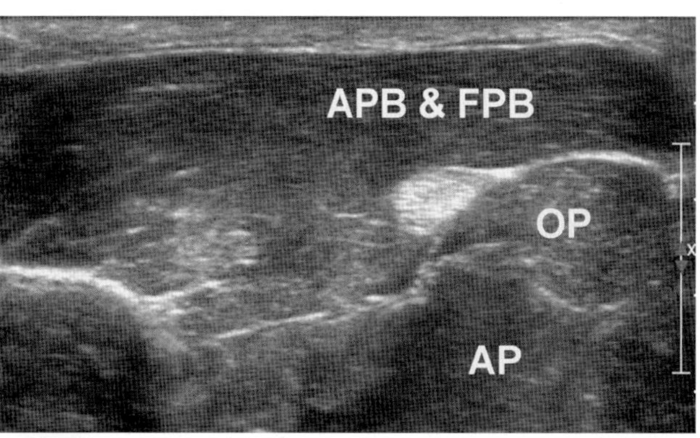

Fig. 4.9 Transverse ultrasound images of the hypothenar **(A)** and thenar **(B)** eminences, and corresponding magnetic resonance image **(C)** showing the relationship of the musculature. APB, abductor pollicis brevis; AP, adductor pollicis; FPB, flexor pollicis brevis; OP, opponens pollicis; ADM, abductor digiti minimi; FDMB, flexor digiti minimi brevis.

aspect, at the level of the first metacarpal bone. The opponens pollicis lies deeper on the radial aspect; the adductor pollicis is on the ulnar aspect. They all insert onto the proximal phalanx, while only the opponens pollicis inserts on the 1st metacarpal. They are all supplied by the median nerve, with the exception of the adductor pollicis, which is supplied by the ulnar nerve.

The opponens pollicis probably has the most important function, which is to oppose the thumb with the other fingers, and also to rotate medially. The ability to oppose provides a myriad of functions of the hand, with the "pinch-grip" allowing us to pick up small objects.

The hypothenar muscles include the abductor digiti minimi (ADM), flexor digiti minimi brevis (FDMB), and the opponens digiti minimi (ODM) (**Fig. 4.9B,C**). The ADM and FDMB muscle bellies contribute the bulk of the hypothenar eminence, with the ODM lying deep. These are all supplied from the ulnar nerve.

Lumbrical and Interossei Muscles

The intrinsic muscles of the hand include the lumbrical and interossei muscles. There are four lumbrical muscles in the palm, and they are unique in the body in that they have no direct bony attachment. They originate from the radial aspects of the flexor digitorum profundus tendons for the first and second lumbricals, and from both the radial and ulnar aspects for the third and fourth lumbricals. They then insert distally onto the lateral bands of the extensor expansion of the fingers, distal to the MCP joints. They are separated from the interossei muscles by the deep transverse intermetacarpal ligament. They function to flex the PIP joints and extend the MCP joints (**Fig. 4.10A,C**).

The four dorsal interossei muscles are bipennate, with each muscle originating from both of the adjacent metacarpals. Their insertions onto the proximal phalanges are different in each finger, attaching only to the radial aspect of the index finger, both radial and ulnar aspects of the middle finger, and only on the ulnar aspects of the ring and little fingers. This asymmetrical attachment allows abduction and spreading of the other fingers away from the middle finger (**Fig. 4.10B,C**).

There are only three palmar interossei, which are all unipennate. They arise from the second, fourth, and fifth metacarpals, and insert onto their respective proximal phalanges, on the ulnar side for the index finger and radial side for the ring and little fingers. Their actions result in adduction, bringing the other fingers toward the middle finger.

Vessels

The structures of the hand are supplied by the radial and ulnar arteries, which anastomose in the palm, forming the superficial and deep palmar arteries.

The superficial palmar arch is formed by the terminal branch of the ulnar artery and a superficial branch of the radial artery. It gives off three branches that run in between

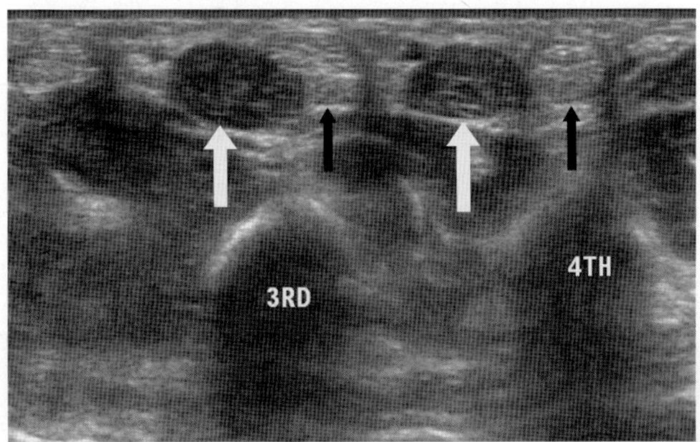

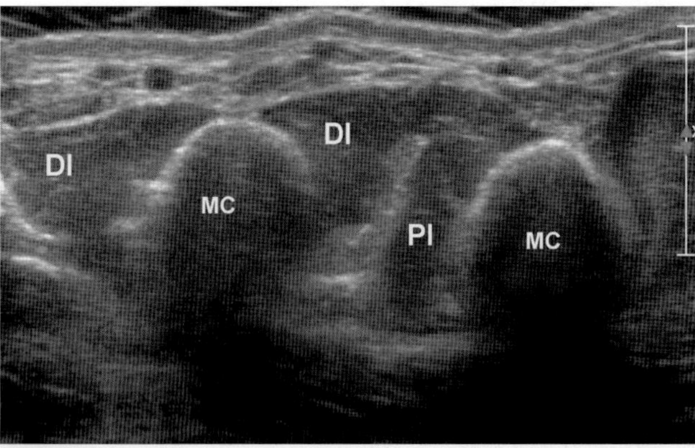

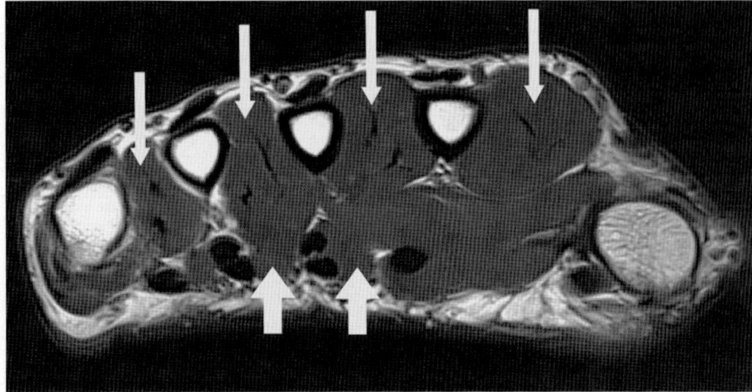

Fig. 4.10 Transverse ultrasound images of the palm from the palmar aspect **(A)** show the lumbrical muscles (*thick white arrows*) in between the flexor tendons (*thin black arrows*). Transverse ultrasound images of the dorsum of the hand **(B)** show the dorsal interossei (DI) and palmar interossei (PI) in between the metacarpals (MC). Corresponding magnetic resonance image **(C)** of the palm shows the lumbricals (*short white arrows*) and interossei (*long white arrows*).

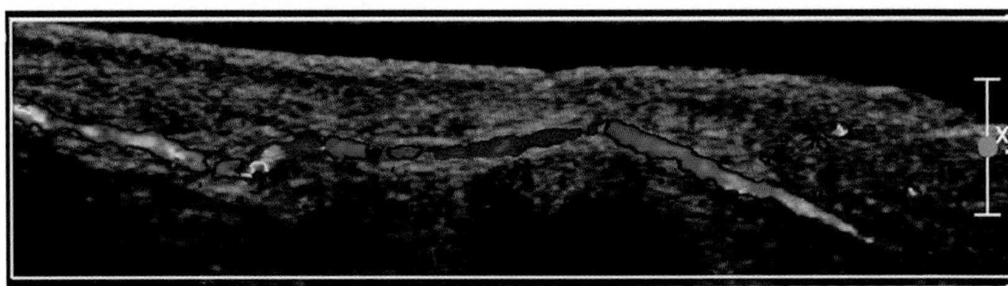

Fig. 4.11 Longitudinal ultrasound color Doppler image of the normal radialis indicis artery on the radial side of the index finger.

the second to fifth metacarpals and bifurcate at the web spaces to form the digital arteries to each finger on the radial and ulnar sides. There is also a single branch, which runs on the ulnar side of the little finger.

The deep palmar arch arises from the terminal branch of the radial artery and a deep branch of the ulnar artery. The arch lies slightly more proximal to the superficial arch, at the level of the carpometacarpal joints. The arch gives off branches that contribute to the digital arteries of the fingers, together with the arteries from the superficial palmar arch.

In addition, the radial artery also winds dorsal to the base of the first metacarpal as it enters the palm from the wrist. At this location within the first web space, it gives off the princeps pollicis artery, which continues distally as the digital artery to the thumb. The princeps pollicis artery terminates as the radialis indicis artery, which runs on the radial side of the index finger as the digital artery (**Fig. 4.11**).

Joints

Carpometacarpal Joints

Thumb

This joint is formed by the concave distal surface of the trapezium and the opposing base of the first metacarpal. The exact bony configuration may vary, but it is primarily a saddle-shaped joint. This allows the joint to have a very wide range of movement, which is particularly useful in opposition of the thumb to the other fingers. As such, the stability of the joint depends mainly on the joint capsule and collateral ligaments.

The ulnar collateral ligament is the strongest ligament in the joint, and extends from the tubercle of the trapezium to the palmar aspect of the base of the first metacarpal. It prevents hyperextension and radial subluxation (**Fig. 4.12**).

The radial collateral ligament lies on the dorsoradial side of the joint, and lies just proximal to the abductor pollicis longus tendon insertion on the first metacarpal.

Both collateral ligaments blend with the joint capsule, which encases the joint space. The capsule is relatively lax to allow for the wide range of movement. There are other smaller supporting ligaments at the first carpometacarpal joint, but these are usually not discernable with ultrasound.

Fingers

The carpometacarpal joints of the fingers form a continuous synovial space extending from the trapezoid-second metacarpal articulation to the hamate-fifth metacarpal articulation. There are short carpometacarpal and intermetacarpal ligaments present.

Metacarpophalangeal Joints

The metacarpophalangeal joints are condyloid in configuration, with a convex or flat head at the metacarpal, and a shallow concave surface at the base of the proximal phalanges.

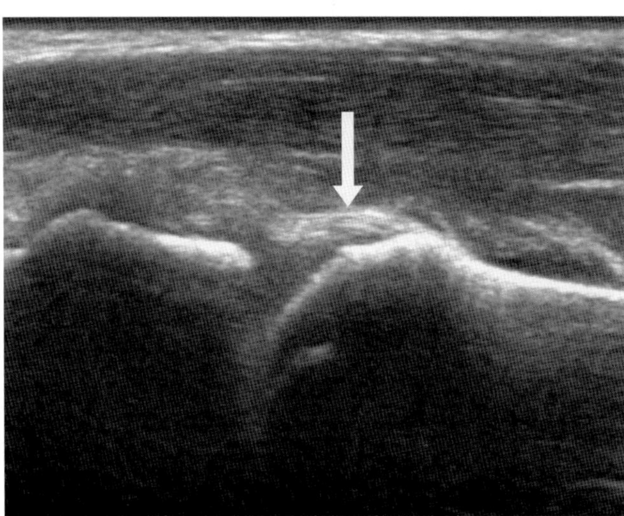

A

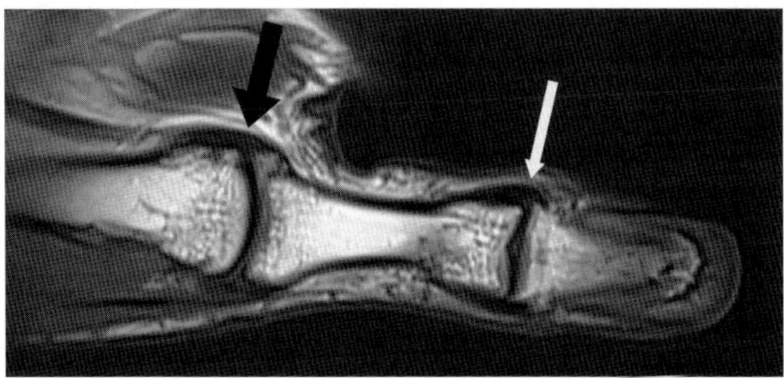

B

Fig. 4.12 Longitudinal ultrasound image of the ulnar collateral ligament at the first carpometacarpal joint (*white arrow*) **(A)**. Corresponding magnetic resonance image **(B)** of the thumb showing the ulnar collateral ligaments of the first carpometacarpal joint (*thick black arrow*) and interphalangeal joint (*thin white arrow*).

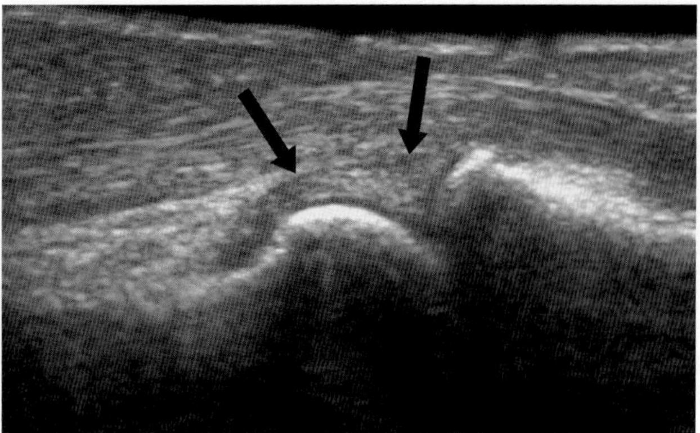

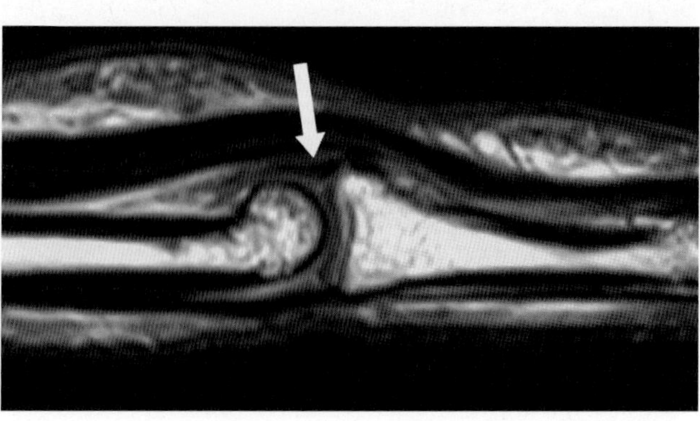

Fig. 4.13 Longitudinal ultrasound image of the volar plate at the metacarpophalangeal joint demonstrating its normal triangular configuration (*black arrows*) **(A)**. Corresponding magnetic resonance image shows similar appearance of the volar plate as well (*white arrow*) **(B)**.

Although the main axis of movement is flexion—extension, abduction—adduction with limited rotation is also possible.

The radial and ulnar collateral ligaments have a broad and thick configuration, with the ulnar ligament being stronger than the radial. They originate from the lateral and medial condyles of the metacarpal heads, run distally and in a slightly volar direction to insert onto the palmar surface of the proximal phalanx and adjacent distal portion of the volar plate. Due to this slight obliquity in their course, they are taut in flexion of the MCP joint and slightly lax in full extension.

The fibrocartilaginous volar plate is triangular in the sagittal cross-section, with the thickest central portion measuring up to 3 to 4 mm in size (**Fig. 4.13**). It has proximal attachments to the palmar surface of the metacarpal neck via the thick radial and ulnar checkrein ligaments, with thinner central band between the checkrein ligaments. The strong distal insertion is onto the cartilage-bone interface at the palmar aspect of the base of the proximal phalanx. Its main function is to provide stability and prevent hyperextension at the joint, and it also merges with the palmar aspect of the joint capsule. There is also a slight groove on the palmar/superficial surface for the adjacent flexor tendon. At the MCP joint of the thumb, there are two sesamoid bones, one each on the radial and ulnar sides of the volar plate. These function as attachments for the thenar muscles.

The joint capsule is lax dorsally with the joint in extension, and there may also be a large proximal bursa. Any significant joint effusion or synovial hypertrophy may be most easily visible on the dorsal aspect. The articular cartilage layer over the head of the metacarpals can be visualized (**Fig. 4.14**).

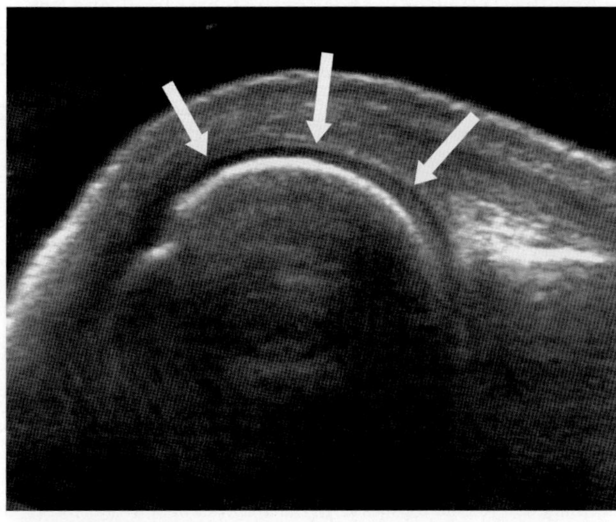

Fig. 4.14 Longitudinal ultrasound image of the metacarpal head with the metacarpophalangeal joint in flexion, showing the hypoechoic layer of normal articular cartilage (*white arrows*).

Interphalangeal Joints (Proximal and Distal)

The interphalangeal joints have a similar appearance and configuration as the metacarpophalangeal joints on ultrasound, with stability provided by the radial and ulnar collateral ligaments, volar plate, and joint capsule in a similar manner. Overall, the interphalangeal joints are smaller in size.

■ Pathologies

Degenerative

Within the hand, the majority of the joint movement occurs in flexion and extension, with a limited degree of abduction and adduction at the metacarpophalangeal joints. The main exception to this is at the carpometacarpal joint of the thumb. Because of its position and plane of movement set off from the rest of the fingers, as well as the wide range of mo-

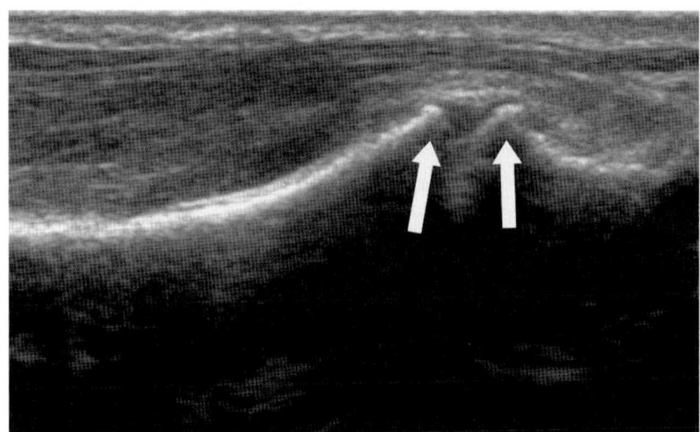
A

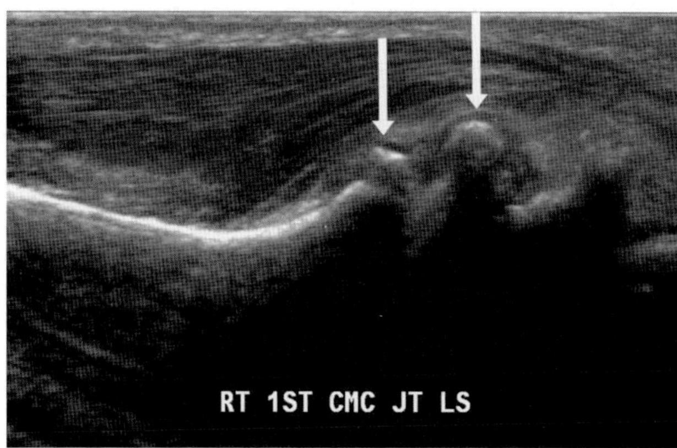

B

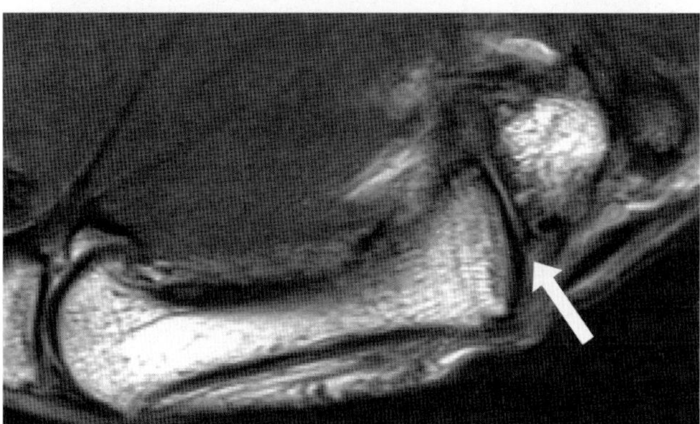
C

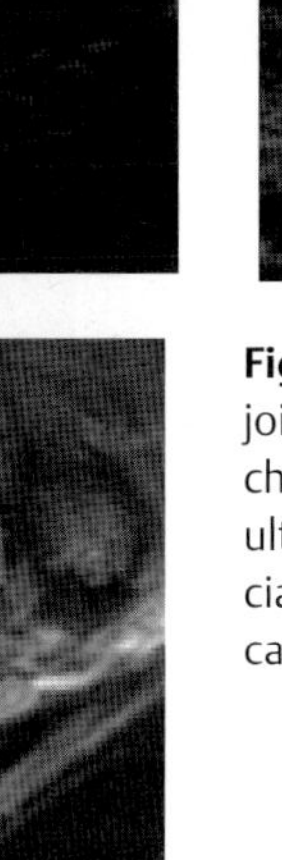

Fig. 4.15 Degenerative osteoarthritis of the first carpometacarpal joint. Early changes with small osteophytes (*white arrows*) **(A)** and later changes with prominent osteophytes (*white arrows*) **(B)** are shown on ultrasound. Corresponding magnetic resonance image shows associated narrowing of the joint space and eburnation of the articular cartilage (*white arrow*) **(C)**.

tion at the joint, the thumb is able to perform the action of opposition to the rest of the fingers, allowing for a pinch grip and also the development of fine motor skills. This range of movement arises from the saddle-shaped configuration of the joint. However, it also means that there is more stress applied to the first carpometacarpal joint as compared with the rest of the carpometacarpal joints in daily use and function, with resulting degeneration at an earlier age.

Subtle findings may be difficult to visualize, and it is only when there is joint space narrowing, osteophyte formation, and possible subluxation that osteoarthritis of the joint can be confirmed (**Fig. 4.15**).

Ganglion cyst formation occurs commonly around the hand and wrist, but the actual connection with the joint space may not always be demonstrable on ultrasound. In the hand, ganglion cysts may be associated with the tendon sheath as well. The ganglion should be anechoic with none or minimal septation, and lack of vascularity (**Fig. 4.16**).

There can also be palpable lesions at the joint margin simulating osteophyte formation. The thumb almost invariably has two sesamoid bones at the first metacarpophalangeal joint, which lie in the flexor tendons. The presence of sesamoid bones at the other metacarpophalangeal joints is not as common, but may present as a palpable lump (**Fig. 4.17**).

Fig. 4.16 Flexor tendon ganglion cyst (between calipers) lying superficial to the associated tendon. No fluid is seen in the tendon sheath.

Inflammatory/Infective

The imaging of rheumatoid arthritis with ultrasound has grown rapidly due to technical advances in small-parts scanning, and its subsequent increase in use of ultrasound by rheumatologists. Many rheumatology clinics have their own ultrasound equipment, and ultrasound imaging of inflammatory joint disease has become an extension of the clinical examination.

Rheumatoid arthritis is probably by far the most common rheumatologic disease studied. One of the more commonly encountered clinical scenarios is a swollen joint in the rheumatoid patient. Ultrasound allows a quick and accurate differentiation between the causes of the joint swelling, which include joint effusion, synovial hypertrophy, and capsular thickening (**Fig. 4.18**).

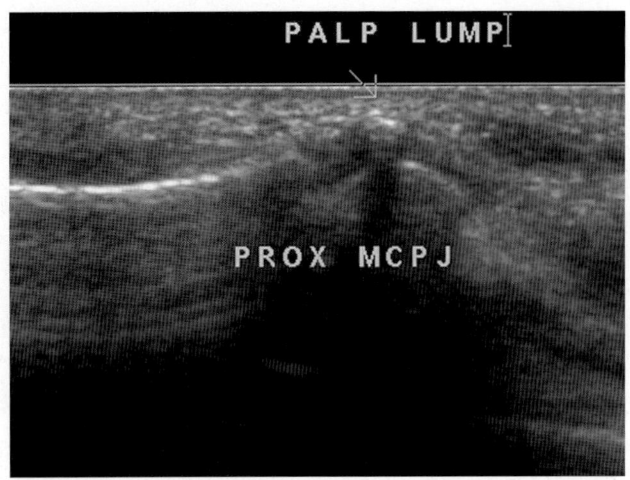

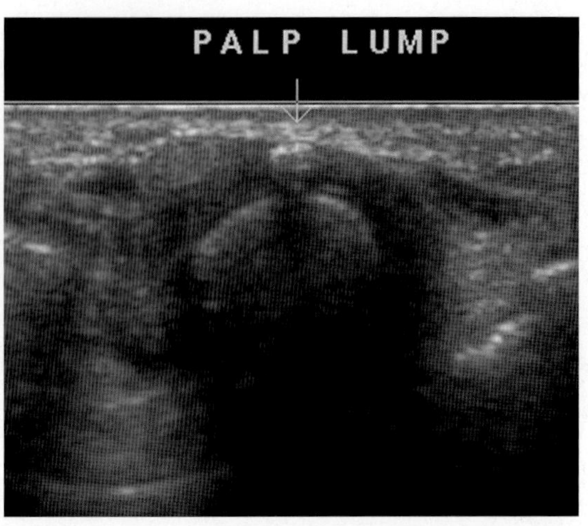

Fig. 4.17 Small sesamoid bone seen over the volar aspect of the fifth metacarpal presenting as a palpable lump. Longitudinal **(A)** and transverse **(B)** sections show no associated soft tissue lesion or capsule thickening.

At a later stage of the disease, bony erosions are a common feature, which occur due to erosion by pannus. Although the erosions can be visible on radiographs, they are harder to detect in the carpal bones as compared with the metacarpophalangeal and interphalangeal joints. Both ultrasound and magnetic resonance imaging (MRI) have the advantage of allowing cross-sectional imaging in multiple planes, which helps to increase clinical confidence in the diagnosis of carpal bone erosions (**Fig. 4.19**).

Tendon sheath thickening and tenosynovitis is also part of the rheumatoid disease picture. Assessment on ultrasound is made easier by being able to compare with other normal tendon sheaths in the same hand or the contralateral hand. Color Doppler or power Doppler ultrasound imaging also demonstrates increased vascularity within the thickened tendon sheath, as opposed to tendon sheath fluid, which does not reflect increased vascularity (**Fig. 4.20**).

Other causes of inflammatory joint disease can be imaged in a similar fashion. However, the features of these are not specific and differentiation of the underlying pathophysiology is usually not possible based on the ultrasound study alone (**Fig. 4.21**). Inflammatory tenosynovitis can also arise from overuse, in a form similar to De Quervain tenosynovitis, but not being limited to the tendons at the radial side of the wrist (**Fig. 4.22**).

Crystal deposition disease can also manifest in the hand, with a similar appearance of joint erosion and synovial hypertrophy. However, in gout, the uric acid crystals may manifest with the tendon substance itself, putting the tendon at risk for rupture (**Fig. 4.23**).

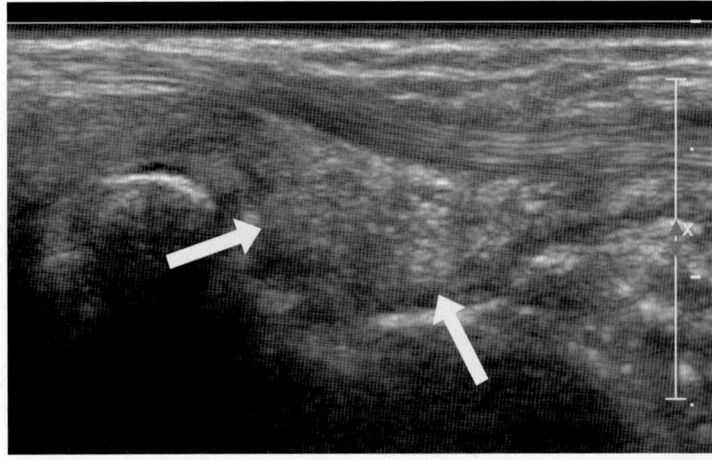

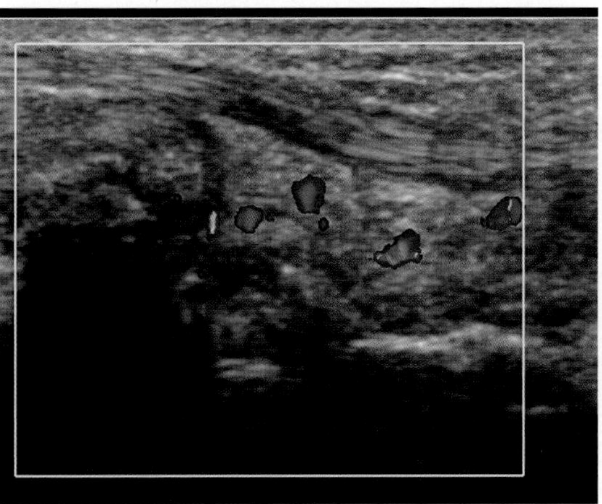

Fig. 4.18 Rheumatoid arthritis showing synovial hypertrophy over the dorsum of the hand (*white arrows*) with displacement of the overlying extensor tendons **(A)**. Color Doppler ultrasound imaging shows increased vascularity with the area of synovial hypertrophy **(B)**.

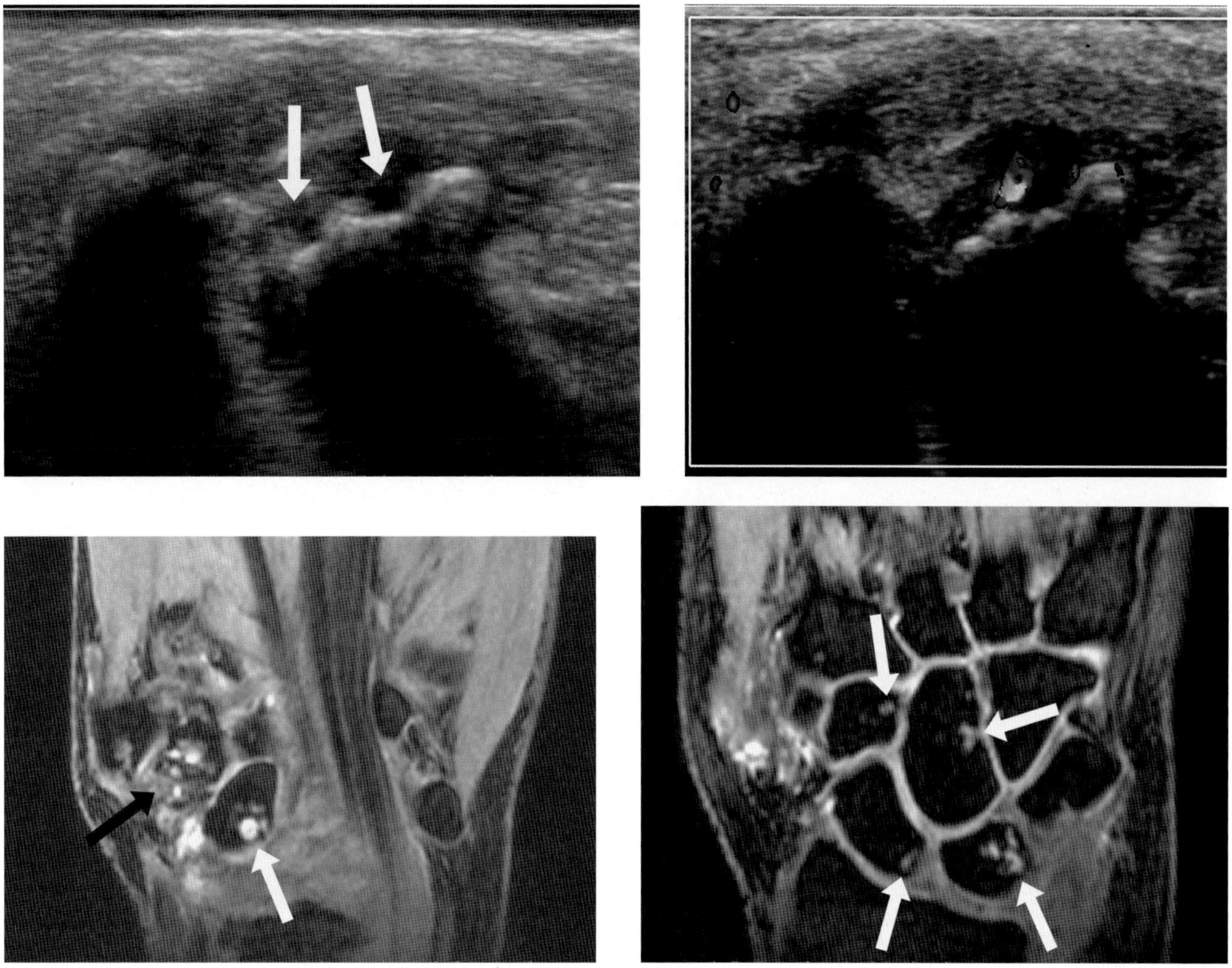

Fig. 4.19 Extensive rheumatoid arthritis affecting the carpal bones of the wrist, with bony erosions seen at the trapezium (*white arrows*) **(A)**, and vascular flow seen within the overlying pannus **(B)**. Corresponding magnetic resonance images **(C,D)** show deformity and loss of configuration of the trapezium (*black arrow*), with smaller erosions in the scaphoid, lunate, trapezoid, and capitate bones (*white arrows*).

Infection in the hand is usually clinically obvious, given the superficial location and relative lack of soft tissue space to expand. The range of infective change can be imaged, from cellulitis to fluid in the fascial plane to overt abscess formation. Ultrasound can also be used in follow-up to assess for resolution, as well as for complications such as sinus formation (**Fig. 4.24**). Paronychia at the fingers may also be related to chronic irritation or eczema, or sometimes there

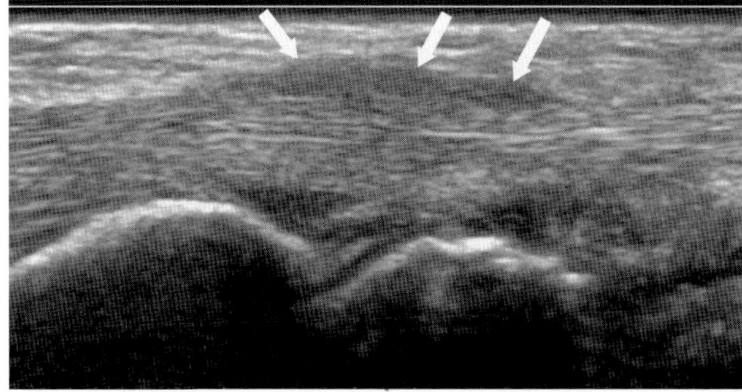

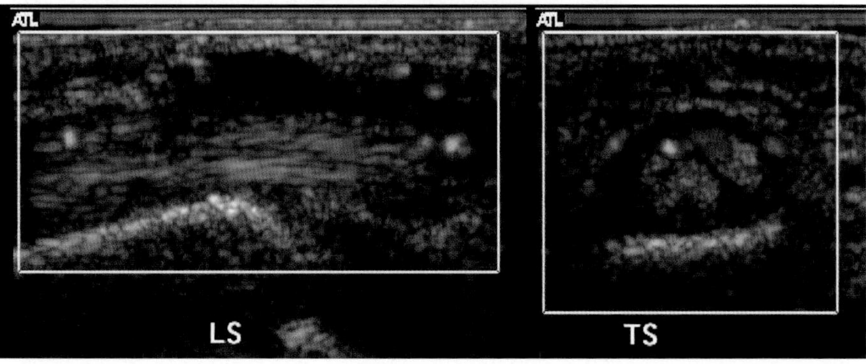

Fig. 4.20 Inflammatory tenosynovitis due to rheumatoid arthritis with a mild degree of tendon sheath thickening (*white arrows*) **(A)** and increased vascular flow on power Doppler imaging **(B)**.

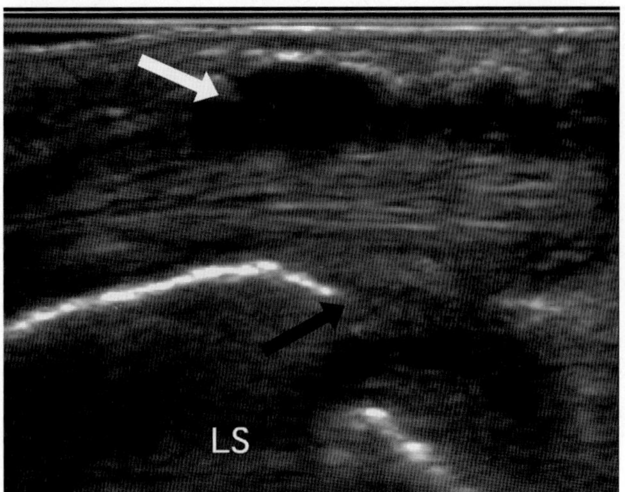

Fig. 4.21 Psoriatic arthropathy in the hand showing fluid in the tendon sheath due to tenosynovitis (*white arrow*) and synovial thickening (*black arrow*). (Courtesy of Dr. Kok-Ooi Kong.)

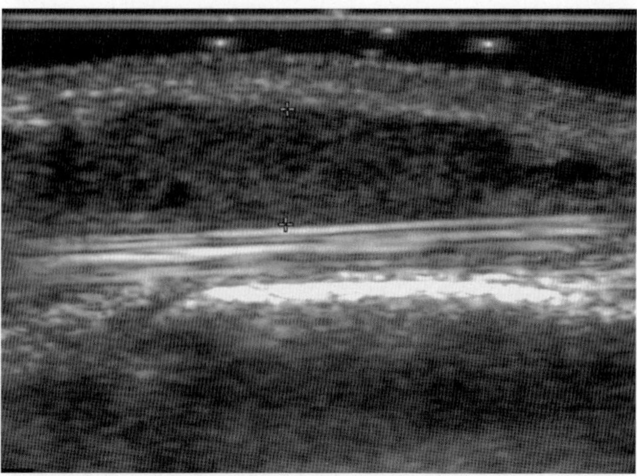

A

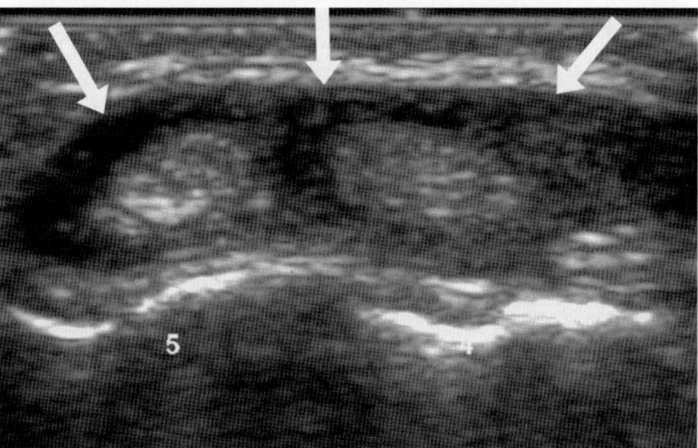

B

Fig. 4.22 Extensor tendon tenosynovitis with thickening over the dorsum of the hand in the longitudinal **(A)** and transverse (*white arrows*) **(B)**, possibly related to repetitive stress injury.

can be an underlying cause such as an ingrown fingernail (**Fig. 4.25**).

Traumatic

Traumatic injuries to the hand which require ultrasound imaging usually involve the tendons or ligaments. Bony injuries such as fractures or dislocations would utilize radiographs as a first line of imaging.

Rupture of the extensor or flexor tendons may be due to direct local injury from a laceration or indirectly from sudden muscle contraction (usually against resistance). The

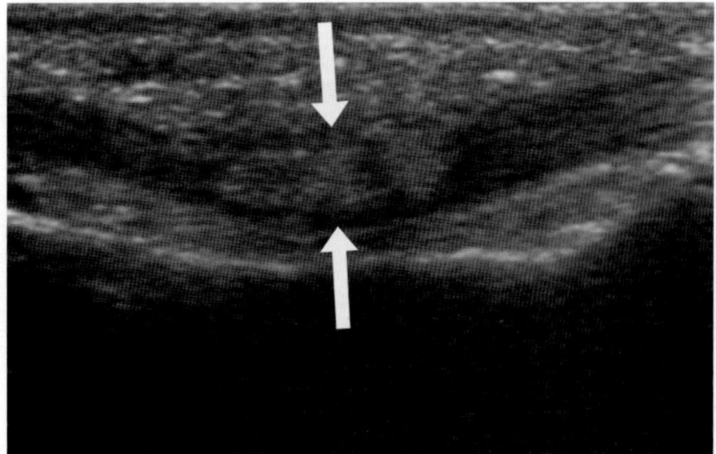

A

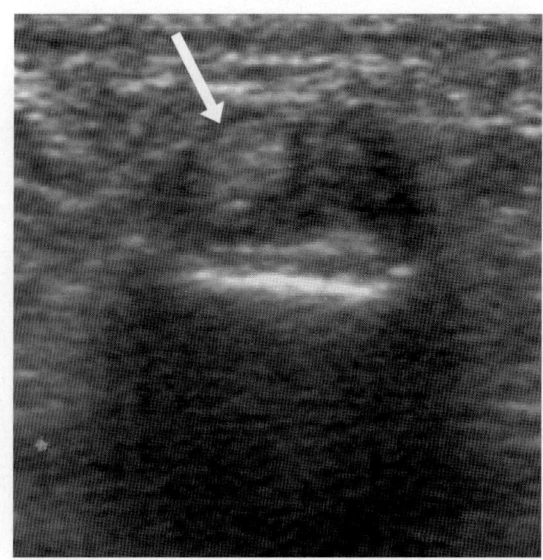

B

Fig. 4.23 Uric acid crystal deposition (*white arrows*) eccentrically within the substance of the flexor tendon on longitudinal **(A)** and transverse **(B)** ultrasound images, in a patient with known gout.

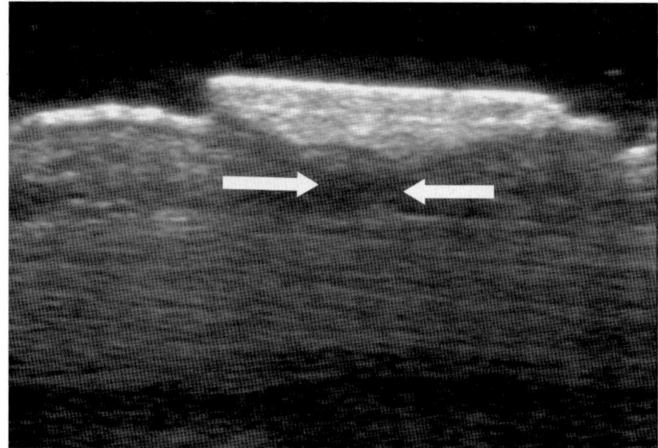

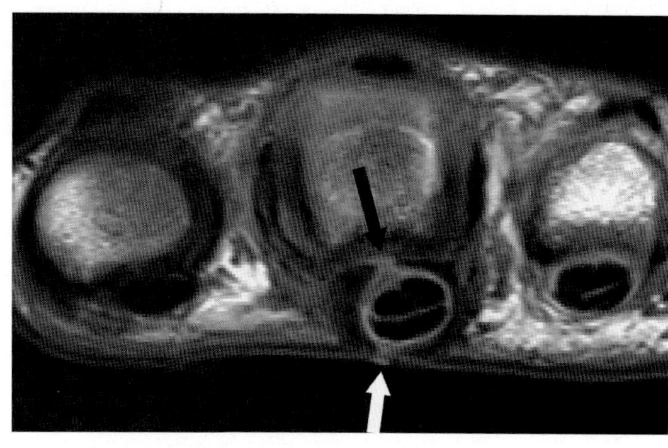

Fig. 4.24 Persistent discharge from a sinus opening for 4 months after cat bite. Ultrasound **(A)** shows the sinus opening (*between white arrows*) under a waterproof dressing. Magnetic resonance imaging **(B)** shows both the skin sinus opening (*white arrow*) as well as a deep track (*black arrow*) leading to the third metacarpal head, which had changes of osteomyelitis (not shown).

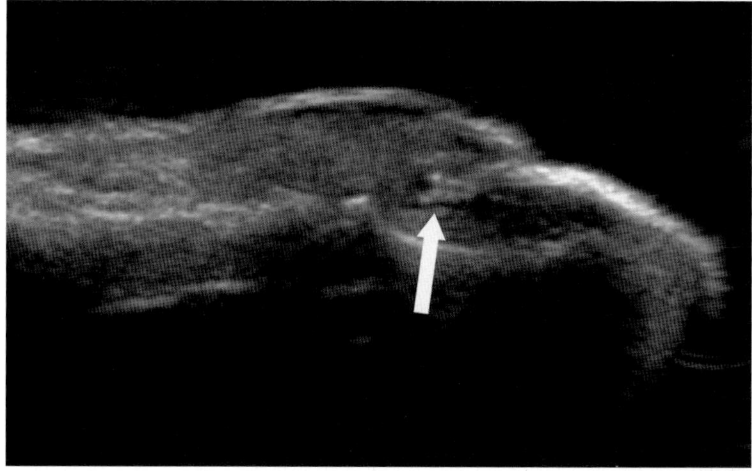

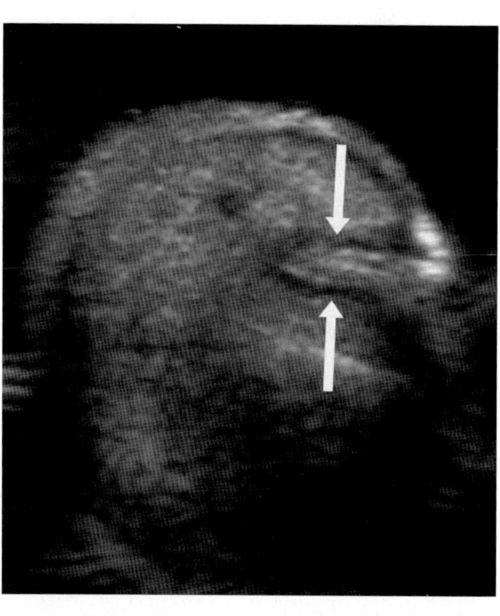

Fig. 4.25 Paronychia of the finger with redness and swelling. Ultrasound in the longitudinal **(A)** and transverse **(B)** planes show the portion of the ingrown fingernail (*white arrows*) as the underlying cause.

clinical diagnosis of a complete tendon rupture is usually not difficult, given the history and clinical findings. Where ultrasound plays an important role is to identify and localize the site of the retracted tendon ends, which have an influence on surgical management (**Fig. 4.26**). This aids the surgeon in planning the site of incision and amount of exposure.

Re-tear of a repaired tendon can also be imaged with ultrasound, although it is comparatively harder to evaluate given the presence of postsurgical change and scarring. However, a complete re-tear can usually be identified with some degree of certainty.

Injury to the collateral ligaments at the metacarpophalangeal and interphalangeal joints are also common (**Fig. 4.27**). Most of these are managed conservatively and usually by themselves may not require ultrasound imaging. The ulnar collateral ligament of the thumb is occasionally put at risk due to a valgus force applied at the metacarpophalan-

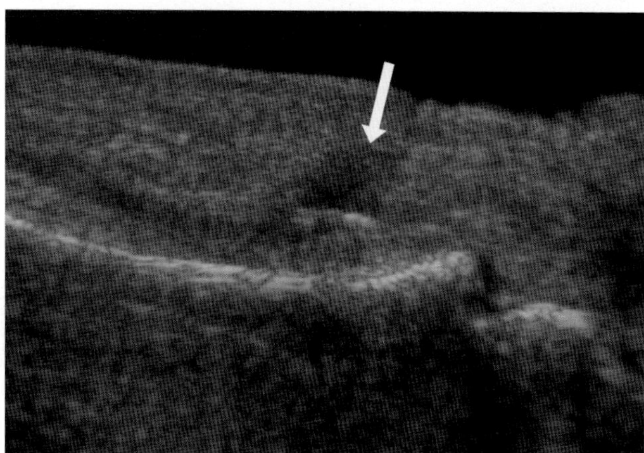

Fig. 4.26 Rupture of the flexor digitorum profundus tendon to the ring finger at the level of the proximal interphalangeal (PIP) joint, with fluid seen in the gap (*white arrow*).

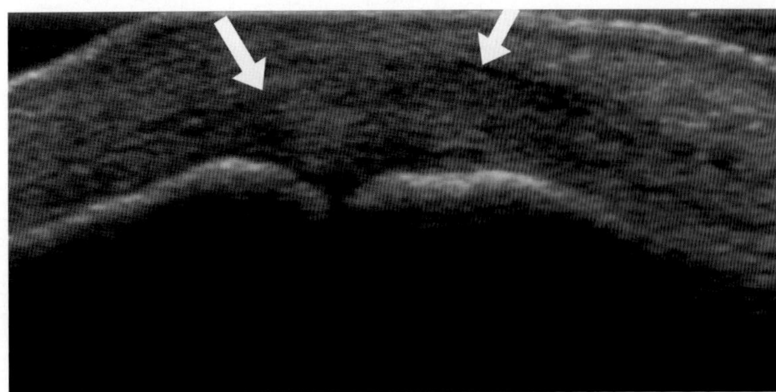

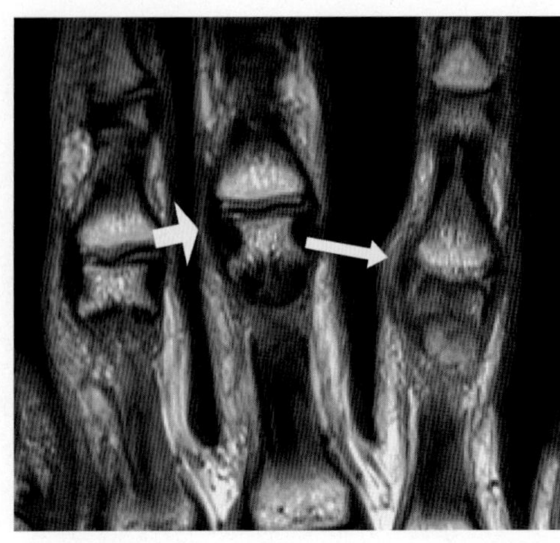

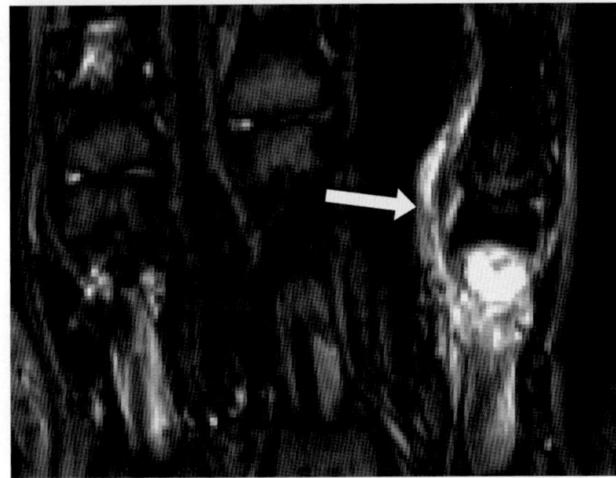

Fig. 4.27 Strain injury without tear to the radial collateral ligament of the proximal interphalangeal (PIP) joint of the index finger. Ultrasound **(A)** shows diffuse thickening (*white arrows*). Corresponding proton-density **(B)** and inversion recovery **(C)** magnetic resonance images show diffuse soft tissue edema and tendon thickening without avulsion (*long white arrows*). The normal radial collateral ligament in the middle finger is shown for comparison (*short white arrow*).

geal joint of the thumb (gamekeeper's thumb as originally described, or skier's thumb in the modern day).

In addition, a complete tear of the ulnar collateral ligament of the thumb may be complicated by interposition of the adductor aponeurosis between the avulsed distal end of the ligament and the base of the proximal phalanx. This is known as a Stener's lesion, and the interposition will prevent healing of the ligament if surgical correction is not done. Ultrasound can be used to identify a Stener's lesion.

Ultrasound is also widely used for confirmation and localization of radiolucent foreign bodies in the hand. Penetrating injuries to the soft tissues of the hand and fingers

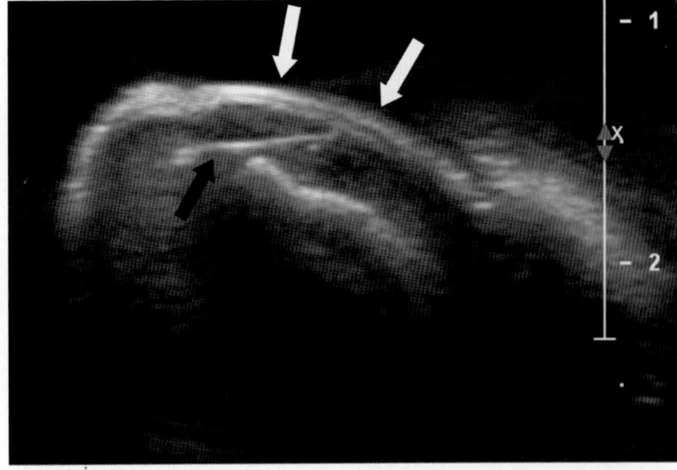

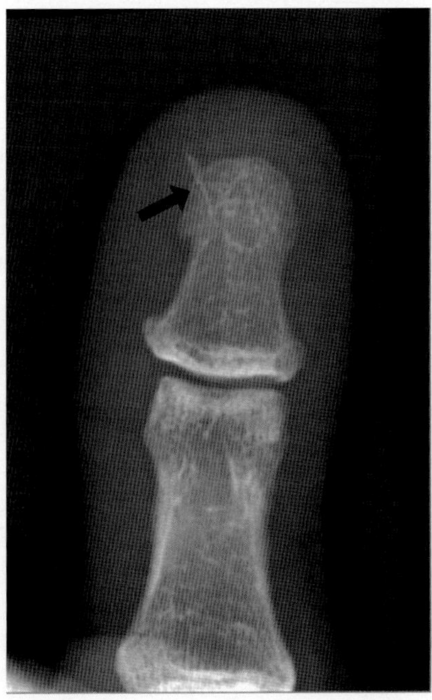

Fig. 4.28 Penetrating injury from fish fin with retained foreign body. The initial foreign body was removed from the skin but there was persistent pain for 1 week. Ultrasound **(A)** showed the foreign body to lie in the soft tissues (*black arrow*) beneath the nail plate (*white arrows*), making it nonpalpable. Correlation was made with a subsequent radiograph **(B)**, confirming the location of the foreign body (*black arrow*).

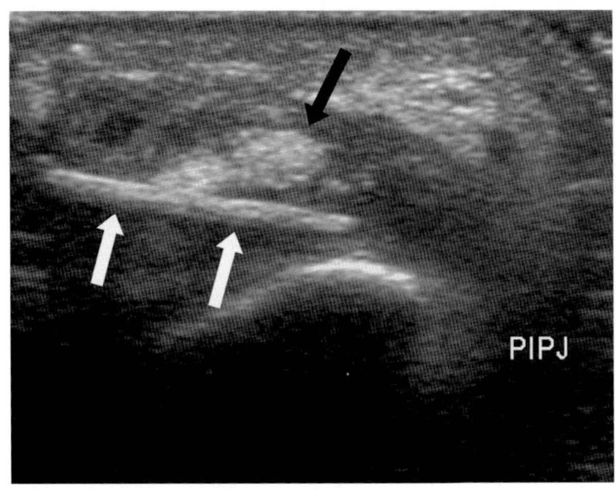

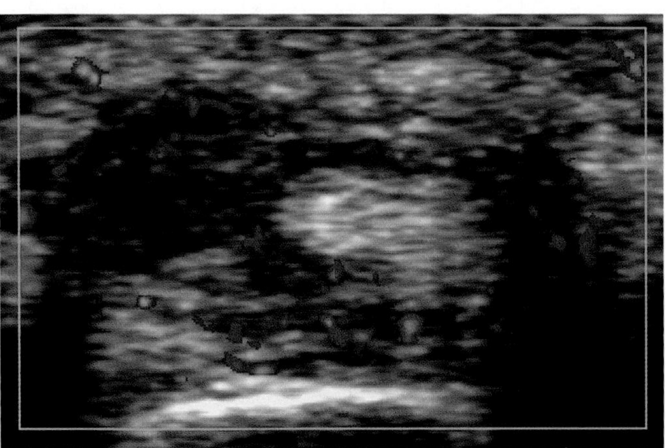

A B

Fig. 4.29 Penetrating injury from wooden foreign body (*white arrows*) lying just beneath flexor tendon (*black arrow*) on ultrasound **(A)**. Moderate amount of granulation tissue with increased vascularity also demonstrated on color Doppler imaging **(B)**.

are common, as the hand is used in many activities such as catching and grasping; some particular occupations such as gardeners or fishmongers are also at risk. Common foreign bodies include thorns, fish bones, glass fragments, wooden splinters, etc.

The position of the retained foreign body may not lie directly under the site of the skin puncture wound, and any external portion of the foreign body may have been broken off or removed incompletely (**Fig. 4.28**). Ultrasound is able to directly visualize the foreign body, and to provide information to the number, size/length, configuration and orientation of the foreign body (**Fig. 4.29**). This will give the surgeon a "road-map" to plan the appropriate surgery.

Ultrasound can also demonstrate the granulation tissue formed in response to the foreign body, if it has been some time since the injury. On occasion, the granulation tissue may be easier to see than the foreign body itself (**Fig. 4.30**).

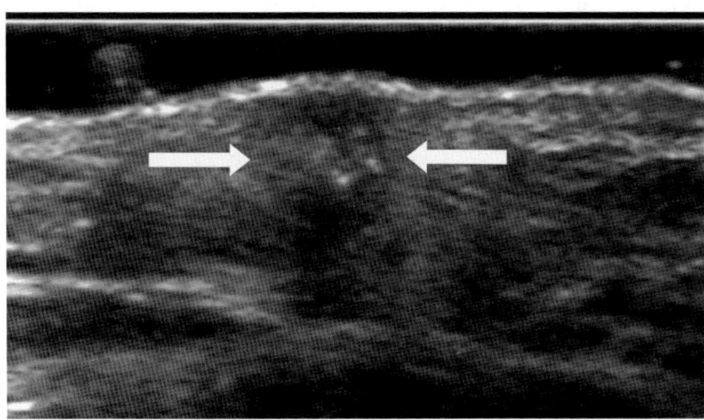

Fig. 4.30 Prior penetrating injury with glass fragments in wound. The hypoechoic granuloma (*between white arrows*) is easily seen, while the actual foreign body glass material is seen only as small echogenic foci within the granuloma.

The germinal matrix at the nail bed, which produces the nail plate, is also prone to injury, and hypertrophy of either the matrix tissue or granulation tissue can produce swelling or a skin lesion. The external appearance is usually obvious, and ultrasound can assist in delineating the extent and depth of the lesion, in planning for excision (**Fig. 4.31**).

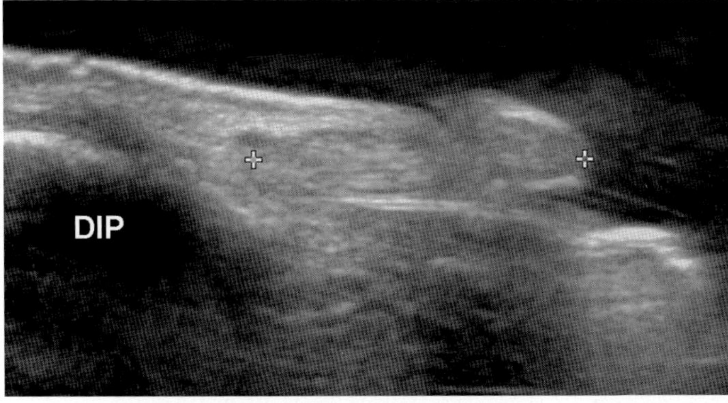

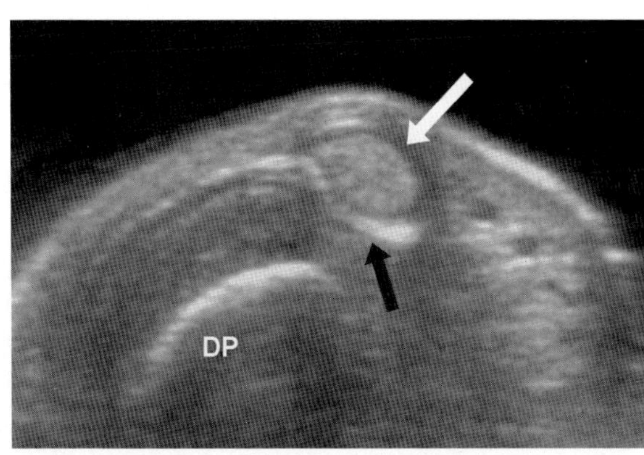

A B

Fig. 4.31 Prominent polyp or granulation tissue emerging from the nail fold, with history of prior trauma. Longitudinal image **(A)** shows the lesion between the calipers, not extending to the level of the distal interphalangeal joint (DIP). The transverse image **(B)** shows the lesion (*white arrow*) indenting on the nail plate (*black arrow*) at the level of the distal phalanx (DP).

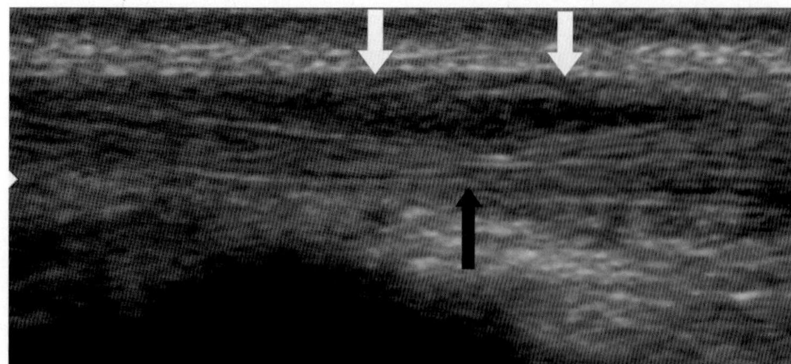

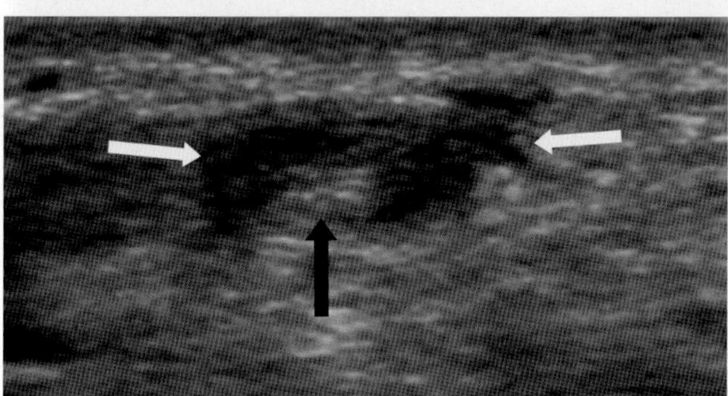

Fig. 4.32 Prior episode of dorsal hand surgery performed. Longitudinal **(A)** and transverse **(B)** ultrasound images show eccentric thickening of the tendon sheath (*white arrows*), encasing the underlying intact tendon (*black arrow*).

Posttraumatic or postsurgical scarring can also cause encasement or involvement of the tendons or tendon sheaths. Patients may present with restriction of movement or triggering (**Fig. 4.32**).

Tumoral

Glomus tumors are a benign vascular tumor with a predilection for the fingers. They are thought to arise from the arterial portion of the glomus body, which in the dermis affects temperature regulation. The glomus tumors in the fingers are found in the subungual region or distal pulp of the finger. These may originate from perivascular cells that develop to form the glomus tumor. Their exact etiology is unknown. Patients usually present with exquisite localized pain.

On ultrasound, the glomus tumor is variable in size, and when large, may have pressure effects on the adjacent tissues, nail plate, and distal phalanx (**Fig. 4.33**). More commonly, they are small (1 to 3 mm) in size, and demonstration

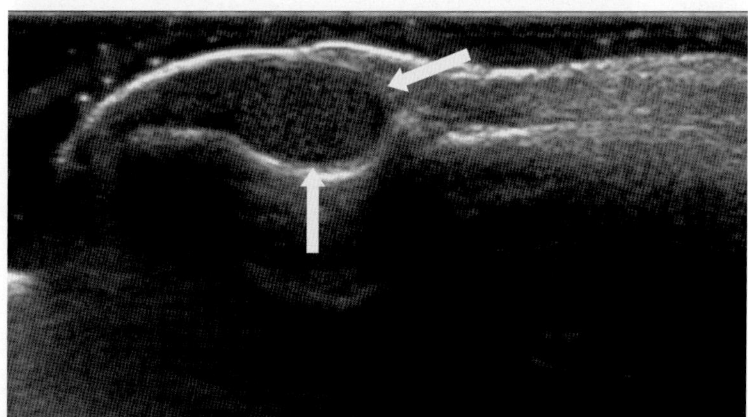

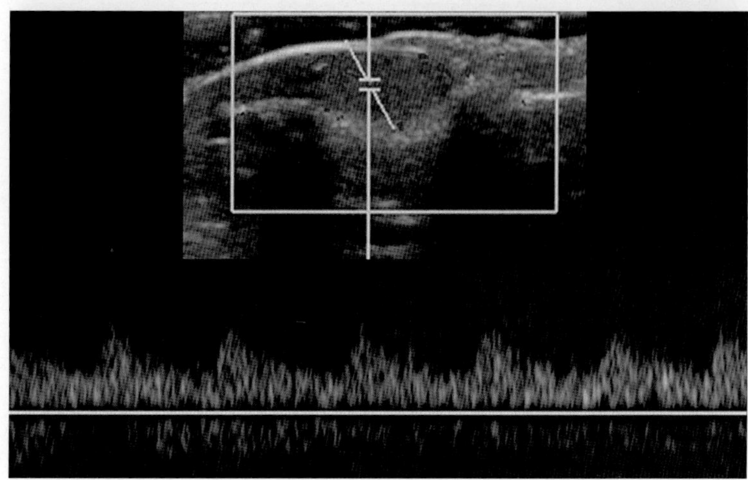

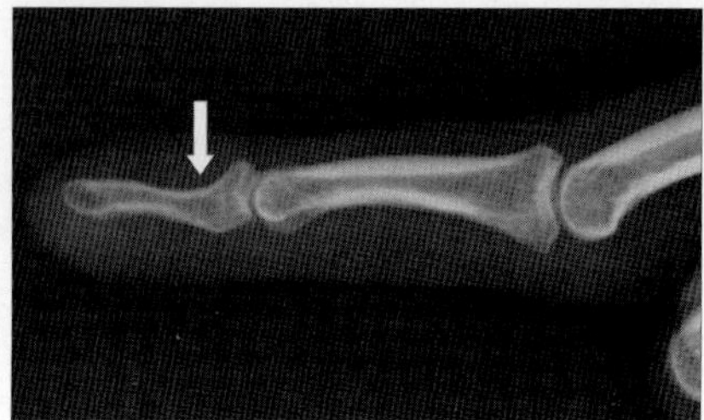

Fig. 4.33 Large glomus tumor demonstrated under the nail plate on the dorsal aspect of the distal phalanx, seen as an ovoid homogeneous echogenic lesion (*white arrows*) **(A)**. It demonstrates vascular flow with an arterial waveform **(B)** and causes a smooth deformity without erosion on the adjacent bony cortex (*white arrow*) **(C)**.

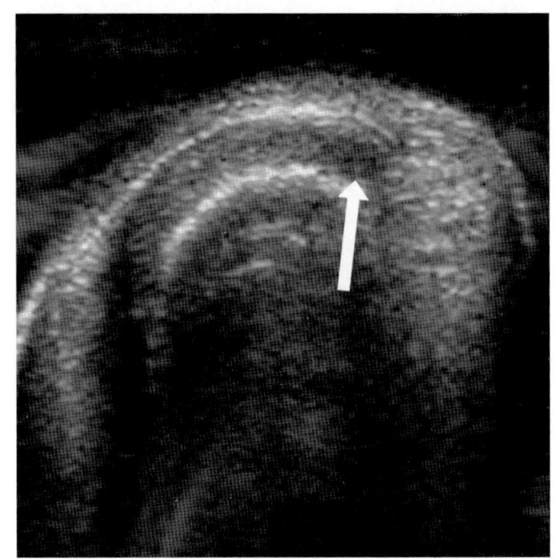
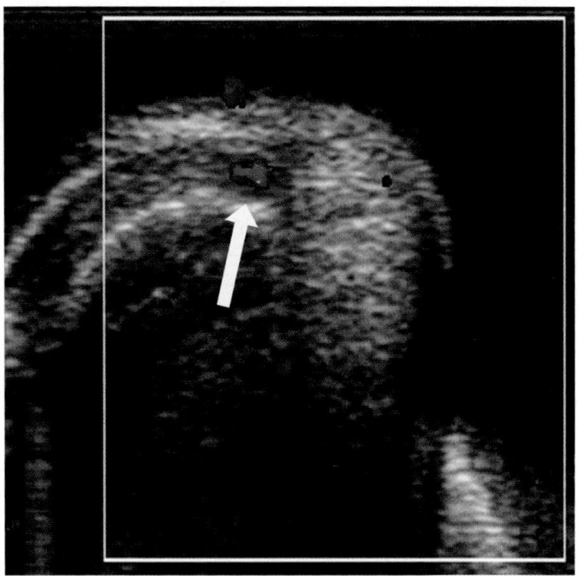

Fig. 4.34 Small glomus tumor (*white arrow*) in the thumb seen as a hypoechoic nodule **(A)** with increased color flow under the nail plate toward the radial side **(B)** on transverse ultrasound.

of these tumors require highly sensitive Doppler color/power imaging. They can be seen as an area of increased vascularity corresponding to the focus of pain (**Fig. 4.34**).

Giant cell tumor of the tendon sheath (GCTTS) is the second most common tumor found in the hand, only less frequently than the ganglion cyst. They are usually slow-growing and are more common on the volar side than the dorsal side. They may be related to pigmented villonodular synovitis (PVNS), and this may be an extra-articular variant of PVNS.

They are seen on ultrasound as solid, lobulated masses with variable vascularity (**Fig. 4.35**). On dynamic movement of the finger, they do not move together with their associated tendons.

Benign peripheral nerve sheath tumors are the most often encountered neurogenic tumor in the hand. Neurilemomas or schwannomas arise from the Schwann cells in the myelin sheath, and are usually well encapsulated and slightly lobulated (**Fig. 4.36**). The normal nerve may be seen within, without separation of the nerve fascicles.

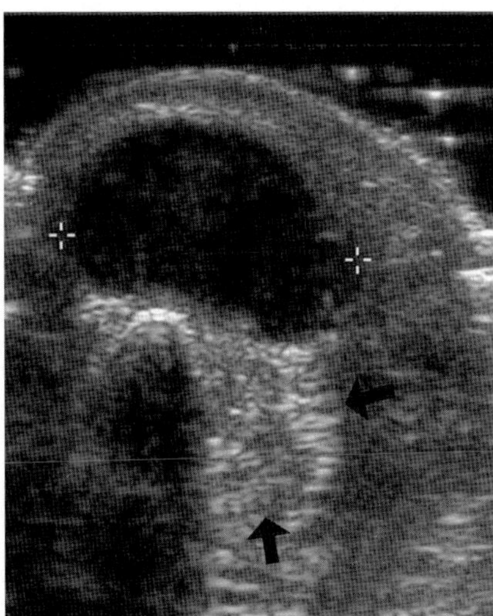
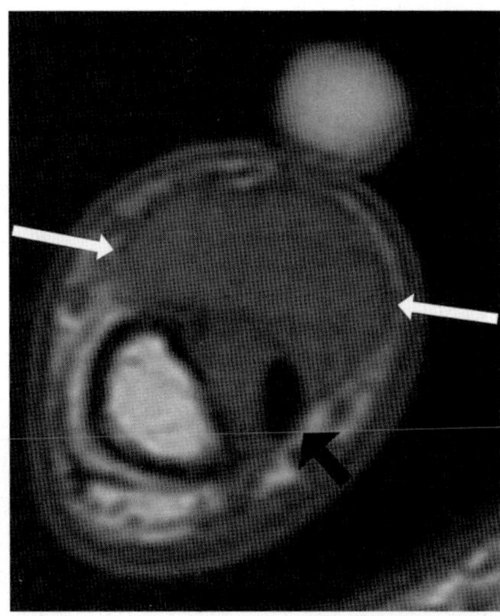
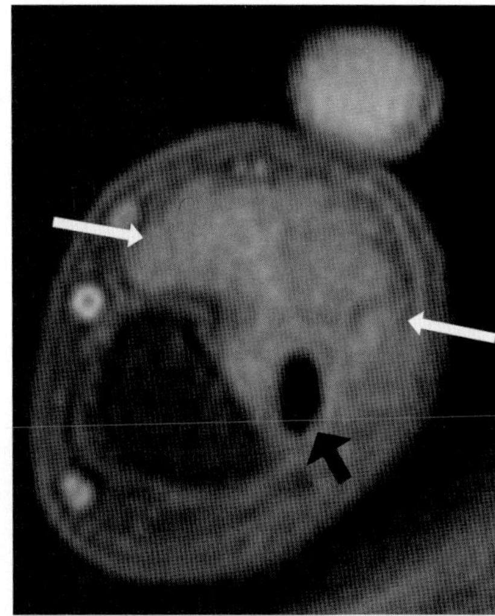

Fig. 4.35 Prominent giant cell tumor of the tendon sheath (GCTTS) seen on ultrasound **(A)** as a hypoechoic nodule (*between calipers*), adjacent to and inseparable from the flexor tendon (*short black arrow*). Axial magnetic resonance (MR) images at the same level with T1-weighted imaging **(B)** and T1-postcontrast **(C)** confirm the presence of a lobulated enhancing soft tissue mass (*white arrows*), displacing the flexor tendon of the thumb (*short black arrows*). Overlying MR skin marker present.

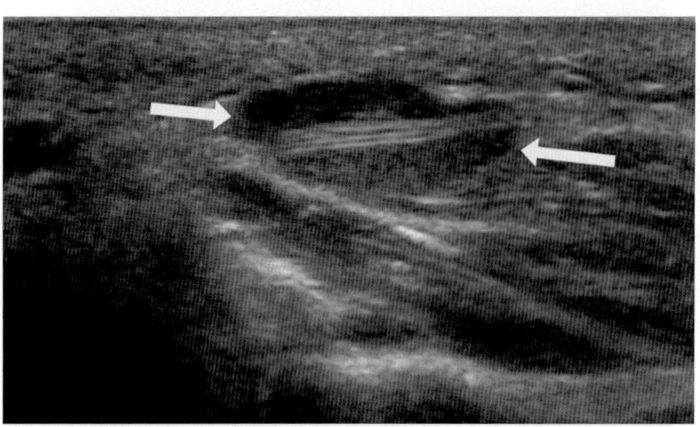

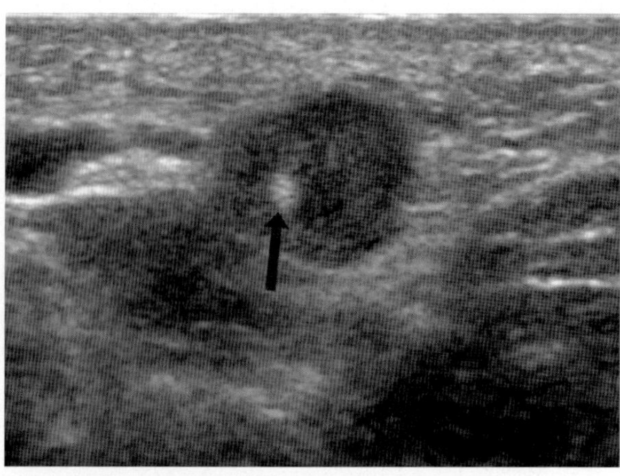

Fig. 4.36 Ulnar nerve sheath tumor arising in the region of the hypothenar eminence shows a well-defined lobulated mass (*white arrows*), with an eccentric echogenic nerve with fascicular pattern within (*black arrow*) on longitudinal **(A)** and transverse **(B)** views.

Fibrolipomatous hamartoma is a benign proliferation of perineural and endoneural fibrosis, resulting in thickening of the neural fascicles, interspersed with fatty tissue. The majority occurs in the median nerve, and present with painless swelling, usually without neurogenic symptoms. On ultrasound imaging, the nerve is diffusely enlarged due to both fascicular enlargement and increased fat deposition within the nerve (**Fig. 4.37**).

Fibromas are benign condensations of fibrous tissue within the palmar fascia, which may be related to Dupuytren contracture. They have a relatively echogenic appearance on ultrasound due to their high cellularity, and are well defined with no invasive component (**Fig. 4.38**).

Miscellaneous

There are a large number of normal variants in the hand, often asymptomatic and these do not present for imaging. Ultrasound is well-suited for the first-line examination of any lumps and bumps in the hand, or for a rapid functional assessment of the muscles and tendons.

There can be atypical courses of the tendons on both the dorsal and palmar aspects, as well as anomalous muscle development or insertion (**Fig. 4.39**).

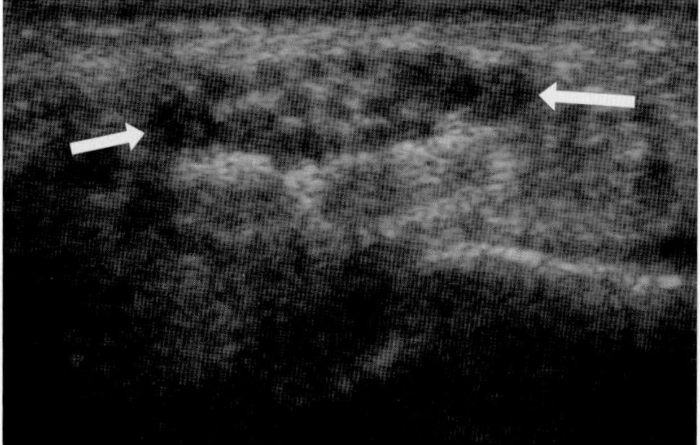

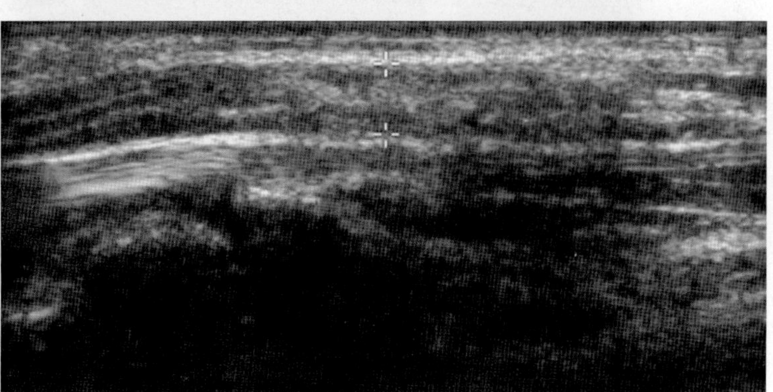

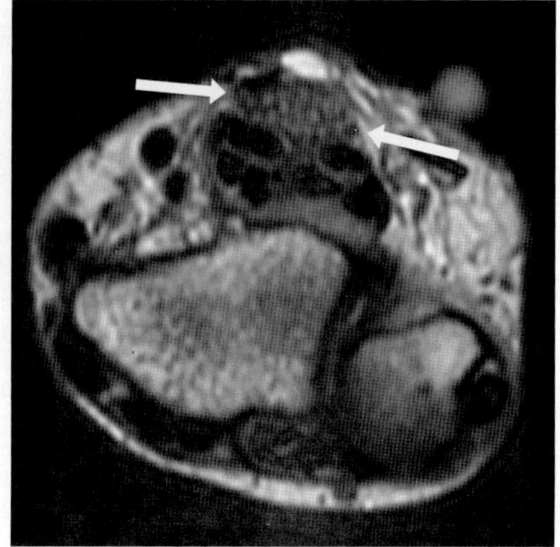

Fig. 4.37 Fibrolipomatous hamartoma of the median nerve in the palm. Transverse **(A)** (*white arrows*) and longitudinal **(B)** images show enlargement of the nerve fascicles and diffuse thickening of the entire nerve. **(C)** Corresponding axial T2-weighted magnetic resonance image shows separation of the nerve fascicles of the median nerve (*white arrows*).

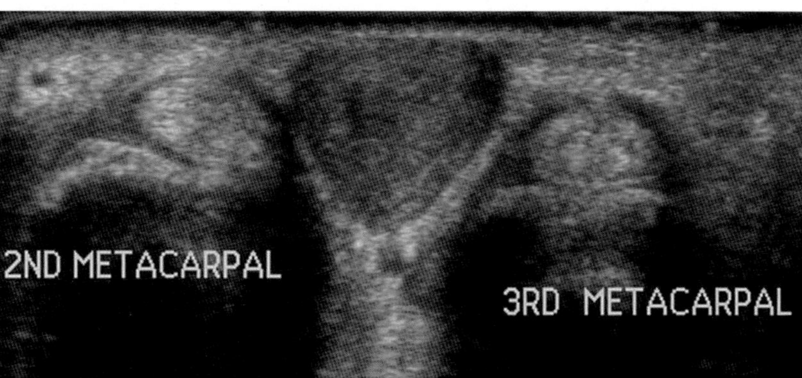

A

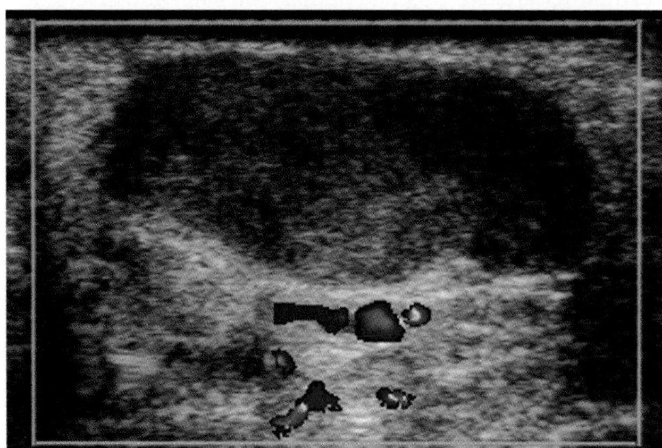

B

Fig. 4.38 Palmar fibroma arising in the plane of the palmar fascia, in between the second and third flexor tendons in the palm **(A)**. No increased vascularity is seen on color Doppler imaging **(B)**.

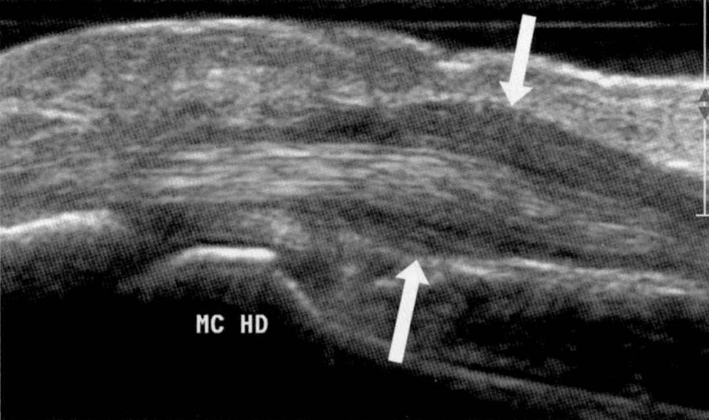

A

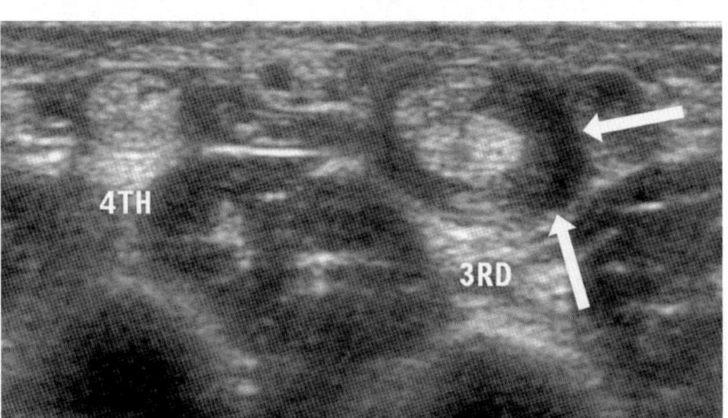

B

Fig. 4.39 Diffuse eccentric swelling is due to an anomalous distal insertion of the lumbrical muscle seen at the radial aspect of the flexor tendon to the middle finger (*white arrows*) on longitudinal **(A)** and transverse **(B)** images. The patient presented with a form of trigger finger, with inability to achieve full extension.

Pearls and Pitfalls

- The use of dynamic movement and its direct visualization with ultrasound is an extremely useful tool, particularly in evaluation of tendon and tendon sheath pathology. It is used both in the identification of normal anatomy as well as to look at abnormal movement of these structures.
- The use of a water bath is a simple and efficient option of maintaining sonographic contact, particularly with flexion of the finger joints and during dynamic movement.
- A good history will go a long way to directing the ultrasound examination to answer the clinical question or problem. It may not be time-efficient to scan every anatomic structure in the hand, or even each finger.
- The choice of an appropriate ultrasound probe is important, as there may need to be a compromise between the larger size of the linear probes, which provide a larger field of view, or the smaller "hockey-stick" probe, which is smaller and more maneuverable.
- The problem of anisotropy is particularly evident with the palmar flexor tendons in the finger, but imaging short segments at a time with proximal or distal tilt of the probe will allow accurate evaluation of the tendons.

Suggested Readings

Jacob D, Cohen M, Bianchi S. Ultrasound imaging of non-traumatic lesions of wrist and hand tendons. Eur Radiol 2007;17(9):2237–2247

Joshua F, Lassere M, Bruyn GA, et al. Summary findings of a systematic review of the ultrasound assessment of synovitis. J Rheumatol 2007;34(4):839–847

Lee JC, Healy JC. Normal sonographic anatomy of the wrist and hand. Radiographics 2005;25(6):1577–1590

Lin J, Jacobson JA, Fessell DP, Weadock WJ, Hayes CW. An illustrated tutorial of musculoskeletal sonography: part 2, upper extremity. AJR Am J Roentgenol 2000;175(4):1071–1079

Scheel AK, Hermann KG, Ohrndorf S, et al. Prospective 7 year follow up imaging study comparing radiography, ultrasonography, and magnetic resonance imaging in rheumatoid arthritis finger joints. Ann Rheum Dis 2006;65(5):595–600

5 Imaging of the Knee

Ian Beggs

Ultrasound examination of the knee is an excellent imaging method that answers specific questions quickly and accurately. It is particularly effective in assessing the extensor mechanism, demonstrating if masses are present—especially in the popliteal fossa, and confirming if mass lesions are cystic or solid. Magnetic resonance imaging (MRI) remains the imaging modality of choice for the menisci, cruciate ligaments, bony abnormalities, and cases with nonspecific clinical features.

Technical Guidelines and Normal Anatomy

Ultrasound of the knee requires a high-frequency linear array transducer. The knee can conveniently be considered as having four separate quadrants: anterior, posterior, lateral, and medial. Ultrasound examinations are usually targeted and directed at one or two quadrants to answer specific clinical questions. It is unusual to perform an examination that looks at all four quadrants.

The anterior knee structures include, from superior to inferior, the quadriceps muscle, quadriceps tendon, patella, and patellar tendon (**Fig. 5.1**). The suprapatellar recess lies deep to the quadriceps tendon and patella and the infrapatellar fat deep to the patellar tendon. Examination of the anterior knee is performed with the patient supine. The hip should be extended. The knee should be slightly flexed. This is best achieved and most comfortable for the patient if a small pad or roll of paper towels is placed under the knee.

The deepest of the quadriceps muscles is the vastus intermedius muscle (**Fig. 5.2**). It lies in the midline immediately anterior to the femur. The rectus femoris muscle is midline and is superficial to vastus intermedius. The vastus medialis and vastus lateralis muscles are also superficial to vastus intermedius and lie on the medial and lateral aspects, respectively, of the rectus femoris muscle. Distally, the quadriceps muscles narrow, form tendons, and contribute to the quadriceps tendon. The rectus femoris tendon forms relatively proximally followed by the vastus intermedius tendon whereas the vastus medialis and vastus lateralis muscles extend more distally before forming their tendons, which run obliquely. The quadriceps tendon inserts into the upper pole of the patella. The patella has an echogenic, slightly convex anterior surface. Variable, frequently negligible, amounts of tendon run superficial to the patella in continuity with the quadriceps and patellar tendons. The retinacula are thin and hypoechoic and run medially and laterally from the patella on transverse images.

The patellar tendon extends from the lower pole of the patella to the tibial tuberosity (**Fig. 5.1**). The patellar tendon has a generally uniform caliber and texture, but the ends are slightly expanded and tendon narrows at the medial and lateral margins, which are convex (**Fig. 5.3**). The ends of the patellar tendon may appear slightly hypoechoic on long axis scans due to anisotropy, but this can be corrected by altering the angulation of the transducer or by beam-steering and confirmed by performing short axis scans. The normal patellar tendon is 10 to 15 mm wide and 3 to 6 mm deep.

The suprapatellar recess extends proximal to the patella and is deep to the quadriceps tendon (**Fig. 5.1**). The normal recess is dry or contains a small amount of fluid. A dry recess appears as a thin echogenic line.

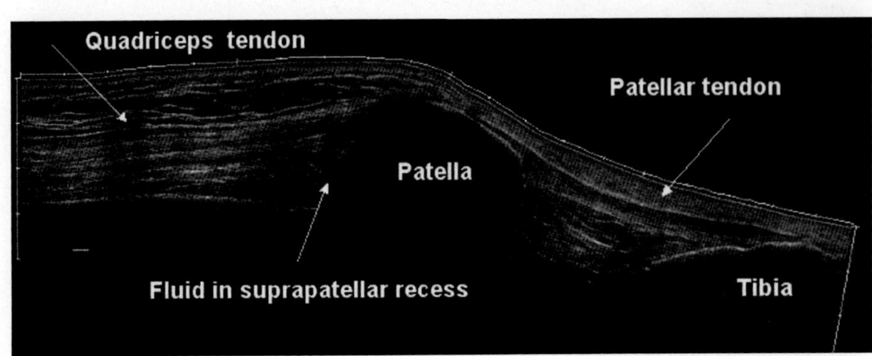

Fig. 5.1 Extended field of view long axis ultrasound scan of extensor mechanism.

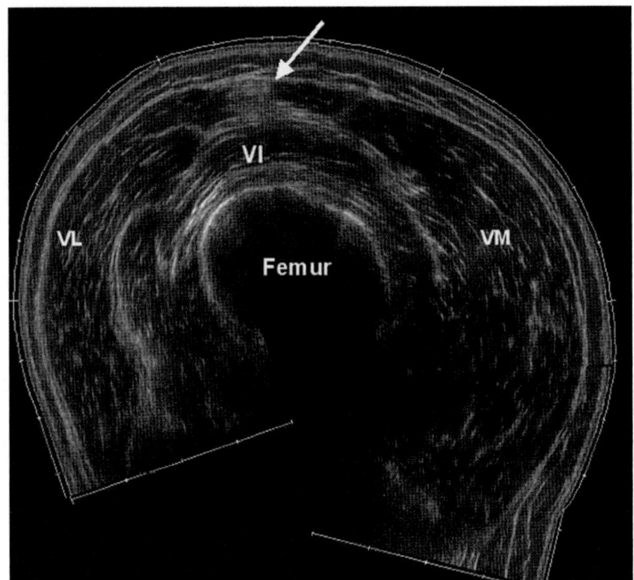

Fig. 5.2 Extended field of view short axis ultrasound scan of distal quadriceps muscle at level of proximal rectus femoris tendon (*arrow*). VL, vastus lateralis; VI, vastus intermedius; VM, vastus medialis muscles.

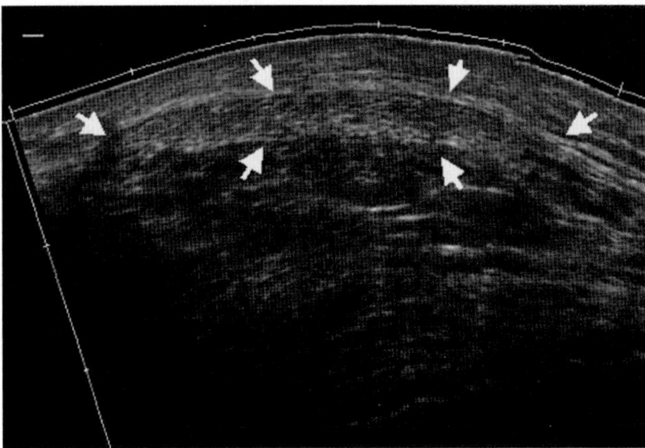

Fig. 5.3 Transverse ultrasound scan of patellar tendon (*arrows*). The tendon is echogenic and is uniform in texture and size. It tapers at the edges.

The infrapatellar fat lies deep to the patellar tendon and has a heterogeneous appearance, although fluid-filled cysts or bursae may be present.

If the knee is fully flexed the patellar sulcus or trochlea can be examined. The articular cartilage is thick and hypoechoic and immediately superficial to the cortical bone (**Fig. 5.4**).

The posterior knee and popliteal fossa are examined with the patient prone. The knee should be minimally flexed or extended. The gastrocnemius muscle has separate heads that originate from the medial and lateral femoral epicondyles. The popliteal neurovascular bundle lies between the medial and lateral heads of gastrocnemius. The popliteal artery is the deepest structure. The popliteal vein lies between the popliteal artery and the more superficial tibial nerve. The common peroneal nerve comes off the tibial nerve and extends distally on the lateral border of the lateral head of gastrocnemius, to run laterally around the neck of the fibula. On the other side of the posterior knee, the semimembranosus and semitendinosus tendons lie on the medial aspect of the medial head of gastrocnemius (**Fig. 5.5**). Semitendinosus is superficial to semimembranosus. Both tendons appear hypoechoic if the transducer is not perpendicular to the tendons and may be mistaken for cysts. Altering transducer angulation or employing beam-steering will correct this artifact.

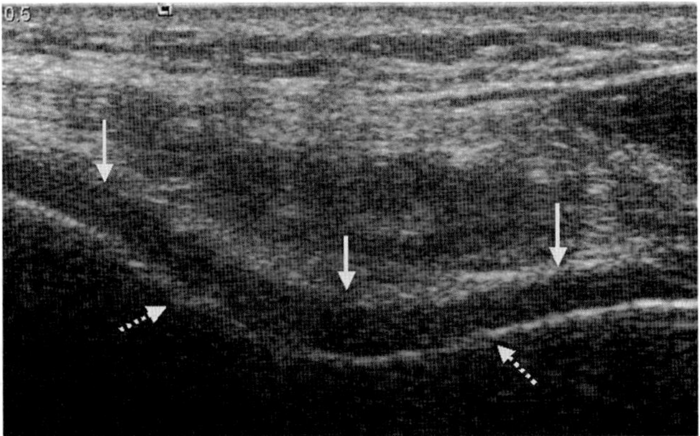

Fig. 5.4 Transverse ultrasound scan of patellar sulcus of distal femur with knee flexed. The hypoechoic articular cartilage (*solid arrows*) is superficial to the cortex of the femur (*broken arrows*).

The medial knee is examined with the patient supine, the hip extended, the knee extended or slightly flexed and the leg slightly externally rotated. The medial collateral ligament runs between the medial femoral epicondyle and the medial surface of the proximal tibia and has uniform texture (**Fig. 5.6**). The distal ligament is slightly expanded. A small bursa is sometimes seen between the deep and superficial layers of the ligament. The medial meniscus lies immediately deep to the medial collateral ligament. The pes anserinus tendons, from anterior to posterior, sartorius, gracilis, and semitendinosus lay posteromedial to the medial collateral ligament and insert on the proximal tibia.

The lateral structures are examined with the patient supine, the hip extended, the knee slightly flexed, and the leg slightly internally rotated. The most anterior structure is the iliotibial band, which inserts on the Gerdy tubercle on the anterolateral aspect of the proximal tibia. The lateral collateral ligament lies posteriorly and runs obliquely from the lateral femoral epicondyle to the fibular head. It forms a conjoined tendon with biceps femoris, which has a more vertical orientation and is the most posterior of the lateral structures.

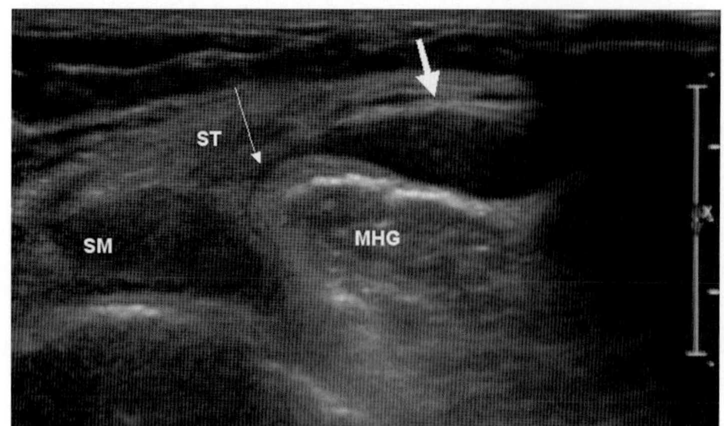

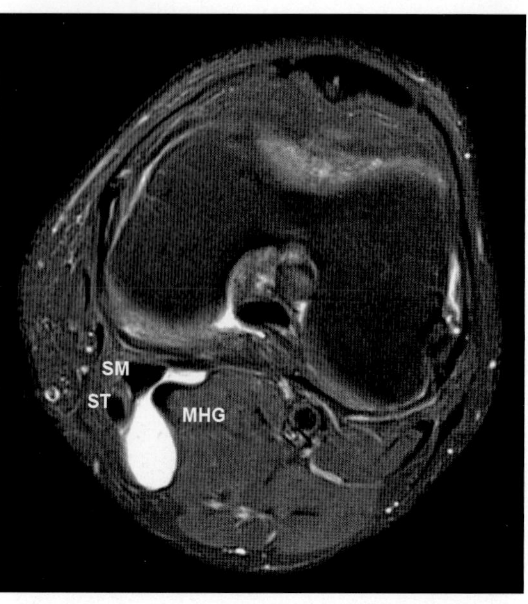

Fig. 5.5 **(A)** Transverse ultrasound scan of popliteal fossa showing small, anechoic Baker cyst (*wide arrow*). Its narrow stalk (*narrow arrow*) emerges between the medial head of gastrocnemius (MHG) and the semimembranosus (SM) and semitendinosus (ST) tendons. The tendons are hypoechoic due to anisotropy. **(B)** Axial fat-saturated proton-density-weighted magnetic resonance image showing small Baker cyst. Its stalk lies between the medial head of gastrocnemius (MHG) and the semimembranosus (SM) and semitendinosus (ST) tendons.

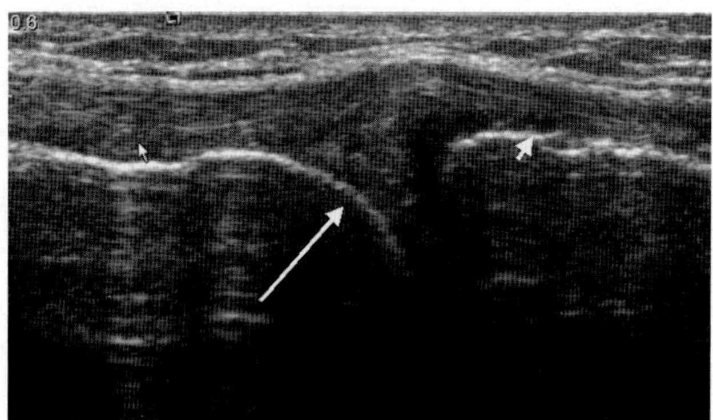

Fig. 5.6 Long axis ultrasound scan of medial collateral ligament (*short arrows*). The triangular, echogenic medial meniscus (*long arrow*) lies immediately deep to the ligament.

Pathologies

Anterior Knee

Tears of Quadriceps and Patellar Tendons and Quadriceps Muscle

Quadriceps tendon tears are relatively uncommon. They are caused by a sudden contraction of the extensor mechanism. Most patients are middle-aged or older. Systemic diseases such as chronic renal failure, gout, systemic lupus erythematosus, diabetes mellitus, rheumatoid arthritis, and hyperparathyroidism may predispose to quadriceps tears. The patient typically presents with swelling and an inability to extend the knee following injury. The diagnosis of a quadriceps muscle or tendon tear is usually clinically obvious, particularly if there is a palpable defect in the quadriceps muscle (**Fig. 5.7**), but a tense joint effusion or a prepatellar hematoma without tendon damage may have a similar clinical presentation. Straight leg raising may be possible with partial tears.

Quadriceps tears are usually incomplete and mostly affect the rectus femoris component of the tendon. Tears occur either in the distal 1 to 2 cm of the tendon or at its insertion into the patella. Ultrasound examination identifies a gap in the tendon fibers. The gap is more conspicuous when filled

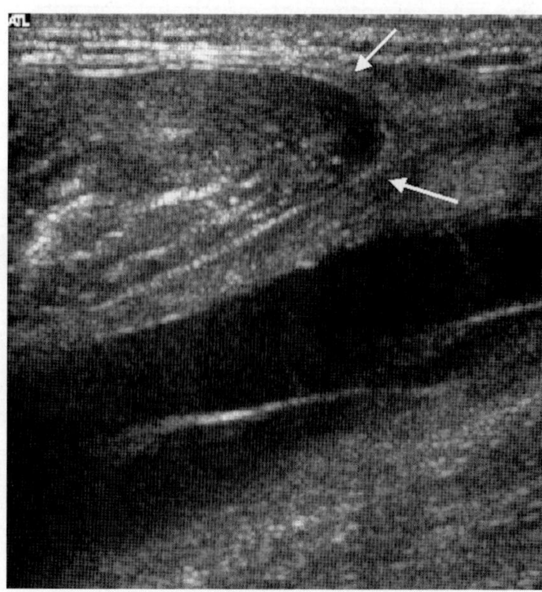

Fig. 5.7 Long axis ultrasound scan of complete tear of rectus femoris muscle. It has a convex inferior margin (*arrows*). There is a large anechoic hematoma deep to the tear.

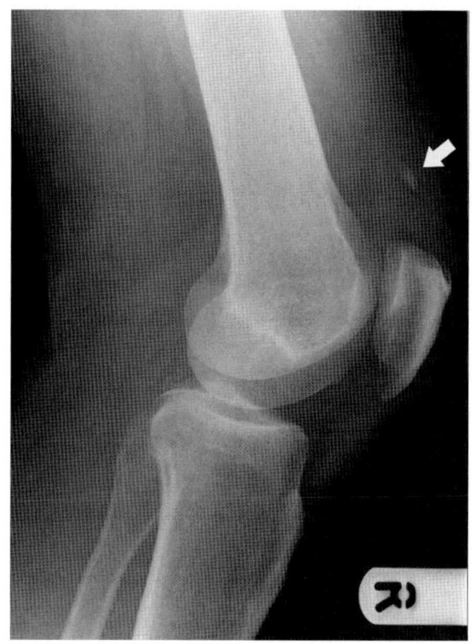

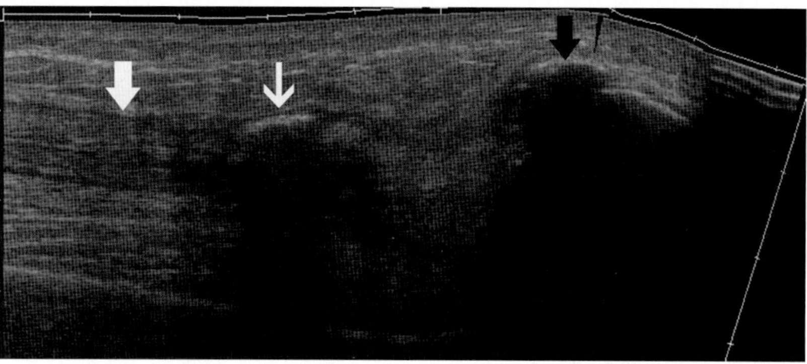

Fig. 5.8 **(A)** Lateral radiograph of knee showing avulsed proximal pole of patella (*arrow*). **(B)** Extended field of view ultrasound scan showing that the quadriceps tendon (*broad white arrow*) is still attached to the avulsed proximal pole of patella (*narrow white arrow*). There is hematoma in the gap between the avulsed fragment and the patella (*black arrow*).

by hematoma, which is hypoechoic. The blood may extend between layers of muscle and tendon and also into subcutaneous tissues. Retraction of the proximal edge of the tendon may be made more obvious by passively flexing the knee.

The distal quadriceps tendon is also involved in complete tears. The tear involves all layers of the tendon. The torn tendon edges are swollen and irregular and the gap is occupied by hypoechoic hematoma that may extend into surrounding soft tissues. Traction on the patella helps to improve conspicuity of the tendon defect and to differentiate complete from incomplete tears. Occasionally, the proximal pole of the patella is avulsed with the tendon still attached (**Fig. 5.8**).

The sensitivity of ultrasound is 100% for partial and complete quadriceps tendon tears and the specificity is 100% for complete tears. Ultrasound is therefore an excellent way to confirm the diagnosis.

Rupture of the patellar tendon involves the proximal tendon. Patellar tendon tears are less frequent than quadriceps tears. They usually occur in younger patients due to sporting injuries, although preexisting tendinosis may be present. Patients present with pain, swelling, and an inability to extend the knee. Proximal retraction of the patella may be obvious on radiographs. Ultrasound shows a defect in the tendon that is occupied by hypoechoic hematoma (**Fig. 5.9**). The distal patellar tendon may have an irregular, redundant appearance. Flexing the knee may make the tear more obvious.

Sometimes, patients present with a clinically obvious tear of the extensor mechanism, but the clinician is uncertain of the level of the tear or if it is complete or incomplete. Ultrasound is an accurate method of confirming the diagnosis, the extent of damage, and the precise site of the tendon injury. It helps to mark the skin at the site of the tear.

Tears of the quadriceps muscles are usually diagnosed clinically at the time of injury and heal spontaneously. Occasionally, patients present with an apparent mass lesion in the anterior thigh due to an unrecognized, chronic quadriceps muscle tear, usually of rectus femoris. The typical presentation is of an anterior thigh mass that enlarges when the quadriceps muscle is contracted. A mass can be palpated and there may be a focal depression distal to the mass. Long axis ultrasound examination shows that the proximal edge of the torn muscle has a convex inferior margin (**Fig. 5.10**). The fibroadipose septae may converge or lie parallel to the tear margin. As the muscle contracts the convex margin,

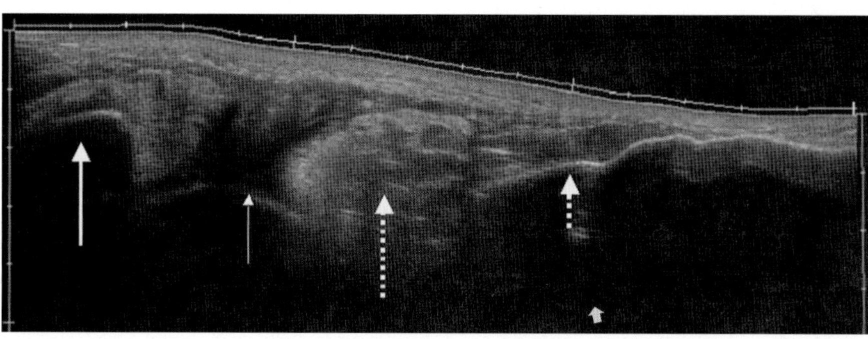

Fig. 5.9 Long axis ultrasound scan of complete midsubstance tear of patellar tendon. Residual tendon is attached to the patella (*large solid arrow*) and the tibial tuberosity (*small broken arrow*). The gap is occupied by liquid hematoma (*small solid arrow*) and echogenic thrombus (*large broken arrow*).

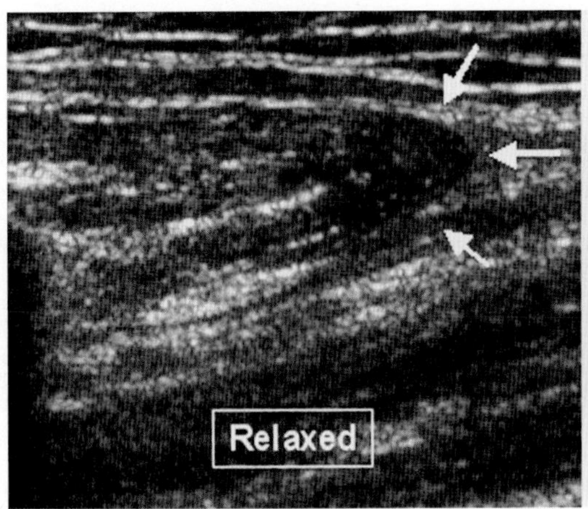

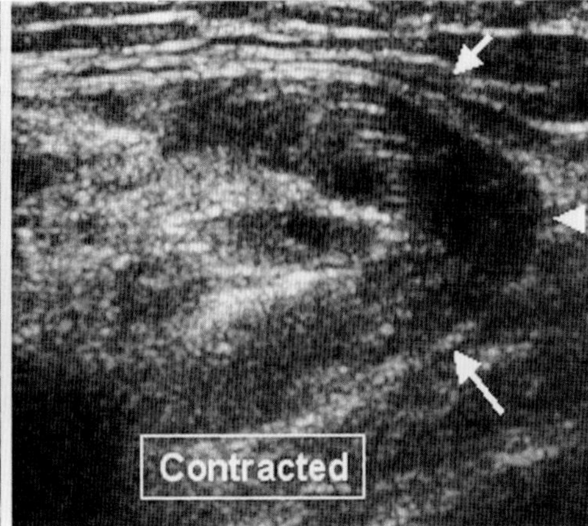

Fig. 5.10 Long axis ultrasound scans of chronic rectus femoris tear. With the patient supine, the knee extended and the muscle relaxed, the inferior margin of the tear is convex (*arrows*). When the muscle is contracted, by asking the patient to elevate the foot while keeping the knee extended, the torn muscle retracts and its inferior edge becomes more rounded and prominent.

and with it the fibroadipose septae, becomes rounder and retracts making the apparent mass more prominent. On short axis scans, a tear can be recognized because the muscle suddenly disappears instead of incrementally becoming smaller (**Fig. 5.11**). Patients are frequently concerned that the mass is a tumor. They readily understand the real nature of the mass and are reassured when the ultrasound appearances are explained. It is particularly helpful to demonstrate the changes during contraction and relaxation of the muscle.

Patellar Tendinosis/Tendinopathy

Patellar tendinosis, which usually involves the proximal patellar tendon, is also known as "jumper's knee." Occasionally the distal tendon is involved. Several etiologic theories have been suggested, but patellar tendinosis is postulated to be a chronic overuse injury. Histologic examination shows disruption of the usual organized bundles of collagen and increased mucoid ground substance and cellular infiltrates, especially of tenocytes. Vascular proliferation and deposits of cartilage and bone may also be seen, but there are no inflammatory changes.

Ultrasound examination demonstrates hypoechoic swelling of the proximal 2 to 3 cm of the patellar tendon adjacent to the lower pole of the patella (**Fig. 5.12**). The swelling does not involve the full width of the tendon. It is focal and usually posterior (**Figs. 5.13** and **5.14**). The affected segment is ill-defined particularly on the deep surface. Echogenic foci in the tendon are due to areas of ossification or calcification (**Fig. 5.15**). Hyperostosis at the enthesis at the lower pole of the patella occurs in long-standing cases and it may be difficult to distinguish between hyperostosis and intratendinous calcification or ossification. Thickening of the paratenon may be present. The ultrasound and MRI assessment of the extent of patellar tendinosis are generally well correlated, although gradient echo images tend to exaggerate the extent of changes. However, asymptomatic morphologic changes are frequently seen with both examinations. Neovascularity may be shown on color or power Doppler in the affected segment of tendon and in adjacent soft tissues (**Fig. 5.16**) and this correlates strongly with pain. Abnormal Doppler signal is less conspicuous when the tendon is under tension so the knee should be relaxed when searching for neovascularity. Exercise may make an abnormal Doppler signal more conspicuous. The presence of abnormal vessels suggests a

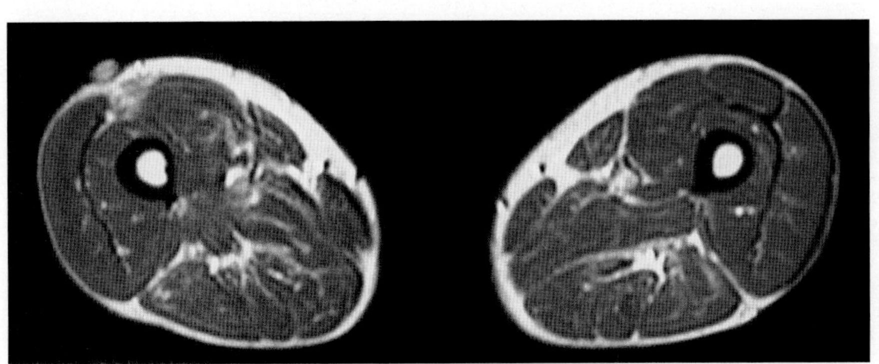

Fig. 5.11 Short axis T1-weighted magnetic resonance images of thighs. The skin marker on the right lies at the edge of a chronic, complete tear of the rectus femoris muscle (cf. opposite side).

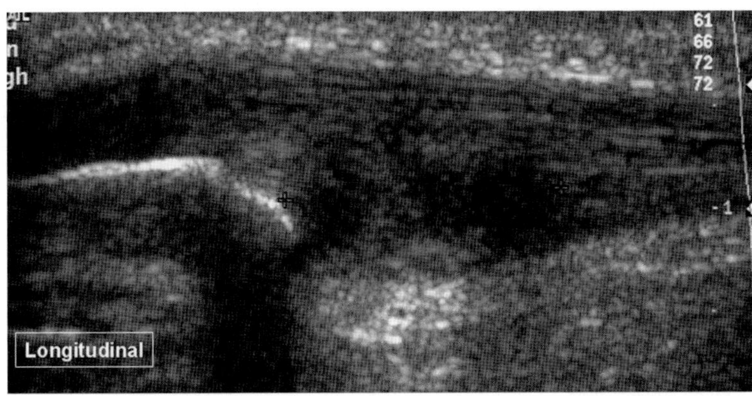

Fig. 5.12 Long axis ultrasound scan of proximal patellar tendinosis (jumper's knee). The affected segment (*between the caliper marks*) is posterior, swollen, hypoechoic and ill-defined.

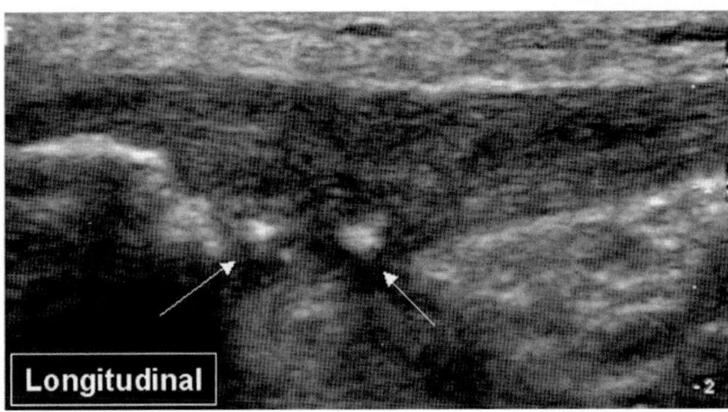

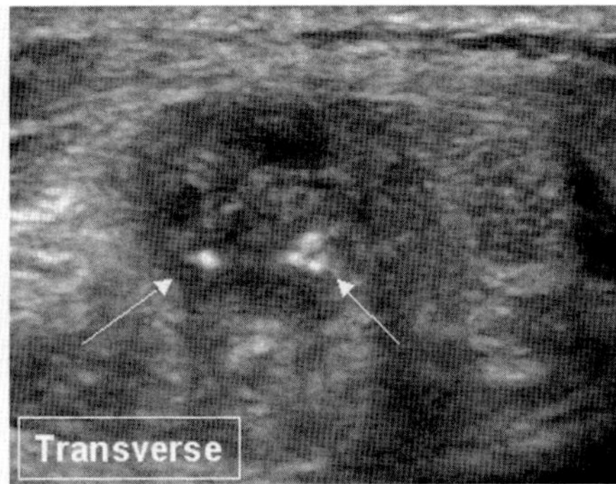

Fig. 5.13 Long and short axis ultrasound scans of chronic proximal patellar tendinosis. The posterior segment of the tendon adjacent to the inferior pole of the patella is swollen, ill-defined, hypoechoic, and contains echogenic foci of calcification or dystrophic ossification (*arrows*).

better prognosis; an inhomogeneous tendon texture is associated with a poorer outcome. Progression from tendinosis to a full-thickness tear is rare.

The usual treatment of jumper's knee is conservative and involves physical therapy although dry needling or injections of autologous blood or sclerosants have been suggested. Dry needling is performed by repeated to-and-fro needle perforations of the tendon. Paradoxically, the aim of dry needling is to induce new vessels to grow into the segment of tendinosis and relieve symptoms. Autologous blood or sclerosant injections are advocated as reducing neovascularity and consequently pain.

Osgood–Schlatter Disease

Patients with Osgood–Schlatter disease are adolescents who present with pain, tenderness, and swelling due to chronic avulsive stress at the insertion of the patellar tendon into the tibial apophysis. The primary insult is to the apophysis. Tendon changes are secondary.

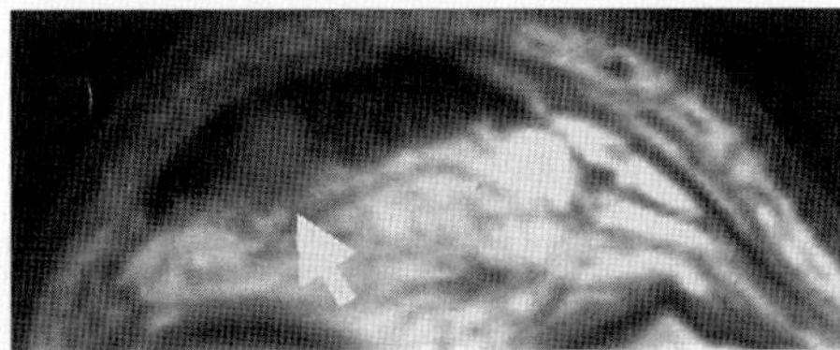

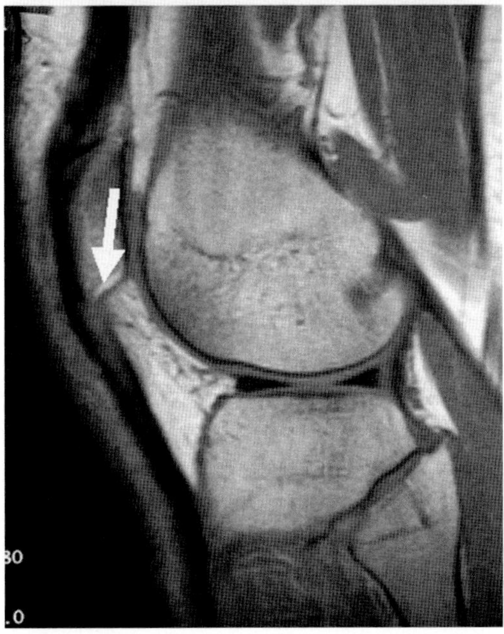

Fig. 5.14 Short and long axis proton-density T1-weighted magnetic resonance images of jumper's knee. A small segment of the tendon is bright, swollen and ill-defined (*arrows*).

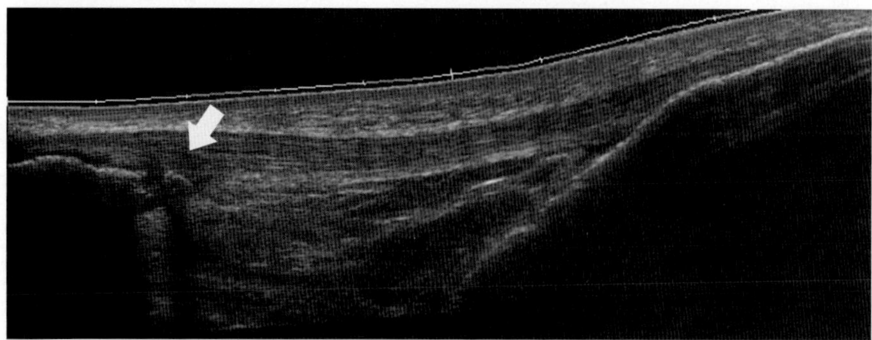

Fig. 5.15 Extended field of view long axis ultrasound scan of jumper's knee. An echogenic focus of calcification (*arrow*) adjacent to the lower pole of the patella casts an acoustic shadow.

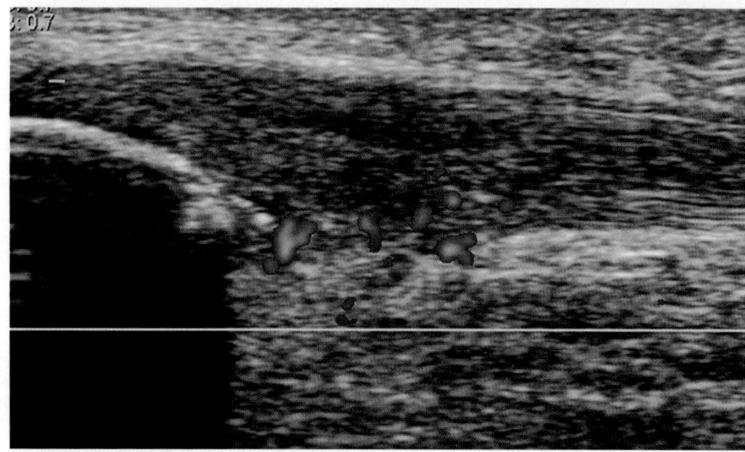

Fig. 5.16 Long axis power Doppler ultrasound scan of jumper's knee shows neovascularity in proximal patellar tendon and adjacent soft tissues. Neovascularity correlates with pain and suggests a good prognosis.

Ultrasound is not frequently required as the diagnosis is usually clinically obvious. Ultrasound shows swelling of the distal patellar tendon, the cartilage at the apophysis, and the pretibial soft tissues. The ossification center is fragmented and the infrapatellar bursa is distended. Neovascularity in both tendon and bursa may be present. Similar changes occur at the inferior pole of the patella in Sinding–Larsen–Johansson disease.

Joint Effusion

Very small amounts of fluid in the suprapatellar recess can be detected by ultrasound. The best places to look are in the recesses on either side of the patella or just proximal to the upper pole of the patella. As an effusion enlarges, it fills the suprapatellar recess (**Fig. 5.17**) proximal to the patella and may be mistaken clinically for a solid mass. Uncomplicated synovial fluid is anechoic. Infection and a chronic effusion may result in fluid that is hypoechoic rather than anechoic. Hypoechoic fluid, possibly with echogenic thrombi, also occurs with a posttraumatic hemarthrosis. Fluid-fluid levels are characteristic of a lipohemarthrosis (**Fig. 5.18**), which is due to an intraarticular fracture and escape of medullary fat into the joint. Early ultrasound shows fat, which is echogenic, floating on the hypoechoic blood and separated by a fluid-fluid level. Within 3 hours or so the serum and red blood cells (RBCs) separate and this may result in three layers and two fluid-fluid levels. The RBCs sink to the bottom and are hypoechoic. The

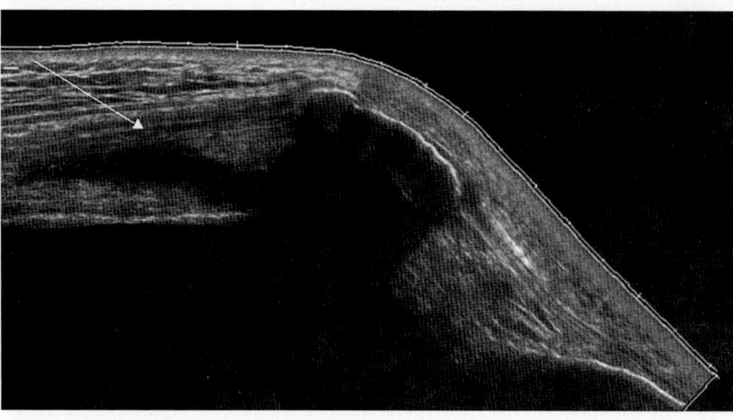

Fig. 5.17 Extended field of view long axis ultrasound scan of anterior knee showing effusion in suprapatellar recess (*arrow*).

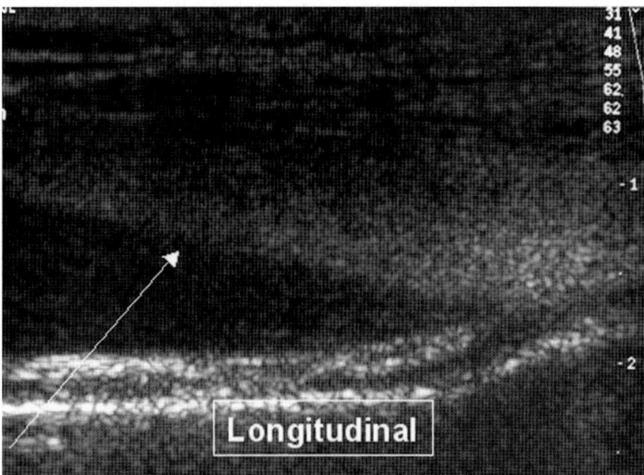

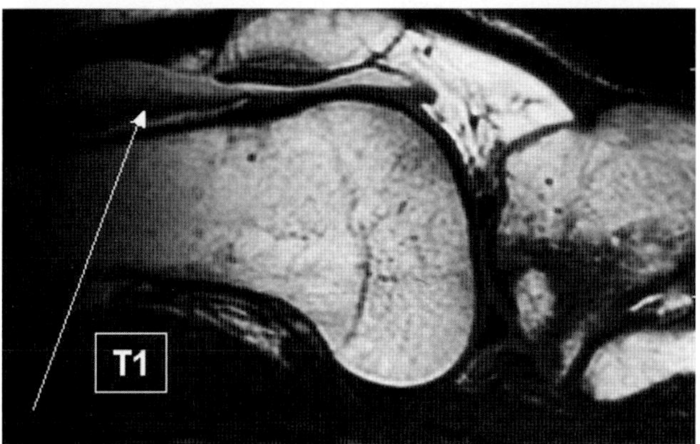

Fig. 5.18 Long axis ultrasound scan (*top*) and sagittal T1-weighted magnetic resonance image (MRI) of lipohemarthrosis due to intraarticular fracture of lateral tibial plateau. The fat separates from the blood and synovial fluid and floats to the top forming a fluid-fluid level (*arrows*). The fat is echogenic on ultrasound and hyperintense on T1-weighted MRI.

fat forms the superior band and is echogenic. The middle layer contains serum and synovial fluid and is almost anechoic. Thin fluid-fluid levels lie between the layers. Ultrasound is superior to radiographs in the detection of a lipohemarthrosis.

Synovial hypertrophy initially produces thickening of the wall of the suprapatellar recess that is hypoechoic. In chronic synovitis the recess may be enlarged and contain solid pannus. Color or power Doppler may be of value in differentiating between active and fibrous pannus. Active pannus is vascular; fibrous pannus is hypovascular. Although the role of contrast agents is not established, reduced perfusion may be seen with contrast-enhanced power Doppler in response to treatment.

Bursae

The deep infrapatellar bursa lies deep to the distal patellar tendon. A small amount of fluid is normal. Deep infrapatellar bursitis can be seen in association with distal patellar tendinopathy, but it may not be possible to distinguish between normal and pathologic bursae.

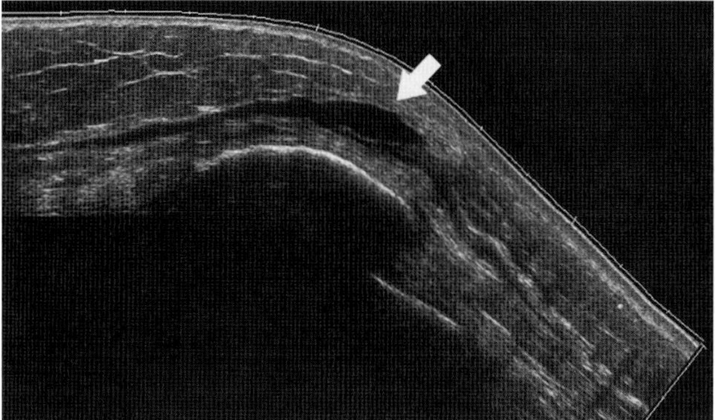

Fig. 5.19 Long axis ultrasound scan showing prepatellar bursa (*arrow*).

Two prepatellar bursae are described. The bursa in "housemaid's knee" lies superficial to the patella (**Fig. 5.19**), but in "clergyman's knee" it is superficial to the patellar tendon. Fluid in the prepatellar bursa may be symptomatic, but small amounts of fluid may be without clinical significance. Bursitis is thought to be due to prolonged kneeling. It is painful and the bursa is tender to palpation. The bursa contains anechoic fluid. Its wall may be thickened and abnormal signal may be seen on color or power Doppler. Synovial hypertrophy may be seen.

Muscle Hernia

Muscle hernias occur in the lower leg and usually involve the tibialis anterior muscle. The herniated muscle bulges into the subcutaneous fat through a defect in the fascia that is thought to be due to trauma, chronic compartment syndrome, or weakness at the site of perforating vessels. Patients are usually adolescents or young adults and present with a mass that enlarges when the patient stands or contracts the muscle, and reduces when the patient is supine or the muscle is relaxed, although occasionally a hernia is effaced by contraction of the muscle.

If a muscle hernia is suspected, the patient should be asked how best to increase conspicuity of the mass. This may mean examining the patient erect, after exercise, or during muscle contraction. The skin should be marked as the mass may be impalpable during the examination. The transducer should be applied lightly as the hernia may be reduced and effaced by heavy pressure.

Ultrasound may show thinning and possibly slight elevation of the deep fascia overlying the muscle. As the muscle herniates, it overlaps the margins of the fascial defect and may assume a mushroom shape (**Fig. 5.20**). Herniated muscle tends to be hypoechoic relative to the remainder of the muscle due either to anisotropy or to atrophy as a result of chronic trauma. The fibroadipose septa are constricted as they run through the defect resulting in a spoke-like appearance and vessels may run through the defect alongside the hernia.

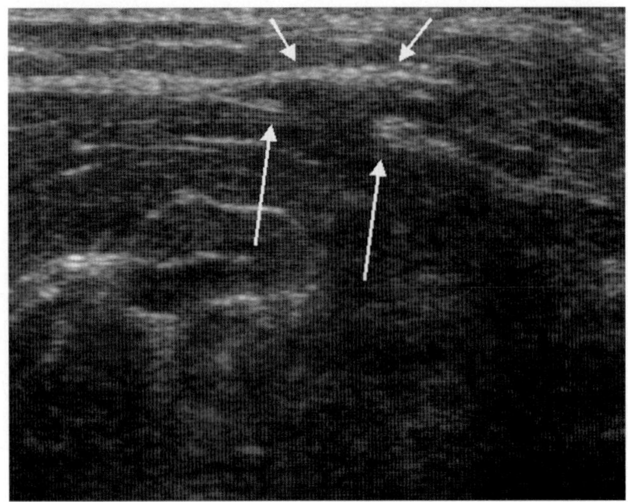

Fig. 5.20 Short axis ultrasound scan of small tibialis anterior muscle hernia (*short arrows*) during muscle contraction. The herniated muscle is hypoechoic and overlaps the markings of the fascial defect (*long arrows*) giving a mushroom-like appearance.

Patients are frequently concerned about the possibility of neoplasia. Ultrasound confirms the diagnosis and can reassure patients particularly when they see the hernia appearing and reducing on dynamic examination.

Posterior Knee

Baker Cyst

Patients frequently present with a swelling or discrete mass in the popliteal fossa. Ultrasound confirms if there is a mass, defines its exact location, and shows if it is cystic or solid. The usual cause of a swelling in the popliteal fossa is a Baker cyst, but not infrequently a patient presents with an apparent swelling that is due to a normal prominence of the medial or lateral head of the gastrocnemius muscle. Ultrasound is particularly valuable as it not only confirms that the swelling is due to normal muscle but this can be demonstrated to the patient, providing immediate reassurance.

A Baker cyst, or semimembranosus-gastrocnemius bursa, is the most frequent cause of a space-occupying lesion in the popliteal fossa. Many produce pain, discomfort, or swelling. However, many Baker cysts are incidental findings of no clinical significance. Small Baker cysts occur in up to 20% of knees. They are generally anechoic and well defined, although hypoechoic fluid contents may be present.

The critical diagnostic feature of a Baker cyst is to demonstrate the neck of the cyst. This lies between the semimembranosus and semitendinosus tendons medially and the medial head of gastrocnemius laterally (**Fig. 5.5**). The best way to show the neck is to perform a transverse scan with the knee slightly flexed. The neck of the cyst is narrow. It may contain fluid, which may be effaced when the knee is fully extended. The cyst itself is well defined and contains fluid that can be anechoic or hypoechoic, but it may contain echogenic foci of synovial osteochondromatosis (**Fig. 5.21**) or be replaced by hypoechoic pannus. The neck of the cyst may function as a one- or two-way valve resulting in a cyst that may enlarge or deflate. Uncomplicated cysts may extend distally or proximally.

A ruptured Baker cyst presents clinically with a painful, swollen calf and may be mistaken for a deep vein thrombosis (DVT). As a ruptured cyst and a DVT may coexist both

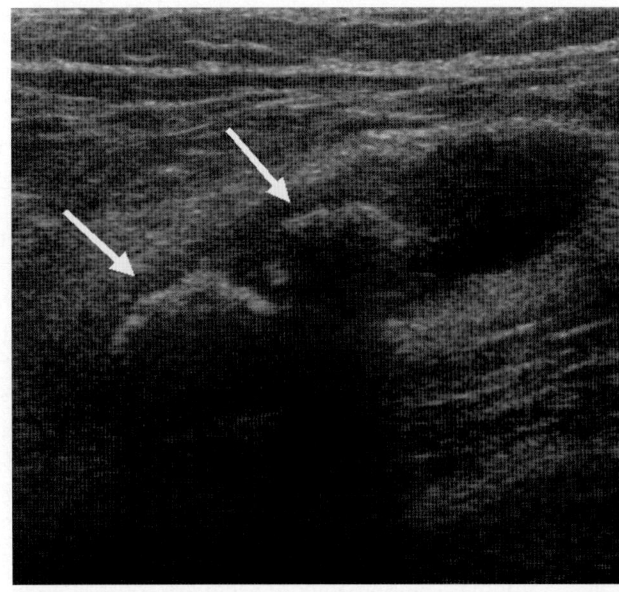

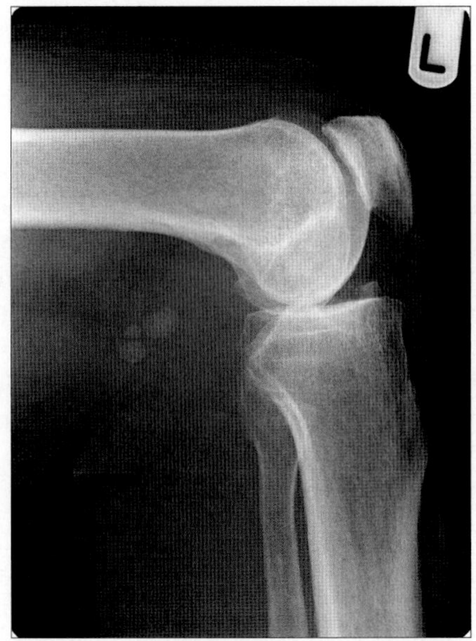

Fig. 5.21 **(A)** Transverse ultrasound scan of Baker cyst that contains echogenic foci of synovial osteochondromatosis (*arrows*). **(B)** The lateral radiograph of the knee shows the ossified foci of osteochondromatosis in the popliteal fossa.

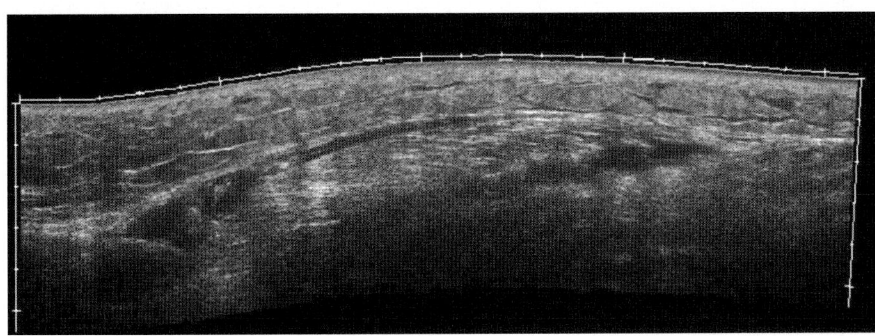

Fig. 5.22 Extended field of view ultrasound scan of calf following rupture of a Baker cyst. Fluid tracks along fascial planes superficial and deep to muscles. Subcutaneous edema is present.

should be looked for on ultrasound. Rupture usually occurs distally and results in the shape of the distal margin of the cyst changing from convex to a more pointed appearance. The fluid tracks along tissue planes, including fascial planes, between muscles and also into subcutaneous tissues (**Fig. 5.22**). Although rupture results in deflation of the cyst a sizeable cyst may still be visible. The cyst reexpands when the leak seals. Hemorrhage into a Baker cyst may be due to trauma or anticoagulation and presents with a swollen, painful calf. The cyst fluid is hypoechoic rather than anechoic and echogenic clots may be present. Cyst hemorrhage and rupture may coexist.

If no abnormality is found in a patient who presents with an acutely swollen, painful, and tender calf, the examination should be extended distally to look for a tear of the medial head of gastrocnemius or a "tennis leg." This is an injury that usually affects "weekend warriors" and occurs between the aponeuroses of the soleus and medial head of gastrocnemius muscles resulting in a focal hematoma (**Fig. 5.23**). Tennis leg usually resolves slowly over several weeks or months, but occasionally results in chronic scar or hematoma formation causing chronic pain and a feeling of tightness (**Fig. 5.24**).

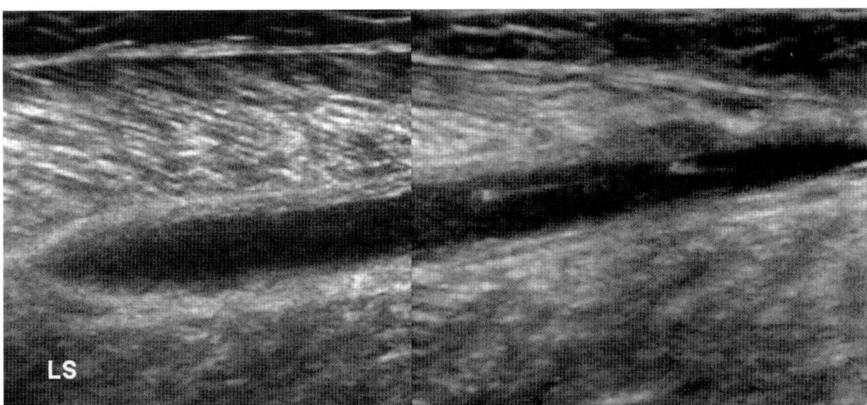

Fig. 5.23 Long axis (composite) ultrasound image of tennis leg. There is a hematoma between the gastrocnemius and soleus muscles.

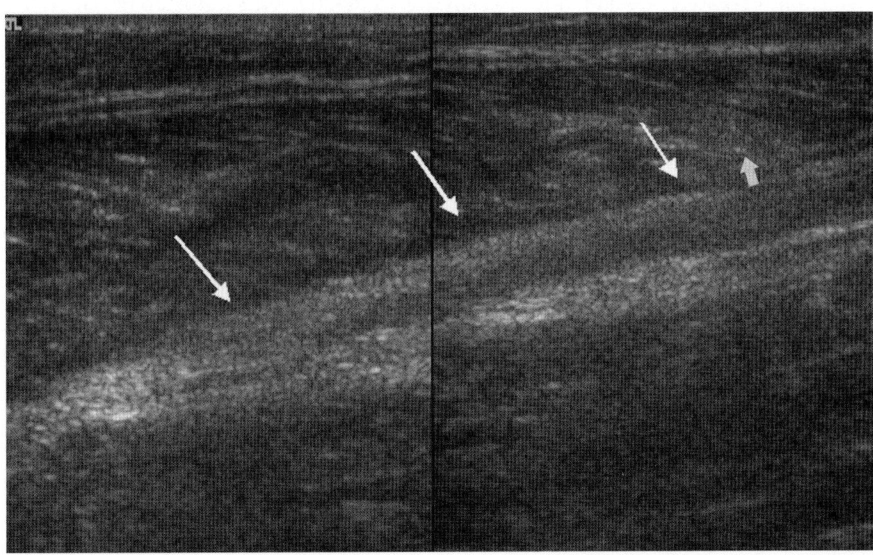

Fig. 5.24 **(A)** Long axis (composite) ultrasound image of chronic tennis leg shows an echogenic scar/chronic hematoma. (*Continued*)

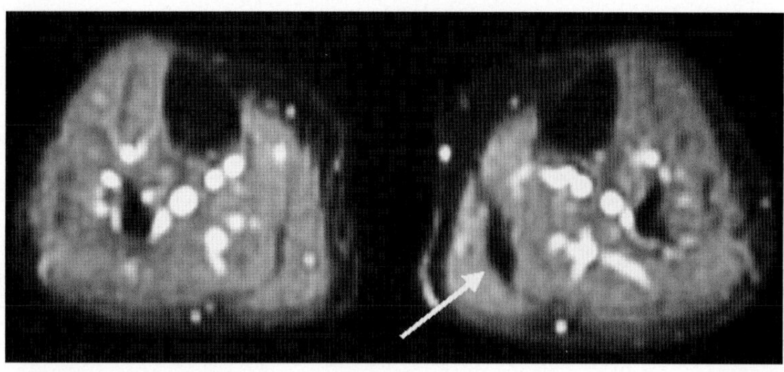

Fig. 5.24 (*Continued*) **(B)** Axial short T1 inversion recovery (STIR) magnetic resonance sequence of calves showing hypointense scar/chronic hematoma (*arrow*) between gastrocnemius and soleus.

Cruciate Ligaments

The cruciate ligaments are not well seen on ultrasound because of their oblique orientation and the effect of anisotropy. MRI is the technique of choice to examine the cruciate ligaments, particularly as tears of the cruciate ligaments are frequently associated with other bone and soft tissue injuries. However, the ultrasound appearances of cruciate injuries have been reported.

An intact posterior cruciate ligament (PCL) is seen on long axis scans as a hypoechoic band that runs obliquely to its insertion on the posterior margin of the tibia. Tears result in focal discontinuity or in diffuse swelling when compared with the opposite PCL.

The anterior cruciate ligament (ACL) is not normally shown by ultrasound, but a tear of ACL may result in a hematoma that is hypoechoic and lies on the lateral wall of the intercondylar notch. This may be demonstrated on a posterior transverse scan.

Ganglion cysts are occasionally seen in or adjacent to the cruciate ligaments. They are well defined and anechoic.

Medial Knee

Medial Collateral Ligament

Injuries to the medial collateral ligament (MCL) are due to valgus stress. Isolated MCL injuries are usually treated conservatively and imaging is not required except in professional or high-level athletes. MRI is performed if more complex injuries are suspected.

Injuries of the MCL usually involve the proximal ligament and affect the deep layer more frequently than the superficial layer. A grade I sprain does not cause instability. It results in hypoechoic fluid and swelling adjacent to the MCL. There are no changes in the MCL itself. A grade II sprain is a partial tear. It produces instability and swelling of the MCL. A grade III injury is a complete tear with gross instability. There is a defect in the deep and superficial layers and this is occupied by hypoechoic fluid or hematoma. Chronic or old injuries cause thickening of the MCL. Calcification adjacent to the medial epicondyle, the Pellegrini–Stieda lesion, can be seen on radiographs or ultrasound and is due to a previous injury.

Medial Meniscus

Ultrasound is not usually the recommended imaging examination for the menisci. MRI is the examination of choice. However, the medial meniscus may be seen during ultrasound examination of the medial knee. The meniscus is normally triangular and echogenic (**Fig. 5.6**). Tears are anechoic or hypoechoic defects, occasionally hyperechoic, or produce an absent or truncated meniscus (**Fig. 5.25**). Meniscal degeneration may produce swelling, reduced echogenicity, or extrusion of the meniscus. Chondrocalcinosis causes focal echogenic areas in the meniscus. A discrete gap between the

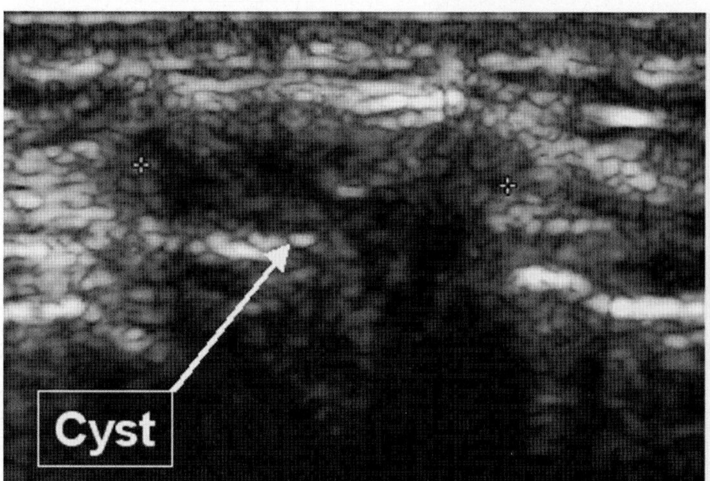

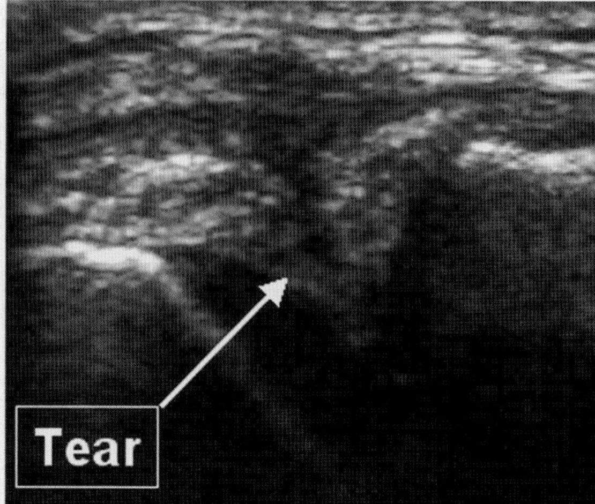

Fig. 5.25 Coronal scans of medial knee joint line showing multiloculated meniscal cyst and meniscal tear.

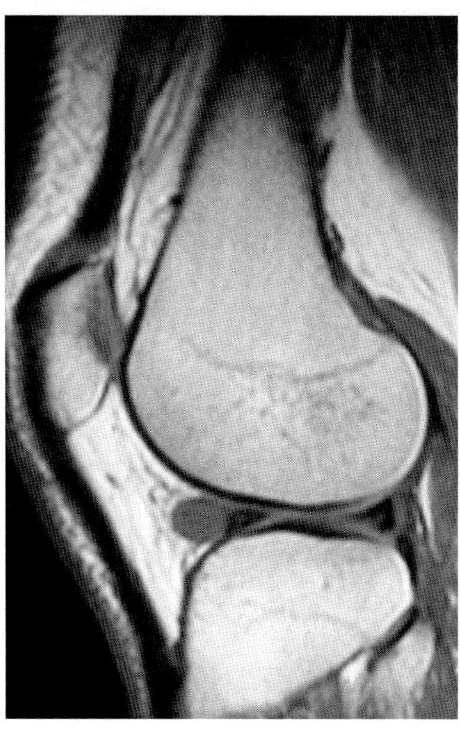

Fig. 5.26 Sagittal proton-density-weighted magnetic resonance image showing lateral meniscal tear and anterior horn cyst.

meniscus and the MCL indicates probable meniscocapsular separation.

Meniscal cysts are frequently asymptomatic or present with pain and swelling at the joint margin. They are due to leakage of joint contents through meniscal tears into the parameniscal tissues. Cysts vary in appearances. They may be uni- or multilocular and contain anechoic or hypoechoic fluid (**Fig. 5.25**), but they may appear solid and hypoechoic. The diagnostic feature is that the cyst or mass is contiguous with the meniscus (**Fig. 5.26**).

Pes Anserinus Bursa

The pes anserinus bursa lies deep to the pes anserinus tendons, sartorius, gracilis, and semitendinosus, running to their insertion on the medial aspect of the tibia. Bursitis presents with localized pain and swelling. Ultrasound shows a well-defined, fluid-filled bursa deep to the tendons and superficial to the tibia.

Lateral Knee

Lateral Collateral Ligament

Isolated sprains of the lateral collateral ligament (LCL) are uncommon. They are usually part of a complex injury and are investigated by MRI. Sprains result in discontinuity or focal swelling on ultrasound.

Iliotibial Band

Iliotibial band friction syndrome is the consequence of chronic friction where the iliotibial band runs over the lateral femoral condyle and is due to sporting activities. The iliotibial band is thickened and there is reduced echogenicity. A deeper hypoechoic area may be due to bursitis or soft tissue inflammation.

In older patients iliotibial band tendinopathy may cause anterior or lateral knee pain. It results from osteoarthritis or a knee prosthesis and is a consequence of altered stresses due to angular deformity or friction against the edge of the tibial component. Ultrasound demonstrates reduced echogenicity, swelling, and loss of the normal architecture of the affected segment. Alterations may be subtle and it may help to compare with the opposite side.

Lateral Meniscus

Lateral meniscal tears and cysts appear identical to those in the medial meniscus. Fluid in the popliteus tendon sheath at the posterior horn of the meniscus may simulate a cyst.

Biceps Femoris and Popliteus Tendons

Tendinopathy of the biceps femoris or popliteus tendons is uncommon and results in swelling and reduced echogenicity of the tendon. A superficial bursa may be seen.

Proximal Tibiofibular Joint

A synovial cyst or ganglion of the proximal tibiofibular joint is often asymptomatic, particularly if it emerges from the posterior joint margin. An anterior cyst may present as a painless swelling on the anterior or lateral aspect of the fibular neck and may extend into the tibialis anterior or peroneus longus muscles. Ultrasound shows a well-defined cyst that is anechoic and has a thick wall. Typically, the cyst is pear-shaped, wider distally, and has a narrow stalk that communicates with the tibiofibular joint.

The common peroneal nerve may be compromised by a ganglion cyst of the proximal tibiofibular joint. The nerve runs obliquely from the popliteal fossa around the lateral surface of the fibular neck, where it runs in a narrow tunnel deep to the peroneus longus muscle, to emerge on the anterior aspect of the fibula. A cyst may compress the nerve in the tunnel causing focal swelling, foot drop, and sensory alteration. Ultrasound shows the cyst adjacent to the nerve (**Fig. 5.27**). Ultrasound-guided aspiration to decompress the cyst may relieve symptoms. A wide-gauge needle is needed as cyst contents are jelly-like. Occasionally, a cyst invades the common peroneal nerve or its deep or superficial branches. The nerve is thickened and nerve fascicles are displaced around the cyst. Compromise of the common peroneal nerve by extra- and intraneural ganglia may produce fatty infiltration, identified as increased echogenicity in the tibialis anterior muscle.

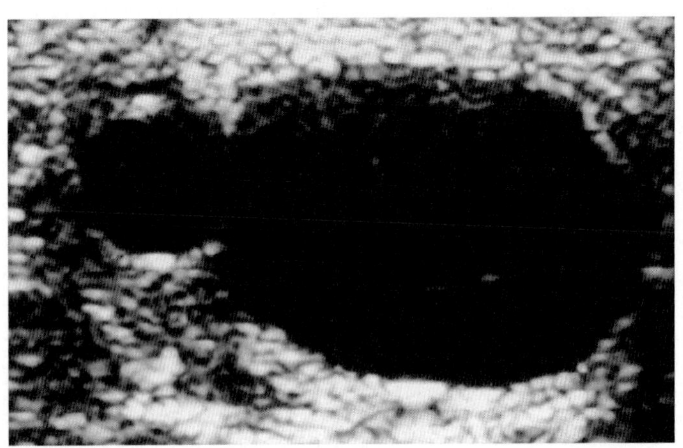

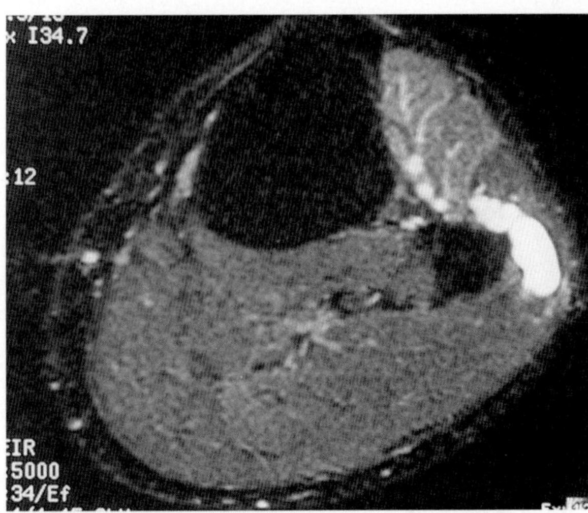

Fig. 5.27 **(A)** Ultrasound scan shows a multiloculated cyst in the line of the common peroneal nerve. **(B)** The axial short T1 inversion recovery (STIR) magnetic resonance sequence shows the ganglion on the anterolateral aspect of the fibular neck in the line of the common peroneal nerve. From Beggs I. Pictorial review: imaging of peripheral nerve tumors. Clinical Radiology 1997;52:8–17.

Masses

Most soft tissue masses at the knee are cystic. Chronic muscle tears, muscle hernias, joint effusions, and thrombosed varicose veins (**Fig. 5.28**) also present as soft tissue masses. All are accurately diagnosed by ultrasound. Ultrasound is valuable when MRI images are distorted by artifact due to metal (**Fig. 5.29**) and can be used for aspiration or biopsy, although biopsy of soft tissue masses should always be preceded by appropriate staging investigations.

Conclusion

Ultrasound is an excellent method of examining the knee for specific, targeted indications. It cannot supplant MRI in investigating bone or internal structures such as the menisci, cruciate ligaments, or articular surfaces. Ultrasound accurately delineates muscle and tendon tears, tendinopathy, and mass lesions; discriminates between solid and cystic masses; and can be used to guide interventional procedures.

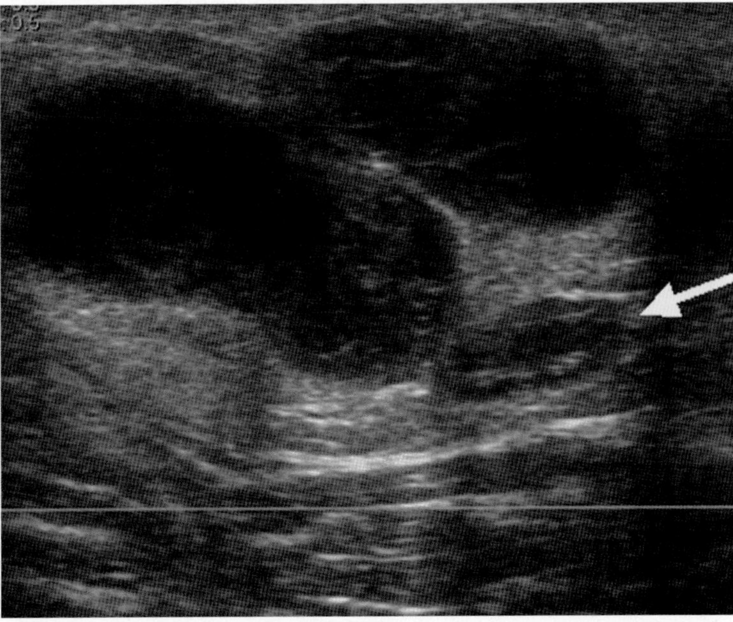

Fig. 5.28 Transverse power Doppler ultrasound image shows a thrombosed long saphenous varix that presented as a painful, enlarging soft tissue mass. The adjacent segment of long saphenous vein is also thrombosed (*arrow*). The varix and vein are incompressible and show no flow on Doppler.

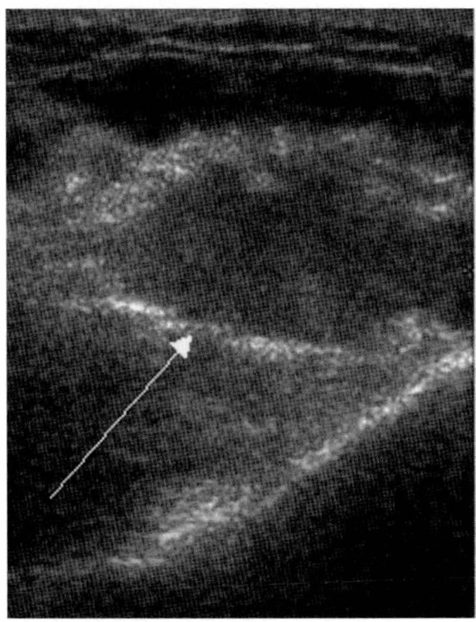

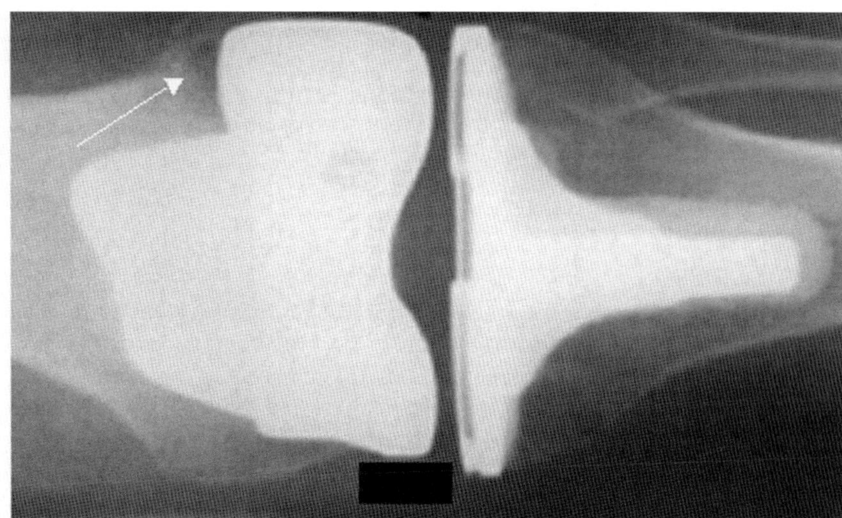

Fig. 5.29 Ultrasound and anteroposterior radiograph showing, respectively, soft tissue mass (*arrow*) and osteolysis (*arrow*) at lateral femoral epicondyle in patient with knee prosthesis. Ultrasound-guided biopsy confirmed granulocytic reaction to wear debris from the prosthesis.

Knee Algorithm

1. Plain radiographs
2. Ultrasound first imaging examination for
   - Soft tissue mass
   - Tear/tendinosis of quadriceps/patellar tendons
   - Acutely painful/swollen calf
   - Muscle hernia/tear
3. Computer tomography to assess extent of tibial plateau fractures
4. Magnetic resonance imaging for meniscal/cruciate tears, occult fracture, spontaneous osteonecrosis of the knee (SONK), ill-defined symptoms

Pearls and Pitfalls

- Most soft tissue masses at the knee are cystic—easily confirmed by ultrasound.
- A Baker cyst is defined by demonstrating the neck of the cyst between the medial head of gastrocnemius and the semimembranosus and semitendinosus tendons.
- Asymptomatic morphologic abnormalities are common in the patellar tendons of athletes.
- Neovascularity in the patellar tendon correlates with pain. Neovascularity may be missed if the tendon is examined while under tension.
- DVT, ruptured Baker cyst, and tennis leg all present clinically with an acutely painful and swollen calf.

Suggested Readings

Beggs I. Sonography of muscle hernias. AJR Am J Roentgenol 2003;180(2):395–399

Bianchi S, Zwass A, Abdelwahab IF, Banderali A. Diagnosis of tears of the quadriceps tendon of the knee: value of sonography. AJR Am J Roentgenol 1994;162(5):1137–1140

Bonnefoy O, Diris B, Moinard M, Aunoble S, Diard F, Hauger O. Acute knee trauma: role of ultrasound. Eur Radiol 2006;16(11):2542–2548

Carr JC, Hanly S, Griffin J, Gibney R. Sonography of the patellar tendon and adjacent structures in pediatric and adult patients. AJR Am J Roentgenol 2001;176(6):1535–1539

Cook JL, Malliaras P, De Luca J, Ptasznik R, Morris ME, Goldie P. Neovascularization and pain in abnormal patellar tendons of active jumping athletes. Clin J Sport Med 2004;14(5):296–299

Costa DN, Cavalcanti CFA, Sernik RA. Sonographic and CT findings in lipohemarthrosis. AJR Am J Roentgenol 2007;188(4):W389

Delgado GJ, Chung CB, Lektrakul N, et al. Tennis leg: clinical US study of 141 patients and anatomic investigation of four cadavers with MR imaging and US. Radiology 2002;224(1):112–119

European Society of Muskuloskeletal Radiology. Muskuloskeletal Ultrasound Technical Guidelines. Available at: http://essr.org/html/img/pool/knee.pdf. Accessed February 27, 2010

Friedman L, Finlay K, Jurriaans E. Ultrasound of the knee. Skeletal Radiol 2001;30(7):361–377

Peace KAL, Lee JC, Healy J. Imaging the infrapatellar tendon in the elite athlete. Clin Radiol 2006;61(7):570–578

Tschirch FT, Schmid MR, Pfirrmann CW, Romero J, Hodler J, Zanetti M. Prevalence and size of meniscal cysts, ganglionic cysts, synovial cysts of the popliteal space, fluid-filled bursae, and other fluid collections in asymptomatic knees on MR imaging. AJR Am J Roentgenol 2003;180(5):1431–1436

Warden SJ, Kiss ZS, Malara FA, Ooi AB, Cook JL, Crossley KM. Comparative accuracy of magnetic resonance imaging and ultrasonography in confirming clinically diagnosed patellar tendinopathy. Am J Sports Med 2007;35(3):427–436

6 Imaging of the Foot and Ankle

Gervais K. L. Wansaicheong, Ian Yu-Yan Tsou, and Seng Choe Tham

The ankle and foot bear the day-to-day locomotive burden of the biped human. As an intricate set of bones held together by uniquely placed ligaments and moved by the many sets of muscular tendons, the complexity of the ankle and foot exceeds that of all other structures in the musculoskeletal system.

Clinical Indications

Trauma

Radiographs are frequently the first modality utilized in the assessment of foot and ankle trauma where most significant fractures and dislocations can be detected.

In the clinical setting, foot and ankle ultrasound is used in the assessment of ligament, tendon, and muscular injuries. An experienced operator can confidently evaluate many of the medial and lateral ligaments of the ankle, as well as the long tendons traversing the ankle joint with ultrasound. The availability of dynamic real-time evaluation of the body part also provides ultrasound with an advantage that other modalities currently do not possess.

Sometimes exposed to the perils of the surroundings, traumatic injuries to the foot and ankle may introduce foreign bodies. Radiopaque foreign bodies such as glass, gravel, or metal are detected 98% of the time with radiographs. However, ultrasound will detect nonradiopaque foreign bodies that are made of wood or plastic which radiographs will miss.

Infection

Infections of the foot and ankle are commonly seen in diabetic patients with poor podiatric care. Ultrasound can be used in the confirmation of soft tissue swelling and edema in cases of cellulitis, while concomitantly aid in the detection of abscess collections to guide drainage.

Masses

Covered with minimal soft tissue, the evaluation of masses within the foot and ankle may be performed with ultrasound. Ultrasound can provide a close-up, detailed examination of the relationship of the mass with the surrounding structures, while allowing for dynamic evaluation of the mass with respect to the neighboring tendons, muscles, and ligaments.

Technical Guidelines

The foot and ankle should be evaluated with ultrasound while the patient is in a relaxed position. In our practice, we frequently position the patient on either an examination bed or a reclining couch with the ankle and foot hanging over the edge. This allows for unimpeded passive and active movement of the foot and ankle during the examination.

The ultrasound probe should be a high frequency probe, preferably with a small footprint to allow for better contact with the ankle and foot surface during scanning.

Normal Anatomy

A systematic approach to an ultrasound study of the foot and ankle is provided below.

Lateral-Sided Ankle Structures

Structures at the lateral ankle are some of the most commonly injured. A Lauge-Hansen supination–adduction type injury frequently results in disruption of the lateral-sided ligaments.

From the anterior to posterior, the anterior talofibular, calcaneofibular, and posterior talofibular ligaments stabilize the ankle joint by holding the lateral malleolus to the talus and calcaneus.

The anterior talofibular (**Fig. 6.1**) and the calcaneofibular ligaments can be visualized with ultrasound (**Fig. 6.2A,B**). The posterior talofibular ligament is deep and overlaid by multiple structures making sonographic evaluation difficult.

The pair of peroneal tendons run and course through the lateral ankle (**Fig. 6.2A,C**). The peroneus brevis inserts into the lateral aspect of the base of the fifth metatarsal (**Fig. 6.3**); the peroneus longus inserts into the lateral margin of the plantar surface of the first cuneiform and the proximal end of the first metatarsal.

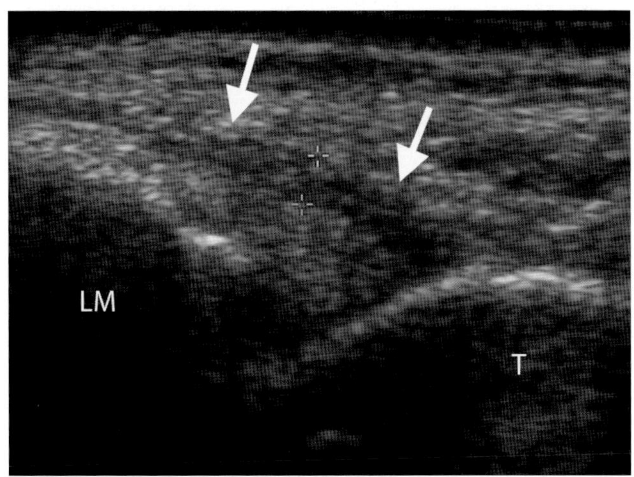

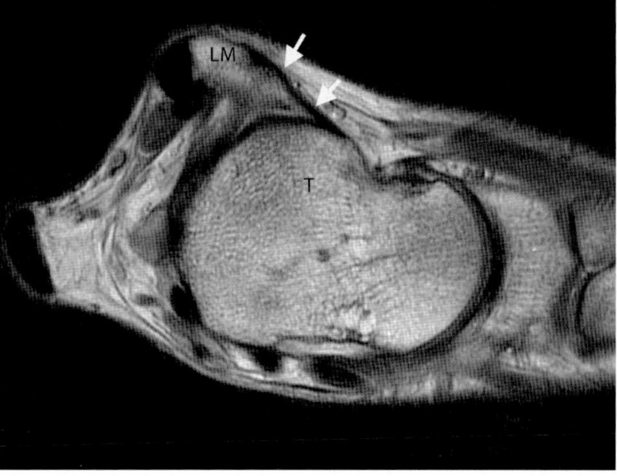

Fig. 6.1 **(A)** The anterior talofibular ligament (*white arrows*) is seen running between the lateral malleolus (LM) and the lateral aspect of the talus (T). This is best demonstrated with the ankle in a supinated and internally rotated position. **(B)** A comparable proton-density axial magnetic resonance image of the ankle showing the anterior talofibular ligament (*white arrows*) between the lateral malleolus (LM) and talus (T).

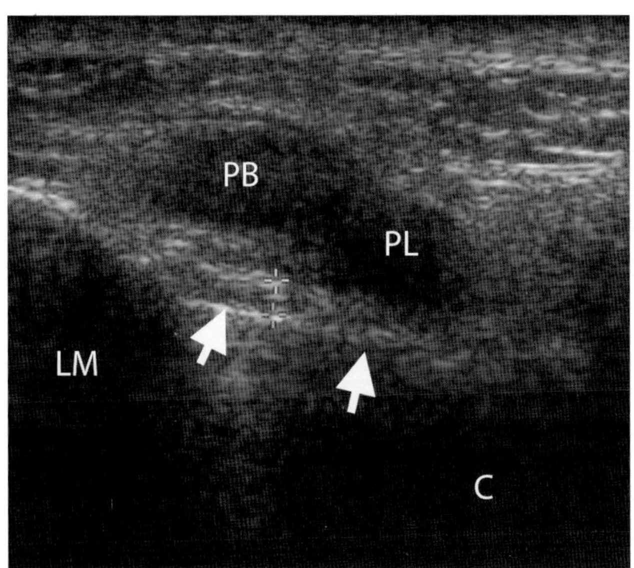

Fig. 6.2 **(A)** The calcaneofibular ligament (*white arrows*) is seen running between the lateral malleolus (LM) and the lateral aspect of the calcaneum (C). The peroneus brevis (PB) and peroneus longus (PL) tendons are seen coursing posterior and inferior to the tip of the lateral malleolus. At this position, the peroneus longus is posterior and inferior to the peroneus brevis. **(B)** A comparable proton density coronal magnetic resonance image (MRI) of the ankle showing the calcaneofibular ligament (*white arrows*). This is typically seen across several coronal images as the ligament travels in an inferoposterior direction from the lateral malleolus to the lateral surface of the calcaneum. The obliquity of this ligament should be borne in mind during sonography. **(C)** A comparable proton density axial MRI of the ankle rotated to match the ultrasound scanning plane showing the peroneus brevis (PB) and peroneus longus (PL) tendons in their short axis, as they course posteroinferior to the lateral malleolus.

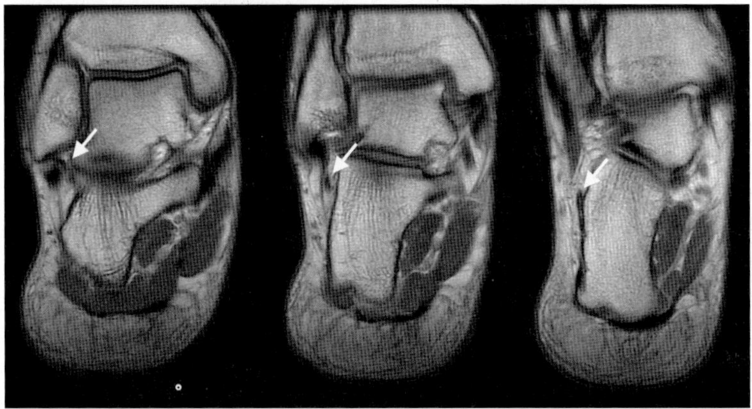

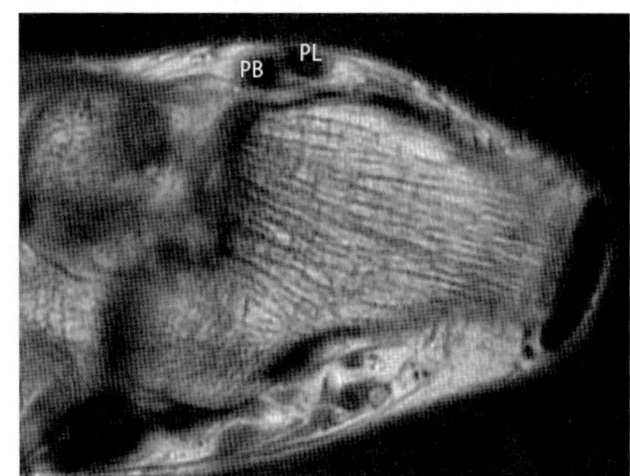

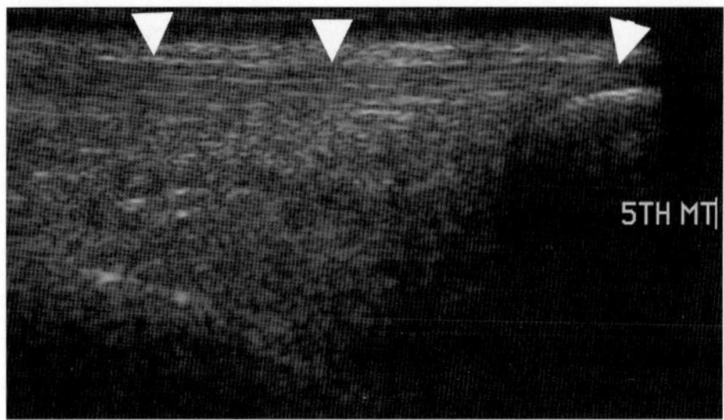

Fig. 6.3 The peroneus brevis (*white arrowheads*) is seen inserting into the base of the fifth metatarsal (5TH MT).

Medial-Sided Ankle Structures

Ligaments in the medial ankle are less commonly injured. Frequently described as having superficial and deep components, the deltoid ligament is a strong ligament. The superficial component comprises the talonavicular, calcaneotibial, and posterior talotibial ligaments (**Fig. 6.4**). These arise from the deep surface of the medial malleolus and insert into the navicular, sustentaculum tali of the calcaneus and posterior talus, respectively. The deep component is made of only the anterior talotibial ligament.

A trio of tendons course through the tarsal tunnel in the medial ankle. From medial to lateral, they are the tibialis posterior, flexor digitorum, and flexor hallucis longus tendons (**Fig. 6.5**). The posterior tibial artery with its accompanying veins and the tibial nerve are also found within the tunnel (**Fig. 6.6**).

Anterior Ankle Structures

Three extensor tendons traverse the anterior ankle. From medial to lateral, they are the tibialis anterior, extensor hallucis, and extensor digitorum tendons (**Fig. 6.7**). The dorsalis pedis artery is also situated here and can be easily studied.

Posterior Ankle Structures

The stout Achilles tendon is located at the posterior ankle and is the main extensor of the foot. This conjoint tendon with contributions from both the soleus and gastrocnemius muscles inserts into the posterior surface of the calcaneus. It has a crescenteric cross-sectional profile and inserts into the posterior surface of the calcaneus (**Fig. 6.8**).

Plantar Structures

The plantar fascia, otherwise known as the plantar aponeurosis, runs from the medial calcaneal tubercle to the proximal

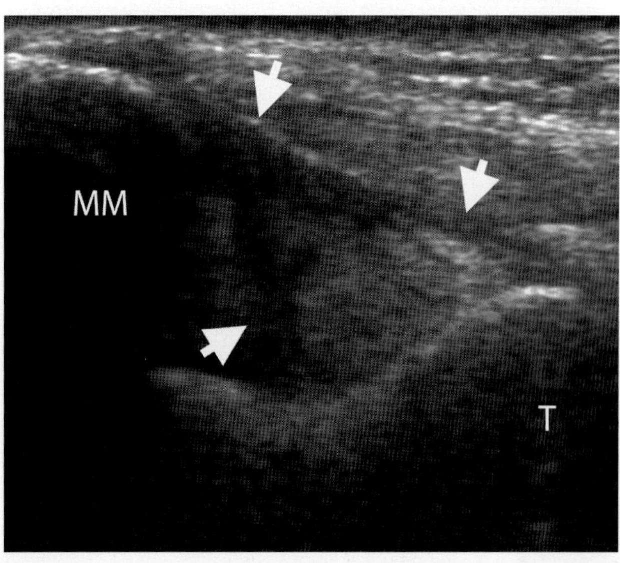

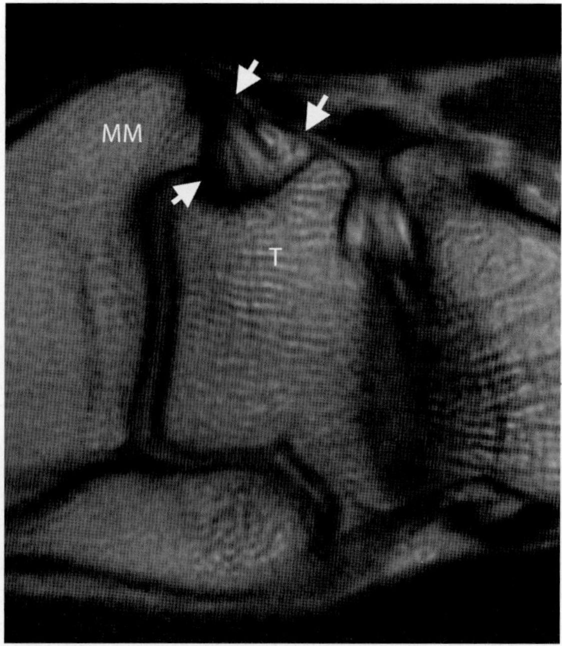

Fig. 6.4 **(A)** The deep and superficial components of the deltoid ligament (*white arrows*) is seen fanning out from the medial malleolus (MM) and the lateral talus (T). **(B)** A comparable proton density coronal magnetic resonance image rotated to match the scanning orientation of ultrasound. This shows the deltoid ligament (*white arrows*) between the medial malleolus (MM) and talus (T). This ligament has superficial and deep components and it fans out as it courses toward the talus.

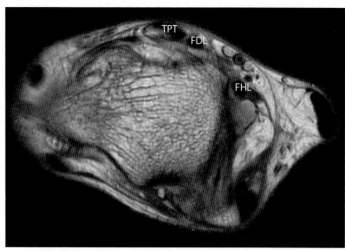

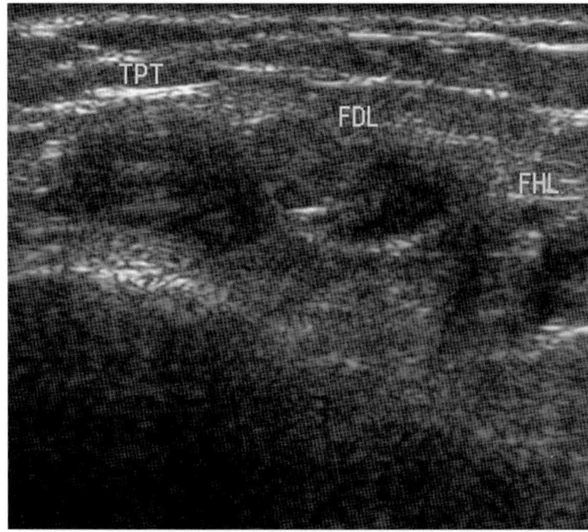

B

Fig. 6.5 **(A)** The trio of tendons within the tarsal tunnel. From anteromedial to posterolateral, the tibialis posterior (TPT), flexor digitorum (FDL), and the flexor hallucis longus (FHL). **(B)** A comparable proton density axial magnetic resonance image rotated to match the ultrasound scanning orientation. The trio of long flexors running within the tarsal tunnel are seen. From medial to lateral they are the tibialis posterior (TPT), flexor digitorum (FDL), and flexor hallucis longus (FHL).

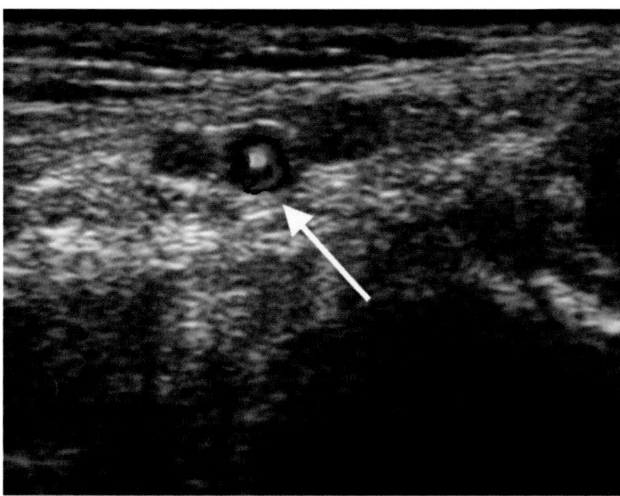

Fig. 6.6 The tibialis posterior artery (*white arrow*) showing flow on color Doppler with the two accompanying veins on each of its side.

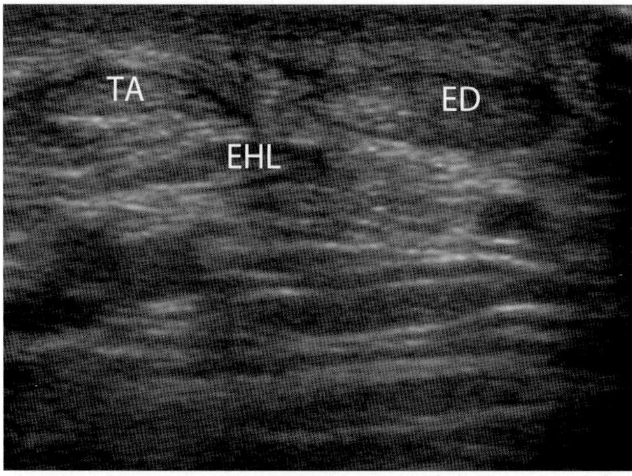

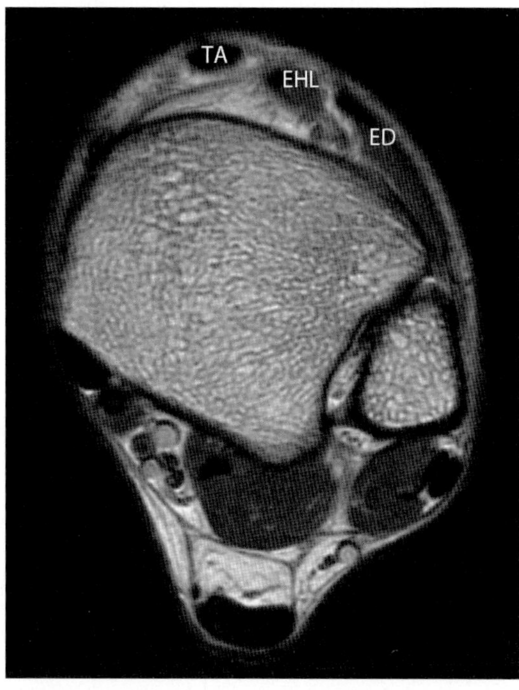

Fig. 6.7 **(A)** The three extensor tendons from medial to lateral on the anterior aspect of the ankle joint, the tibialis anterior (TA), extensor hallucis longus (EHL), and extensor digitorum (ED). **(B)** A comparable proton density axial magnetic resonance image showing the three long extensors anterior to the ankle joint. From medial to lateral, they are the tibialis anterior (TA), extensor hallucis longus (EHL), and extensor digitorum (ED) tendons.

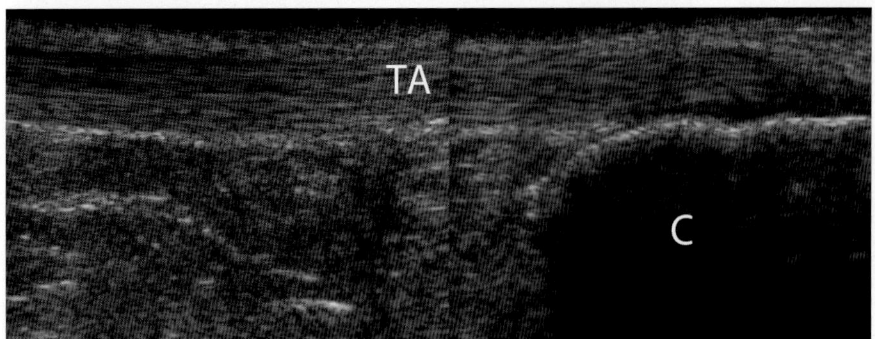

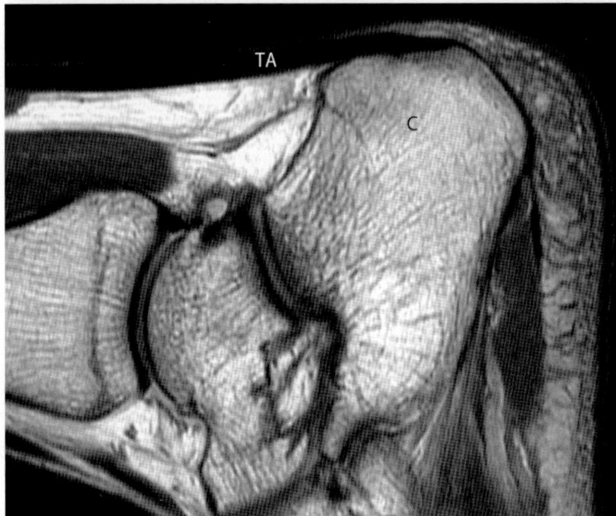

Fig. 6.8 **(A)** The Achilles tendon (TA) inserting into the posterior surface of the calcaneum (C). **(B)** A comparable proton density sagittal magnetic resonance image rotated to match the ultrasound scanning orientation. The Achilles tendon (TA) is seen to insert into the posterior aspect of the calcaneum (C).

phalanges of the toes (**Fig. 6.9**). Three components exist in this broad structure namely the medial, central, and lateral components; with the central being the most prominent.

The plantar fascia contributes to the support of the foot arch by acting as a tie-rod under tension during weight bearing. It also dynamically stretches maintaining the arch of the foot as well as contributing to the degree and timing of supination and pronation of the foot during gait.

Forefoot Structures

Metatarsophalangeal and interphalangeal joints as well as their surrounding structures may be evaluated with ultrasound. The usage of a small footprint probe such as a "hockey stick" probe allows for optimal contact during scanning. A water bath may also be utilized in patients with a more undulating surface anatomy (see Chapter 4: Imaging of the Hand).

Pathologies

Degenerative

Subjected to large forces and stress, joints in the foot and ankle are susceptible to degenerative changes such as osteoarthritis. These changes are primarily evaluated via plain radiographs. Sonographic examination of a degenerate foot and ankle may yield findings of osteophytes (**Fig. 6.10**).

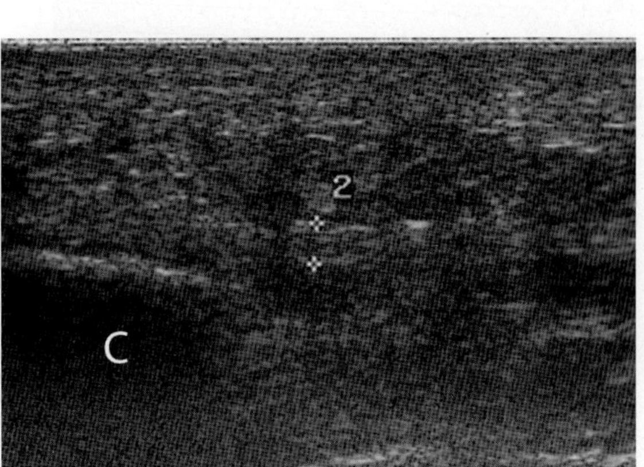

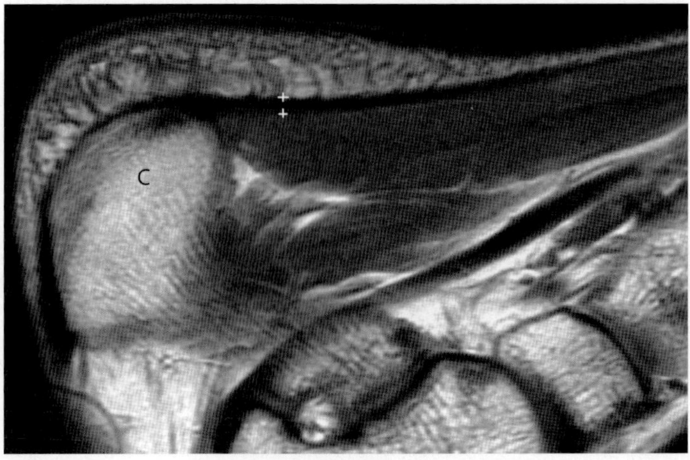

Fig. 6.9 **(A)** The plantar fascia (between calipers) is seen on this ultrasound image arising from the medial calcaneal tubercle. **(B)** A comparable proton density sagittal magnetic resonance image rotated to match the ultrasound scanning orientation. This shows the plantar fascia (between calipers) arising from the medial aspect of the calcaneum (C).

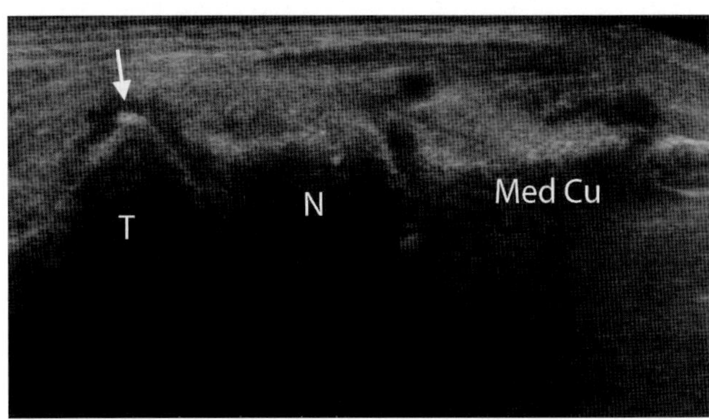

Fig. 6.10 A large osteophyte (*white arrow*) in this patient at the talonavicular joint is causing a palpable lump on the dorsum of the foot, which is the primary complaint of this patient. Talus (T), navicular (N), and medial cuneiform (Med Cu) bones.

Overuse leading to tendinous pathologies of the long tendons running through the foot and ankle will also show up in a variety of ultrasound appearances. These include fluid within the tendon sheaths, tendinopathy, and tendon ruptures (**Fig. 6.11**).

Inflammatory

Infections

Infections of the foot and ankle are encountered in patients with peripheral neuropathy. Pathologies are wide ranging spanning from abscesses, cellulitis, and osteomyelitis. With most of the soft tissue structures being relatively superficial, many of these changes may be easily accessed with ultrasound (**Fig. 6.12**). Nevertheless, bony lesions such as osteomyelitis are still better evaluated via radiography, computed tomography (CT), or magnetic resonance imaging (MRI). Postoperative infective complications can also commonly be assessed (**Fig. 6.13**).

Plantar Fasciitis

Overuse as well as abnormal biomechanics of the foot and ankle may result in the development of plantar fasciitis. Sonographic evaluation reveals a thickened plantar fascia as well as reduction in the echogenicity of the fascia (**Fig. 6.14**).

Traumatic

Trauma frequently occurs due to "twisting" of the ankle. Lauge-Hansen described a classification of malleolar fractures (**Table 6.1**). The most common ligament injury in the ankle joint is to the anterior talofibular ligament (**Fig. 6.15**). Associated injuries to the calcaneofibular ligament at the lateral ankle can also be picked up on ultrasound. Deltoid ligament injuries are less common. Similar to ligaments, the long tendons that traverse the ankle and foot can be injured (**Fig. 6.16**).

A

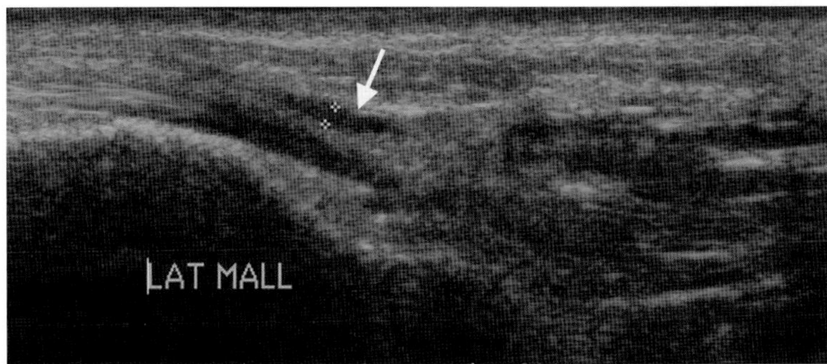

B

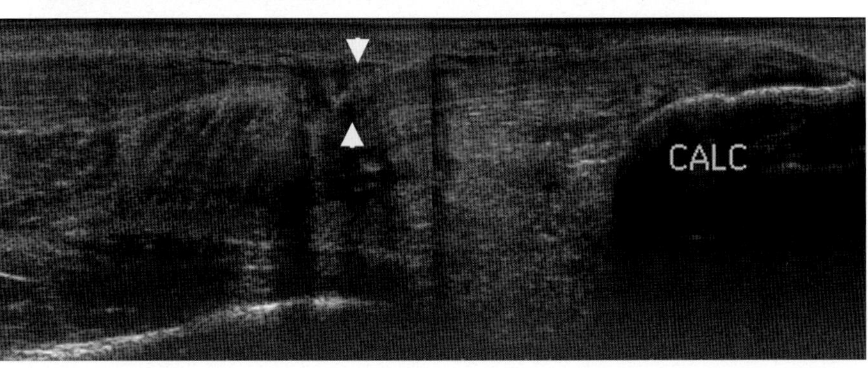

Fig. 6.11 **(A)** Fluid as indicated by the anechoic region between the calipers is seen to surround the peroneus brevis tendon in this patient with peroneus brevis tendinitis. **(B)** An almost complete tear of the Achilles tendon (*white arrows*). This commonly occurs at the musculotendinous junction of the Achilles tendon and is frequently associated with an increase in physical activity of a previously sedentary individual.

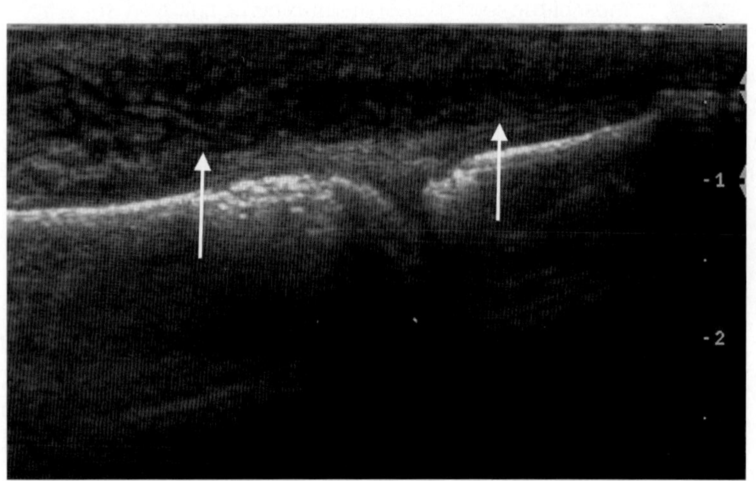

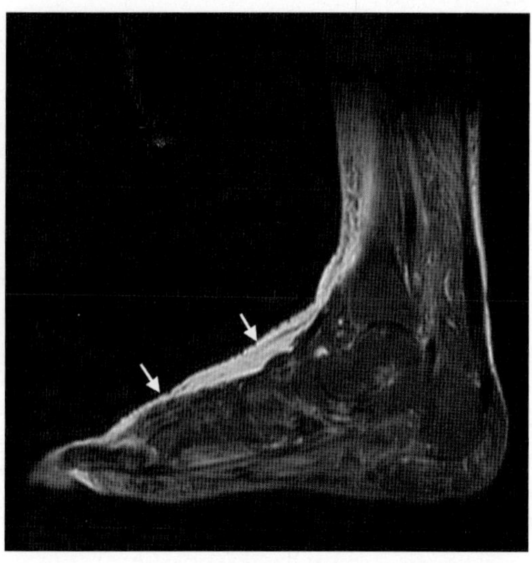

Fig. 6.12 **(A)** Examination of the forefoot reveals a thickened and edematous subcutaneous tissue (*white arrows*). The overlying skin was observed to be erythematous during scanning. Features are compatible with cellulitis. **(B)** An inversion recovery sagittal magnetic resonance image of the foot shows subcutaneous tissue thickening with T2 prolongation (*white arrows*) compatible with cellulitis of the foot and ankle.

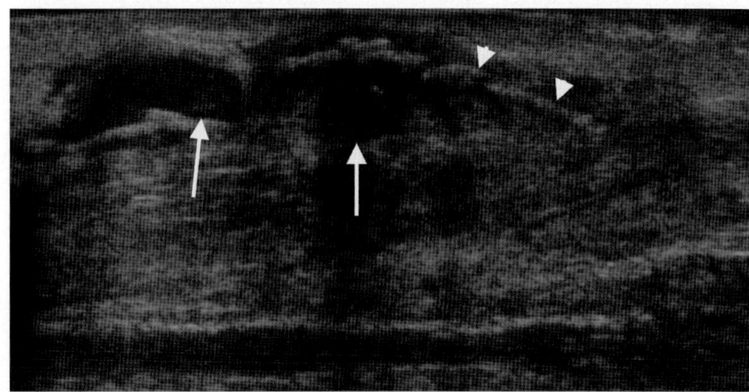

Fig. 6.13 Ultrasound over a tender region of an Achilles tendon repair showing collections (*white arrows*) in the region of the repair site. The tendon repair sutures (*white arrowheads*) can be visualized.

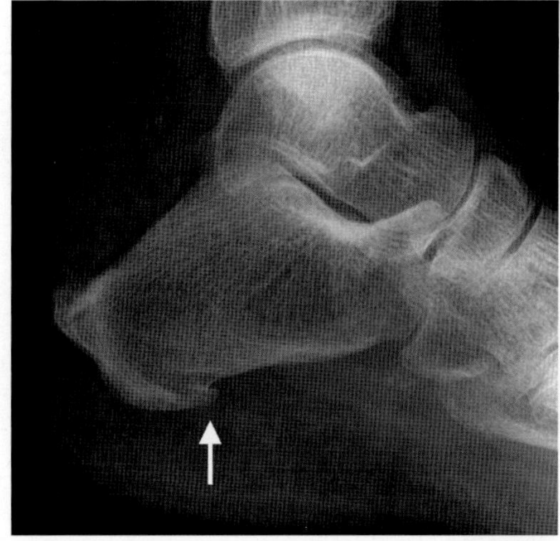

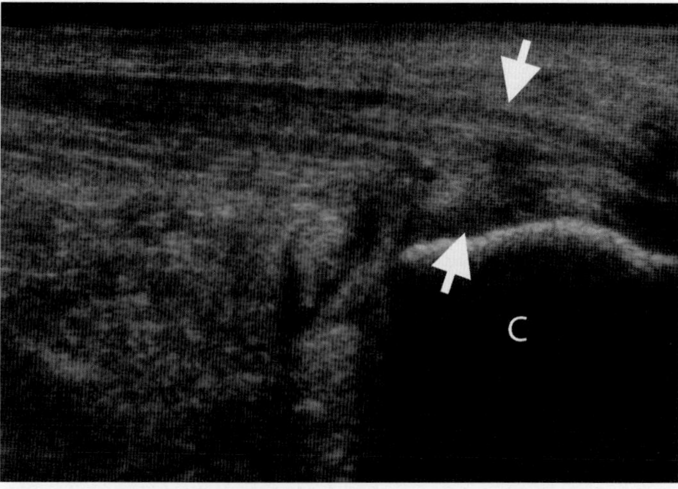

Fig. 6.14 **(A)** A plain radiograph of the calcaneum showing a prominent calcaneal spur of this patient with plantar fasciitis. **(B)** Sonographic examination showing thickening of the plantar fascia at its origin near the medial tubercle of the calcaneum (C).

Table 6.1 Lauge-Hansen Classification of Ankle Injuries

Type	
1	Supination–Adduction
2	Supination–External rotation
3	Pronation–Adduction
4	Pronation–Eversion
5	Pronation–Dorsiflexion

Fractures are conventionally detected via radiographs, but may be incidentally picked up on ultrasound. Fractures can either appear as a step in the cortical outline or as a raised hump in the cortical outline when periosteal new bone formation has occurred (**Fig. 6.17**).

Nonradiopaque foreign bodies such as wood and plastic are better detected on ultrasound (**Fig. 6.18**). Left unextracted, granulation tissue can surround these foreign bodies.

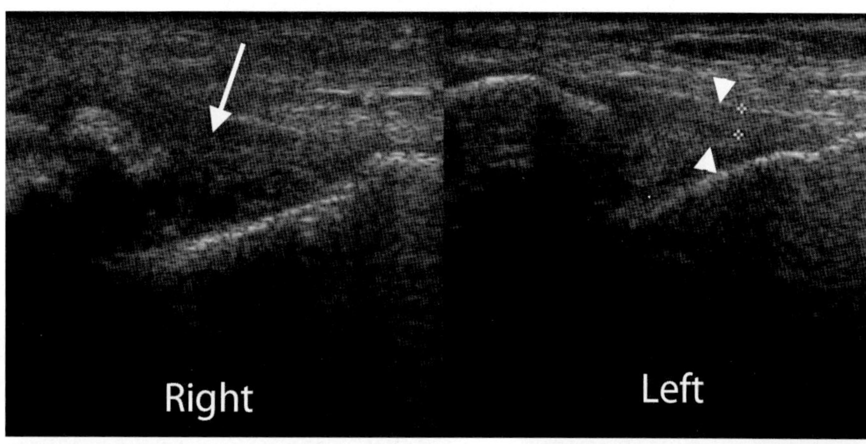

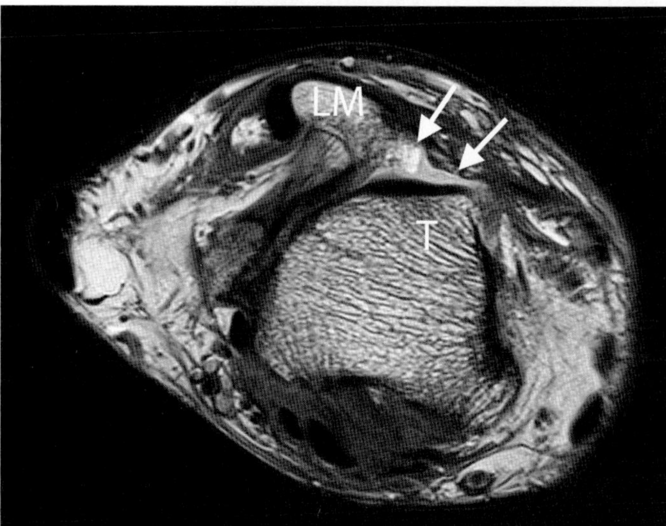

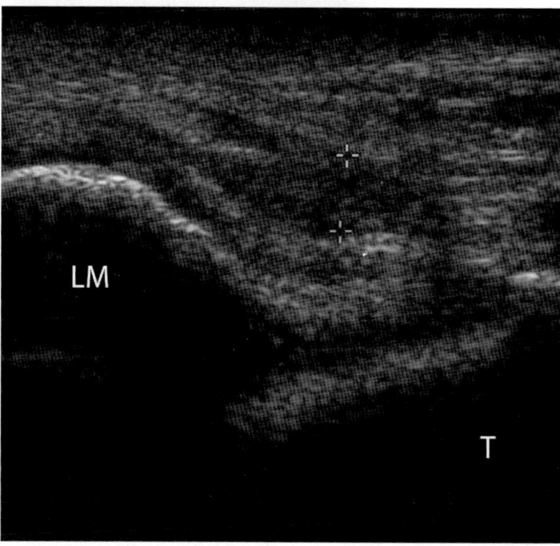

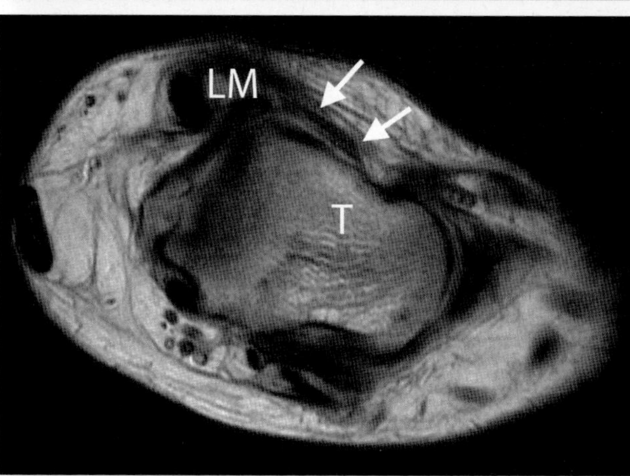

Fig. 6.15 **(A)** The right ankle of this patient showing an absent anterior talofibular ligament (*white arrow*) where it is expected to be found, indicating a complete tear of the ligament. Ultrasound examination of the contralateral normal ankle reveals a normal anterior talofibular ligament (*white arrowheads*) at its expected location. **(B)** A comparable proton density axial magnetic resonance image of the ankle rotated to the ultrasound scanning orientation showing the absence of the normal anterior talofibular ligament (*white arrows*) where it is normally expected between the lateral malleolus (LM) and talus (T). **(C)** The anterior talofibular ligament (between calipers) is markedly thickened, indicating chronic injury with scarring of the ligament. LM, lateral malleolus; T, talus. **(D)** A comparable proton density axial magnetic resonance image rotated to match the ultrasound scanning orientation showing a thick anterior talofibular ligament (*white arrows*) indicating an old or chronic injury.

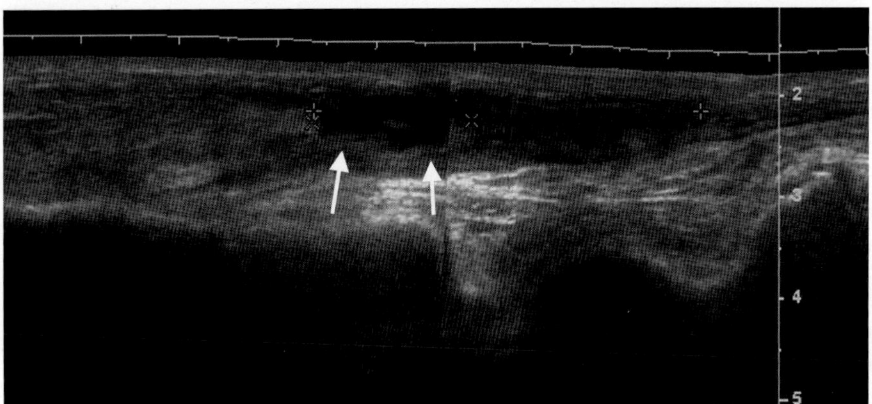

Fig. 6.16 The tibialis anterior tendon is seen with a hypoechoic gap (*between white arrows*) indicating a tear of the tendon with the torn ends not in apposition with each other.

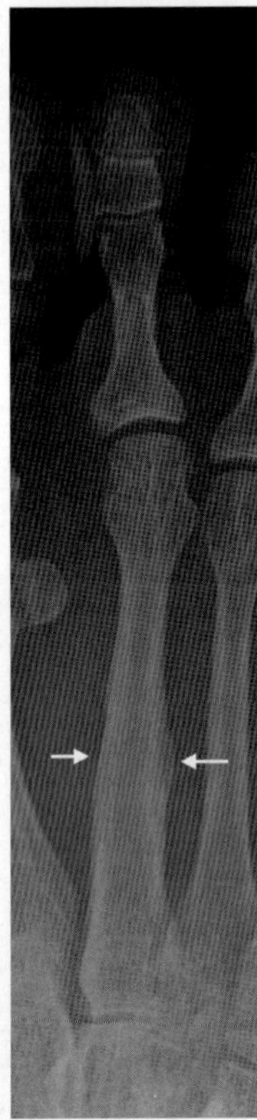

A

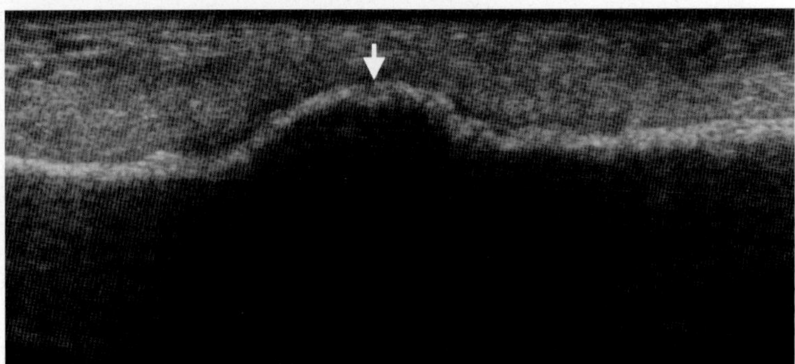

B

Fig. 6.17 **(A)** Plain radiograph of the second metatarsal shows a stress fracture at the shaft with surrounding periosteal new bone formation (*white arrows*). **(B)** Ultrasound over this site of tenderness reveals a hump (*white arrow*) in the cortical outline depicting the periosteal new bone formation.

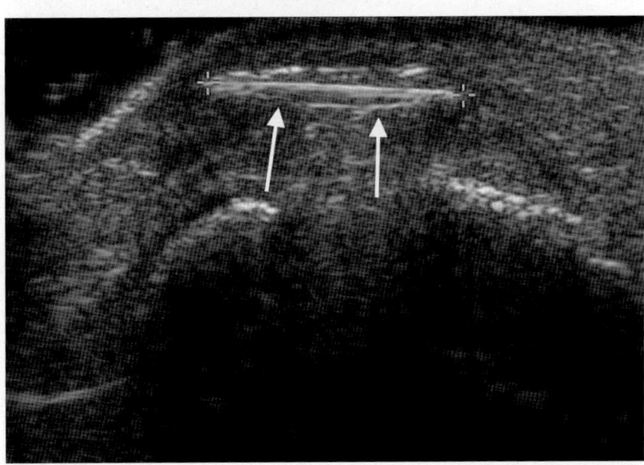

A

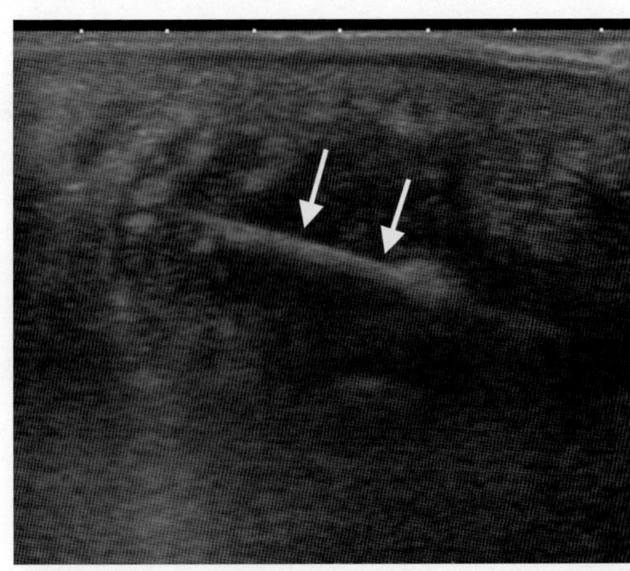

B

Fig. 6.18 **(A)** A glass foreign body in the sole of the foot showing up as a linear hyperechoic structure (*white arrows*). **(B)** A wooden kebab stick foreign body shows up as a linear hyperechoic structure on ultrasound (*white arrows*). There is adjacent soft tissue edema and pus as indicated by the surrounding hypoechoic region.

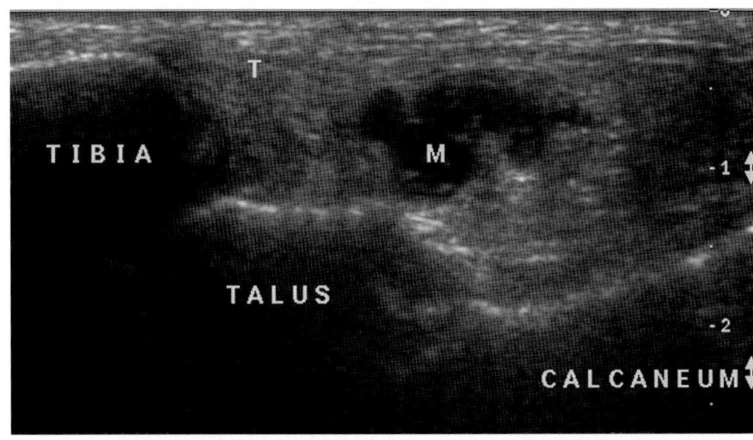

Fig. 6.19 A multiloculated hypoechoic lesion (M) at the medial aspect of the ankle joint just adjacent to the tibialis posterior tendon (T), which was surgically proven to be a multiloculated ganglion cyst.

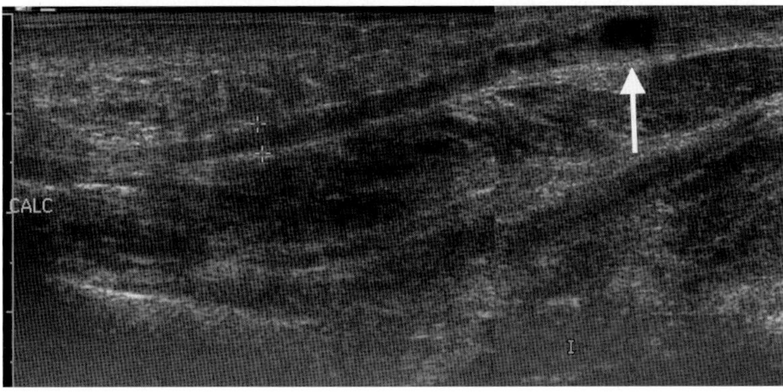

Fig. 6.20 The plantar fascia (*between calipers*) is traced from the calcaneum (calc) to one of the palpable lumps in the sole (*white arrow*) representing a plantar fibroma.

Tumoral and Tumorlike Masses

Ganglion Cyst

A ganglion cyst is the most common mass of the foot and ankle. Ultrasound can aid in assessing the internal structure of these cysts to distinguish it from a complex mass, which will need further evaluation (**Fig. 6.19**). The intimate relation of these ganglion cysts with the surrounding tendons and other structures can also be studied with ultrasound to guide the surgeon should removal be contemplated.

Plantar Fibromatosis

Plantar fibromatosis is a relatively uncommon condition of an unencapsulated fibromatosis of the plantar fascia. This can present with either a solitary mass or as multiple nodules, which are typically located at the central and medial components of the plantar fascia (**Fig. 6.20**).

This is a benign condition and surgery is usually considered should the patient be symptomatic. However, the high rate of local recurrence may result in extensive surgeries over time in some patients.

Morton Neuroma

This is a benign perineural fibroma of the intermetatarsal plantar nerve, frequently of the third and fourth metatarsal spaces. Symptoms include a “shooting” pain in the contiguous halves of the two neighboring toes, although a numbness or paresthesia may also be encountered.

Sonographically, the lesion is usually hypoechoic to muscle and demonstration of a noncompressible hypoechoic mass is often considered diagnostic (**Fig. 6.21**).

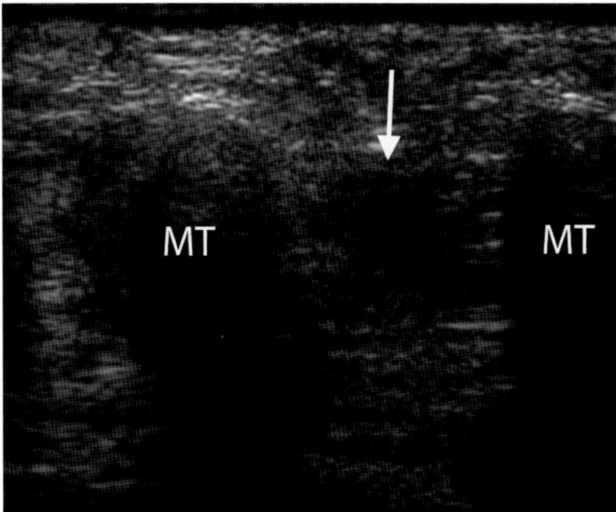

Fig. 6.21 A hypoechoic mass (*white arrow*) is located in between two metatarsals (MT) compatible with a neuroma of the common plantar digital nerve, otherwise known as a Morton neuroma.

Artifacts

Anisotropy is an issue for evaluation of the foot and ankle, especially for the long tendons which traverse and curve past the ankle joint. The operator should adhere to proper scanning technique to prevent anisotropy. It should be remembered that the tendons and ligament may not run parallel to the skin surface and the transducer may need to be adjusted accordingly. For example, the anterior talofibular ligament often runs at an oblique angle to the skin surface.

The foot and ankle has an undulating surface. The usage of sufficient coupling gel or a water bath can help create better sonographic coupling.

Pearls and Pitfalls

- A systematic approach to sonographic evaluation of the foot and ankle will help the evaluation of this complex anatomic part.
- A targeted sonographic evaluation may be used when the patient has focal symptoms or signs. Scanning the site of symptoms while reproducing the situation in which they occur is helpful in identifying the problem.
- The easiest place to start identifying the tendons is behind the malleoli in the short axis. After that, following the tendons is relatively easy so long as the transducer is kept perpendicular to the tendon to avoid anisotropy.
- A combination of a linear transducer with a small footprint for short axis views and a long footprint for longitudinal axis views is ideal. Extended field of view imaging with software that can reconstruct a larger image based on smaller images is helpful.

Suggested Readings

Cardinal E, Chhem RK, Beauregard CG, Aubin B, Pelletier M. Plantar fasciitis: sonographic evaluation. Radiology 1996;201(1):257–259

Lauge-Hansen N. Fractures of the ankle. II. Combined experimental-surgical and experimental-roentgenologic investigations. Arch Surg 1950;60(5):957–985

Manthey DE, Storrow AB, Milbourn JM, Wagner BJ. Ultrasound versus radiography in the detection of soft-tissue foreign bodies. Ann Emerg Med 1996;28(1):7–9

Ortega R, Fessell DP, Jacobson JA, Lin J, Van Holsbeeck MT, Hayes CW. Sonography of ankle ganglia with pathologic correlation in 10 pediatric and adult patients. AJR Am J Roentgenol 2002;178(6):1445–1449

Quinn TJ, Jacobson JA, Craig JG, van Holsbeeck MT. Sonography of Morton's neuromas. AJR Am J Roentgenol 2000;174(6):1723–1728

7 Imaging of the Hip

Ahmet Tuncay Turgut, Elif Ergun, Pinar Koşar, and Vikram S. Dogra

Based on its wide availability, noninvasiveness, no need for patient preparation, portability, and the absence of ionizing radiation, ultrasound is the primary imaging method for hip disorders. This is especially true for pediatric patients, whose motion or lack of cooperation presents a contraindication for other imaging modalities, and for infants because of the inability to image cartilage by radiography at this age. The management of some clinical problems can usually be performed by the imaging data provided by ultrasound alone. Moreover, the relatively lower cost of the ultrasound equipment compared with other cross-sectional methods like computed tomography (CT) or magnetic resonance imaging (MRI) makes this method an essential tool for hip evaluation for cases in which close follow-up or an extensive screening may be required.

Clinical Indications

The main clinical indication for an ultrasound evaluation of the hip is the investigation of developmental dysplasia of the hip (DDH) or the follow-up of the pediatric cases with DDH. Another indication is the evaluation of the cases with hip pain, mostly having a joint effusion. The technique is also used as an adjunct to other alternative imaging modalities for the diagnosis of Legg–Calve–Perthes disease, usually presenting with the complaint of hip pain. Moreover, it is useful for the diagnosis of proximal femoral focal deficiency. It can also be used to guide percutaneous aspiration of the articular and/or extraarticular fluid collections.

Pathologies

Developmental Dysplasia of the Hip

DDH includes a wide spectrum of pathologic conditions, from the stable acetabular dysplasia to irreducible dislocations. Since Hippocrates, the term congenital dysplasia was used to describe hip dysplasia and displacement in infants because it was thought to be of congenital origin. Since the 1980s, the developmental nature of the disease has been clearly understood as some infants with a normal hip examination at birth developed dysplasia of the hip during the first months after birth. Acetabular dysplasia and ligamentous laxity are the key factors in the pathophysiology of DDH.

Pathophysiology of Developmental Dysplasia of the Hip

- Acetabular dysplasia and the ligamentous laxity are the key features.
- Adequate development of the hip joint necessitates a balanced interaction of the acetabulum and femur.
- Dysplastic acetabulum causes incomplete support for the femoral head and allows its movement freely in and out of the socket resulting in hip instability.
- Acetabular development deteriorates in the lax hip where the femur moves freely in and out of the socket, resulting in acetabular dysplasia.
- DDH is three times more common on the left side due to the left occiput anterior positioning of the nonbreech fetus, in which the left hip lies against the mother's spine and hip abduction is limited.
- There are two types of dislocation: typical dislocation (98%) and teratologic dislocation (2%) with all parts of the hip joint being abnormal.

To prevent long-term complications of the disease, an early and correct diagnosis as well as an effective treatment strategy is very important. Ultrasound is an excellent diagnostic tool for the evaluation of infants with hip dysplasia; both clinically and radiographically undetected abnormalities can be easily demonstrated by ultrasound examination alone. Graf, an Austrian pediatric orthopedic surgeon, first introduced the use of ultrasound in the diagnosis of pediatric hip dysplasia in 1980. For 30 years, it has been used to examine the hips of infants in clinical practice.

Incidence

There is no gold standard for the diagnosis of DDH in the newborn period. Both physical examination and various imaging studies, such as radiography and ultrasound, have false-positive and false-negative results. Although MRI and arthrography demonstrate the precise anatomic details of the hip, these techniques are not suitable as screening methods; instead, they are used for problem solving in selected cases. Moreover, various factors such as the age of the child at the time of the examination, genetic and racial factors, diagnostic criteria and methods, influence the incidence of

DDH. Therefore, it is not possible to give a true incidence of DDH: its incidence can only be estimated. In the newborn period, the reported incidence of DDH varies from 1 to 5%. The incidence of frank dislocations is 1 to 1.5 per 1000 newborns.

Normal Sonographic Anatomy of the Hip

Knowledge of the sonographic hip anatomy is crucial for an accurate diagnosis of DDH (**Fig. 7.1**).

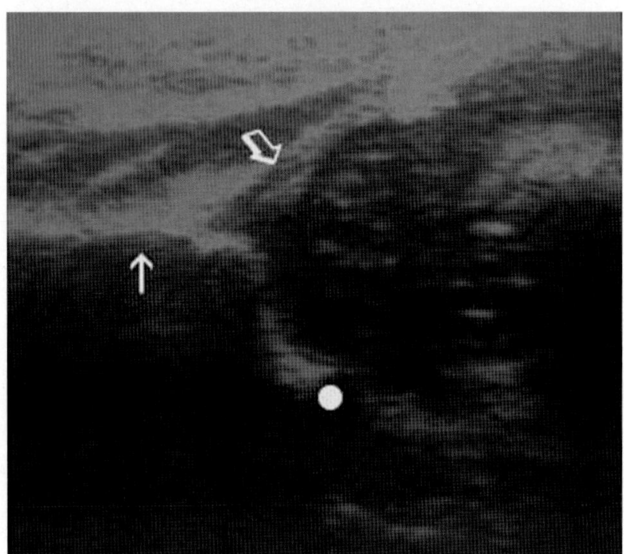

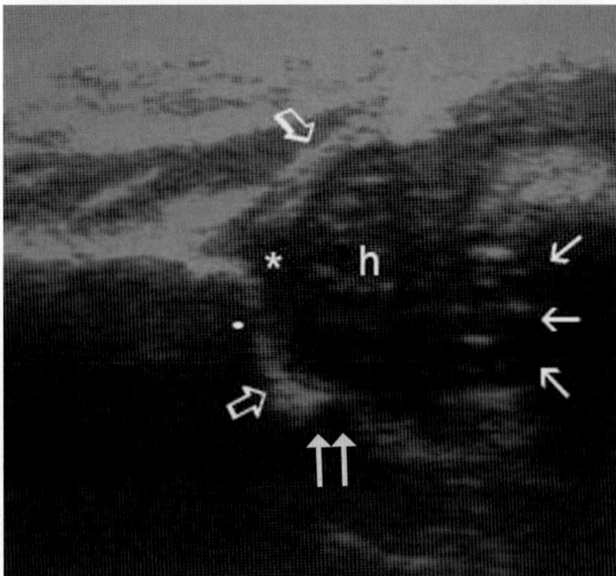

Fig. 7.1 Standard coronal plane. **(A)** Presence of the three landmarks, which are the lower limb of os ilium (*circle*), midportion of the acetabular roof accompanied by straight iliac wing parallel to the horizontal plane (*arrow*), and labrum (*open arrow*) should be checked. **(B)** Anatomic structures to be identified adjunct to the ultrasound landmarks are the chondroosseous junction (*arrows*), joint capsule (*oblique open arrow*), head of the femur (h), hyaline cartilage roof (*), bony acetabular roof (*straight open arrow*), bony rim (*white dot*), and triradiate cartilage (*double arrow*) are shown.

Sonographic Anatomy

- The ilium, ischium, and pubis converge to form the acetabulum.
- At the junction of these three bones a cartilaginous structure called the triradiate cartilage is situated, which is the most central and the deepest part of the acetabulum. It appears hypoechoic on ultrasound and allows through transmission of the sound beam.
- Acetabulum has a bony and cartilaginous portion in the newborn.
- The cartilaginous portion has a triangular hyaline cartilage roof appearing hypoechoic on ultrasound and fibrocartilaginous acetabular labrum with triangular hyperechoic ultrasound appearance.
- The base of the hyaline cartilage roof triangle is in contact with the femoral head and the apex is located superiorly on the iliac wing.
- In the well-developed bony acetabulum, the base of cartilaginous triangle is narrow; in the immature bony acetabulum, it is broad.
- The os ilium extends superiorly from the upper part of the acetabulum to form the iliac wing.
- At birth, the femoral head, greater trochanter, and proximal portion of the femoral neck—as they are made up of hyaline cartilage and are separated from the bony shaft by the chondroosseous border—appear hypoechoic on ultrasound, whereas the chondroosseous junction is highly echogenic. The femoral shaft is also seen as a highly echogenic linear structure below the chondroosseous junction.
- The ossification center of the femoral head, which may be present at birth, is seen as an echogenic structure on ultrasound. It appears on ultrasound 3 to 4 weeks earlier than it appears on plain x-ray. The center is not round and it is not always in the center of the head, so it cannot be used to assess the position of the head sonographically. It is not possible to determine the size of the ossification center by ultrasound.

Technical Guidelines

Ultrasound's real-time capability allows evaluation of the dynamics of the instability as well as morphology of the hip. Soon after Graf's initial publications about the use of hip ultrasound for the diagnosis of DDH, a different technique was developed by Novick et al and Harcke et al known as the "dynamic method"; it is an imaging mimic of a clinical hip examination. Moreover, other techniques such as a modified Graf technique (Rosendahl), the Morin technique, and the modified Morin technique (Terjesen) are routinely used in the diagnosis of the hip. Whatever method is used, it is apparent that ultrasound is more sensitive than a clinical examination.

Graf's Static Technique

Graf's static technique is based on a morphologic evaluation of the hip in a coronal neutral view. In this technique, no emphasis is given to the position of the femoral head. The

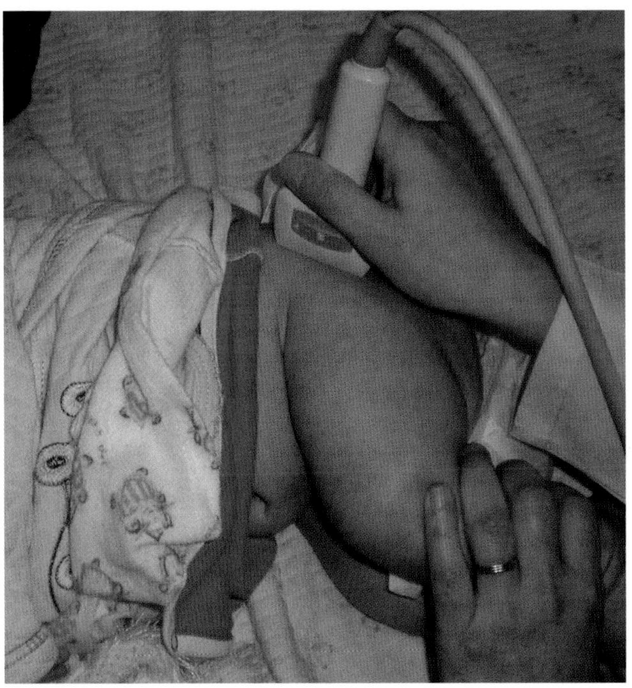

Fig. 7.2 Patient is in lateral decubitus position with the leg in neutral position and the transducer oriented longitudinally.

patient lies in the lateral decubitus position with the leg in neutral position slightly flexed at the hip and knee. The transducer is longitudinally oriented from a lateral approach to the hip (**Fig. 7.2**). Graf designed a positioning device placing the infant in the desired position, but the use of this device is optional. The highest frequency linear ultrasound probe should be used to permit an optimal penetration of the soft tissues.

From a technical point of view, obtaining images in the same section through the hip is crucial for a correct and reproducible ultrasound examination. Graf described a standard coronal plane for this purpose.

Standard Coronal Plane

- Involves the lower limb of the bony ilium in the depth of the acetabular fossa, midposition of the acetabular roof, and the acetabular labrum (**Fig. 7.1A**)
- The iliac wing above the bony roof should be straight and parallel to the transducer to make sure that the sectional plane through the midposition of the acetabular roof is obtained (**Fig. 7.1A**).
- Anatomic structures to be identified as ultrasound landmarks are the chondroosseous junction, femoral head, synovial fold, joint capsule, acetabular structures from lateral to medial (labrum, hyaline cartilage, and bony acetabular roof), and the osseous rim (the point where concavity of the bony acetabulum changes to the convexity of ilium) (**Fig. 7.1B**).

After subjective evaluation of the bony acetabular modeling, the bony rim, the cartilage roof triangle acetabular inclination angle (α), and the cartilage roof angle (β) are measured.

Measurement of α and β Angles

- To define these angles, three measurement lines are drawn on the image.
- Bony roof line is tangential to the bony roof drawn from the inferior limb of os ilium laterally to the promontory (**Fig. 7.3A**).
- Baseline originates at the apex of the cartilaginous roof triangle and it is tangential to the lateral surface of the iliac wing (**Fig. 7.3B**).
- Cartilage roof line is drawn from the bony rim through the center of the acetabular labrum (**Fig. 7.3C**).
- α is the angle between the bony roof line and baseline and is the measurement of the maturity of the bony roof (**Fig. 7.3D**).
- β is the angle between the cartilage roof line and baseline and indicates the degree of cartilaginous roof coverage (**Fig. 7.3D**).

Graf classified the hips into five main groups.

Graf's Classification

- Type I is mature hip (**Fig. 7.4A**) with α ^{3}60 degrees. It is divided into two subgroups as type Ia and type Ib having a β angle greater than and less than 55 degrees, respectively.
- Type IIa is the physiologic immature hip (**Fig. 7.4B**): the α angle is between 50 and 59 degrees in an infant younger than 12 weeks of age.
- If type IIa morphology persists beyond 12 weeks, it is termed as type IIb (acetabular dysplasia): α angle is between 50 and 59 degrees.
- Type IIc is the hip in critical range (α = 43 to 49 degrees). It is divided into two subgroups: type IIc stable and type IIc unstable.
- In type IId hips, the α angle is in the same range as in the type IIc hip; however, decentering of the hip starts and $\beta >$ 77 degrees in type IId hips.
- Type III and type IV hips are both decentered hips, $\alpha < 43$ degrees and $\beta > 77$ degrees in both of them. Determination of the position of the cartilaginous roof is crucial for their differentiation, which is pushed cranially in type III hips (**Fig. 7.4C**) and caudally in type IV hips (**Fig. 7.4D**).
- Type III hip is further divided into two subgroups according to the echogenicity of the cartilaginous roof. In type IIIa hips it is hypoechoic, whereas in type IIIb hips the hyaline cartilage is deformed and appears hyperechoic.

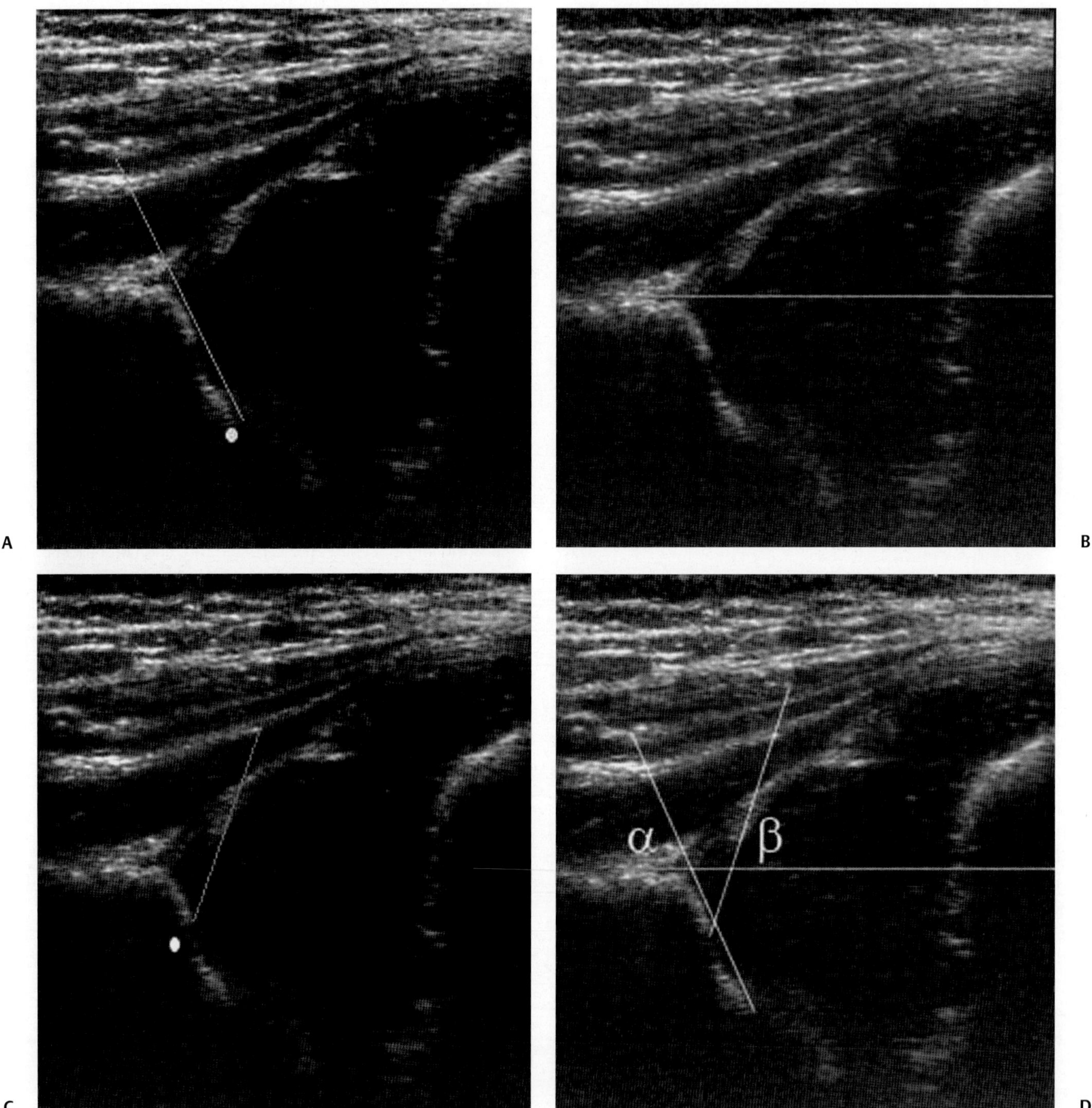

Fig. 7.3 **(A)** Bony roof line; tangential to the bony roof and drawn from the inferior limb of os ilium (*white dot*) laterally. **(B)** Baseline; tangential to the lateral part of the iliac wing and drawn from the uppermost part of the hyaline cartilage roof caudally. **(C)** Cartilaginous roof line; drawn from the bony rim (*white dot*) through the center of the labrum. **(D)** α angle between baseline and bony roof line and β angle between baseline and cartilaginous roof line are shown.

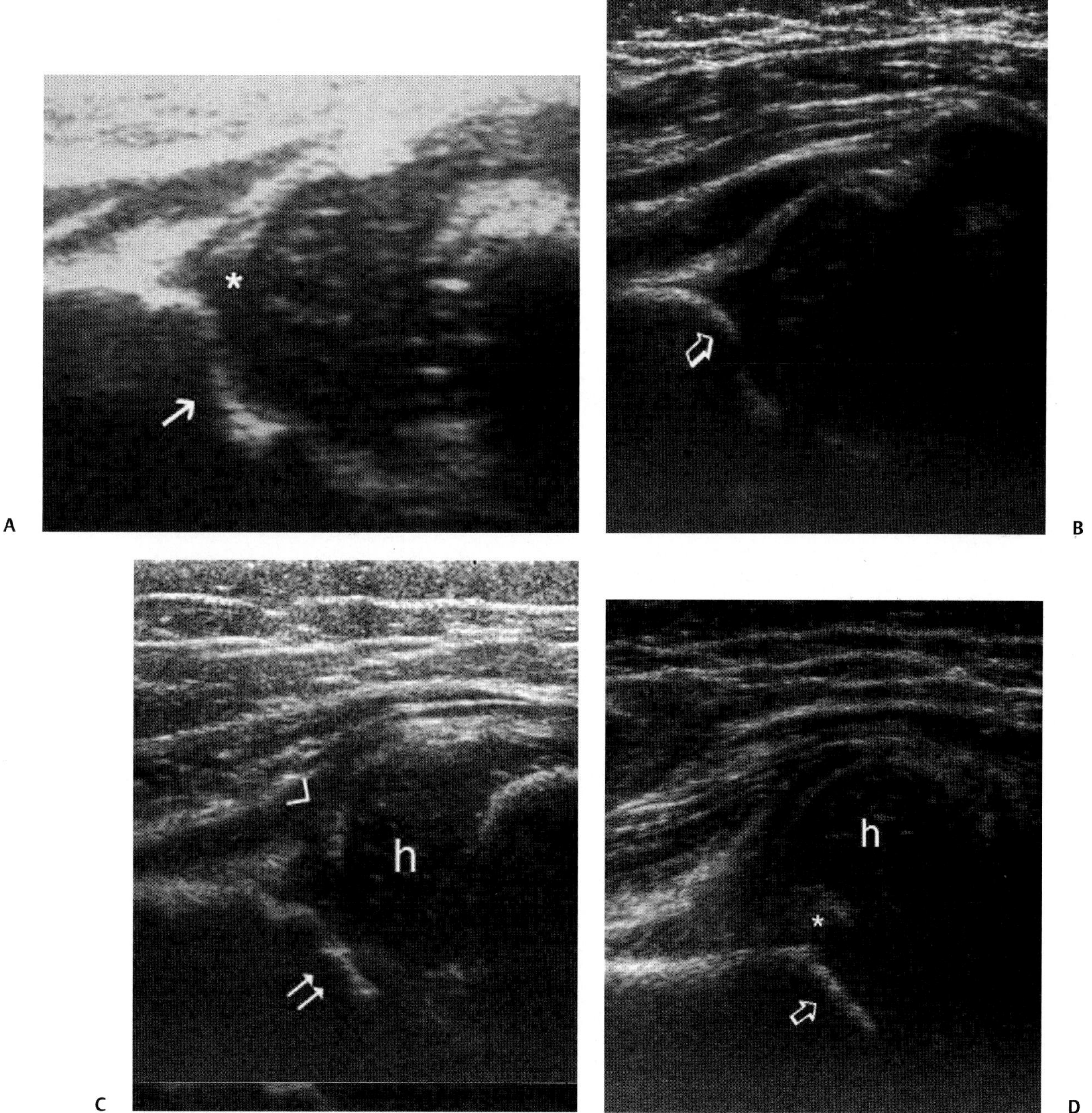

Fig. 7.4 **(A)** Type I hip with a well-developed bony roof (*arrow*), angular bony rim and a covering cartilaginous roof (*) is shown. **(B)** Type IIa hip with a round bony rim (*open arrow*) is depicted. **(C)** Type IIIa: bony roof (*double arrow*) is poorly developed, bony rim is flattened and the cartilage roof (*arrowhead*) is pressed upward by the superolaterally displaced femoral head (h). **(D)** Type IV: bony roof is poor (*straight open arrow*), bony rim is flattened and cartilage roof (*) is pushed downward by the displaced femoral head (h).

Harcke's Dynamic Method

In this method, emphasis is given to the position of the femoral head and the stability of the hip. A visual assessment of the acetabular morphology and the degree of acetabular maturity is also made. The patient lies in a supine or a slight decubitus position with a towel placed under the hip being examined. While examining the right hip, the transducer should be in the left hand and the hip should be positioned by the right hand and the opposite is done for the left hip. The images are obtained in four planes using a lateral approach.

Harcke's Imaging Planes

- Transverse neutral view enables the assessment of the position of the femoral head of the femur, which should be well centered over the triradiate cartilage in a normal hip.
- Transverse flexion view obtained by stress application via Barlow maneuver (gentle posterior push to the hip which is flexed and adducted) provides the assessment of hip stability.
- The degree of posterior, lateral, or posterolateral instability is best assessed by the aforementioned transverse views.
- Coronal views are used to assess acetabular morphology; they are most useful for observing displacement of the femoral head with a superior component.

1. Transverse neutral view (**Fig. 7.5**)
2. Transverse flexion view (**Fig. 7.6**)
3. Coronal neutral view
4. Coronal flexion view (**Fig. 7.7**)

In patients younger than 2 weeks old, a displacement of the femoral head up to 6 mm is considered normal. Nevertheless, the head should always be in its normal position at rest and after 2 weeks there should be no displacement. If the hip is dislocated, the reducibility should be checked by the Ortolani maneuver performed under ultrasound visualization, involving abduction and external rotation of the hip. Harcke classifies the hip as normal, subluxated, or dislocated when evaluating the position of the femoral head in the transverse neutral view and as lax, dislocatable, reducible, or not reducible by ultrasound evaluation under stress maneuvers.

Graf's static method has been criticized for requiring a higher level of experience, whereas Harcke's dynamic method mandates a certain operator skill to achieve a correct sectional plane.

Morin et al proposed another method of hip ultrasound in DDH in 1985, which was modified slightly by Terjesen et al in 1989.

Morin and Modified Morin (Terjesen) Technique

- A static method based on the assessment of the lateralization degree of the femoral head.
- On Harcke's coronal flexion view two lines are drawn parallel to Graf's baseline, one tangent to the lateral part of femoral head and the other tangential to the medial junction of the head and acetabular fossa.
- The ratio of the distance between the medial and iliac lines (d) and between the medial and lateral lines (D) multiplied by 100 indicates the percentage of femoral head covered by the bony acetabulum; with a value of >0.55 for the normal hip (**Fig. 7.8**).
- In Terjesen's method instead of the Graf's baseline, a line through the lateral bony rim of the acetabulum that is parallel to the long axis of the transducer is used. The "bony rim percentage," which is termed "femoral head coverage," is measured. The normal lower limit of this parameter is 47% for boys and 44% for girls.

In European countries, Graf's ultrasound technique or its modification is commonly used; in some areas of Europe, a modified Morin's method is frequently used, whereas Harcke's method is preferred occasionally in Europe. In North America, however, Harcke's dynamic method is widely used.

Recently, a guideline was developed by American Institute of Ultrasound in Medicine (AIUM) and the American College of Radiology (ACR) regarding the use of hip ultrasound for the detection of DDH. The guideline incorporates the basic principles of the Harcke, Graf, and Clarcke techniques in its recommended "Dynamic Standard Minimum" examination.

Dynamic Standard Minimum Examination

- Both acetabular morphology and stability of the hip are assessed.
- Morphologic assessment is performed in the coronal neutral view.
- Stability is determined by applying stress, while scanning in the transverse plane; the application of stress in the coronal plane is optional.
- Angular measurements of the acetabular landmarks are optional.

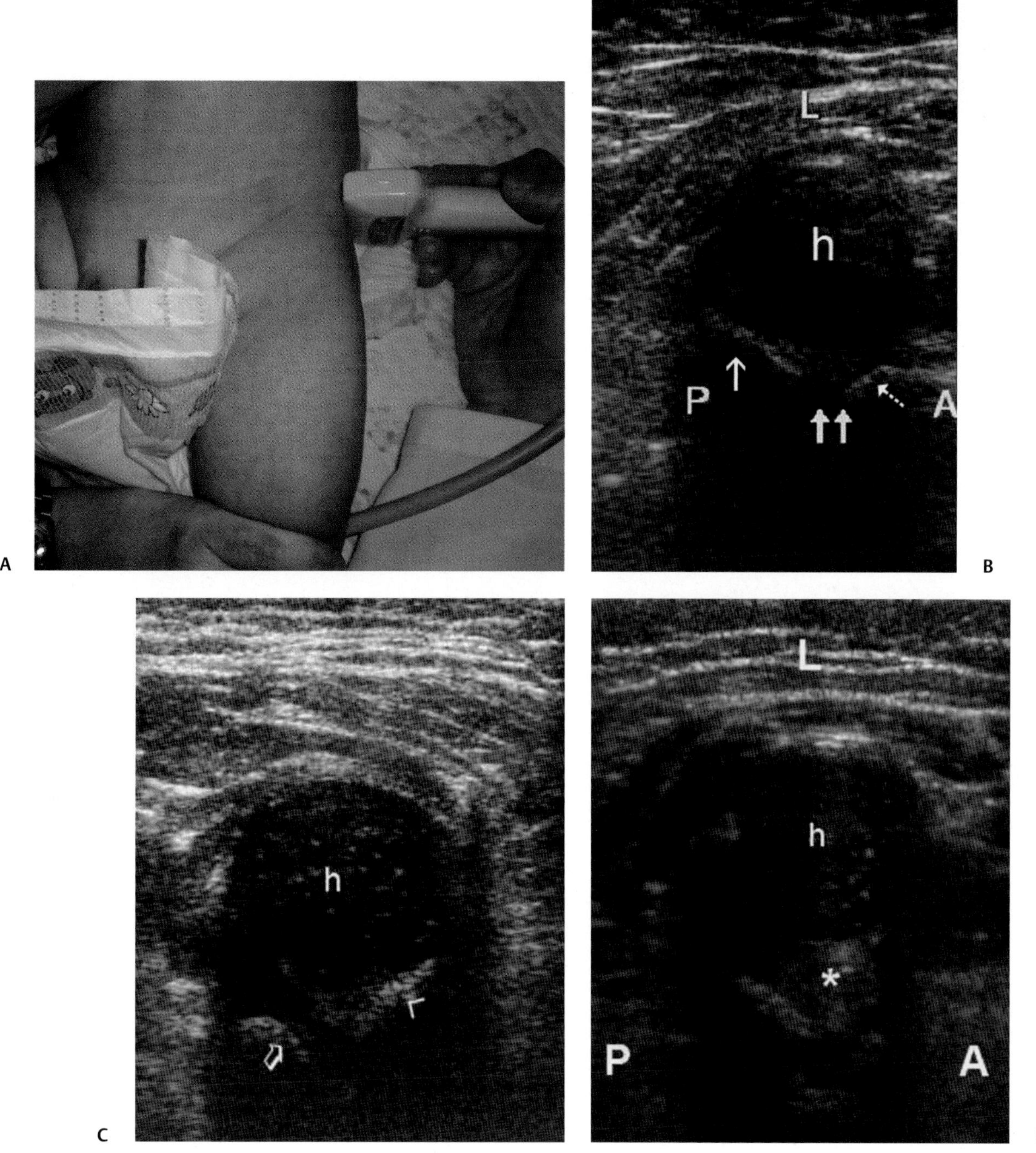

Fig. 7.5 Transverse neutral view. **(A)** Patient lies supine with the leg extended and the transducer is oriented in a transverse position. **(B)** Normal right hip with the femoral head (h) centered over the triradiate cartilage (*double arrow*), ischium (*arrow*) located posteriorly (P) and pubis (*dashed arrow*) seen anteriorly. **(C)** Sonogram revealing a subluxated hip with the posterolaterally displaced femoral head (h), which is not situated over the triradiate cartilage but still in contact with the ischium (*arrowhead*). Pubis (*open arrow*) is seen anteriorly. **(D)** Laterally (L) dislocated hip where femoral head (h) is not in contact with the acetabulum and echogenic pulvinar (*) is seen in between. A, anterior; P, posterior.

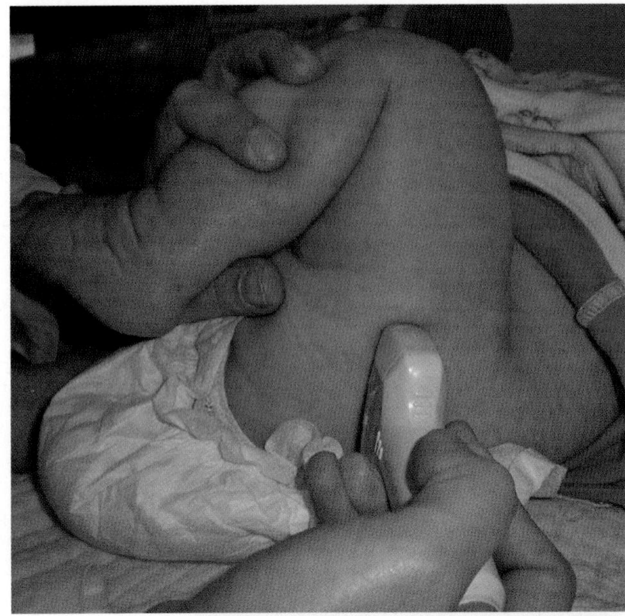

A

Fig. 7.6 Transverse flexion view. **(A)** Patient lies supine with flexed hip and knee and the transducer is oriented in a transverse position. **(B)** Sonogram of the abducted normal hip showing the femoral metaphysis (*arrow*) located anteriorly (A) and ischium (*double arrow*) located posteriorly (P) forming a smooth U shape and the femoral head (h) is situated in between. **(C)** Dislocated hip with laterally displaced femoral head (h) where there is no contact between femoral head (h) and ischium (*open arrow*). The U shape formed by the femoral metaphysis (*arrow*) and ischium (*open arrow*) is disturbed.

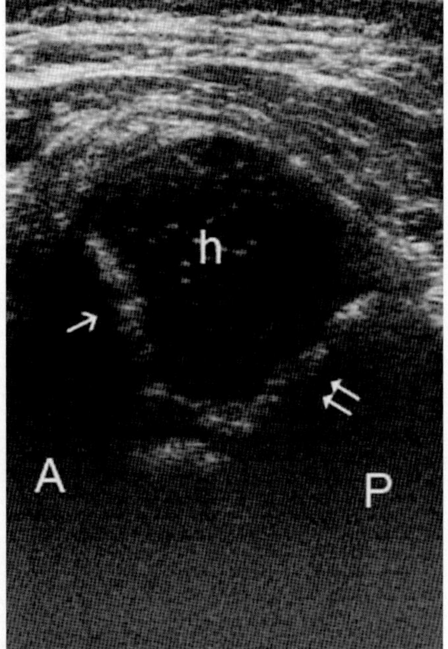

B

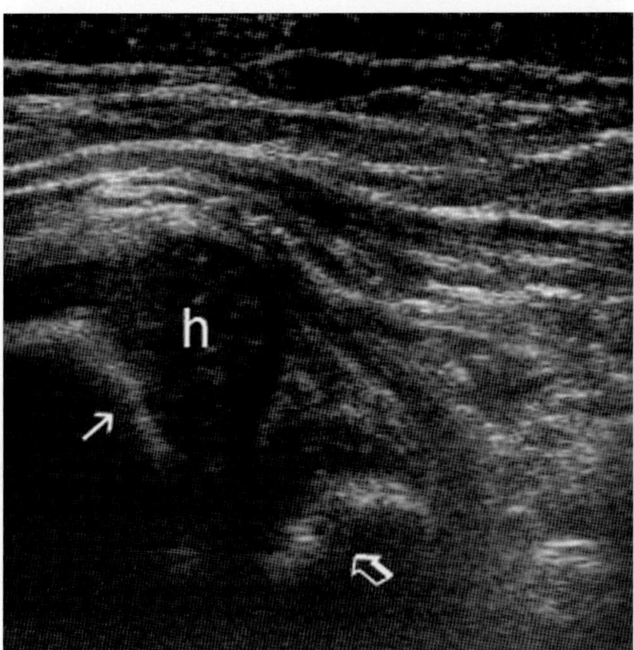

C

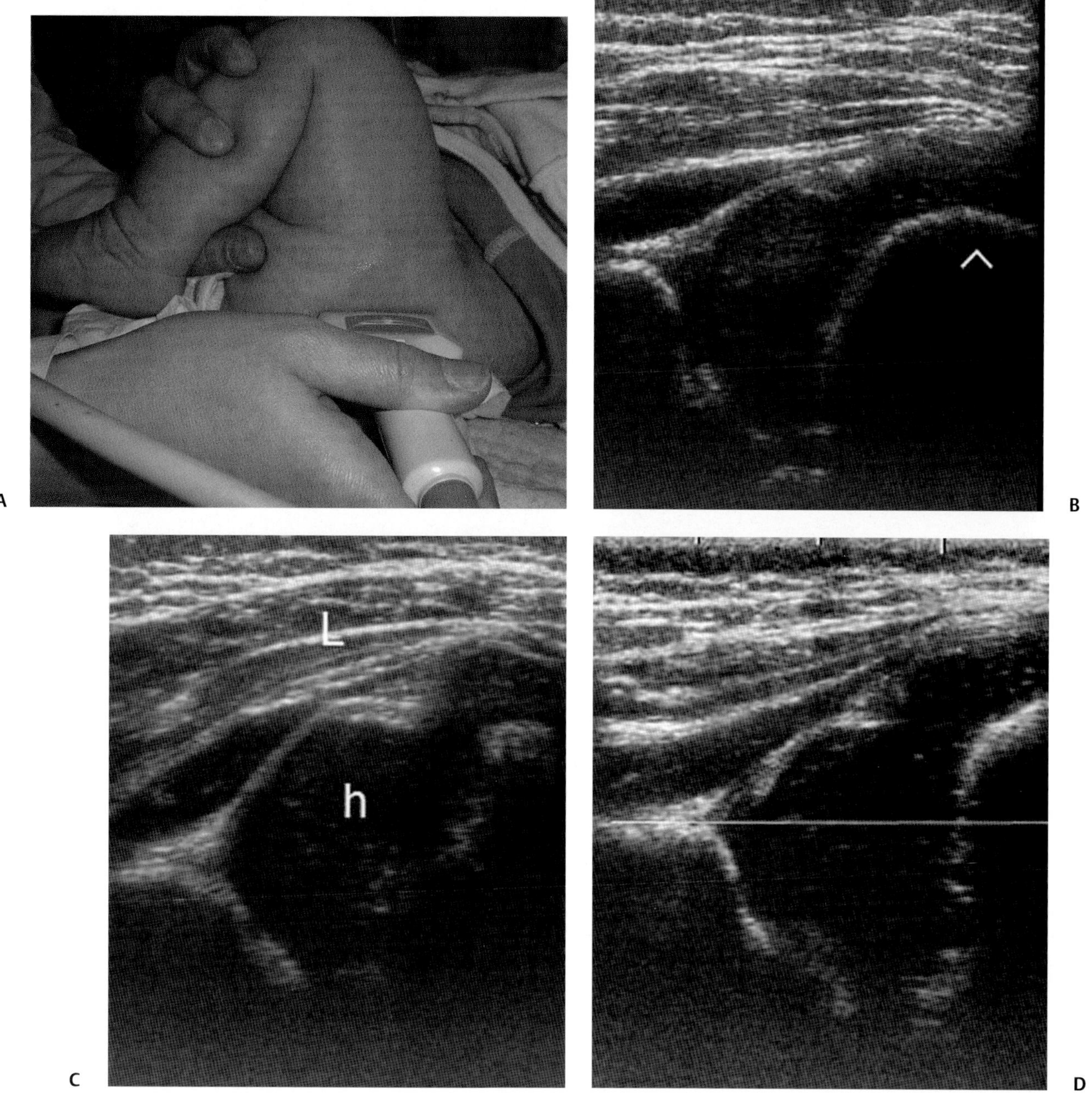

Fig. 7.7 Coronal flexion view. **(A)** Patient lies supine, flexed at hip and knee and the transducer is in longitudinal orientation. **(B)** The appearance of the anatomic structures is identical to the coronal neutral view except for the femoral shaft (*arrowhead*), which is seen as a curvilinear echogenicity. **(C)** Stress is applied to the hip shown in B with a gentle posterior push while the hip is adducted. The femoral head (h) is displaced laterally (L). **(D)** Equator sign demonstrated with a line drawn along the lateral border of the iliac bone and requiring the identification of at least 50% of the femoral head within the acetabulum is shown.

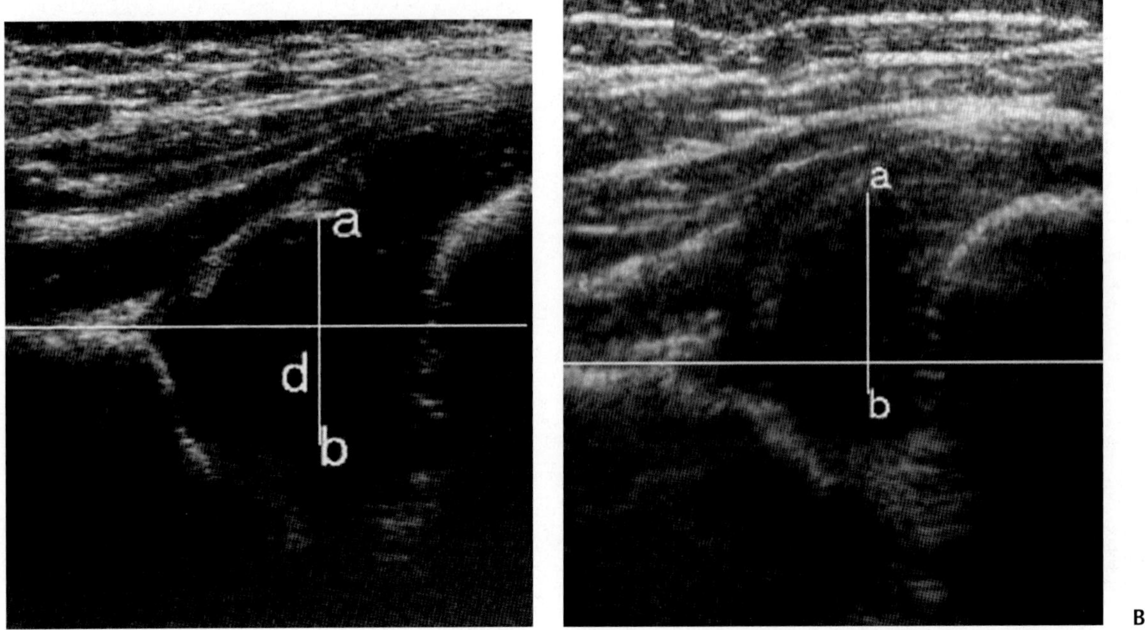

Fig. 7.8 **(A)** Morin ratio in a normal hip; d/D x 100 is greater than 0.55 [d = distance between iliac line and medial junction of the head and acetabular fossa (b), D = distance between lateral part of femoral head (a) and (b)]. **(B)** Morin ratio in a dislocated hip is less than 0.55.

Reporting the Sonographic Signs

Proper procedure is the key to an accurate imaging evaluation of the pathology, but the documentation of the different ultrasound signs is also very important. The aforementioned report of the AIUM and ACR suggests that acetabular morphology should be described in every report. Graf shares the same emphasis and recommends the usage of some basic terms to aid in the reporting process.

Description of Acetabular Morphology According to Graf

- First describe the bony roof.
- If it is well developed and mature like in type I hips "good" is the term used to describe the bony roof.
- If it is not developed enough with respect to the age of the child like in type IIb and type IIc hips "deficient" is the appropriate term.
- For type IIa hips, the term "adequate" is preferred.
- Bony rim can be described as angular (type I), rounded (type II hips), or flat (decentered joints).
- Acetabular cartilage roof should be described in every report and it may be
  - "covering" as in centered hips where the cartilage roof overlaps femoral head and helps to hold it in the socket.
  - "displaced" as in decentered hips where the cartilage roof is deformed and pushed by the displaced femoral head. It is either pushed cranially with normal hyaline cartilage roof echogenicity (type IIIa) or increased hyaline cartilage roof echogenicity (type IIIb) or pressed caudally (type IV).

Graf suggests mentioning α and β angles in every ultrasound report to define the morphologic evaluation more objectively. According to the AIUM report, the position of the femoral head should be noted at rest and while applying stress, and if the hip is subluxated or dislocated reducibility should be checked by real-time ultrasound imaging under the Ortalani maneuver, and it should be mentioned in the report. However, measurement of the acetabular angles and reporting them are optional.

Screening DDH by Ultrasound

Ultrasound has a high sensitivity in detecting DDH, which is desirable for a screening test. This technique is more sensitive than clinical examination and it is possible to detect clinically silent abnormalities by ultrasound. It is accepted that in infants with a normal ultrasound examination at birth the possibility of the development of DDH later is very low. Although an ideal screening test should be specific for the disease, ultrasound is a poorly specific examination for clinically significant DDH. It has been reported that a majority of cases with abnormal ultrasound findings regarding hip, normalize spontaneously without treatment. Depending on the screening method and the treatment threshold, ultrasound has a potential for increasing rates of overdiagnosis and unnecessary treatment of abnormalities that will resolve spontaneously. In addition, ultrasound may increase the number of unnecessary control examinations. There is no hard evidence that ultrasound screening may help to reduce the rates of cases with late DDH and the need for a surgical intervention.

Taking all these facts into consideration, it is not surprising that the role of ultrasound in screening DDH is still a controversial issue. A variety of screening programs are followed in Europe, Britain, and North America. In Britain and North America, routine screening programs are based on physical examination and selective ultrasound examination is performed for patients having high risk for DDH.

Risk Factors

1. Positive family history (especially a parent or sibling)
2. Breech presentation
3. Mechanical factors restricting space for in utero motion (maternal primiparity, oligohydramnios, bicornuate uterus, increased birth weight, twin birth)
4. Congenital torticollis, clubfoot, or congenital musculoskeletal abnormalities
5. Female gender (more susceptibility to maternal hormone relaxin causing ligamentous laxity)
6. Cultural factors (swaddling the infant)
7. Caesarean section

Ultrasound is currently used as a universal screening test in Europe. In reports published in 2000 and updated in 2005, the American Academy of Pediatrics (AAP) recommended the use of ultrasound as an adjunct to clinical examination. Furthermore, the AAP clearly indicated that ultrasound is the technique of choice for clarifying a physical finding, assessing infants with high risk, and monitoring the cases with DDH during treatment.

As a rule, ultrasound evaluation for screening purposes should be performed in the first 4 to 6 weeks of life.

Monitoring Treatment of DDH by Ultrasound

The Pavlik harness, a device that maintains the hip at 100 to 110 degrees of flexion and 30 to 40 degrees of abduction, is widely used in the treatment of infants with DDH. After 6 months of age, however, treatment becomes more difficult and closed or open reduction under general anesthesia is usually required. Spica casting is generally used to maintain the reduction of the hip after an open or closed reduction procedure is performed. Open reduction is rarely needed in cases with classical DDH owing to widespread application of neonatal clinical or ultrasound screening, contrary to the teratologic dislocation necessitating an open reduction procedure more often.

Ultrasound is a widely used technique in monitoring the treatment of DDH, as well as in the follow-up of borderline cases before a definitive treatment regimen is decided.

Ultrasound is likely to decrease the duration of treatment and the number of necessary radiographs, as well as ensure the quick detection of persistent dislocations. For patients in a spica cast, a limited CT examination with very low mAs (milliamperes/second) or a limited MRI study is routinely used to decide whether the hip is reduced or not.

Scanning the Hip in a Pavlik Harness (Through Lateral Approach)

- Coronal flexion and axial flexion views are obtained through a lateral approach.
- The position of the femoral head is assessed.
- Stress should not be applied unless the physician requires it, or the weaning process begins.
- The assessment of acetabular morphology, which is not always reliable, is under debate.

Scanning the Hip in a Pavlik Harness (Through Anterior Approach)

- There are two reference lines in this view; one is on the pubic bone and the other one is on the femoral metaphysis, both appearing as linear echoes with posterior acoustic shadowing. The femoral head, which appears oval with the long axis perpendicular to the muscular and cutaneous planes, is situated between them.
- If the femoral head is normally positioned, the pubic ramus aligns with the femoral metaphysis.

Pearls and Pitfalls

- To obtain the ultrasound image in an appropriate plane is of crucial importance for correct diagnosis of DDH. Standard coronal plane that is described by Graf is used for morphologic analysis of the hip. Even small movements of the operator's hand may influence the transducer orientation and the production of the image.
- When scanning anteriorly the iliac wing flares laterally (**Fig. 7.9A**) and when scanning posteriorly it recedes medially (**Fig. 7.9B**). The posterior part of the bony acetabular roof is better developed than its middle and anterior parts; as a result of this, when scanning anteriorly, the bony roof may incorrectly appear shallower than it really is and vice versa when scanning posteriorly, it may show a shallow acetabulum deeper than it really is.
- Measurements of both α and β angles are optional. There is a great interobserver and intraobserver variability in measuring these angles. To measure them correctly, one has to be sure that the image is obtained in the standard coronal plane. To draw the bony roof line, the lower limb of bony ilium where the line starts should be seen as a sharp point. The cartilage roof line begins from the bony rim and goes through the center of the acetabular labrum.
- A common mistake is drawing the cartilage roof line from the junction of the iliac wing and the upper part of the bony acetabulum, which is referred as promontory or transition point (**Fig. 7.10**).
- The ossification center of the femoral head cannot be used to evaluate the position of the femoral head by ultrasound. Measurement of the ossification center also is not possible by ultrasound. Therefore, assessment of position and size of the femoral ossification center is not a part of an ultrasound study in DDH cases.

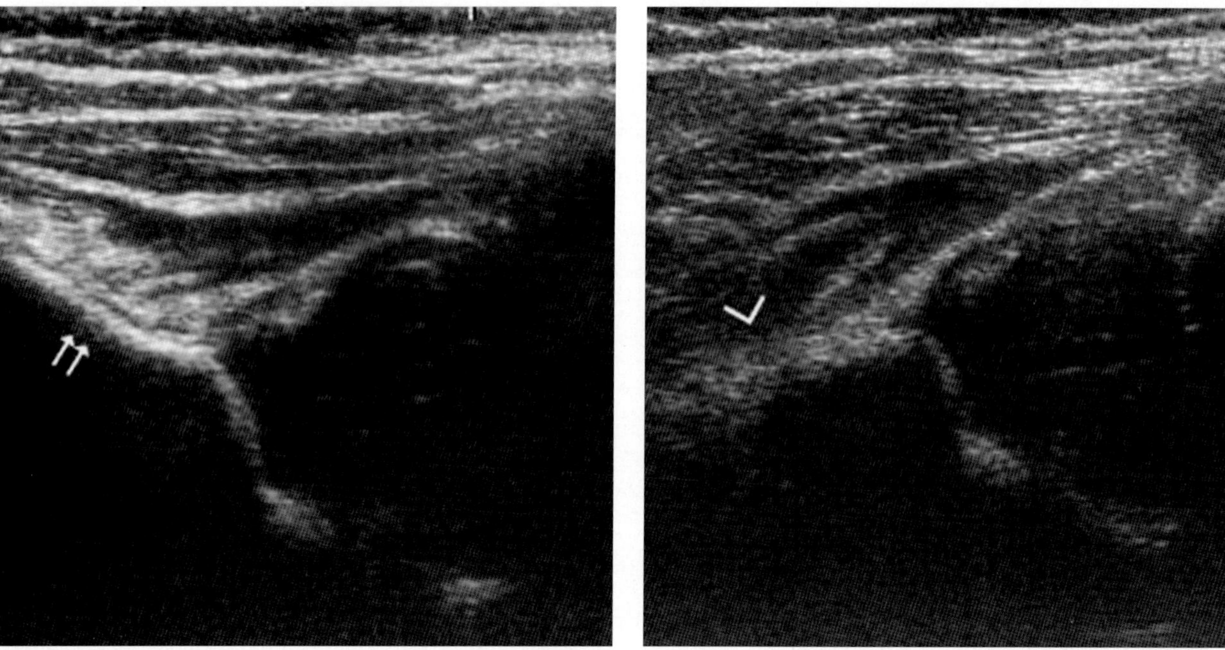

Fig. 7.9 **(A)** Anterior section; iliac wing (*double arrow*) flares laterally, toward the transducer. **(B)** Posterior section; iliac wing (*arrowhead*) flares medially away from the transducer.

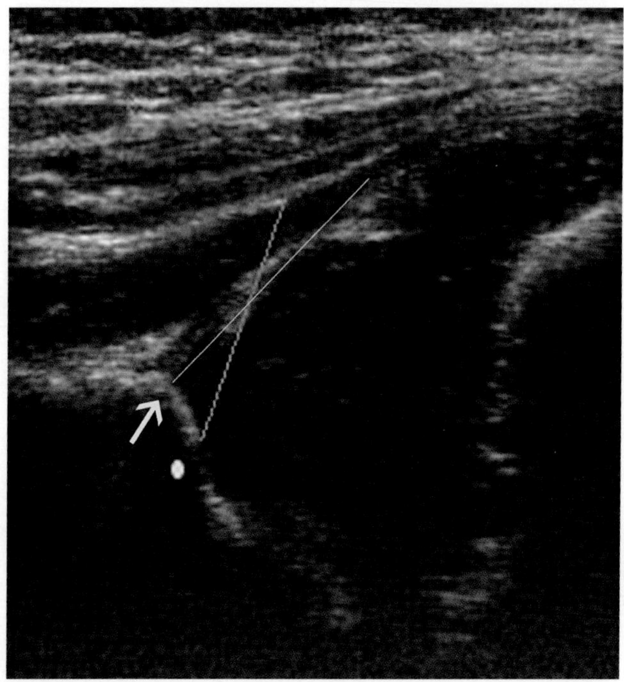

Fig. 7.10 Standard coronal plane. White line is the correct cartilage roof line, whereas the yellow line starting from the promontory (*arrow*) is incorrect.

Artifacts

The acetabular roof should be clearly visualized in the image to decide the level of its maturation and to make a correct morphologic analysis of the hip. Acoustic shadow behind the femoral ossification center interrupts the visualization of acetabular roof by ultrasound. Because of this as the infant gets older, with a larger femoral ossification center, the diagnostic value of ultrasound in detecting DDH decreases. The appearance and development of the femoral ossification center shows variability among infants; therefore, there is not a rigid cutoff regarding the upper limit of age for hip ultrasound.

Hip Effusion

Hip effusion is present in almost half of the pediatric patients with hip pain. Among numerous causes, transient synovitis—toxic synovitis—is the predominating pathology causing intraarticular fluid. The finding can infrequently be detected in patients with Legg–Calve–Perthes disease, rheumatoid arthritis, traumatic hemarthrosis, slipped femoral capital epiphysis, or septic arthritis. From an algorithmic point of view, ultrasound should be preceded by radiography. As a rule, no radiographic finding can be detected in the availability of small amount of hip effusion, whereas lateral displacement of the femoral head suggests the possibility of larger amounts of joint fluid. Furthermore, Doppler ultrasound may have a role in the evaluation of hip effusion. Thereby, an increase in the resistive index and a decrease in diastolic velocities in arteries of the femoral head can be detected in patients with hip effusion (**Fig. 7.11**). Alternatively, CT or MRI can be considered for the imaging of smaller amounts of joint fluid and revealing the etiology, particularly in cases with a normal ultrasound examination (**Figs. 7.12** and **7.13**).

A

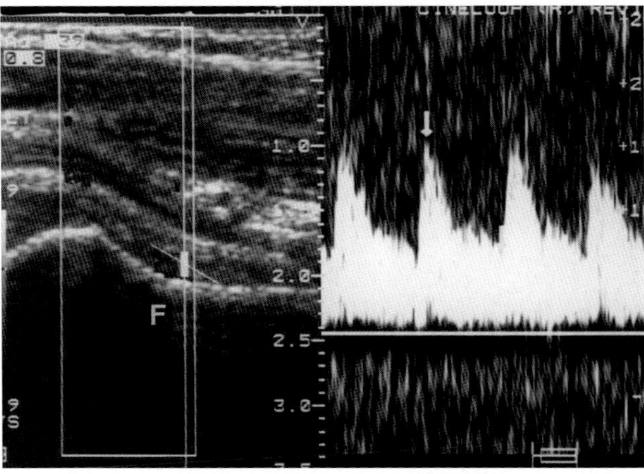

B

Fig. 7.11 Doppler ultrasound study of a patient with transient synovitis. (**A**) Spectral evaluation showed reversal of the diastolic flow with a RI value of 1.33. F, femoral neck; E, effusion. (**B**) Ultrasound of the same hip one month later revealed a normal arterial wave form and a RI of 0.58. No effusion is seen. F, femoral neck. (Used with permission from Robben SGF, Lequin MH, Diepstraten AFM, Hop WCJ, Meradji M. Doppler sonography of the anterior ascending cervical arteries of the hip: evaluation of healthy and painful hips in children. AJR 2000; 174:1629–1634)

Technical Guidelines

Ultrasound has a sensitivity higher than 90% for the determination of hip effusion. The technique enables the detection of joint fluid as small as 1 mL. Fortunately, the false-negative rate of the technique is low, except in infants. Technically, the patient is positioned supine with the hip in neutral position and the probe centered on the epiphysis, including part of the acetabulum superiorly and the femoral neck inferiorly during the investigation for joint fluid. Ultrasound scanning should involve an anterior approach in both longitudinal and transverse planes. The joint fluid accumulates initially anterior to the femoral neck in the inferior, caudal recess of the joint. Therefore, sagittal scanning over the extended hip and rotating the transducer so as to be parallel with the long axis of the femoral neck will enable the evaluation of the joint effusion. Occasionally, transverse views can facilitate the detection of fluid in joint space recesses, which cannot be visualized on sagittal planes. Notably, external rotation of the hip may serve as an adjunct for the detection of lesser amounts of joint fluid by including the most inferior recess. In addition, the relevant ultrasound findings should be compared with those of the contralateral hip. Thus, an identical positioning of both hips is crucial for the accuracy of an ultrasound evaluation.

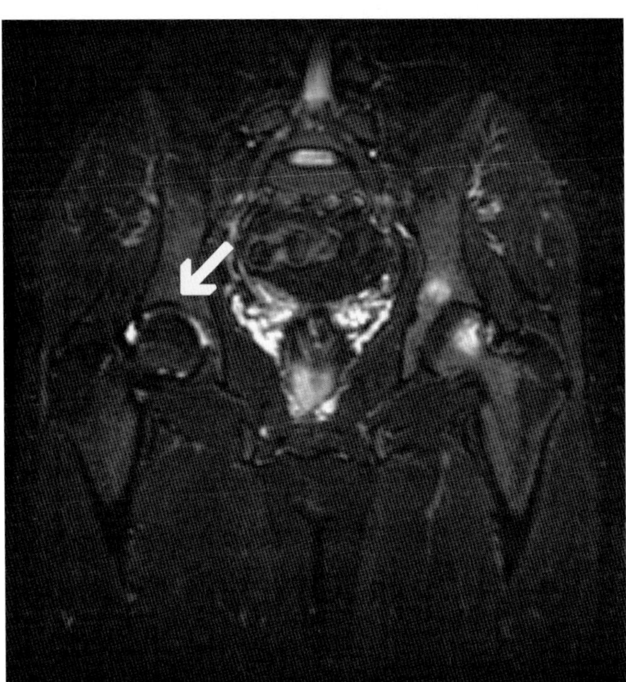

Fig. 7.12 Coronal short T1 inversion recovery (STIR) image in a patient with inflammatory arthropathy showing a small amount of right hip effusion (*arrow*) concomitant with narrowing of the left hip joint and a hyperintensity associated with bone marrow edema in left femoral head and acetabulum (Courtesy of Ali Yıkılmaz, MD, Kayseri, Turkey).

Anatomically, the normal joint capsule which consists of anterior and posterior layers of fibrous tissue lies parallel to the curvature of the femoral neck. Sonographically, the anterior layer is slightly thicker and more echogenic compared with the posterior layer resulting in an anteriorly concave and echogenic capsule appearance. Instead, joint effusion causes bulging of the joint capsule anteriorly resulting in a convex configuration, which can be demonstrated best with the hips extended (**Fig. 7.14**). Normally, the distance between anterior surface of the femoral neck and the joint capsule is less than 3 mm. In addition, the difference between both hips for the relevant distance should be less than 2 mm. Accordingly, a capsular-to-bone distance anterior to the femoral neck at a point halfway between physis and the

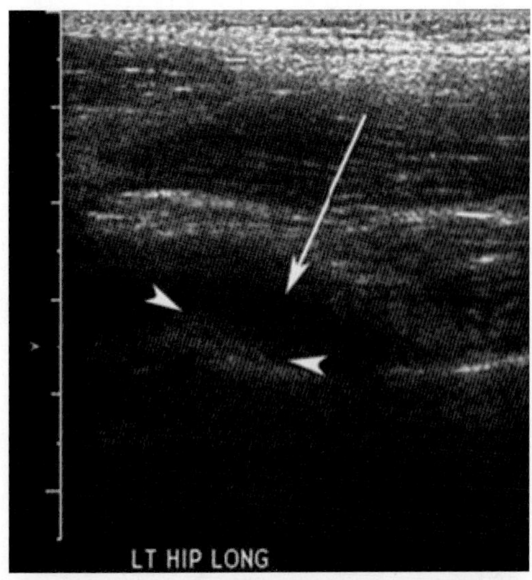

A

Fig. 7.13 Septic hip and osteomyelitis. **(A)** Sagittal sonogram revealed hip joint effusion (*arrow*) concomitant with periosteal reaction (*arrowheads*) in the proximal femur. Arthrocentesis yielding methicillin-resistant *Staphylococcus aureus* was preceded by magnetic resonance imaging (MRI). **(B)** Coronal fast spin-echo (FSE) T2-weighted fat-suppressed (FS) MRI confirms the effusion in left hip joint (*arrow*) and abnormally increased periarticular signal intensity (*arrowheads*). **(C)** Coronal FSE T2-weighted FS image obtained 1 month later revealed new abnormal signal intensity within the femoral head and neck marrow, consistent with osteomyelitis. (Used with permission from Bancroft LW, Merinbaum DJ, Zaleski CG, Peterson JJ, Kransdorf MJ, Berquist TH. Hip ultrasound. Seminars in Musculoskeletal Radiology 2007; 11(2):133)

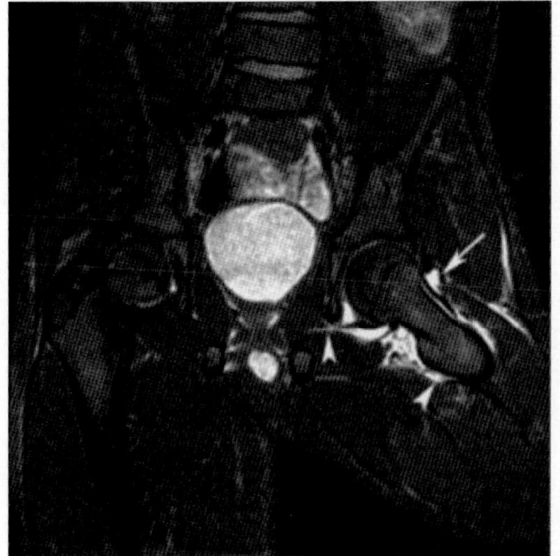

B

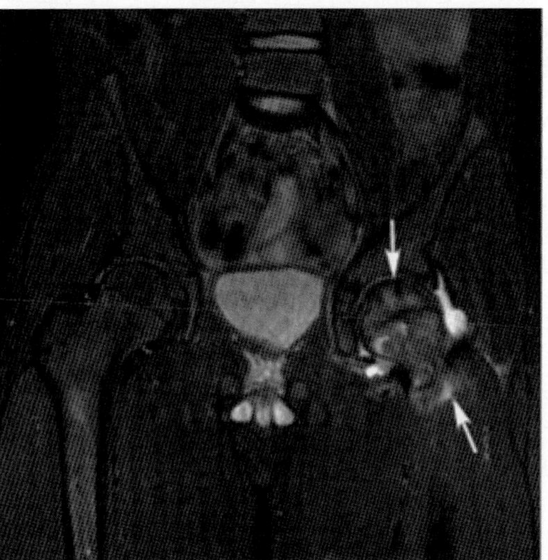

C

L R

Fig. 7.14 Sagittal ultrasound images of both hips revealing distention of the left hip capsule with convex outer border representing joint effusion associated with transient synovitis (*arrows*). R, right hip; L, left hip. (Courtesy of Suat Fitöz, MD, Ankara, Turkey).

caudal insertion of the joint capsule exceeding 3 mm signifies hip effusion. Likewise, a difference greater than 2 mm for the measurement of the relevant distance between the two sides also implies hip effusion.

The composition of the joint fluid has a great impact on its echogenicity. Consistently, a transudate results in an anechoic appearance, whereas an increased echogenicity with low-level echoes is usually associated with exudate or hemorrhagic fluid. Increased echogenicity of the fluid concomitant with the thickening of the articular capsule more than 2 mm suggests the diagnosis of septic arthritis. On the contrary, no significant capsular thickening occurs in patients with transient synovitis. Additionally, increased capsular blood flow can be detected on power Doppler ultrasound in patients with infected effusion, despite having low specificity for joint effusion. Nevertheless, the differentiation of infected hip effusion from a sterile one solely by imaging tools remains a challenge. In this regard, hip joint aspiration which can also be performed by ultrasound guidance is required for both enlightening the etiology of joint effusion and excluding septic arthritis reliably.

Miscellaneous Disorders

The demonstration of focal deficiency involving the proximal femur is a rare application of hip ultrasound in the pediatric age group, whereby the technique is superior to plain radiography owing to its ability for depicting the cartilaginous femoral head, the acetabulum, and the unossified femur. In Legg–Calve–Perthes disease, hip ultrasound may aid in the diagnosis by revealing joint fluid, fragmentation and lateral displacement of the femoral head, and thickening of the synovium and the articular cartilage.

Pearls and Pitfalls

- Importantly, both positioning of the patient and the determination of the scanning planes properly has a great impact on the ultrasound evaluation of hip effusion. Flexion of the hip may cause inaccuracies in the imaging findings by masking the joint effusion, as the distention of the anterior aspect of the joint capsule may be less prominent due to redistribution of the fluid in the aforementioned position.
- Moreover, identical positioning of both hips is vital for the accuracy of ultrasound evaluation because these findings are compared with those of the opposite hip.
- Hip joint effusions may be misdiagnosed as synovitis in obese patients because the poor beam penetration may render joint effusions hypoechoic.
- Hyperemia on power Doppler ultrasound may aid in the differentiation of synovitis from infected joint fluid.

Suggested Readings

American Academy of Pediatrics. Clinical practice guideline: early detection of developmental dysplasia of the hip. Committee on Quality Improvement, Subcommittee on Developmental Dysplasia of the Hip. Pediatrics 2000;105(4 Pt 1):896–905

American Institute of Ultrasound in Medicine; American College of Radiology. AIUM practice guideline for the performance of an ultrasound examination for detection and assessment of developmental dysplasia of the hip. J Ultrasound Med 2009;28(1):114–119

DiPietro MA, Harcke T. Pediatric musculoskeletal and spinal sonography. In: Van Holsbeeck MT, Introcaso JH. Musculoskeletal Ultrasound. St. Louis: Mosby;2001:277–324

El Ferzli J, Abuamara S, Eurin D, Le Dosseur P, Dacher JN. Anterior axial ultrasound in monitoring infants with Pavlik harness. Eur Radiol 2004;14(1):73–77

Graf R. Hip Sonography-Diagnosis and Management of Infant Hip Dysplasia. Berlin/Heidelberg: Springer-Verlag; 2006

Harcke HT, Grissom LE. Performing dynamic sonography of the infant hip. AJR Am J Roentgenol 1990;155(4):837–844

Portinaro NM, Pelillo F, Cerutti P. The role of ultrasonography in the diagnosis of developmental dysplasia of the hip. J Pediatr Orthop 2007;27(2):247–250

Rosendahl K, Toma P. Ultrasound in the diagnosis of developmental dysplasia of the hip in newborns. The European approach. A review of methods, accuracy and clinical validity. Eur Radiol 2007;17(8):1960–1967

Siegel MJ, McAlister WH. Musculoskeletal system and spine. In: Siegel MJ Pediatric Sonography. Philadelphia, PA: Lippincott-Raven; 1996:513–552

8 Bone Imaging

Diana Gaitini, Daniela Militianu, Alicia Nachtigal, and Vikram S. Dogra

The Physics of Bone Imaging

Although the medullary bone cannot be demonstrated on ultrasound, the sharp definition of cortical bone contours enables normal and pathologic bone diagnoses to be performed based on this modality.

According to the physics of ultrasound, the amount of sound reflection (R) or backscatter is determined by the differences in acoustic impedances (Z) of the tissues or materials forming the interface [e.g., (ΔZ) between $Z2$ and $Z1$]. Acoustic impedance of a tissue (Z) is directly proportional to density (p) and sound propagation velocity (c)

$$Z = p \cdot c$$

For different media, the acoustic impedance changes considerably. For example, for air, $Z = 0$ ($p \cong 0$ and $c = 340$ m/s); for muscle, $Z = 1.65$ ($p = 1.06$ g/cc and $c = 1.560$ m/s). The acoustic impedance of bone is much higher than the one for soft tissues

$$Z = 8 \ (p = 2 \text{ g/cc and } c = 4.000 \text{ m/s})$$

Sound reflection (R) is a function of the differences in acoustic impedances of the media at the interface:

$$R = Z2 - Z1 / Z2 + Z1$$

At an air–tissue interface, $R = 1$ ($R = 0 - 1.5 / 0 + 1.5$), which means that all the incident sound is reflected. At a bone–tissue interface,

$$R = 0.7 \ (R = 8 - 1.5 / 8 + 1.5)$$

which means that 70% of the incident sound is reflected.

From these equations, we may infer that the highly reflective tissue–bone interface is seen as a hyperechogenic line with posterior acoustic shadow.

Technical Guidelines and Normal Anatomy

Transducer and Equipment Capabilities

High-resolution broad bandwidth 5 to 12 MHz or 4 to 8 MHz, when the depth of the scanned target exceeds 2 to 3 cm, linear array transducers or 5 to 8 MHz and even 2 to 5 MHz, when depth exceeds 4 to 5 cm, sector array transducers are currently used for bone sonography. With the development of software and hardware new technologies like tissue harmonic and extended field-of-view imaging, sharp definition of bone contours and the surrounding tissues may be achieved.

Patient Positioning

The patient is examined seated or lying down, according to the anatomic region to be scanned, allowing a comfortable positioning for patient and examiner. The examiner is generally seated on a wheeled chair in front of the patient.

Normal Anatomy

Ultrasound examination is able to identify bone contours, cartilage on articular surfaces, tuberosities, grooves, fossae, and other bone structures.

Pathologies

Fractures

On ultrasound, fractures appear as focal breaks of the cortical hyperechogenicity, frequently associated with periosteal thickening and subperiosteal hematoma.

Linear Fracture

Disruption of the normal bone cortex is demonstrated on ultrasound by a step-off deformity or angulation of the fractured bones. Adjacent subperiosteal hemorrhage confirms the diagnosis (**Fig. 8.1**).

Subchondral Compression Fracture

Compression fractures of the humeral head are often hardly visualized on x-ray. A triangular-shaped defect in the cortex of the humeral head is detected on ultrasound. A Hill–Sachs fracture is the result of an impact of the humeral head on the glenoid contour in anterior shoulder dislocation. It is seen at the posterolateral contour of the humeral head (**Fig. 8.2**). A McLaughlin fracture is the homonymous of the previous one at the anterior humeral head contour (**Fig. 8.3**), developing as a result of a posterior shoulder dislocation. Large lesions are associated with a predisposition for recurrent dislocation.

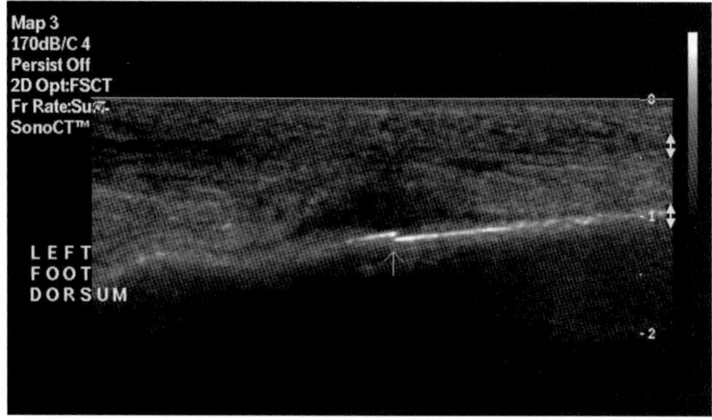

Fig. 8.1 Linear fracture. Step-off discontinuity of a metatarsal bone surface (*small arrow*) in a soldier with acute middle foot pain, compatible with stress fracture. Adjacent to the fracture, a sonolucent hematoma and soft tissue edema are seen.

Fig. 8.2 Hill–Sachs compression fracture. **(A)** On ultrasound, a triangular notch representing an osteochondral fracture is seen at the posterior area of the humeral head (*small arrow*). The bone defect is filled by synovial fluid. The rotator cuff (*large arrow*) is seen above the humeral head. **(B)** Axial proton-density fast spin echo fat-suppressed magnetic resonance image (PD FSE FS MRI) shows the defect in the humeral head (*arrow*).

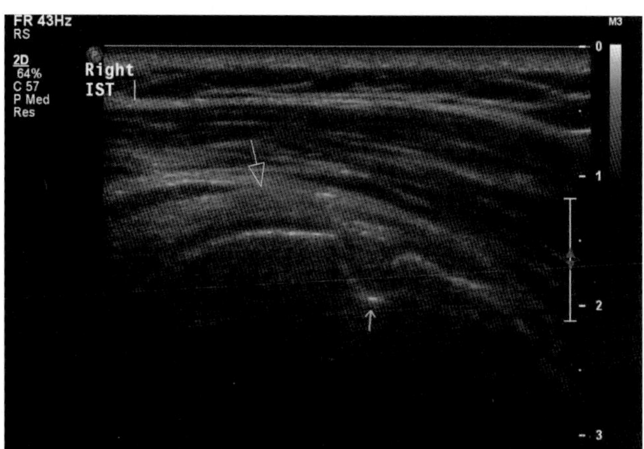

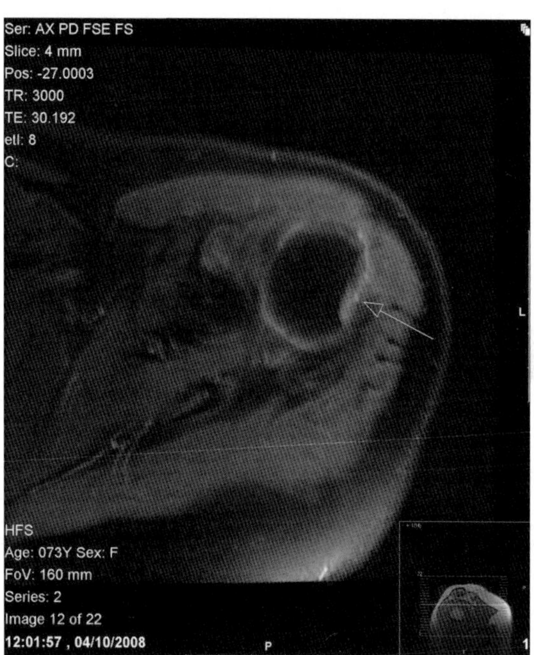

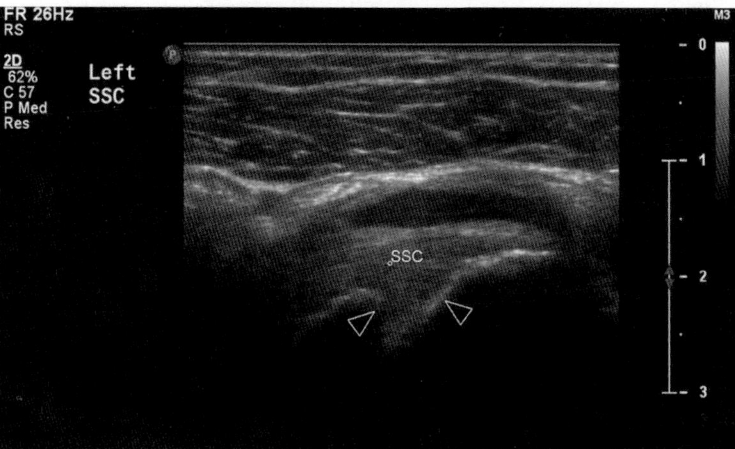

Fig. 8.3 McLaughlin compression fracture. Triangular defect in the anteromedial aspect of the humeral head (*arrowheads*). The bone defect is seen below the subscapularis (SSC) tendon.

Avulsion Fracture

An osteochondral fractured segment may be seen standing free in the proximity of a fractured bone (**Fig. 8.4**).

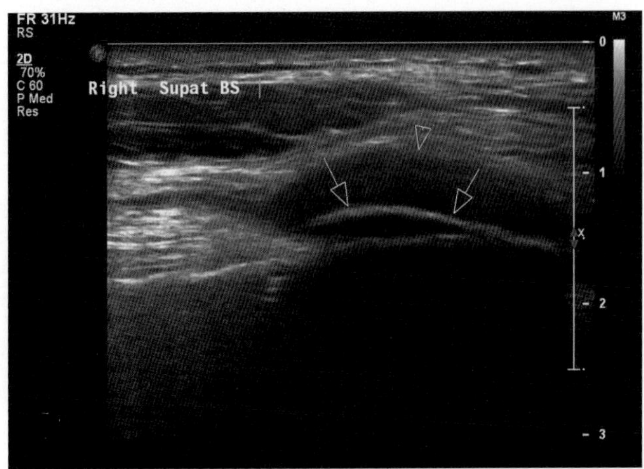

A

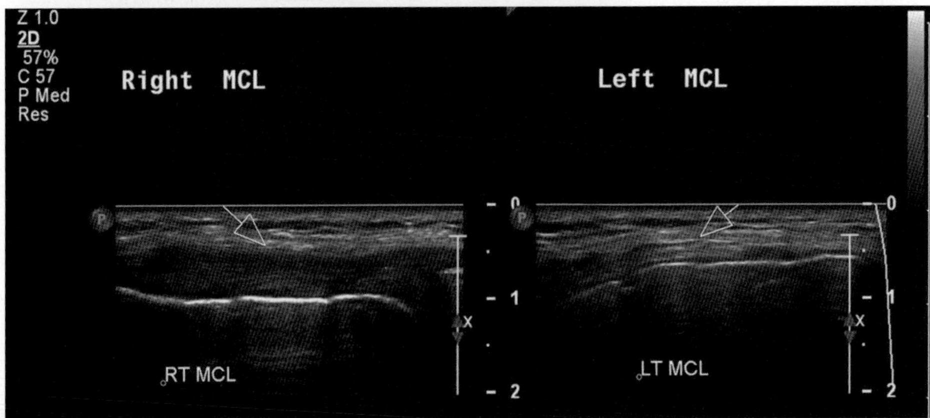

B

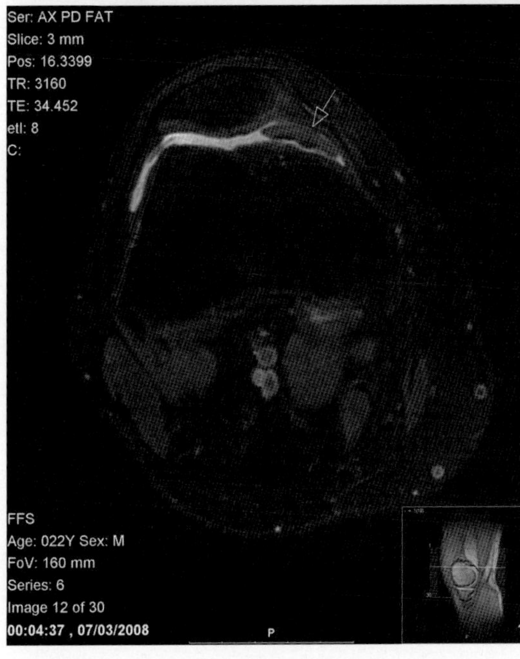

C

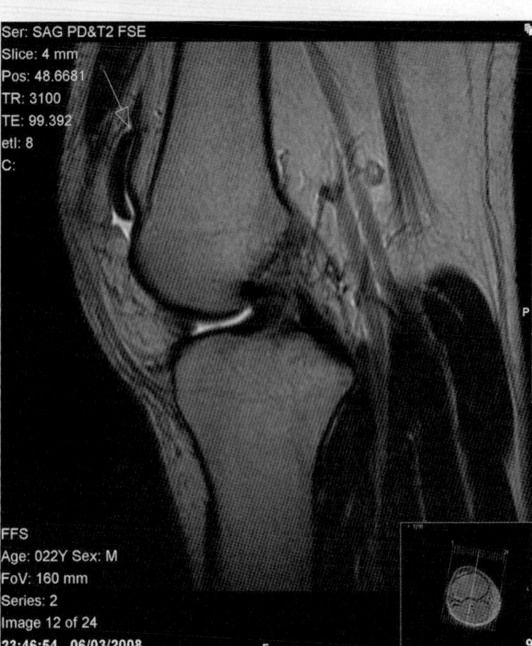

D

Fig. 8.4 Osteochondral avulsion fracture of the patella. **(A)** On ultrasound, a hyperechoic bone fragment is seen at the medial side of the right knee, due to avulsion fracture of the patella (*arrows*) with cranial displacement. Fluid is detected in the suprapatellar bursa (*arrowhead*). **(B)** Ipsilateral middle collateral ligament tear (*arrow*) secondary to trauma is seen on the left plot, opposite to the normal contralateral ligament (*arrow*) on the right plot. **(C)** Axial proton-density fast spin echo fat-suppressed magnetic resonance image (PD FSE FS MRI) shows the loose osteocartilage fragment (*arrow*) in the medial recess of the suprapatellar bursa, surrounded by synovial fluid. **(D)** On sagittal PD FSE MRI, the medially displaced osteocartilaginous fragment (*arrow*) may be seen.

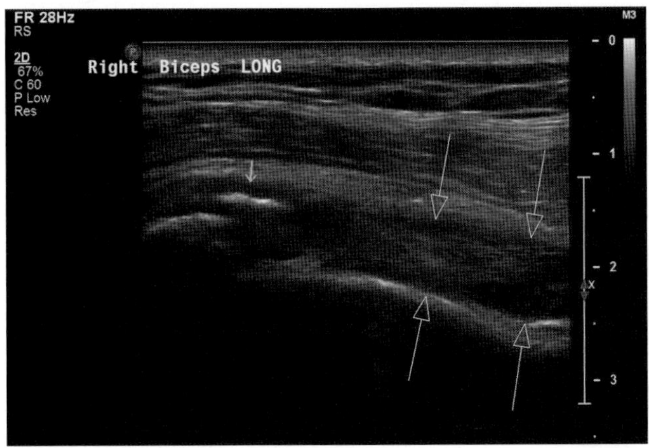

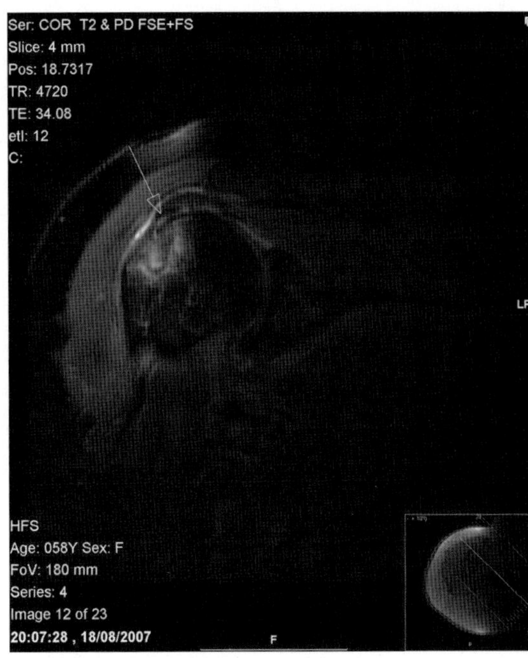

Fig. 8.5 Occult fracture at the humeral greater tuberosity. **(A)** Discontinuity in the normally smooth bony surface and avulsion fracture are seen on sagittal ultrasound. The osteochondral fragment is seen as a hyperechogenic focus (*short arrow*) at the proximal bicipital groove. A large hematoma is seen along the humeral shaft (long arrows), posterior to the long head of the biceps tendon. **(B)** On coronal MRI PD FSE FS a fracture line surrounded by intramedullary contusion and mild compression of the greater tuberosity (*arrow*) is seen.

Occult Fracture

Unsuspected fractures on conventional radiography may be diagnosed on ultrasound. Examples are a humeral greater tuberosity fracture (**Fig. 8.5**), which leads to impingement in the subacromial space, and fractures at ribs. An occult fracture should be looked for in cases presenting with subperiosteal hemorrhage (**Fig. 8.6**). In an appropriate clinical setting, stress fractures at an early stage are suspected on ultrasound by the presence of soft tissue swelling and hyperemia.

Subluxation

Ultrasound is useful in the evaluation of joint subluxation, difficult to evaluate radiographically. Examples are subluxation of the acromioclavicular joint (**Fig. 8.7**), radioulnar and tibiofibular joints, and the symphysis pubis. Comparison with the uninjured side is helpful.

Erosion

Erosions may be detected earlier on ultrasound than on conventional radiographs. Marginal erosions are seen on sonography as rounded cortical breaks; they are early markers of inflammatory arthropathies in particular when associated with synovial effusion. Bone erosions may be secondary to external pressure by a paraosseous process (**Fig. 8.8**).

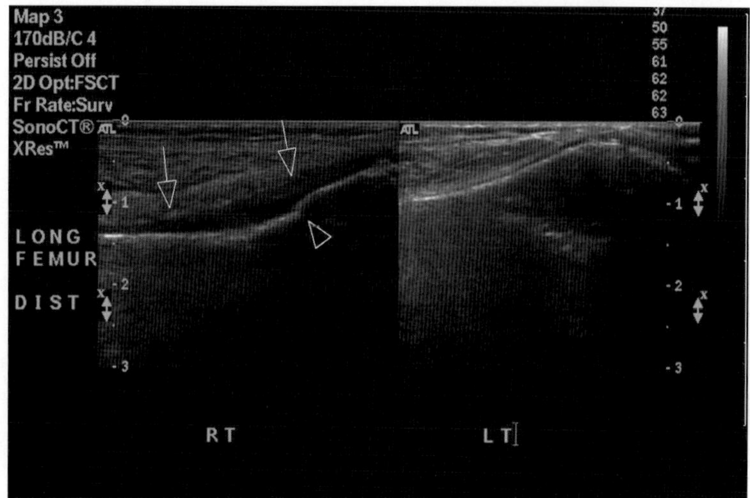

A

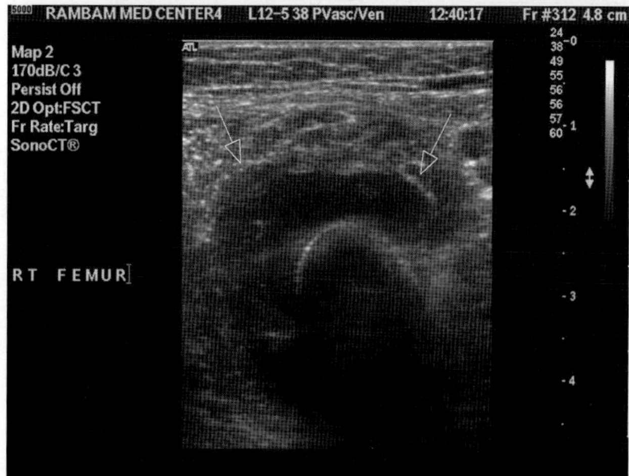

B

Fig. 8.6 Occult fracture at proximal femoral diaphysis with subperiosteal hematoma. A 12-year-old mentally retarded girl with pain and swelling in right thigh. **(A)** Side-by-side longitudinal ultrasound scan. On the left plot, a tiny gap at the right distal femoral shaft (*arrowhead*) compatible with greenstick, an undisplaced fracture, and adjacent subperiosteal fluid (*arrows*) are seen. On the right plot, the normal continuous echogenic line of the contralateral femoral shaft is shown. **(B)** Transverse scan at the level of the swollen thigh, proximal to the fracture, shows a large subperiosteal hematoma (*arrows*). **(C)** Contrast-enhanced computed tomography (CT) scan with soft tissue window shows an enhanced periosteum (*arrow*) surrounding the subperiosteal hematoma. **(D)** CT scan at the distal femoral shaft shows the cortical fracture (*arrow*) with small surrounding soft tissue hematoma. Bone hyperdensity around the fracture line represents intramedullary hematoma. Normal bone and soft tissue structures are seen at the contralateral thigh, useful for comparison.

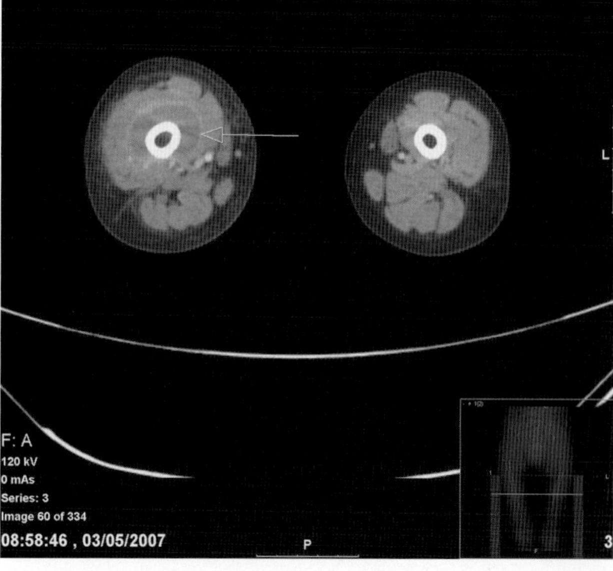

C

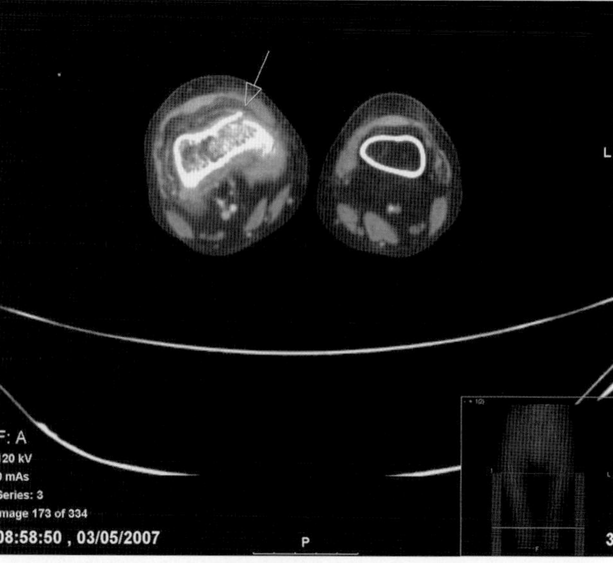

D

Fig. 8.7 Acromioclavicular joint subluxation. **(A)** A widened gap (*cursors*) between the clavicle end (C) and the acromion (A) is seen in this patient, following blunt chest trauma with fracture of the clavicle. **(B)** Coronal T1-weighted fast spin echo magnetic resonance image (T1 FSE MRI) showing a gap (*arrow*) between clavicle (C) and acromion (A) in another patient, as evidence of subluxation.

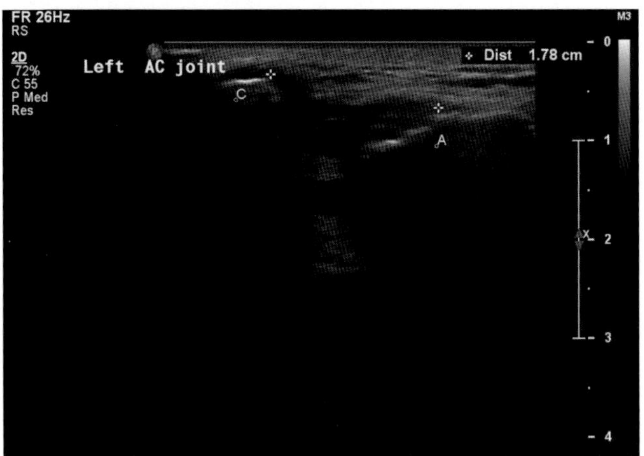

A

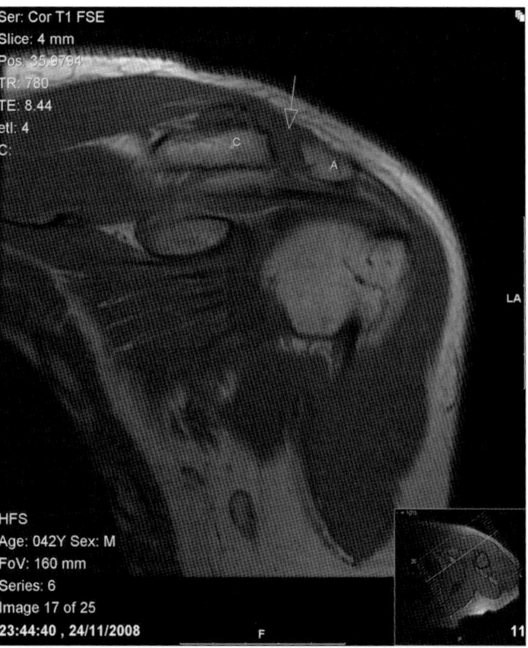

B

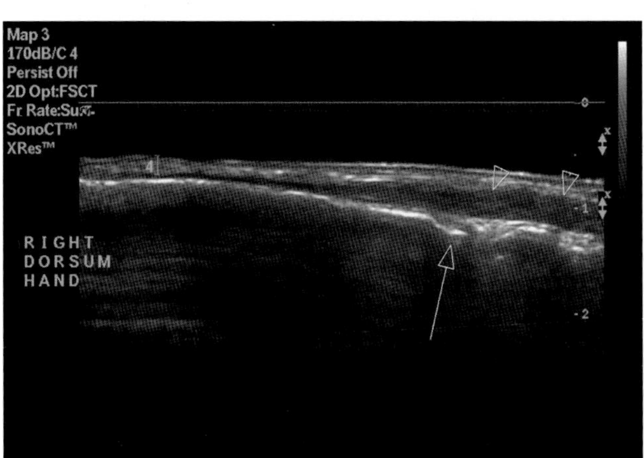

A

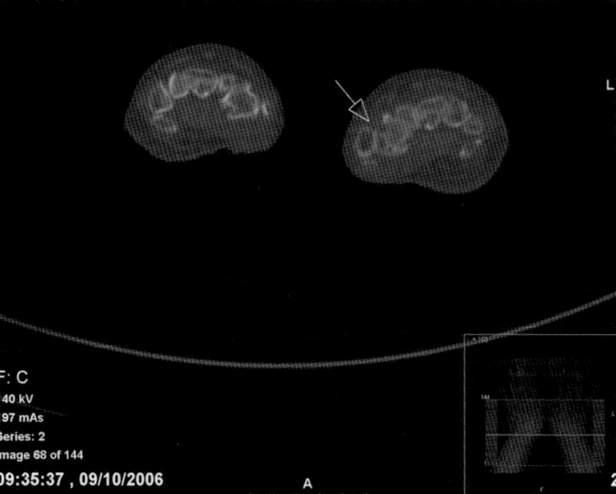

B

Fig. 8.8 Bone erosion. **(A)** Rounded cortical defect (*arrow*) in proximal interphalangeal joint and signs of tenosynovitis of the extensor tendon (*arrowheads*) seen in a longitudinal scan of the finger in a patient with rheumatoid arthritis. The use of a silicon pad allowed definition of near field structures at 0.5 cm depth. **(B)** Erosions at carpal bones (*arrow*) seen in computed tomography (CT) scan at bone windows in severe rheumatoid arthritis.

Exostosis-Osteochondroma

Exostoses or osteochondromas are seen as an echogenic lesion protruding from the cortical bone; at the free margin, the anechoic area represents cartilaginous cap (**Figs. 8.9** and **8.10**). Cartilaginous cap thickness may be accurately measured by ultrasound. A rapidly growing cartilaginous cap raises suspicion of sarcomatous degeneration. Bursitis around the cap of the osteochondroma, fracture of the osteochondroma and pressure on an adjacent structure can be detected by the ultrasound study. Vascular injury to an adjacent artery or pressure on veins may lead to the development of aneurysms and deep vein thrombosis, which also can be easily detected by ultrasound.

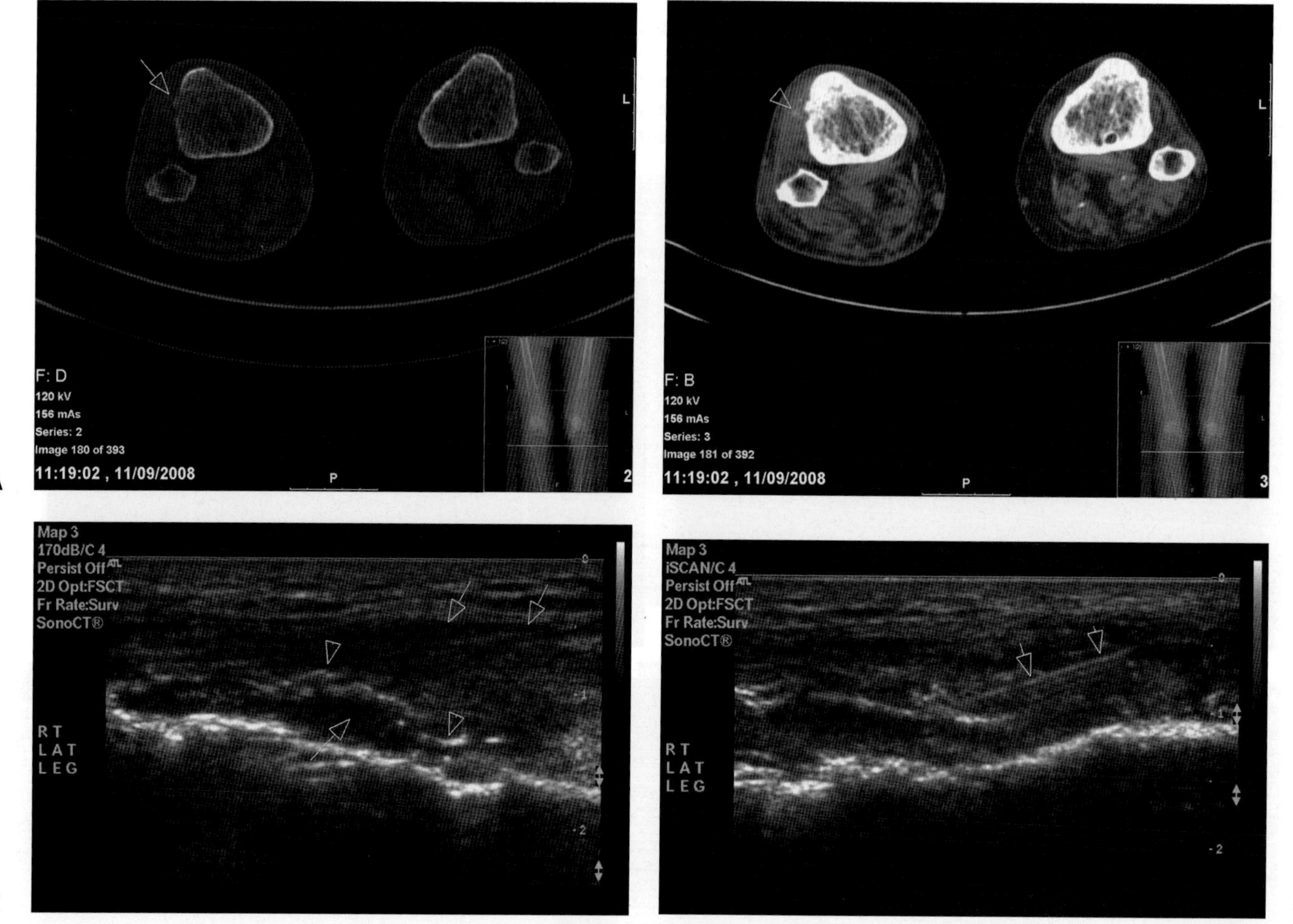

Fig. 8.12 Osteomyelitis at the proximal tibia. **(A)** Erosion in anterolateral tibial cortex (*arrow*) seen on axial computed tomography (CT) scan with bone window, in a patient with known Kaposi sarcoma presenting with local tenderness and erythema. **(B)** CT scan with soft tissue window shows focal bone erosion at the tibial cortex, periosteal detachment (*arrowhead*), and adjacent soft tissue mass. **(C)** Ultrasound at the level of the swollen proximal calf shows an irregular hyperechogenic line representing periosteal reaction (arrowheads) and hypoechoic inflammatory tissue on both sides of the detached periosteum (arrows). **(D)** Ultrasound-guided fluid aspiration with a 20-gauge spinal needle (*arrow*) was performed. Inflammatory cells without signs of malignancy were diagnosed on cytology.

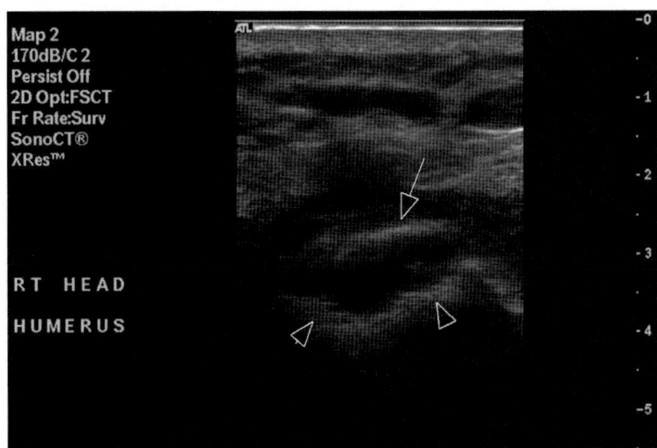

Fig. 8.13 Humeral head osteomyelitis and glenohumeral joint septic arthritis. **(A)** Humeral head erosions (*arrowheads*) and a bone fragment (*arrow*) are seen on ultrasound. **(B)** On color Doppler ultrasound, intense hyperemia is seen at the subdeltoid bursa. **(C)** A computed tomography (CT) scan at bone window shows a lytic lesion in the humeral head with cortical destruction (*arrow*) and surrounding soft tissue swelling. **(D)** A large amount of synovial fluid in the subdeltoid bursa is seen on ultrasound. **(E)** Ultrasound-guided aspiration was performed. The needle (*arrows*) is seen into the synovial fluid. Inflammatory cells and high glucose levels were found in the synovial fluid.

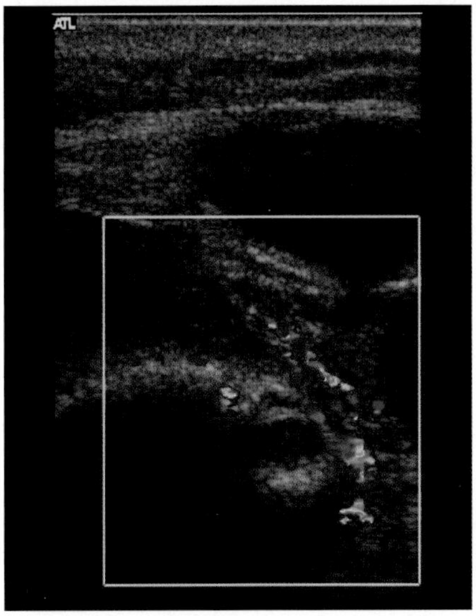

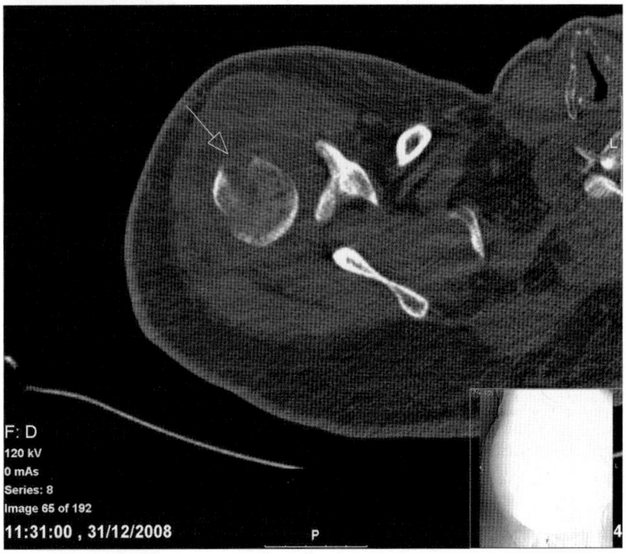

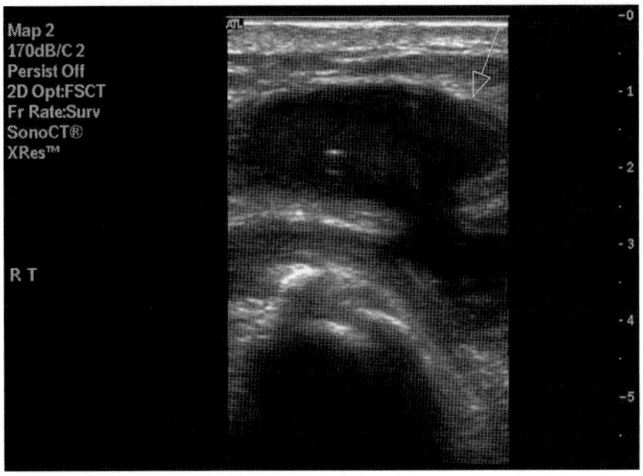

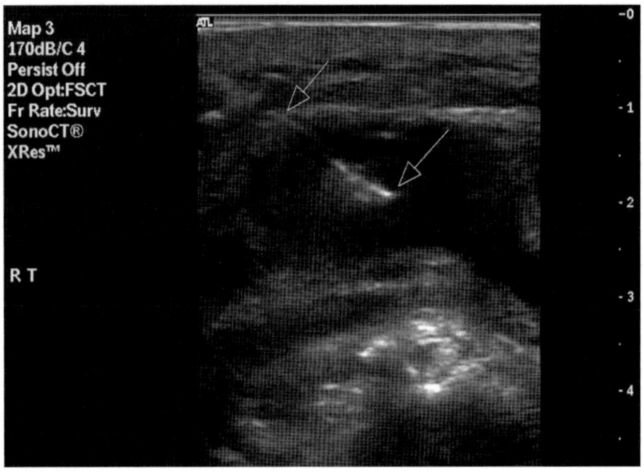

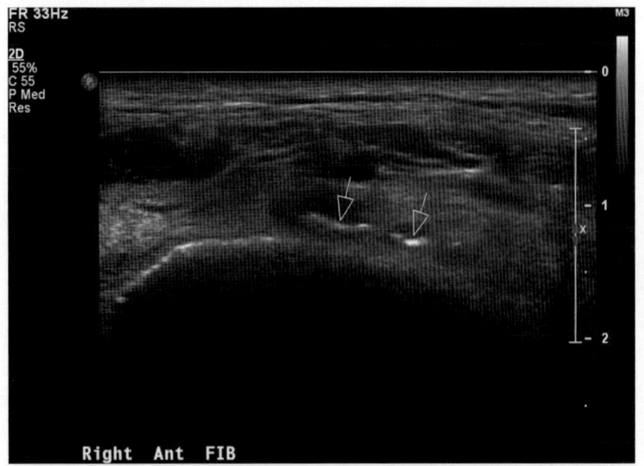

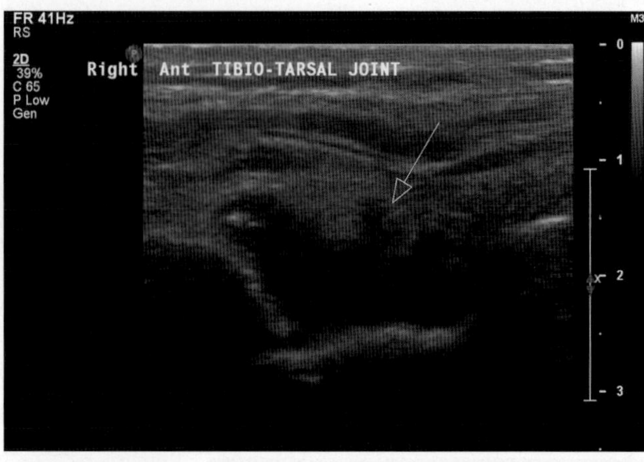

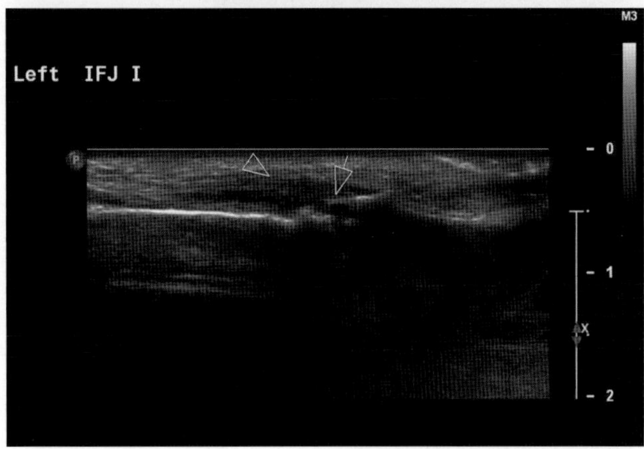

Fig. 8.14 Periostitis in psoriatic arthritis. **(A)** Periostitis (*arrows*) is seen at the fibulotarsal joint. **(B)** Large amount of fluid (arrow) seen in the tibiotarsal joint. **(C)** Periostitis at the first interphalangeal joint of the hand (*arrow*), with adjacent hypoechogenic inflamed tendon (*arrowhead*).

Tumor

Bone tumors may be diagnosed on ultrasound by local invasion to cortical bone and mass effect upon the surrounding soft tissues (**Fig. 8.15**). Color and power Doppler are useful techniques to evaluate tumor vascularization and differentiate a hypoechoic solid mass from a fluid collection. Ultrasound is also of benefit targeting computed tomography (CT) and magnetic resonance imaging (MRI) studies and guiding percutaneously performed biopsies (**Fig. 8.16**).

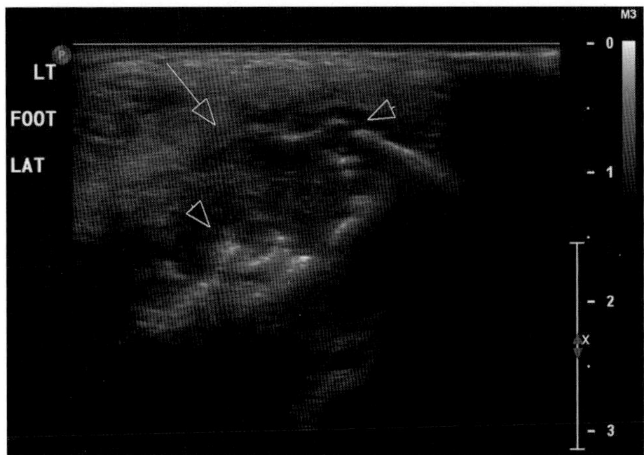

A

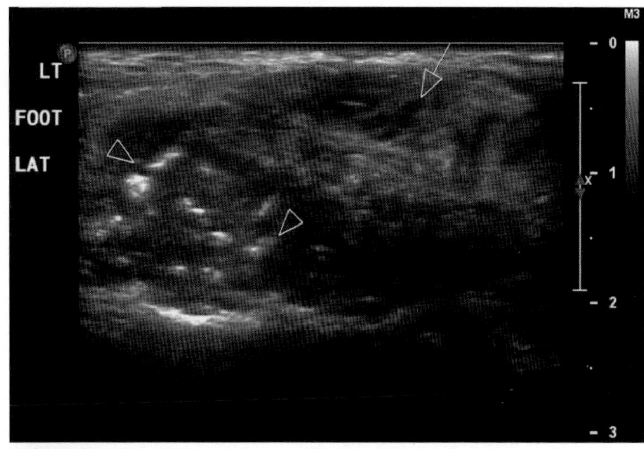

B

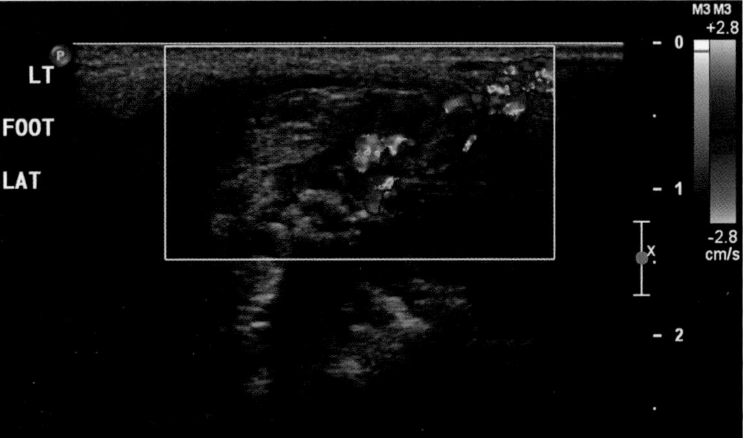

C

Fig. 8.15 Bone tumor in calcaneus. A 14-year-old boy presenting with swelling and pain over posterior ankle and back left foot. **(A)** Ultrasound demonstrates an irregular lytic defect (*arrowheads*) at the calcaneus with an adjacent soft tissue mass (*arrow*). **(B)** Bone fragments (*arrowheads*) and a widely extending soft tissue tumor (*arrow*) are seen at the lateral heel. **(C)** Rich vascularity at the soft tissue mass is seen at color Doppler ultrasound. *(Continued)*

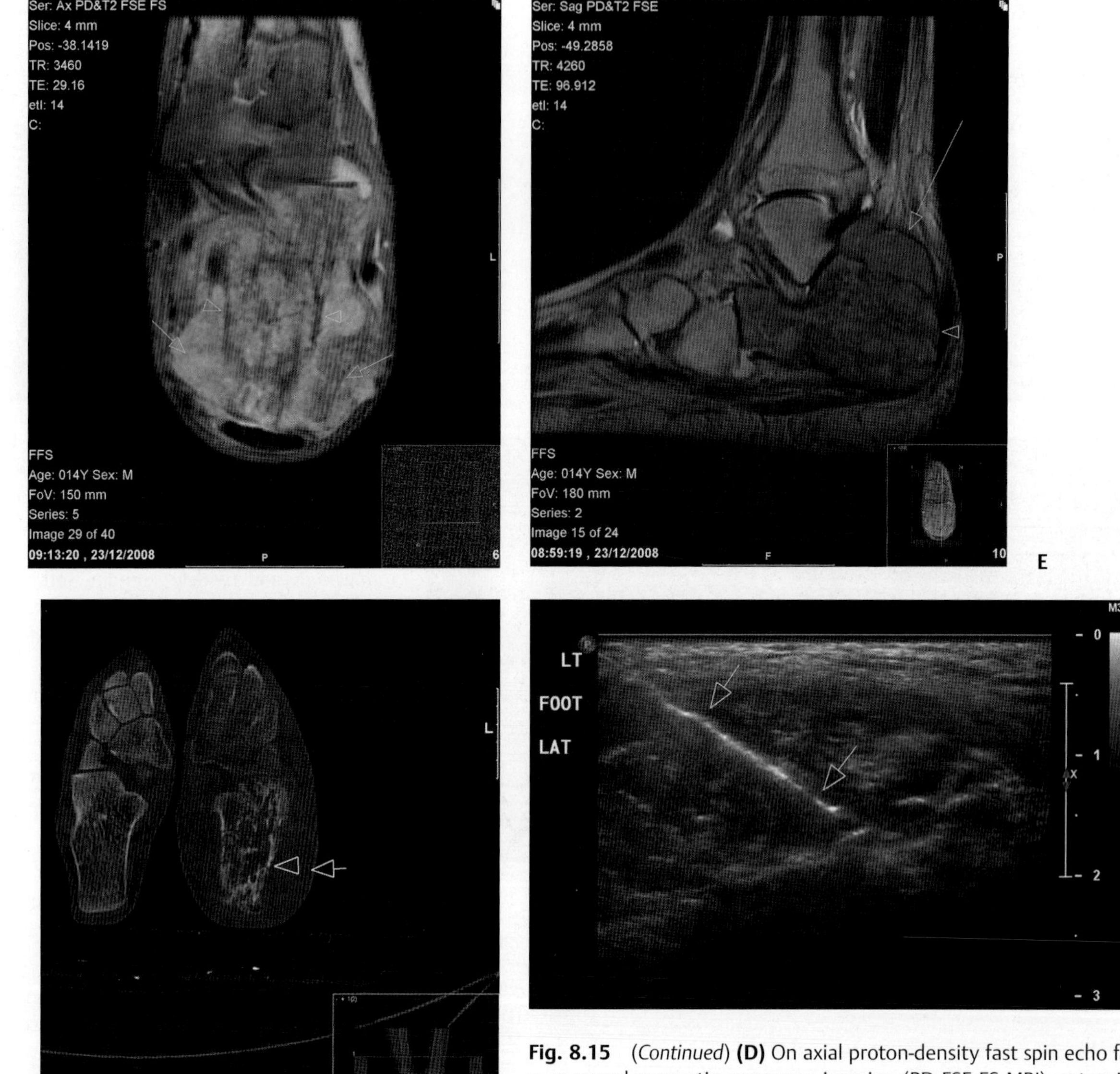

Fig. 8.15 (*Continued*) **(D)** On axial proton-density fast spin echo fat-suppressed magnetic resonance imaging (PD FSE FS MRI), extensive bone destruction (*arrowheads*) is seen surrounded by a soft tissue mass (*arrows*). **(E)** Sagittal T2-weighted FSE MRI shows the extensive bone infiltration (*arrowhead*) with cortical destruction and the soft tissue mass (*arrow*). **(F)** Axial computed tomography (CT) scan with bone window shows the extensive lytic lesion of the calcaneus (*arrowhead*) with surrounding soft tissue involvement by the tumor and osteoporosis of the tarsal bones in the left foot. The normal bone and soft tissue structures in the right foot are shown. **(G)** Ultrasound-guided biopsy was performed with a 16-gauge biopsy needle (*arrows*). The histopathologic diagnosis was Ewing sarcoma.

Conclusion

Bone pathologies involving the cortical bone and the surrounding soft tissues are suitable for ultrasound diagnosis, often in an early stage of the disease. Doppler sonography is invaluable for lesion characterization. Ultrasound-guided interventional procedures, like biopsies, fluid aspiration and abscess drainage, allow rapid and precise diagnosis and therapy. Nevertheless, evaluation of osseous abnormalities requires combined imaging algorithms using conventional radiographs, ultrasound, nuclear medicine, CT, and MRI, specific for each clinical scenario.

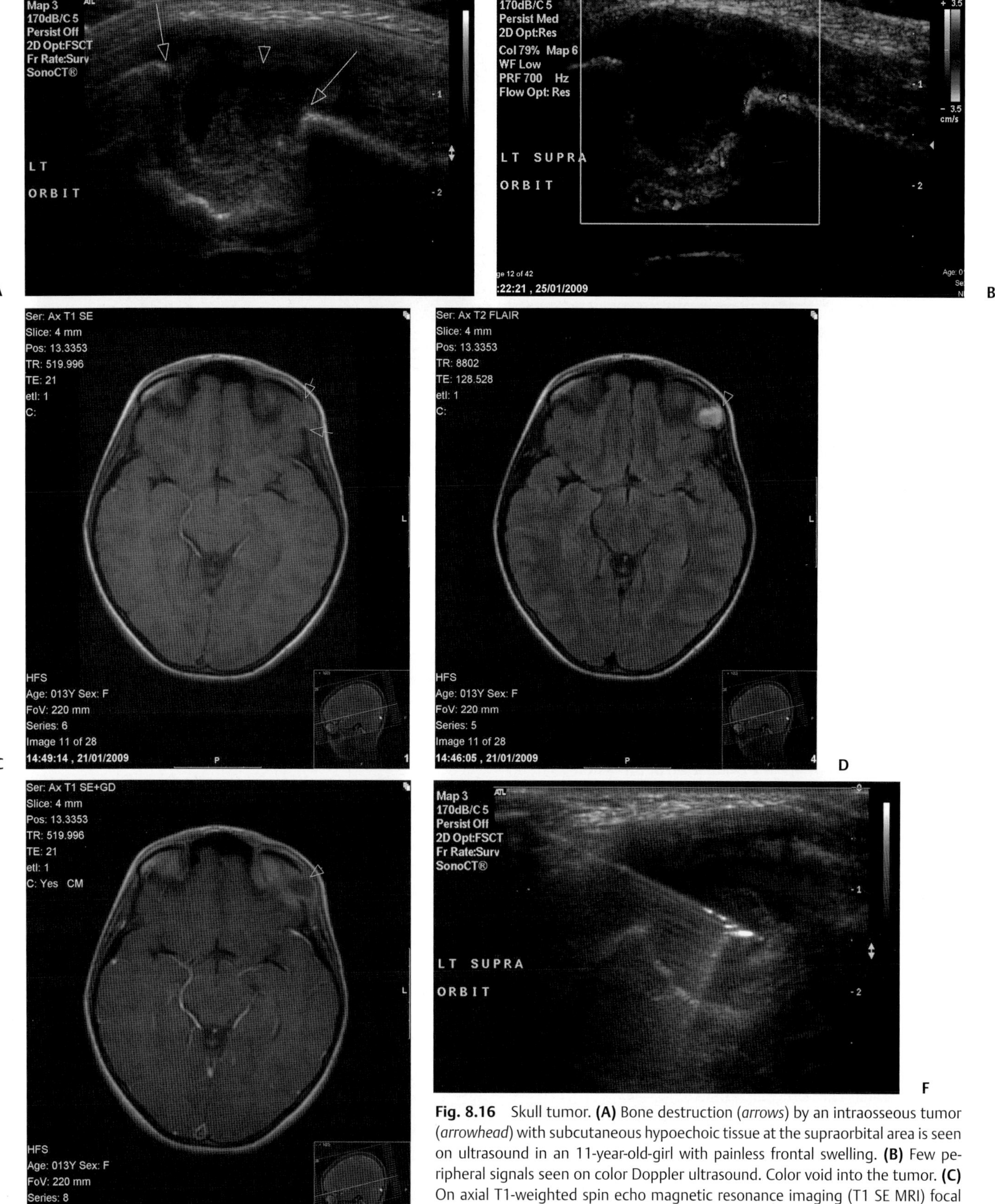

Fig. 8.16 Skull tumor. **(A)** Bone destruction (*arrows*) by an intraosseous tumor (*arrowhead*) with subcutaneous hypoechoic tissue at the supraorbital area is seen on ultrasound in an 11-year-old-girl with painless frontal swelling. **(B)** Few peripheral signals seen on color Doppler ultrasound. Color void into the tumor. **(C)** On axial T1-weighted spin echo magnetic resonance imaging (T1 SE MRI) focal complete destruction of the lateral orbital wall (*arrows*) with surrounding soft tissue mass is seen. **(D)** Axial T2-weighted fluid attenuated inversion recovery (T2 FLAIR) MRI shows high intensity signal in the mass (*arrowhead*). **(E)** Axial T1 SE MRI with gadolinium showing peripheral enhancement of the mass (*arrowhead*). **(F)** Needle biopsy of the mass under ultrasound-guidance was performed. The needle is seen as a bright echo with posterior reverberations. The pathologic diagnosis was eosinophilic granuloma.

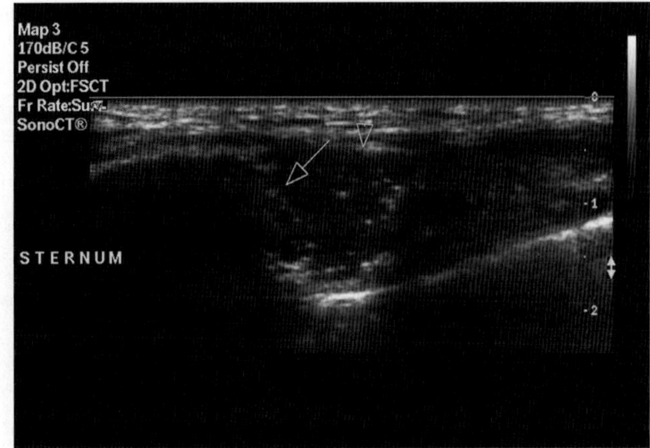

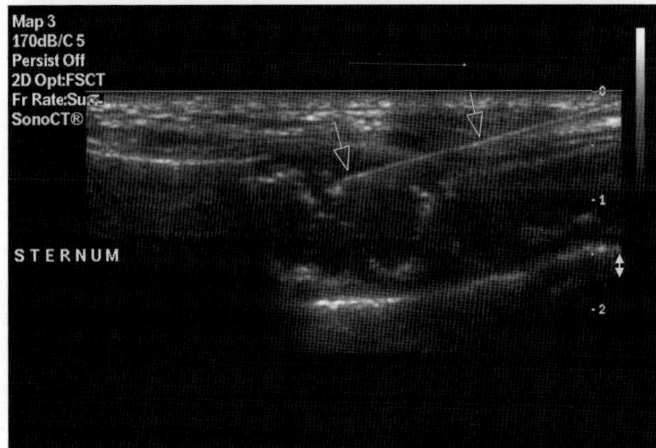

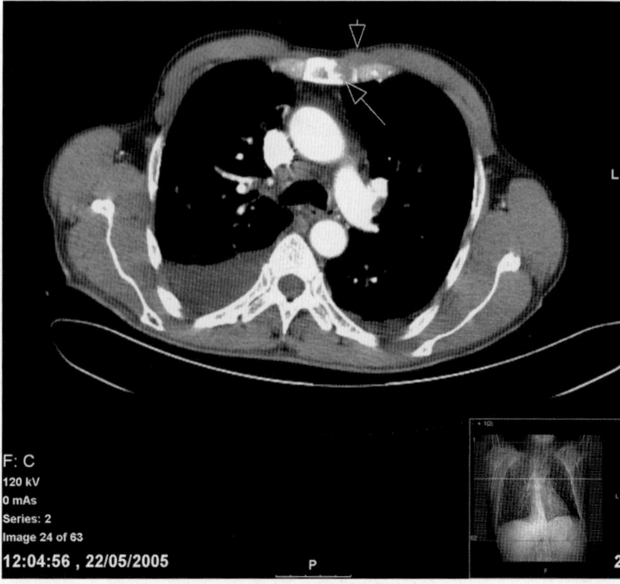

Fig. 8.17 Sternal metastasis. **(A)** Cortical destruction in the sternum (*arrow*) and an adjacent soft tissue mass (*arrowhead*) in a patient with left parasternal chest wall pain seen on an ultrasound axial scan. **(B)** Chest CT scan shows bone lysis at the sternal manubrium (*arrow*) and a parasternal small soft tissue mass (*arrowhead*). Note also right moderate pleural effusion and pretracheal mediastinal lymphadenopathy. **(C)** Ultrasound-guided fine-needle biopsy (FNB) of the parasternal mass; the biopsy needle (*arrow*) is seen in the soft tissue mass. Small cell carcinoma was diagnosed on histology.

Comprehensive Approach to Bone Imaging Diagnosis

1- Plain radiography
2- Bone scintigraphy, for the evaluation of the whole skeletal system
3- CT with and without contrast on bone and soft tissue windows, for bone pathology and soft tissue involvement
4- Ultrasound and color Doppler ultrasound, for definition of surrounding soft tissue findings
5- MRI for precise local anatomic extension

Suggested Readings

Bianchi S, Martinoli C. Ultrasound of the musculoskeletal system. Heidelberg/Berlin/New York: Springer-Verlag;2007

Van Holsbeeck MT, Introcaso JH. Musculoskeletal Ultrasound. St. Louis: Mosby; 2001

Winter TC III, Teefey SA, Middleton WD. Musculoskeletal ultrasound: an update. Radiol Clin North Am 2001;39(3):465–483

Pearls and Pitfalls

- High resolution multifrequency transducers, with advanced imaging capabilities such as real-time compound, tissue harmonic, color and power flow, and extended field of view have improved the diagnostic quality, in particular tissue contrast and spatial resolution, of ultrasound images of the musculoskeletal system.
- Sonographic "palpation" is a valuable technique in localizing the region of interest. Occult fractures may be demonstrated by a step-off bone deformity or angulation.
- Interventional ultrasound is rapidly achieving an important role for the definitive diagnosis and treatment of many musculoskeletal disorders.
- Be aware of "mirror" artifact in large very reflective structures like large extremity bones, which may make structures on the opposite side of a cortical bone appear as real anatomic structures.
- Despite the technologic advances in ultrasound equipment, a good knowledge of anatomy and pathology of the musculoskeletal system and experience in performing the examinations are essential for a precise diagnosis and treatment planning.

9 Skin Imaging

Ximena Wortsman and Jacobo Wortsman

High-resolution ultrasound is a recently added tool used in the evaluation of skin lesions. Ultrasound is able to produce an image of the cutaneous layers along multiple axes; this results in a three-dimensional representation of a lesion that includes size and dimension, morphology, and content.

As a clinical imaging test, ultrasound has obvious differences with conventional histology. A skin biopsy is performed ex vivo, follows an invasive procedure, and examines tissues altered by dehydration and fixation. Although considered the gold standard, histology can be inconclusive, gives sparse information on the extralesional matrix, and the procedure cannot be easily repeated. The shortcomings of skin biopsy may become particularly important when planning subsequent surgical treatment. Precise knowledge of local anatomy is essential to decrease postoperative complications and produce optimal cosmetic outcomes. Ultrasound pinpoints that information and delivers images of lesional and postbiopsy distortions. The best ultrasound scans are obtained when using machines equipped with linear probes of variable frequency capable of generating waves of 15 MHz and greater, making it possible to detect all skin layers separately. The newest probes are compact and hockey-shaped to easily follow contour changes, even in highly irregular areas such as the face or the ears. Given these properties, ultrasound can be used to not only fully characterize skin lesions, but to differentiate lesional from extralesional tissues, and to determine local vascularization and perfusion hemodynamics.

Lastly, ultrasound can guide direct lesional approaches and facilitate the evaluation of therapeutic responses.

Ultrasound was first applied to the study of the skin lesions in 1979, using available probes that could generate waves of only a single (fixed) frequency. That technique, also called fixed high-frequency ultrasound (20–100 MHz; FFUS), provided very low tissue penetration. In ultrasound, a higher frequency generates lower penetration through the skin layers. Even 20 MHz waves can penetrate only 5 or 6 mm, whereas 75 MHz will reach at most 3 mm. In FFUS, the skin layers are ill-defined, depending on tissue thicknesses; and even in the dorsal region, where the dermis is thicker, it may still not be visualized clearly; furthermore, the subcutaneous tissue is barely visible. Deeper structures are beyond the reach of FFUS and blood flow patterns cannot be defined in real time. The newest high-resolution ultrasound machines are instead equipped with variable frequency probes that give—in real time—clear definition of skin layers and of deeper structures such as tendons, nerves, or muscles. Perfusion characteristics can also be assessed in detail.

A comparison of high-resolution ultrasound with the noninvasive soft tissue imaging technique of magnetic resonance imaging (MRI) reveals the clear advantage represented by the live interaction between the patient and sonographer, making it possible to correlate the clinical picture and the ultrasound image instantly, and to modify the views accordingly. Ultrasound promotes the visualization of the superficial perfusion without the need for intravenous contrast. In addition, in its current version MRI is limited in its resolution of lesions in the nail to 3 mm, preventing detection of glomus tumors measuring less than 3 mm in diameter. However, in the same location, ultrasound is capable of detecting tumors that measure 1 mm or slightly less. Other imaging techniques such as computed tomography (CT) and x-rays cannot define the skin layers with clarity, and involve exposure to ionizing radiation.

Musculoskeletal disorders can often present as skin lesions; conversely, skin disorders can secondarily involve musculoskeletal structures. These clinical situations can add complexity to the differential diagnosis.

Clinical Indications

Primary Diagnosis

- Benign nonvascular tumors
- Benign vascular tumors
- Malignant tumors
- Vascular lesions
- Articular and periarticular lesions
- Inflammatory and infectious lesions
- Exogenous skin components
- Nail lesions

Ancillary Diagnosis: Determination of Disease Extension, Activity, or Response to Treatment

- Hemangiomas
- Morpheas
- Plantar warts
- Basal cell carcinoma

Therapeutics: Presurgical Definition of Lesional Anatomy

- Involvement of extralesional tissue structures
- Characterization of lesional and perilesional blood supply and hemodynamics

Limitations

The use of ultrasound in skin imaging requires a trained physician. The large heterogeneity of cutaneous lesions and the distortional effect introduced by uneven pressure from alterations in the compressibility of skin tissues complicates the imaging process. Moreover, lesions of solely epidermal localization, of flat subepidermal lesions, or measuring less than 0.1 mm can give normal ultrasound images (false-negatives). In these cases, ultrasound can help exclude concomitant pathologies, while providing anatomic information on the surrounding tissues. Calcium deposits, foreign bodies, and hair follicle fragments are easily defined on ultrasound, but cutaneous pigment deposits cannot be detected.

■ Technical Guidelines

The ultrasound examination starts with a thorough visual inspection of the lesion to determine the positional approach that would place the affected site closest to the operator. Sedation is administered to children less than 4 years old (chloral hydrate, 50 mg/kg, orally, 30 minutes prior to the exam) to prevent artifacts in the color Doppler spectral curve analysis. Sedation recovery is monitored with a modification of the Aldrete test score.

A copious amount of gel is then applied to the affected skin to serve as a sound conductor, pressure distributor, and focusing agent, thus directing the probe to the most superficial layers of the skin.

Lesions are examined on the screen along all cross-sectional axes (longitudinal, transverse, and oblique), and described with regard to shape, echogenicity, composition, location, and vascularity. Relevant details of the surrounding tissues, including the presence and location of feeding and surrounding vessels are also noted.

To magnify the contrast between lesional and extralesional structures, it may be helpful to perform comparative evaluations examining the contralateral side or different areas in the same corporal segment. Compression maneuvers may help define venous vessels or free-fluid collections.

■ Normal Anatomy

The skin layers can be defined on ultrasound as clearly separated structures: the epidermis appears as a fine hyperechoic line, except in the palm of the hands and sole of the feet where it is thicker and bilaminar. The dermis shows a hyperechoic band of variable thickness, produced by the dense collagen content, which is thicker in the dorsal area and thinner in the ventral forearm. The subcutaneous tissue (hypodermis) contains hypoechoic fat lobules separated by hyperechoic fibrous septa (**Fig. 9.1**).

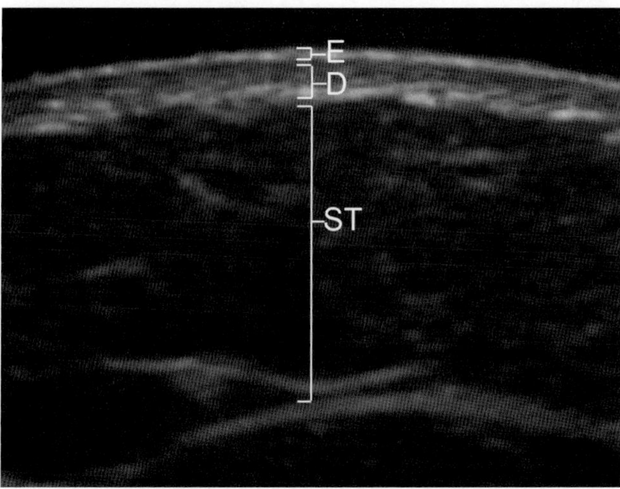

Fig. 9.1 Sonographic anatomy of the skin. E, epidermis; D, dermis; ST, subcutaneous tissue.

The nail unit comprises a hypoechoic nail bed that changes proximally to hyperechoic at the junction where the underlying dermis defines the hypoechoic matrix. The dorsal and ventral plates appear as a bilaminar parallel hyperechoic structure with a narrow, almost virtual space between the plates. The bone margin of the distal phalanx is also visible as a hyperechoic line (**Fig. 9.2**).

Low-flow vessels, venous or arterial, may be detected in the subcutaneous tissue and within the nail bed.

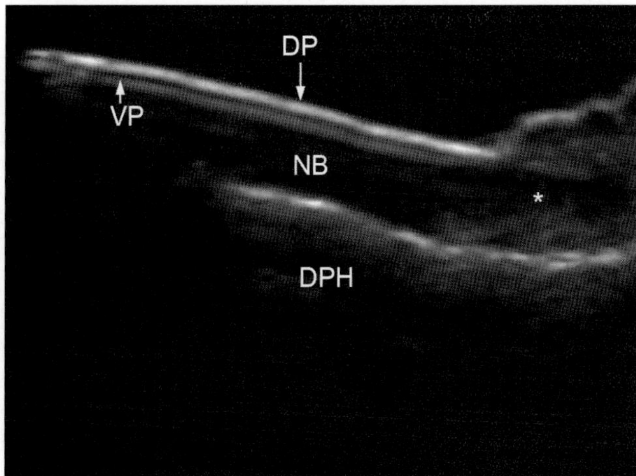

Fig. 9.2 Sonographic anatomy of the nail unit. DP, dorsal plate; VP, ventral plate; NB, nail bed; (*), matrix; DPH, bone margin of the distal phalanx.

Pathologies

Benign Tumors

Skin Cysts

Skin cysts, particularly epidermal, trichilemmal, or pilonidal cysts represent one of the most common requests for ultrasound skin examination. All these cystic lesions are located in the dermis and superficial subcutaneous tissue and present as a cosmetic problem, or as inflammatory lesions containing clear fluid, pus, or cheesy material. On ultrasound, skin cysts vary in their appearance depending on the density of the keratinous component, or the presence of inflammation or wall rupture. Noninflamed cystic lesions are round or oval, with well-defined anechoic or hypoechoic content that may contain hyperechoic hair follicle fragments or calcium deposits. In contrast, in the inflammatory stages or after wall rupture, the lesion outline becomes ill defined with a heterogeneous echo pattern and increased blood vessel signals in the periphery. In these cases, the detection of a posterior acoustic enhancement artifact can help identify the cystic origin of the lesion.

Epidermal cysts, sometimes called sebaceous cysts, originate in the infundibular portion of the hair follicle. They are not related to the sebaceous glands; hence, a "sebaceous cyst" is a misnomer. Epidermal cysts can be congenital or the result of previous trauma, including surgery. They can contain calcium deposits and/or a connecting tract to the skin surface clinically seen as a punctum. Histologically, these cysts are composed of a wall that contains squamous stratified epithelium with a granular layer and a center that contains keratin squames and fluid (**Figs. 9.3** and **9.4**).

Trichilemmal cysts originate in the external sheath of the hair follicle root; they generally do not have a connecting tract to the epidermis and are more common in areas with high hair density such as the scalp. Histologically, they are composed of a wall that contains epithelium without a granular layer and a center that contains fluid, keratin, cholesterol crystals, and sometimes calcium deposits (**Fig. 9.5**).

Pilonidal cysts are located in the intergluteal region. They are presumably related to the development of a sacral dimple that traps hair follicles; they may also be the result of repetitive local trauma. They frequently become inflamed and infected, with purulent matter discharging through a draining fistulous tract. Pilonidal cysts may be large structures; they usually present as hypoechoic fistulous tracts that become enlarged downward and contain multiple and large hyperechoic lines corresponding to a nest with hair follicle fragments (**Fig. 9.6**).

Lipomas

These are the most common soft tissue tumors and are composed of mature adipose cells. On ultrasound, they show variable echogenicity, most frequently hypoechogenicity, but a mixed pattern of hypo-/hyperechogenicity may also be seen. The lipomas may be oval or round and usually run parallel to the main axis of the skin, most often as single tumors, in the subcutaneous tissue, although in 5 to 15% of the cases they may appear as multiple tumors (**Fig. 9.7**).

Pilomatrixomas

Also called calcifying Malherbe epitheliomas, these tumors are derived from the hair matrix. They are most frequently found in children and young adults. Pilomatrixomas appear as single or multiple skin-colored or purplish lesions mainly in the head and neck. Sonographically, they are target round-shaped lesions located in the dermis and subcutaneous tissue composed by a hypoechoic rim corresponding to the tumor capsule that surrounds a hyperechoic center.

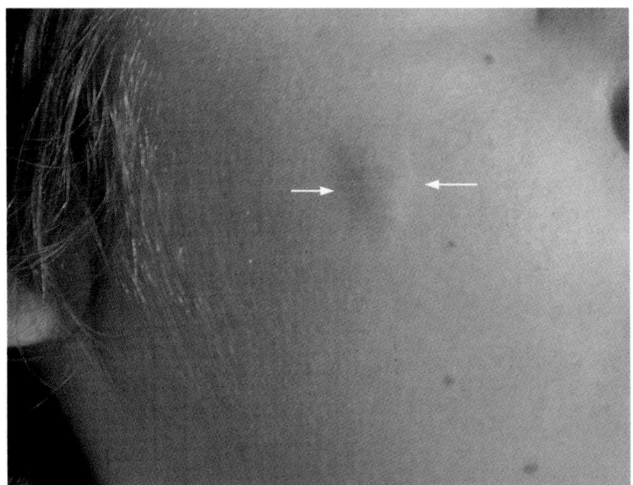

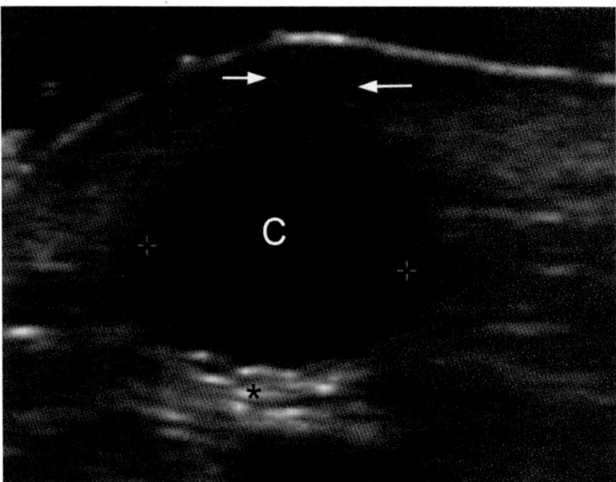

Fig. 9.3 Epidermal cyst. **(A)** Erythematous lesion in the cheek of a child (*arrows*). **(B)** Transverse view shows a round anechoic structure with inner echoes (*between markers*) in the dermis and upper subcutaneous tissue, and connected by a duct to the subepidermal zone (*arrows*). Posterior acoustic enhancement artifact is visible (*). C, cyst.

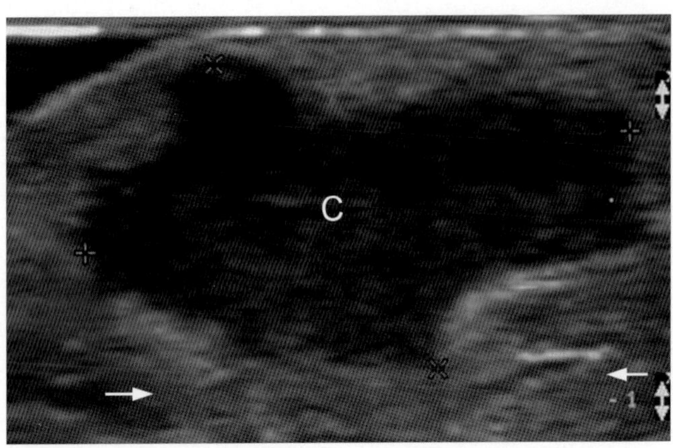

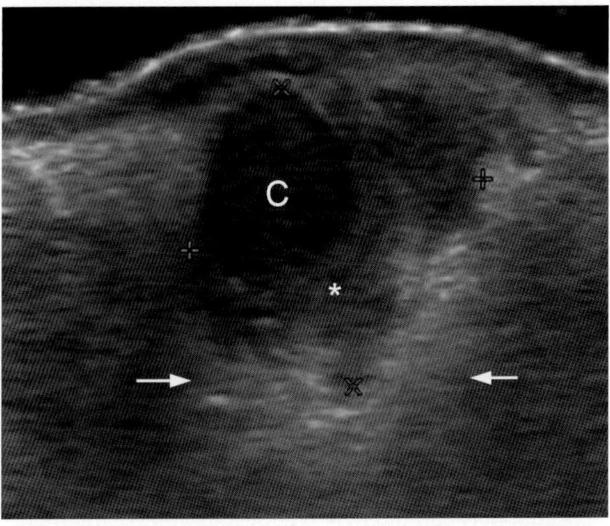

Fig. 9.4 Epidermal cyst complicated with inflammation. **(A)** Transverse view shows a hypoechoic structure of irregular shape (C) that corresponds with the epidermal cyst. A posterior acoustic enhancement artifact, seen in fluid-filled structures, is also present (*arrows*). **(B)** Transverse view shows a cyst with disruption of its capsule and inflammatory reaction to the keratinous component released to the surrounding tissue (*).The posterior acoustic enhancement artifact is still detectable under the cyst (*arrows*).

This center is composed of epithelial cells, and in 75% of the cases, of calcium deposits that appear as hyperechoic dots (**Fig. 9.8**).

Malignant Tumors

Skin cancer affects sun-exposed areas of the skin and is classified into nonmelanoma skin cancer (NMSC) and melanoma. NMSC, the most frequent tumors, include two subtypes: basal cell carcinoma (BCC) and squamous cell carcinoma (SCC).

Basal cell carcinoma is the most common cancer in humans; it is a slow-growing lesion affecting mostly individuals with light colored skin. They may be locally aggressive, but rarely metastasize. The most frequent location is the face; less often, the trunk and extremities. Several subtypes are recognized histologically: nodular, adenoid, and morpheaform, but clinically they have a common presentation as a round pearly nodule covered with telangiectasias, ulceration, and/or bleeding. Rare clinical presentations are as a bluish–gray cystic nodule or as a scarring plaque lesion. On ultrasound, BCCs appear as oval-shaped tumors of heterogeneous hypoechogenicity, with irregular contour and in-

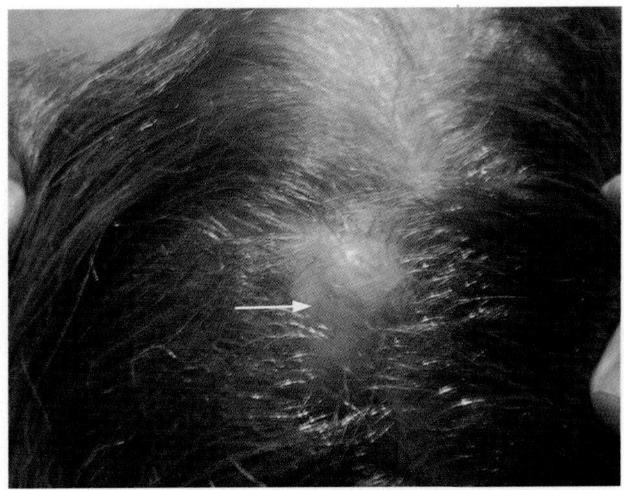

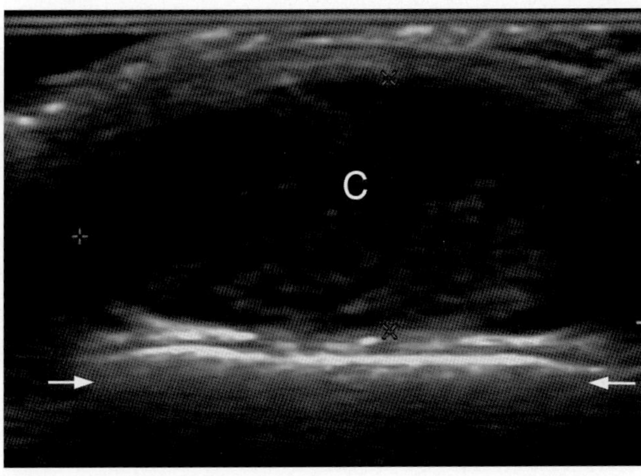

Fig. 9.5 Trichilemmal cyst in the scalp. **(A)** Clinically, there is an area of swelling and alopecia in the scalp (*arrow*). **(B)** Ultrasound (transverse view) in the scalp shows an anechoic cystic lesion (C, *between markers*) with echoes that correspond to the keratinous content. Posterior acoustic enhancement is clearly detectable (*arrows*).

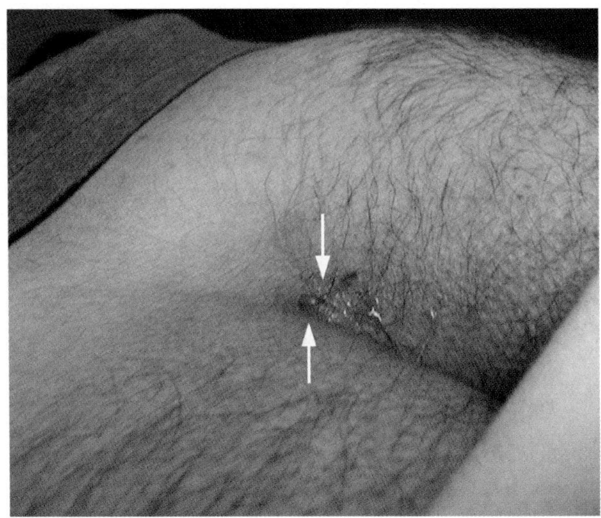

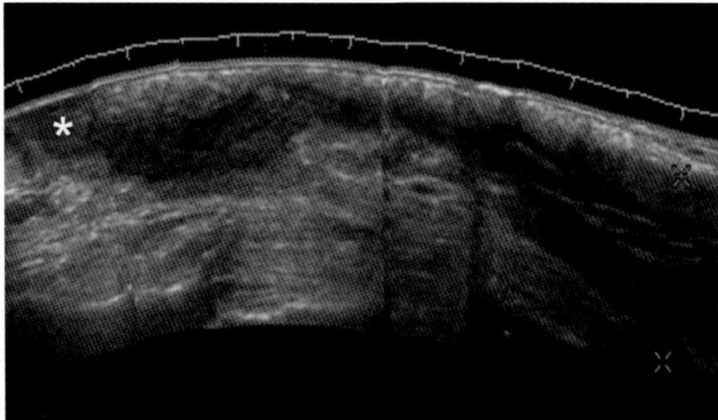

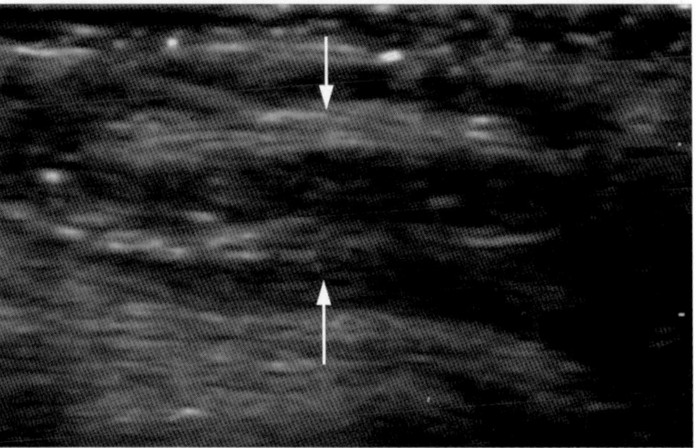

Fig. 9.6 Pilonidal cyst. **(A)** Clinically, there is erythematous swelling in the intergluteal zone (*arrows*). **(B)** Panoramic longitudinal view of the intergluteal region shows an extensive fistulous tract that runs through the cutaneous layers and becomes wider in the sacral region (*between markers*). The clinical cutaneous lesion corresponds to only the upward part of the cyst (*). **(C)** Longitudinal view shows multiple hyperechoic lines inside the cyst that correspond to hair fragments (*arrows*) inside the cyst.

creased arterial vascularization deep within the tumor and at the periphery. Hyperechoic dots inside the tumor have been also described (**Figs. 9.9** and **9.10**).

Squamous cell carcinoma is the second most common cancer of the skin and appears as crusted or scaly patches with a red inflamed base, as a growing nodule, or as a nonhealing ulcer. On ultrasound, they are seen as slightly irregular heterogeneous hypoechoic lesions, or as nodules extending to deeper structures. SCC has tumoral blood vessels on color Doppler that are more prominent than in BCC and also a higher recurrence rate (**Fig. 9.11**).

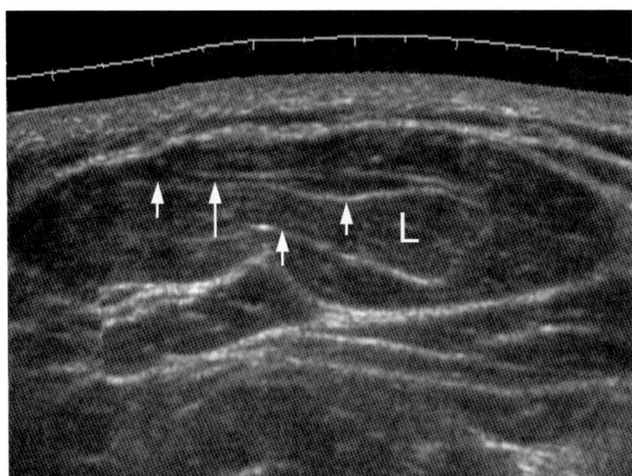

Fig. 9.7 Lipoma. Longitudinal panoramic view shows an oval hypoechoic structure (L) with hyperechoic fibrous septa (*arrows*) in the subcutaneous tissue that runs parallel to the skin layers' axis.

Melanoma is a malignant skin tumor derived from melanocytes. It is the least frequent, but most threatening type of skin cancer, accounting for 75% of all skin cancer deaths. Melanoma thickness is used to calculate the Breslow index from the depth of involvement by the tumor and is used to assess the patient's prognosis. Both sonographic and histologic measurements are strongly and directly correlated. On ultrasound, melanoma lesions have an oval or slightly fusiform shape of hypoechoic and heterogeneous structure, generally accompanied by increased vascularity within the tumor, probably related to increased angiogenesis and a marker for metastatic potential. Locoregional detection of metastases by ultrasound has been reported as significantly more sensitive than physical examination (**Fig. 9.12**).

Vascular Tumors

These are the most common childhood tumors—present in approximately one in three children. In 1992, Mulliken classified these vascular lesions into hemangiomas and vascular malformations, differing in presentation, clinical course, and histologic characteristics.

Hemangiomas are hamartomas composed of small vessels; immediately after birth the tumors grow rapidly and

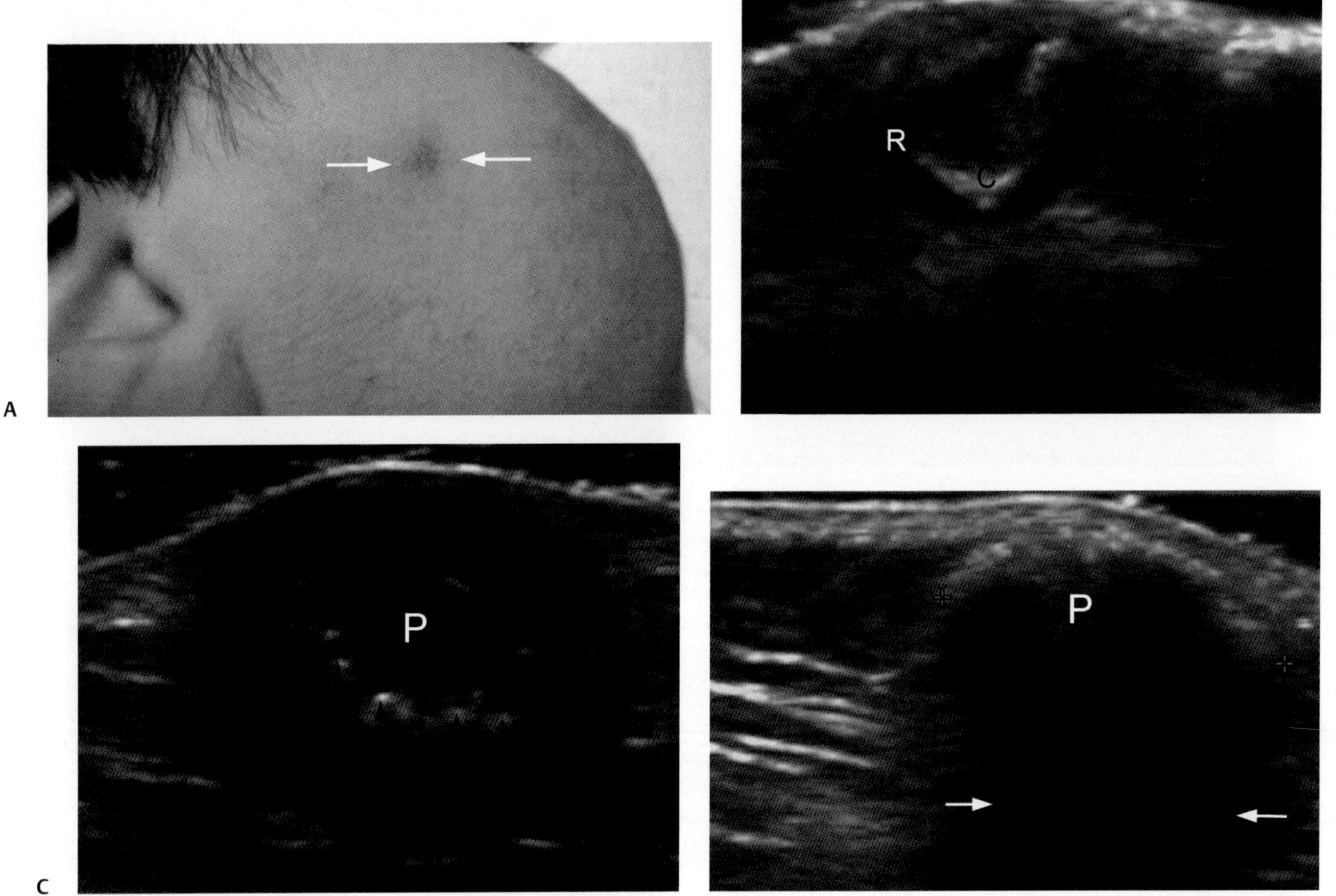

Fig. 9.8 Sonographic appearances of pilomatrixomas. **(A)** Clinical erythematous swelling in the cheek (*arrows*). **(B)** Transverse view shows a lesion with a hypoechoic rim (R) and a hyperechoic center (C), the classical target pattern of pilomatrixomas. **(C)** Transverse view shows a target-shaped nodule in the dermis and upper subcutaneous tissue with a hypoechoic rim (P) and a hyperechoic center. There are inner hyperechoic dots corresponding to calcium deposits (*arrows*). **(D)** Transverse view shows a nodule (P) with high calcium content and intense posterior acoustic shadowing artifact (*arrows*).

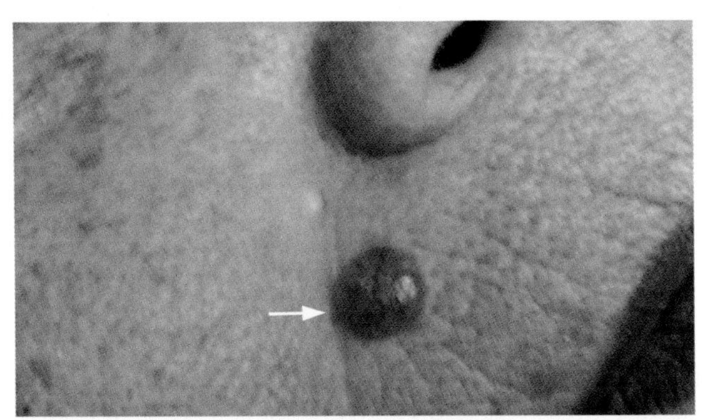

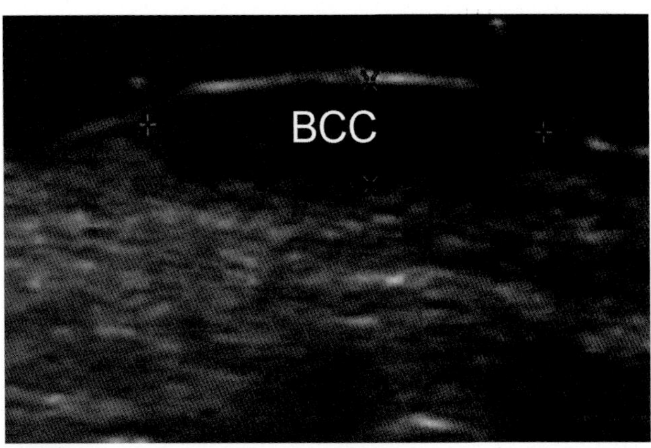

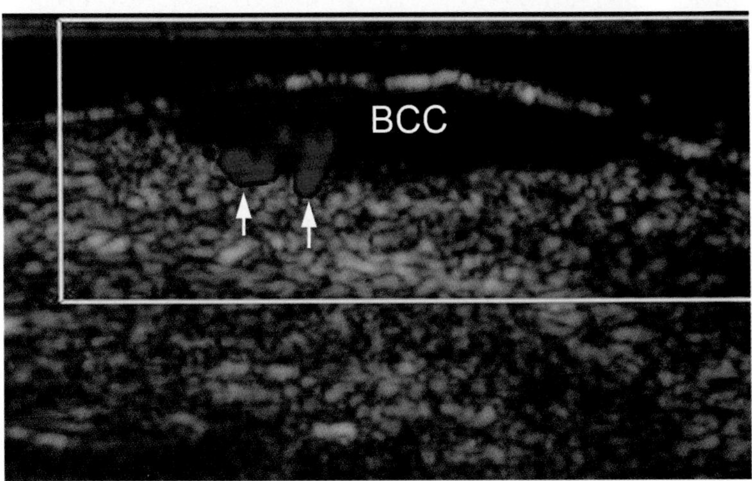

Fig. 9.9 Basal cell carcinoma (BCC). **(A)** Clinical nodular telangiectatic lesion in the upper lip (*arrow*). **(B)** Transverse view shows an oval-shaped hypoechoic lesion (*between markers*) involving epidermis and dermis. **(C)** Color Doppler transverse view shows the presence of blood vessels in the deep portion of the tumor (*colors and arrows*).

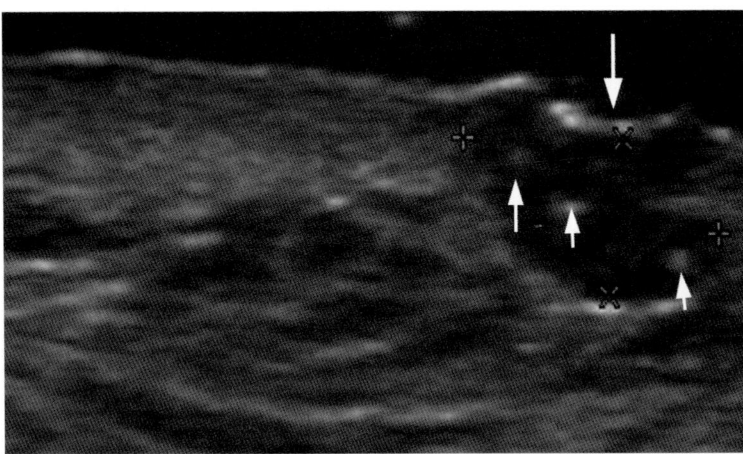

Fig. 9.10 Basal cell carcinoma (BCC). Longitudinal view of a BCC lesion shows a hypoechoic and irregular nodule that involves epidermis, dermis, and the upper subcutaneous tissue (*between markers*). Ulceration is seen in the epidermal area (*long arrow*) and some hyperechoic dots (*short arrows*) are detectable inside the lesion.

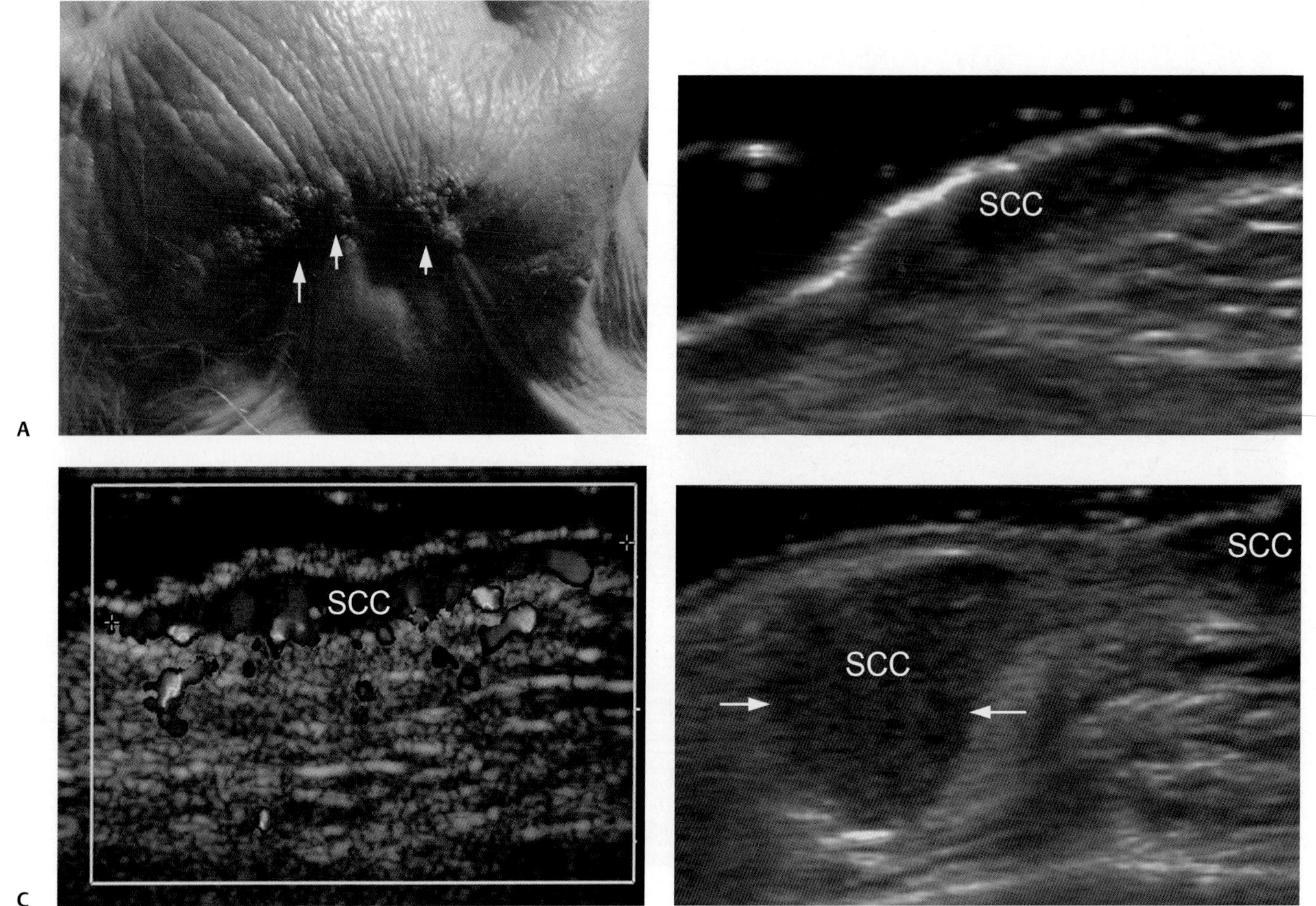

Fig. 9.11 Squamous cell carcinoma (SCC). **(A)** Clinical lesion in the right cheek (*arrows*). **(B)** Longitudinal view shows a hypoechoic and heterogeneous solid lesion involving epidermis and dermis. **(C)** Color Doppler (longitudinal view) shows the moderate presence of blood vessels inside the lesion (*colors*). **(D)** Transverse view shows in the upper right part of the ultrasound image, the original SCC lesion that presents a hidden and satellite deep extension with an oval hypoechoic nodule (*SCC and arrows*) in the subcutaneous tissue.

reach a plateau only at 1 to 2 years of age, to be followed by involution through the following 5 to 6 years. These stages can be separated sonographically, with the growth phase appearing as a solid hypoechoic and highly vascular lesion that contains arterial and venous vessels, and arteriovenous shunts. The vessels progressively decrease in both size and flow, and echogenicity becomes more heterogeneous (**Figs. 9.13** and **9.14**). In the phase of involution, tumors become hyperechoic with scarce blood flow.

Hemangiomas are often treated with corticosteroids when there is periorificial involvement (orbital, nasal, or oral), or when they extend to deeper structures. In these cases, ultrasound is especially useful to monitor the response to treatment.

Vascular malformations (VM) are the result of embryologic abnormalities and are classified according to the dominant vascular channel into arterial, venous, capillary, mixed, and lymphatic lesions. According to the flow pattern, VM have been also grouped into high or low flow lesions, with high flow lesions corresponding to a predominance of arterial vessels. Vascular malformations are already present at birth and tend to grow proportionally with the child, and to become even more noticeable during adolescence or pregnancy. Effective treatments include laser, surgery, or

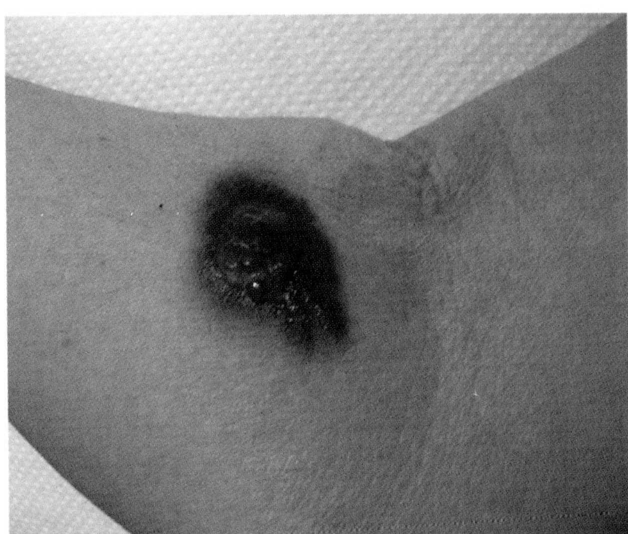

A

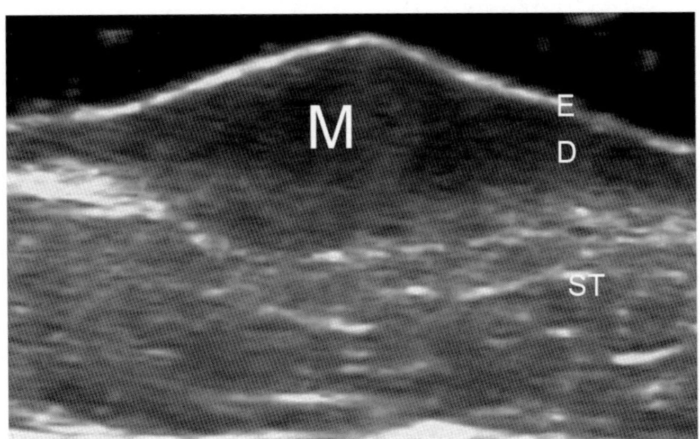

B

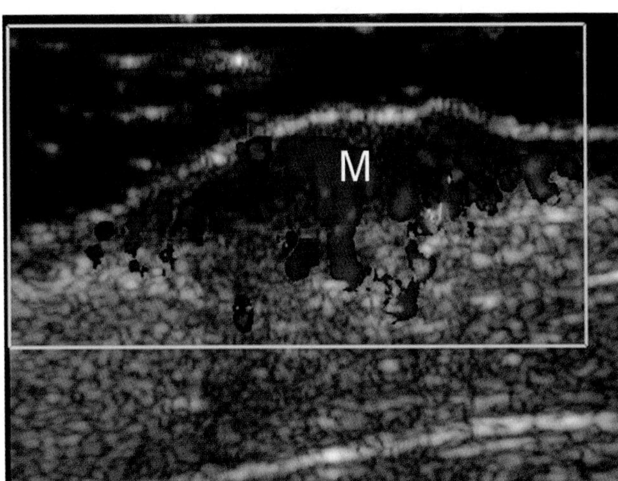

C

Fig. 9.12 **(A)** Melanoma clinical lesion darkly pigmented. **(B)** Melanoma (M). Transverse view shows fusiform and hypoechoic lesion involving epidermis (E), dermis (D), and superficial subcutaneous tissue (ST). **(C)** Melanoma (M). Color Doppler transverse view shows marked vascularity of the lesion.

embolization techniques; the lesions are usually unresponsive to steroids. Sonographically, VM are seen as tubular anechoic structures shaped as a nest, or as anechoic lake-like areas (**Figs. 9.15** and **9.16**). Low-flow capillary malformations may appear as a solid hyperechoic structure when located subcutaneously, or as hypoechoic when located in the dermis.

Vascular malformations are most commonly restricted to the skin layers, although occasionally they involve deeper structures; for example, vascular malformations may be associated with zones of lipodystrophy (focal hypertrophy or atrophy of the fat in the subcutaneous tissue) and misdiagnosed as lipomatous tumors.

Both hemangiomas and vascular malformations may involve musculoskeletal structures or glands, locations that could become critical around natural orifices. Hemangiomas may also be associated with secondary (reactive) enlargement of muscles or adjacent structures.

Nontumoral Vascular Lesions of the Skin

Mondor Disease

Mondor disease, or sclerosing thrombophlebitis of subcutaneous veins, was first described in the breast, but it can affect other sites such as the abdominal or thoracic walls.

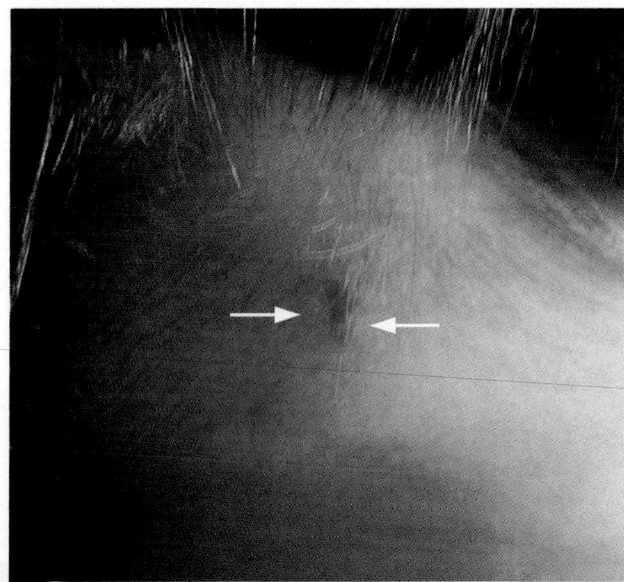

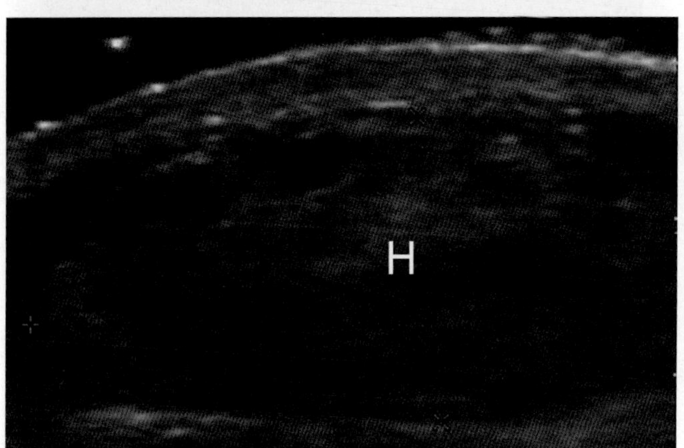

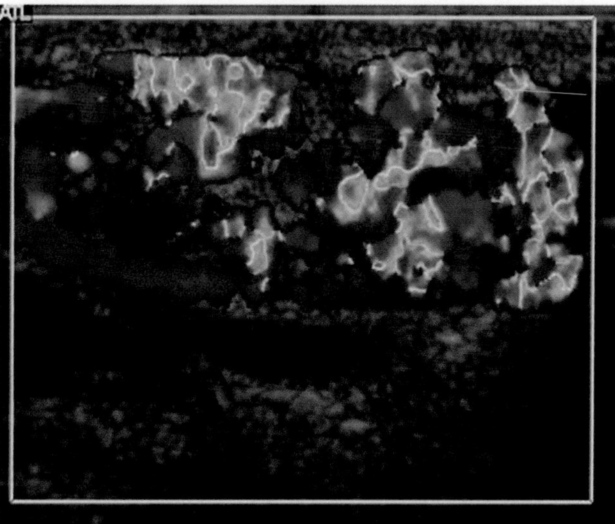

Fig. 9.13 Hemangioma. **(A)** Clinical small erythematous lesion (*arrows*) in the posterior neck of a child. **(B)** Hemangioma (H). Transverse view shows a hyperechoic and heterogeneous solid structure in the subcutaneous tissue (*between markers*), much larger and deeper than clinical appearance. **(C)** Color Doppler transverse view shows marked vascularity (*colors*) inside the solid subcutaneous lesion.

Clinically, they appear as palpable, sometimes painful, cord-like structures. Mondor disease is more common in women and may be related to trauma. Sonography shows a venous vessel with lumen occluded by thrombotic hypoechoic material, without detectable flow (**Fig. 9.17**). On follow-up studies, ultrasound can show actual regression of the venous thrombosis.

Large Vessel Thrombosis

Large vessel thrombosis can elicit sudden changes in the skin, such as telangiectasis (dilatation of capillary skin vessels), erythema. or edema. Affected vessels are most frequently veins, and ultrasound shows thrombotic hypoechoic endoluminal material and absence of compressibility of the vein walls. Color Doppler and spectral curve analysis demonstrates absence of flow in the affected vessel. Compensatory venous dilatation may also be observed (**Fig. 9.18**).

Insufficiency of Perforant Veins

Chronic incompetence of perforant veins that drain into the superficial venous system can elicit pigmentary changes and/or chronic ulcers in the skin. On ultrasound, superficial veins are dilated and tortuous, and are associated with reflux flow during the Valsalva maneuver on dynamic color Doppler examination. The differential diagnosis includes pyoderma gangrenosum, which is an uncommon ulcerative inflammatory condition of unclear etiology that presents as chronic painful ulcerations occasionally associated with inflammatory bowel

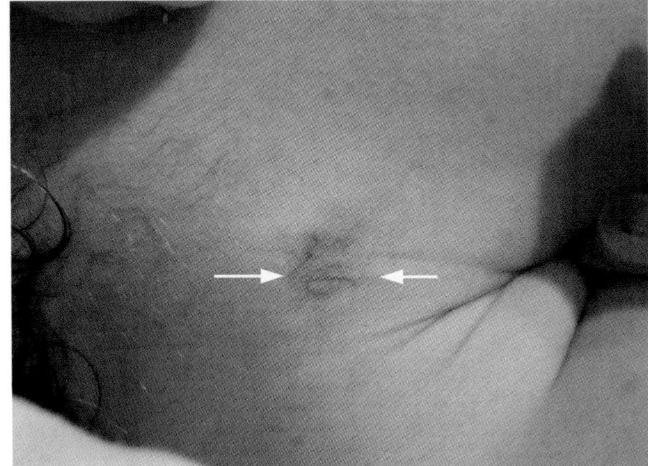

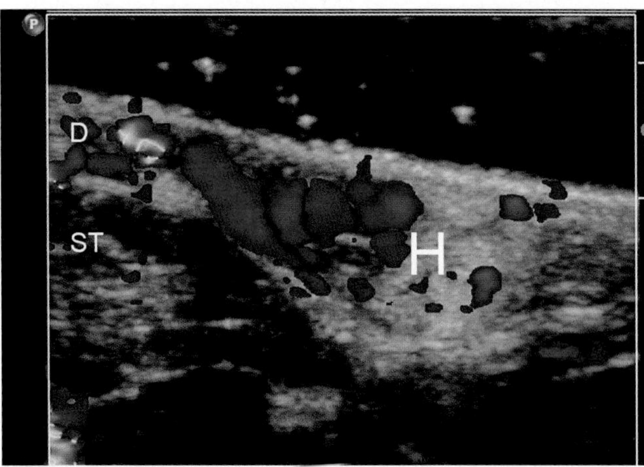

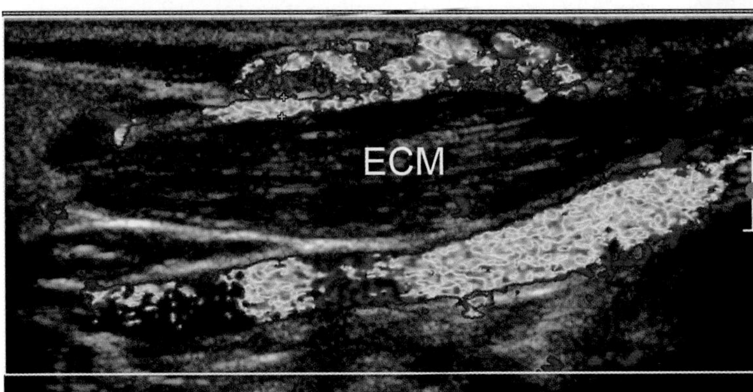

Fig. 9.14 Hemangioma. **(A)** Clinical vascular skin lesion in the anterior aspect of the neck of a child (*arrows*). **(B)** Color Doppler longitudinal view shows a solid and heterogeneous structure in the subcutaneous tissue presenting a highly vascular component (*colors*). H, hemangioma. D, dermis; ST, subcutaneous tissue. **(C)** Hemangioma with secondary muscle hypertrophy. Color Doppler longitudinal view shows enlargement of the sternocleidomastoid muscle (ECM) in the side of the hemangioma. High vascularity in the affected area is also detected.

diseases, arthritis, monoclonal gammopathies, or cancer. On ultrasound of pyoderma gangrenosum lesions, superficial veins are normal and there is significant hyperechogenicity (inflammation) of the subcutaneous layer; more rarely, subcutaneous veins may be inflamed (phlebitis) appearing as venous walls thickening. Occasionally, insufficiency of perforant veins may mimic vascular skin tumors (**Fig. 9.19**).

Pseudoaneurysms

These are commonly the result of incomplete laceration of the arterial wall with formation of an intraparietal hematoma from direct trauma. They usually present as a pulsatile mass and/or superficial swelling. Ultrasound of the pseudoaneurysm affected segment shows turbulent blood flow; hard compression maneuvers to decrease or occlude the lesion could be useful in the early stages. When the pulsatile nature of the pseudoaneurysm is subtle, it may be confused with other causes of swelling such as skin cysts or lipomas and generate major surgical complications (**Fig. 9.20**).

Inflammatory and Infectious Disorders of the Skin

Fistulous Tracts

These present with chronic discharge of pus or exudate through the skin; they are most often located in the mandibular region (odontogenic fistula). Fistulous tracts may

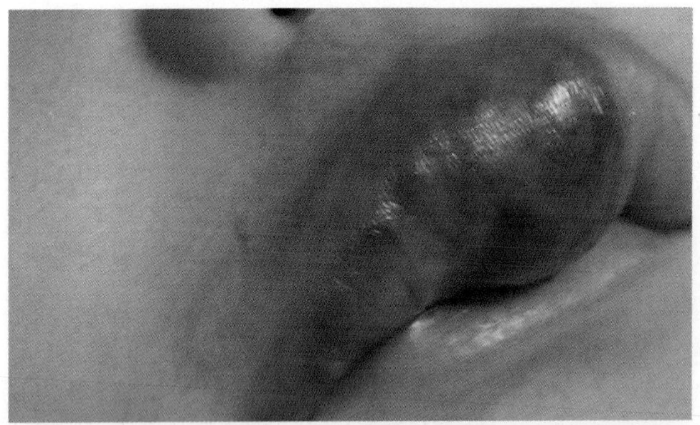

A

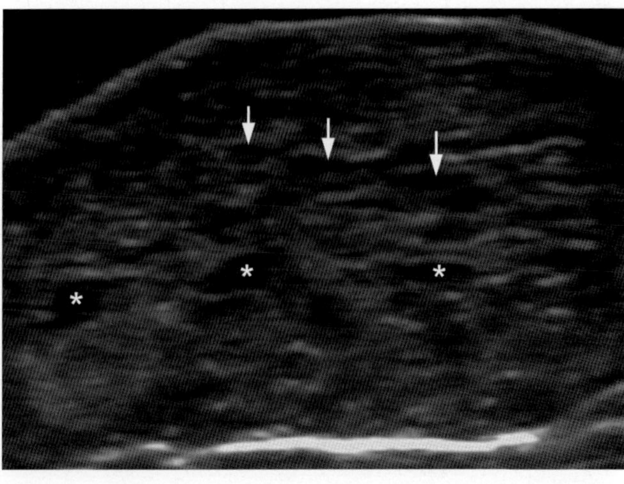

B

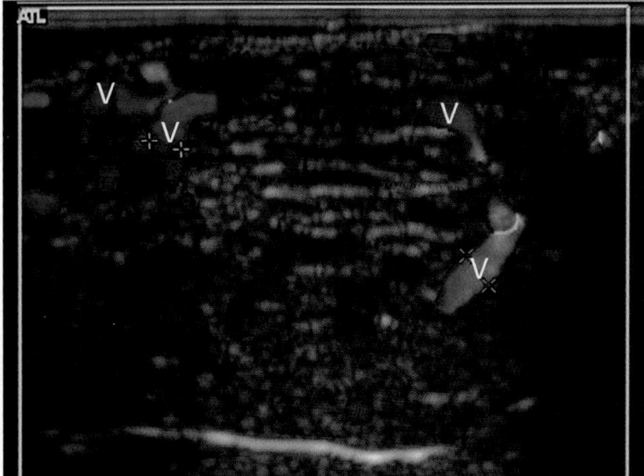

C

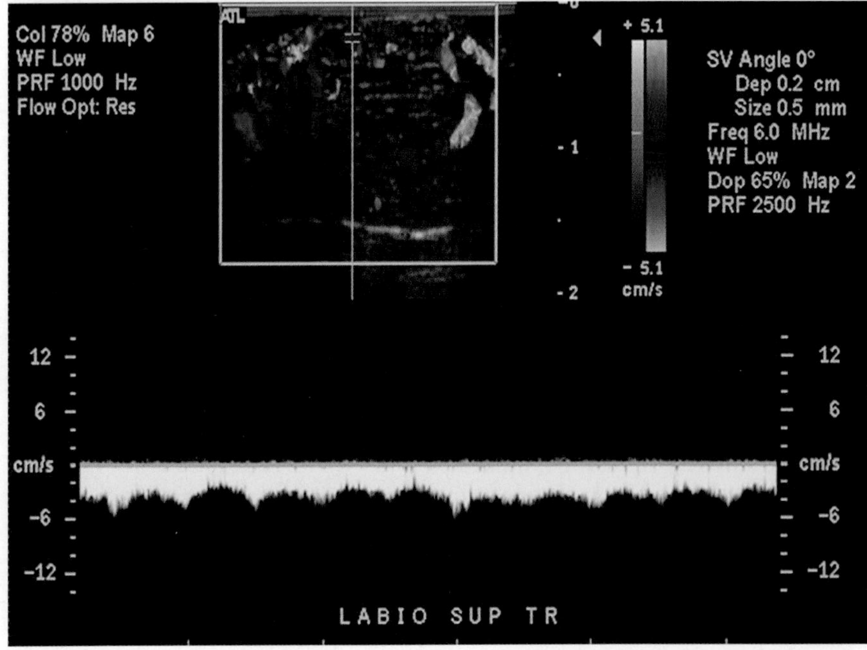

D

Fig. 9.15 Venous vascular malformation. **(A)** Clinical prominence of the upper lip. **(B)** Transverse view shows multiple anechoic tubular structures (*arrows*) and lake-areas (*) in the dermis and subcutaneous tissue of the upper lip, also involving the orbicularis oris muscle layer. **(C)** Color Doppler transverse view shows low vascularity inside the lesion; venous vessels (V) could be compressed easily with the probe. **(D)** Color Doppler spectral curve shows venous blood flow inside the vascular structures.

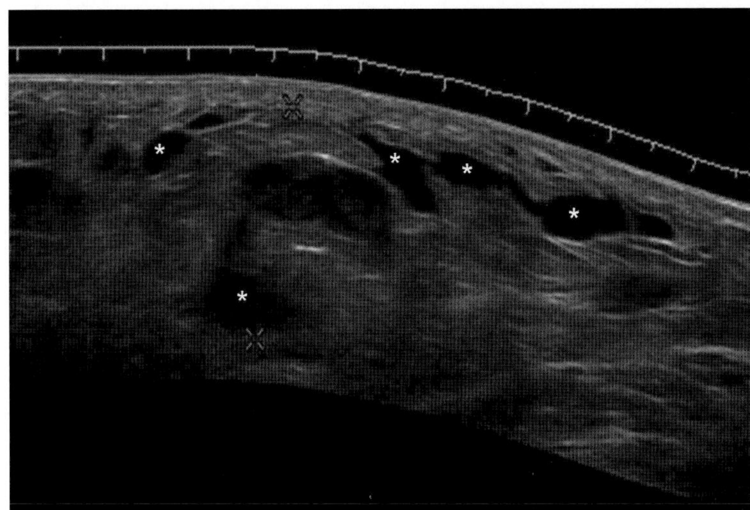

Fig. 9.16 Lymphatic vascular malformation. Transverse panoramic view in the cheek of a child shows multiple anechoic lake-areas in the subcutaneous tissue (*). No flow was detectable in these areas during the color Doppler ultrasound examination.

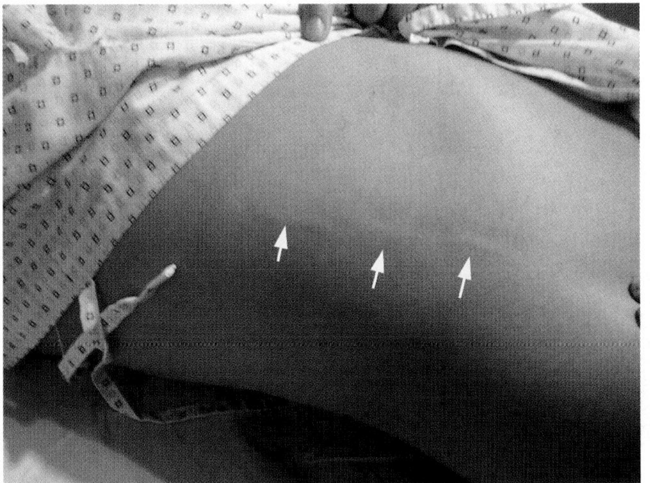

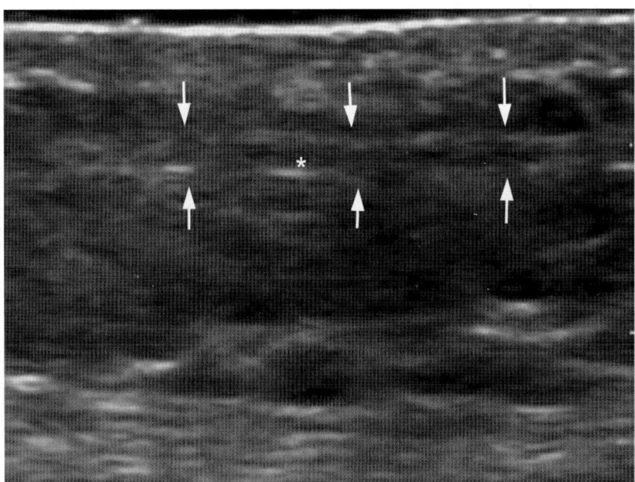

Fig. 9.17 Mondor disease. **(A)** Clinical picture of a woman presenting with a cord-like lesion in the right abdomen (*arrows*). **(B)** Longitudinal view shows a subcutaneous vein filled with hypoechoic thrombosed material (*arrows and* *). **(C)** Color Doppler longitudinal view shows absence of flow inside the subcutaneous vein.

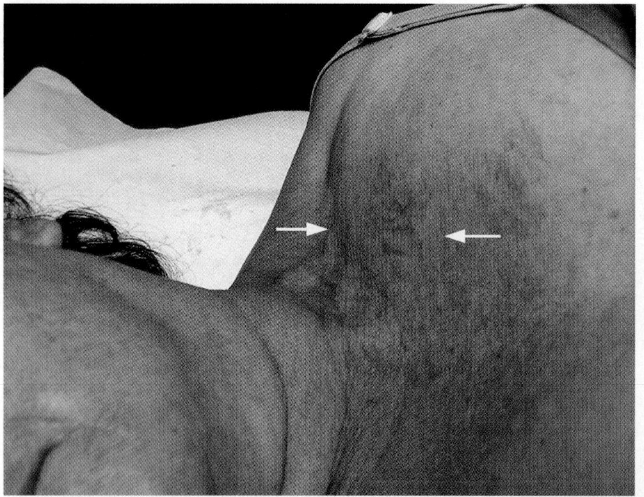

A

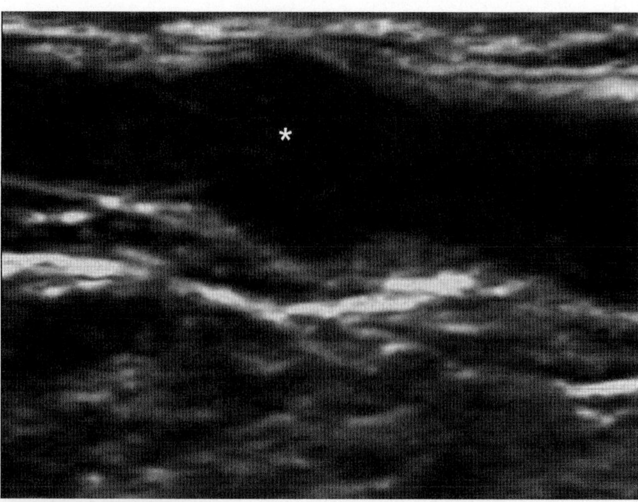

B

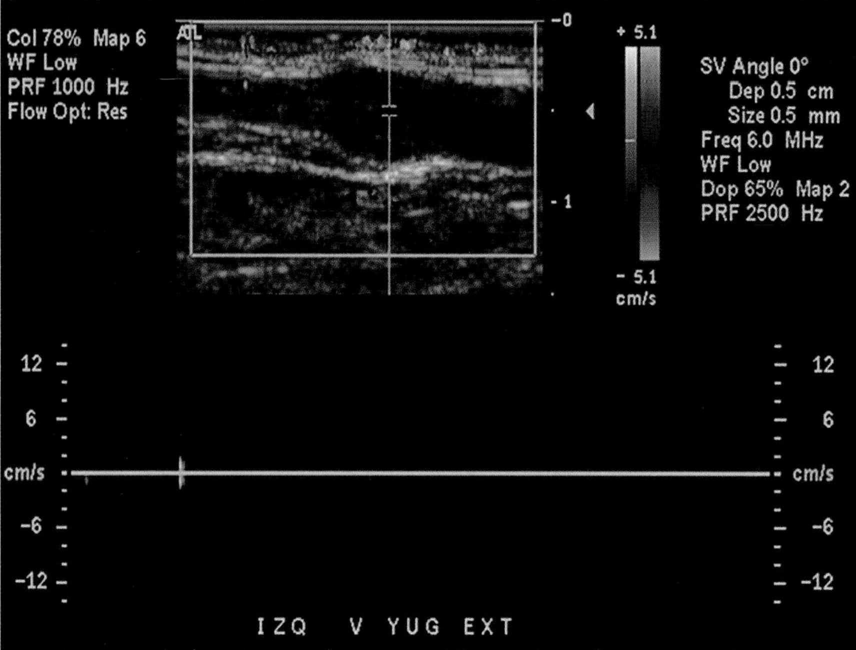

C

Fig. 9.18 External jugular vein thrombosis. **(A)** Female patient presenting with telangiectasias (*arrows*) of sudden onset in the left side of the neck and supraclavicular region. **(B)** Longitudinal view shows the external jugular vein dilated and filled with hypoechoic thrombotic material (*). **(C)** Color Doppler spectral curve analysis shows absence of blood flow inside the vein. The patient also had thrombosis of the common jugular and the subclavian veins.

also be caused by hidradenitis suppurativa, a condition that usually affects the axillae and inguinal areas.

On ultrasound, fistulous tracts appear as hypoechoic channels containing inner rich-debris echoes and/or hair fragments surrounded by blood vessels. Occasionally, fistulous tracts may extend into deeper structures that allow skin layers to communicate with the bone margin (**Fig. 9.21**). Fistulous tracts associated with hidradenitis suppurativa present a chronic course and run through the dermis. These fistulous tracts can be accompanied by large and complex hypoechoic dermal fluid collections and nodular lesions (**Fig. 9.22**).

Fat Necrosis

Fat necrosis is the liquefaction of fatty tissue, most frequently after direct trauma, resulting in the development of subcutaneous nodules. Fat necrosis can be associated with pigmentary changes of the skin as well as musculoskeletal injury. On ultrasound, small anechoic cystic structures are

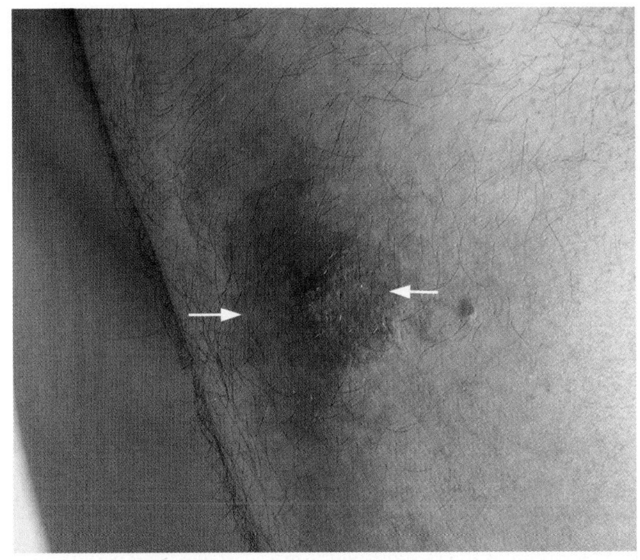

A

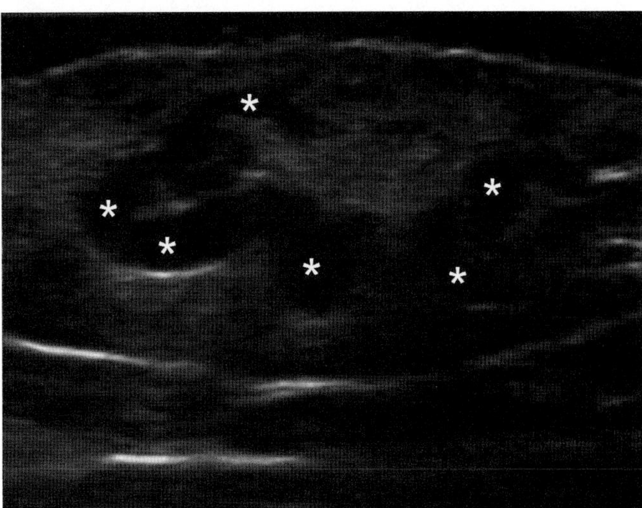

B

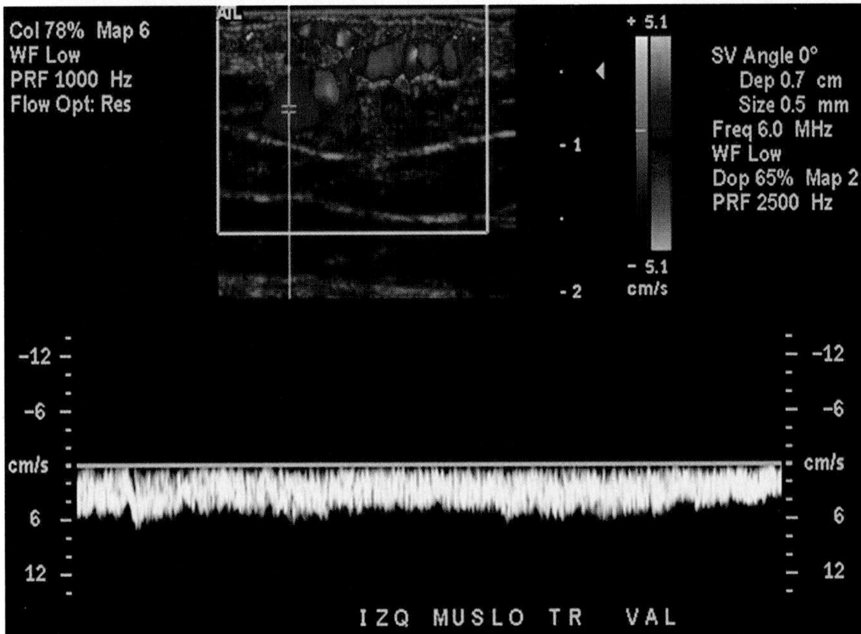

C

Fig. 9.19 Perforant veins insufficiency. **(A)** Clinical erythematous and purple rash with swelling in the right thigh (*arrows*) suspected of angiosarcoma. **(B)** Longitudinal view shows numerous dilated and tortuous vessels in the dermis and subcutaneous tissue (*). There is also hyperechogenicity and thickening of the dermis and superficial subcutaneous tissue. **(C)** Color Doppler spectral curve analysis shows low-flow venous vessels. On a dynamic study, the vessels demonstrated reflux of the blood flow.

detected between areas of edematous hyperechoic fatty lobules in the subcutaneous tissue (**Fig. 9.23**).

Fluid Collections

These are hematomas or abscesses, and represent collections of blood or fibrinous material organized and/or infected. On ultrasound, there is variable echogenicity that depending on the type of fluid collected may range from anechoic to a complex hypoechoic pattern. When infection is present, echogenicity is enhanced and internal echoes or septa can be detected within the fluid collection; color Doppler ultrasound may show hypervascularity in the periphery of the lesions.

Dermatomyositis—Calcinosis

This is a connective tissue disease characterized by myositis and inflammation of the skin layers. On ultrasound, dystrophic calcifications (secondary calcinosis) can be detected within the muscles and cutaneous layers appearing as hy-

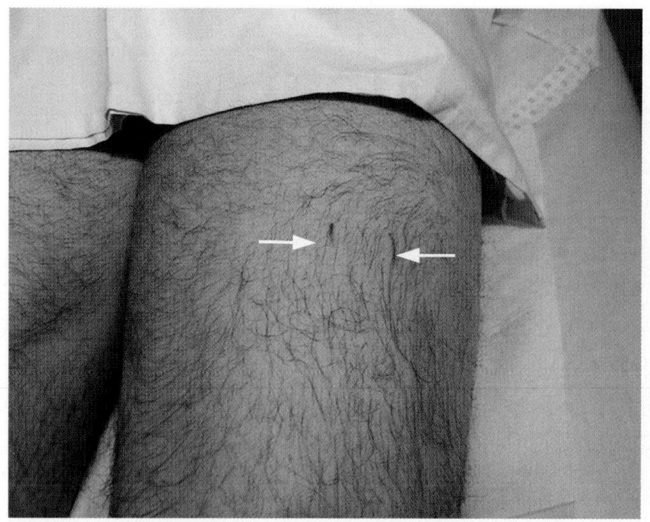
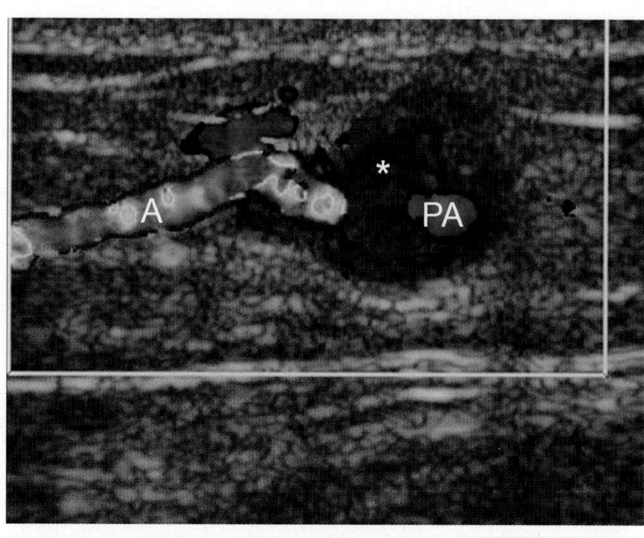

Fig. 9.20 Pseudoaneurysm partially thrombosed. **(A)** Clinical swelling in the upper thigh suggested of lipoma (*arrows*). **(B)** Color Doppler ultrasound shows saccular dilatation (PA) of a subcutaneous artery (A). The lumen of the pseudoaneurysm is partially filled with thrombotic material (*).

perechoic focal deposits with posterior acoustic shadowing (**Fig. 9.24**). Muscular echogenicity can also be increased by the underlying inflammatory process.

Lymphedema

This is characterized by diffuse thickening of the cutaneous layers due to lymphatic obstruction from trauma, surgery, and/or infection. Lymphedema presents with a swollen limb or more localized skin area, associated sometimes with color changes (discoloration or erythema). On ultrasound, there is thickening of the skin layers with hypoechogenicity of the dermis and hyperechogenicity of subcutaneous tissues; anechoic laminar fluid between the subcutaneous fat lobules may also be detected (**Fig. 9.25**). Lastly, blood flow is maintained through superficial and deep venous blood vessels and used to differentiate lymphedema from deep venous thrombosis that can also cause a swollen limb.

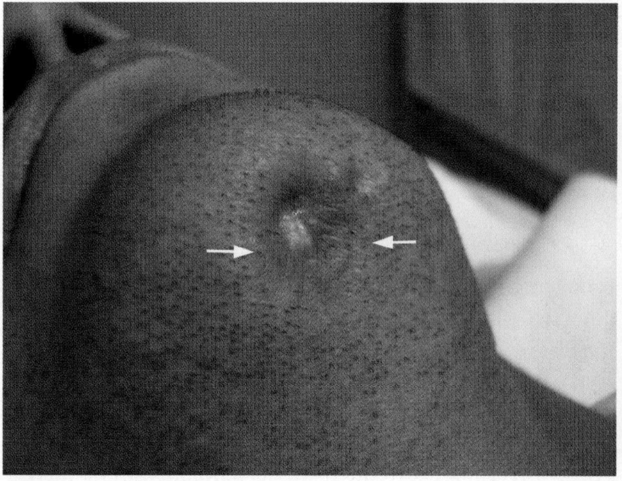
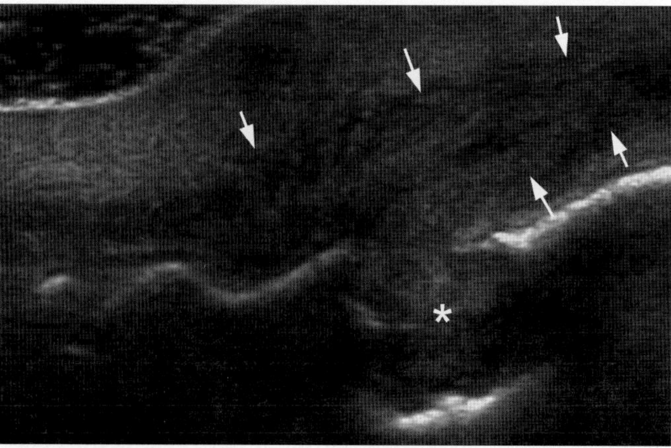

Fig. 9.21 Odontogenic fistula. **(A)** Clinical scarred depressed erythematous lesion in the middle line of the submandibular region (*arrows*). **(B)** Longitudinal view shows a hypoechoic tract (*arrows*) connecting the skin with the mandibular bone margin. There is also erosion and destruction of the mandible bone (*) corresponding to osteomyelitis.

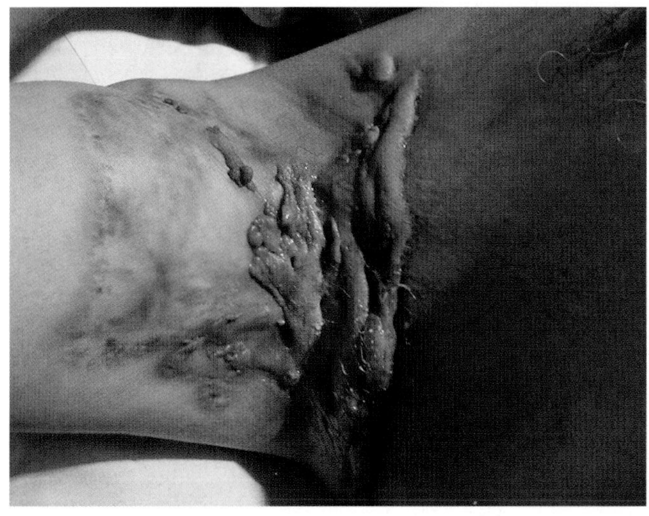
A

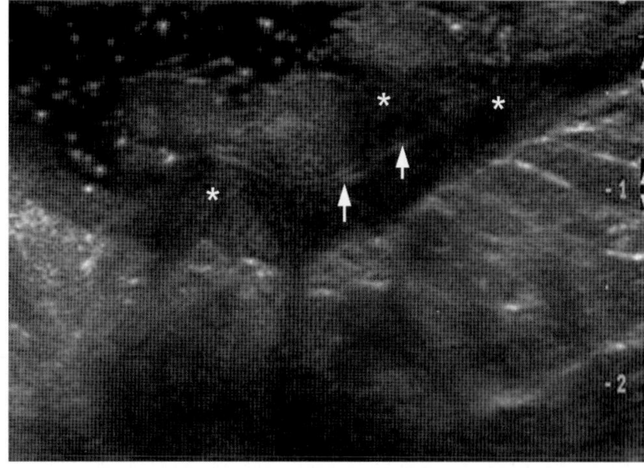

B

Fig. 9.22 **(A)** Hidradenitis suppurativa clinical lesion in the axillary region. **(B)** Hidradenitis suppurativa collection. Transverse view of the axillae shows a large dermal collection (*) with anechoic fluid, echo-rich debris, and a hyperechoic linear structure corresponding to a hair fragment (*arrows*).

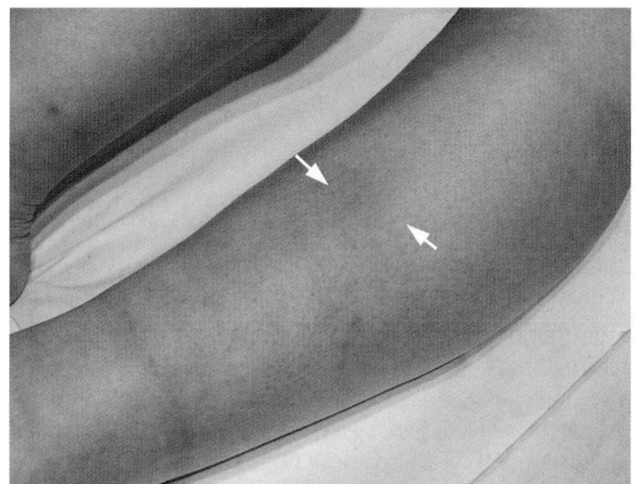
A

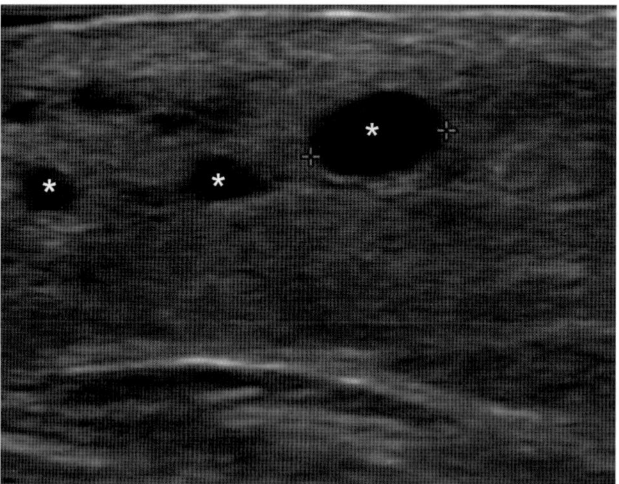

B

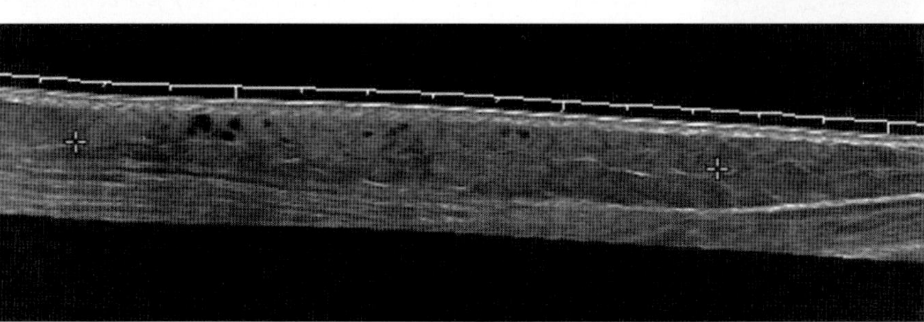
C

Fig. 9.23 Fat necrosis. **(A)** Clinical picture shows subtly pigmented area in the anterior aspect of the left leg (*arrows*). **(B)** Transverse view shows multiple round anechoic cystic structures (*) and increased echogenicity of the subcutaneous tissue. **(C)** Panoramic longitudinal view shows extensive subcutaneous involvement (*between markers*).

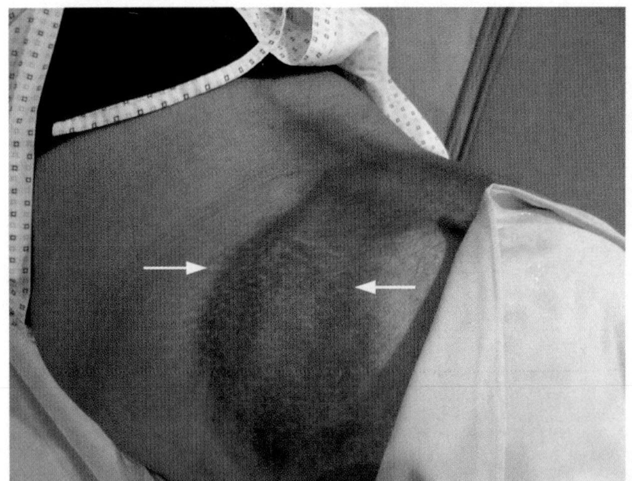

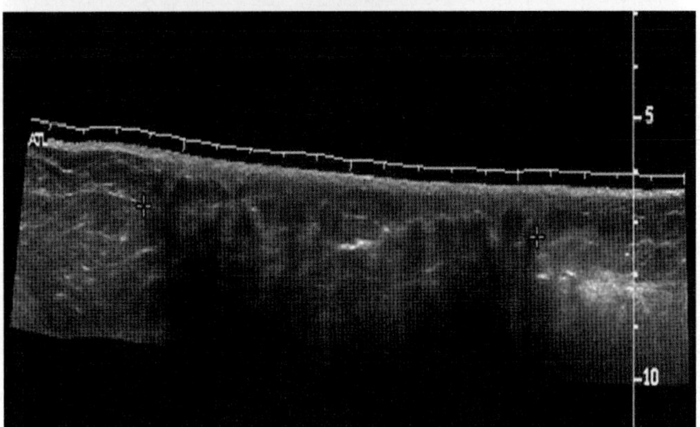

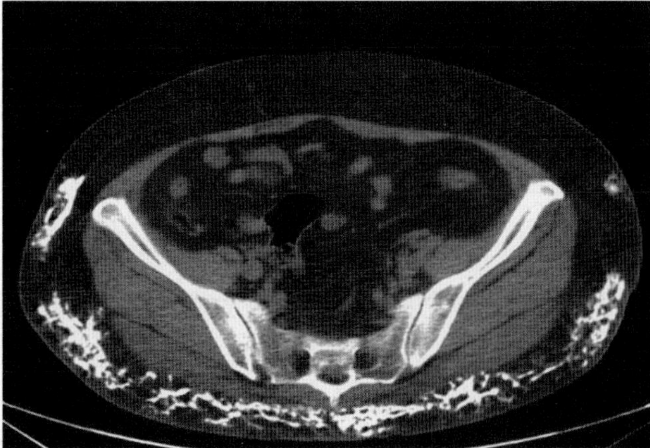

Fig. 9.24 Dermatomyositis. **(A)** Clinical pigmentation and swelling (*arrows*) of the lumbar region in a female patient. **(B)** Longitudinal panoramic view shows presence of multiple hyperechoic calcic deposits in the subcutaneous tissue with posterior acoustic shadowing (*between markers*). **(C)** Computed tomography (CT) axial image shows the large hyperdense calcium deposits.

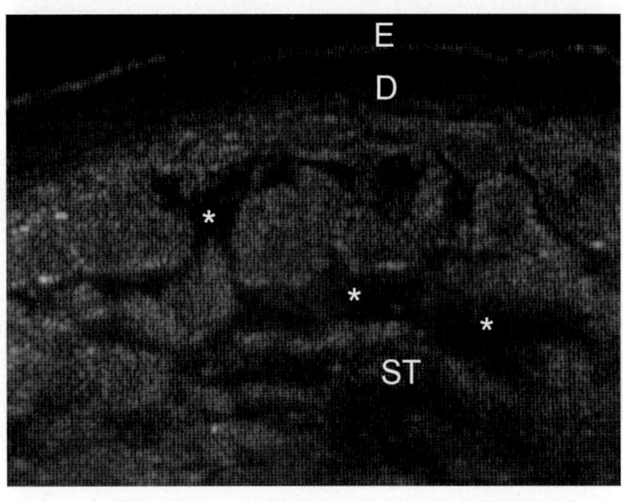

Fig. 9.25 Lymphedema. Transverse view shows thickening of all cutaneous layers. The dermis (D) becomes hypoechoic and the subcutaneous tissue (ST) hyperechoic. Anechoic fluid (*) is visible interspersed between the fat lobules of the subcutaneous tissue.

Chondritis of the Nose and Pinna

Inflammation of the nose cartilage or the pinna of the ear may present as isolated chondritis; or as part of the autoimmune disease relapsing polychondritis. Cartilage is normally seen as a hypoechoic band with regular borders without visible blood vessels in its inner structure. During inflammation the cartilage becomes thicker, acquiring higher echogenicity and prominent vessels (**Fig. 9.26**). In more advanced stages the cartilage has a beaded appearance, and actual dissection of the cartilage by fluid-infected collections has also been reported. When the etiology is relapsing polychondritis, besides pinna and nose, other cartilaginous structures such as the trachea may be involved.

Plantar Warts

These are painful, often recurrent hyperkeratotic lesions on the sole of the feet that are caused by infection with the human papillomavirus (HPV). Ultrasound imaging is useful to differentiate wart recurrences from Morton neuroma, plantar bursitis, synovitis, or tumors. On sonography, warts appear as fusiform hypoechoic lesions affecting the epidermal and dermal layers of the plantar skin. Hypervascularity of the superficial dermis is also described (**Fig. 9.27**). Plantar bursitis in the proximity of the wart is commonly

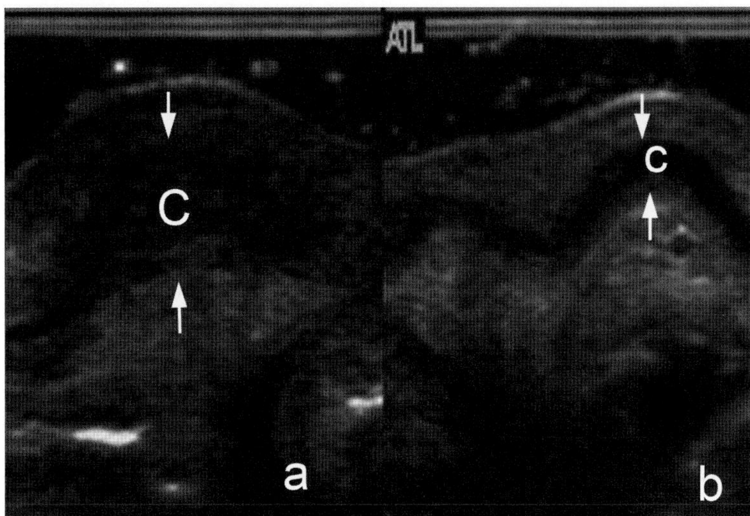

A

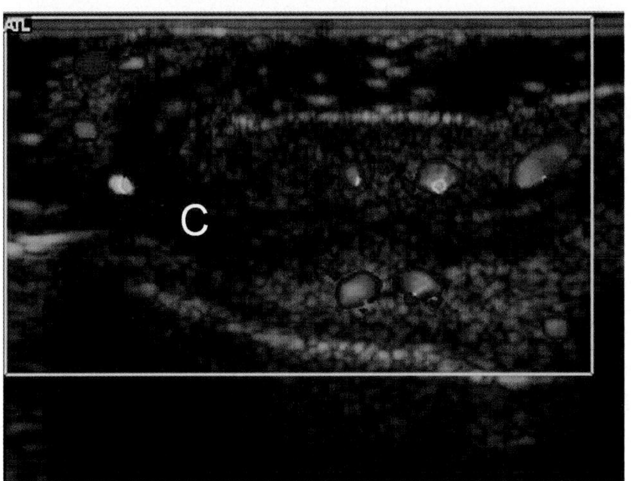

B

Fig. 9.26 Chondritis of the ear cartilage. **(A)** Comparative transverse view shows in the affected side (a) thickening and increased echogenicity of the ear cartilage (C, *long arrows*). In contrast, side (b) shows a normal cartilage (C, *short arrows*). **(B)** Color Doppler transverse view shows high presence of vascularity inside the cartilage (C) and the surrounding skin layers.

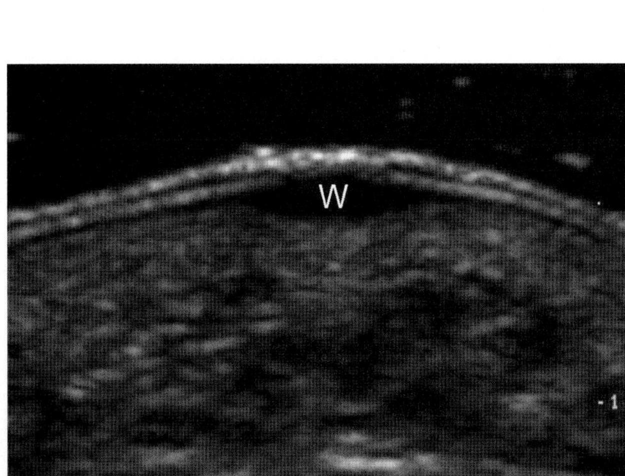

A

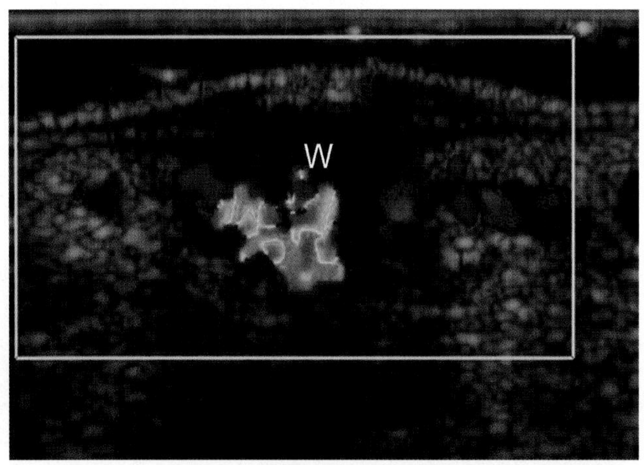

B

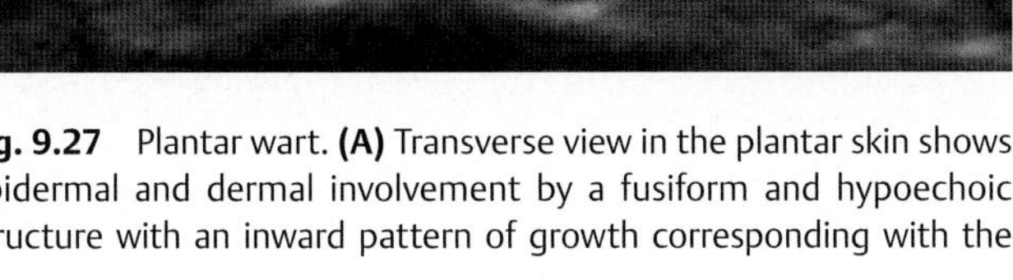

Fig. 9.27 Plantar wart. **(A)** Transverse view in the plantar skin shows epidermal and dermal involvement by a fusiform and hypoechoic structure with an inward pattern of growth corresponding with the wart (W) lesion. **(B)** Color Doppler ultrasound of a fusiform and hypoechoic lesion in the epidermis and dermis corresponding to a wart (W) shows increased dermal vascularity.

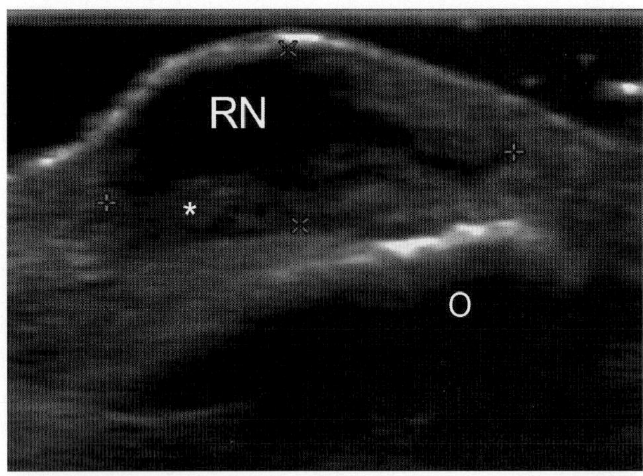

Fig. 9.28 Rheumatoid nodule. Transverse view shows an anechoic cystic lesion (RN, *between markers*) with thick walls and hypoechoic debris in the bottom (*). O, olecranon.

seen, probably representing reactive inflammation in the surrounding tissues.

Periarticular Conditions

Rheumatoid Nodules

These may be present in longstanding rheumatoid arthritis; they consist of a central necrotic area surrounded by epithelioid and chronic inflammatory cells. Sites commonly affected are elbows, forearms, and hands. On ultrasound, they appear as cystic anechoic nodules with a thick hypoechoic wall located in the subcutaneous tissue and dermis (**Fig. 9.28**). Associated joint and bony changes such as proliferative synovitis (pannus) and erosions can be detected in the vicinity of the nodules.

Gout Tophi

These develop in patients with preexistent gout and consist of solid nodules that contain uric acid crystal deposits. On ultrasound, the tophi appearance has been described as "wet sugar clumps"; round-shaped and hyperechoic nodules of periarticular or peritendinous location (**Fig. 9.29**). The nodules are not visible in x-ray projections. Tophi can be associated with other articular and periarticular abnormalities such as joint effusion and synovitis; ultrasound may also show linear hyperechoic uric acid deposits on the surface of hyaline cartilage and bone erosions.

Nail Bed Lesions

Psoriasis

Nail involvement is described in 5% of psoriatic patients, usually in association with arthropathy. On ultrasound, psoriatic changes may affect selectively a deeper structure, producing hyperechoic segments in the nail plates that may not be detectable clinically; alternately, psoriasis can progress to involve both plates, successively appearing as hyperechoic focal zones, blurring of the nail plates, and wavy shape or thickening of both plates, from low to high stages of involvement (**Fig. 9.30**). Also, the ventral nail plate may separate from the bone margin of the distal phalanx (nail bed thickness) because of edema. Commonly, there is associated synovitis of the distal interphalangeal joint.

A

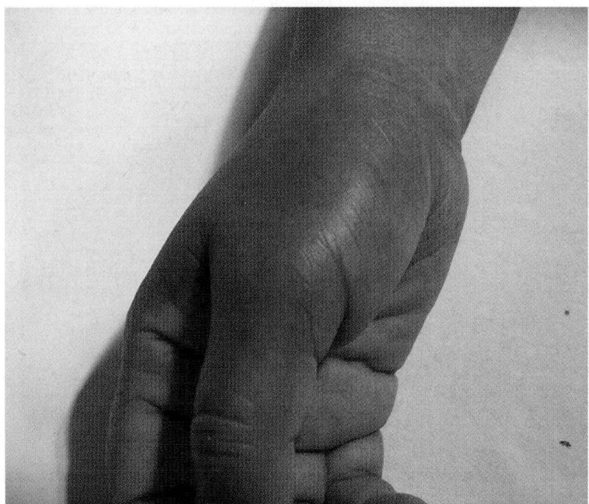

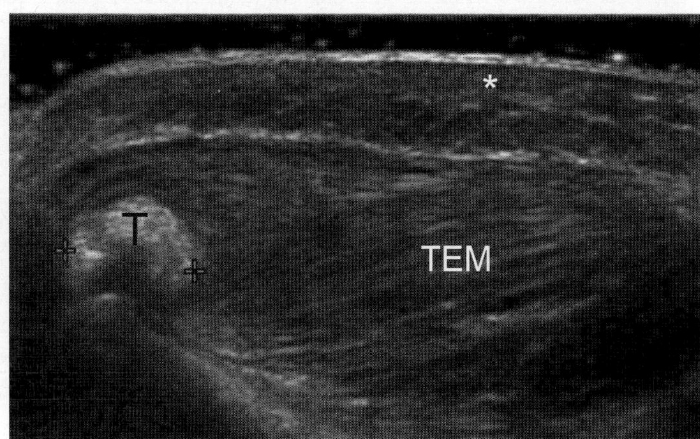

B

Fig. 9.29 Gouty tophi. **(A)** Clinical erythema and swelling in the thenar side of the hand. **(B)** Longitudinal view shows a hyperechoic nodule (*between markers*) corresponding with the tophi. Increased echogenicity and enlargement of the thenar eminence muscles (TEM) is also detected representing a secondary myositis in gout. The skin layers are also thickened (*).

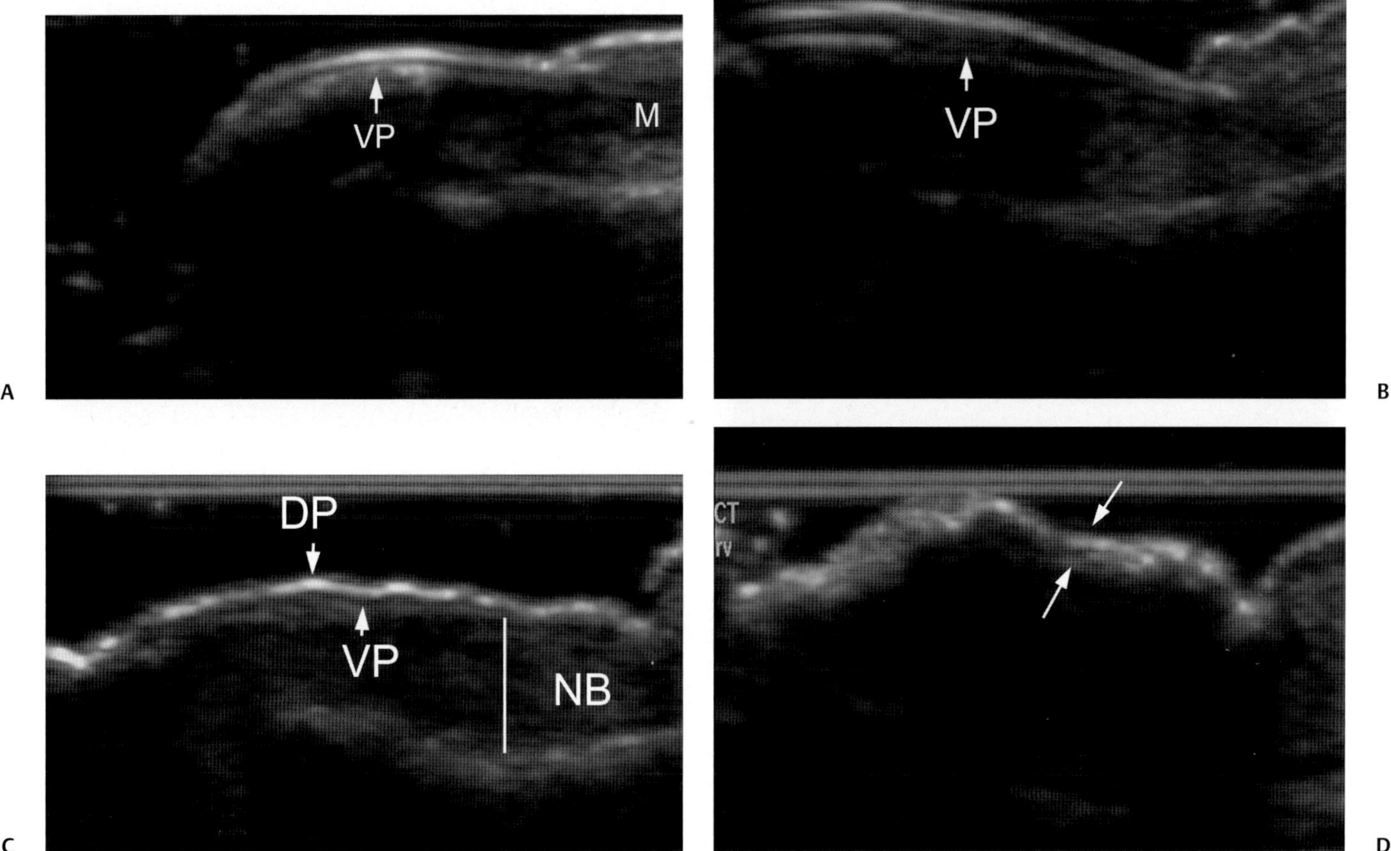

Fig. 9.30 **(A)** Nail psoriasis exclusive involvement of the ventral plate. Longitudinal view of the nailbed shows thickening and hyperechogenicity of the ventral plate (VP and *arrow*). M, matrix. **(B)** Nail psoriasis with loss of definition of the ventral plate. Longitudinal view shows absence of the ventral plate (VP) hyperechoic line in the proximal fingernail (*arrow*). **(C)** Nail psoriasis with wavy plates. Longitudinal view shows a wavy appearance of both plates (*arrows*). Increase of the distance between the ventral plate and the bone margin of the distal phalanx is also detected (*white line*). NB, nail bed; VP, ventral plate; DP, dorsal plate. **(D)** Nail psoriasis with loss of definition of both plates. Longitudinal view shows thickening and loss of definition of both plates (*arrows*).

Glomus Tumor

Small tumors, derived from the neuromyoarterial apparatus, present with pain, tenderness, and hypersensitivity to cold in the fingernails. Nail ridding and/or blue or red spots can also be visible. On ultrasound, glomus tumors appear in most cases as nodular hypoechoic lesions with prominent vascularity (**Fig. 9.31**); they are located more frequently in the proximal nail bed involving the matrix zone. A glomus tumor can also be seen in other portions of the nail or in a periungual location. Ultrasound is extremely useful to locate the tumor, providing information on tumor size, perfusion, and bony alterations. These data are important for the planning of surgery. Ultrasound also helps with prognostic assessment of information on the cosmetic sequels, especially when the nail matrix is affected, resulting in permanent and visible changes in the fingernails. Although a high rate of recurrence has been reported, recurrences have yet to be described in cases of glomus tumors with presurgical ultrasound.

Nail Bed Cysts

The most common cystic lesions in the nail bed are mucous and synovial cysts. Mucous cysts occur inside the nail bed and are filled with degenerated collagen and mucoid viscous fluid. Synovial cysts are lined with synovium and are frequently located on the distal interphalangeal joint; they may secondarily extend to the nail bed and compress the surface of the matrix. Nail bed cysts can also cause permanent changes in the nail plates from compression of the matrix zone. Another clinical presentation is that of indolent periungual swelling. On ultrasound, cystic lesions are anechoic, round or oval in shape, without associated alterations in the vessels of the nail bed. It is often possible to detect a tract

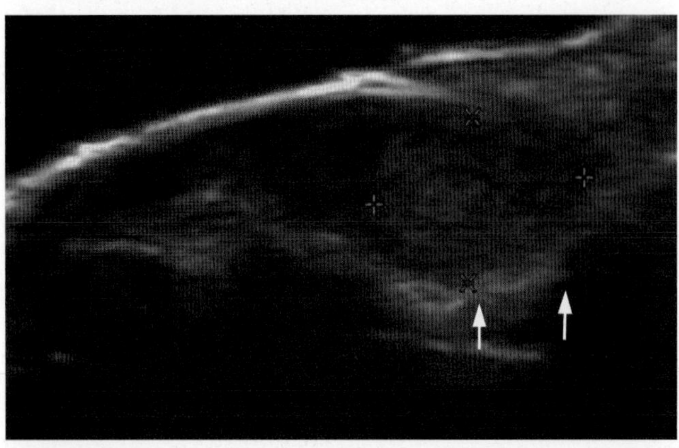

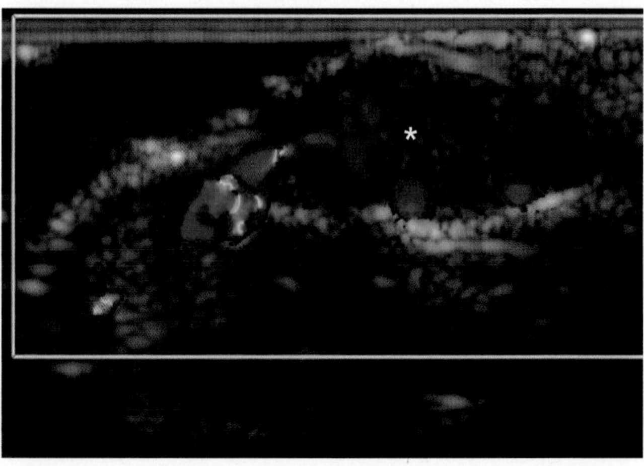

Fig. 9.31 Glomus tumor. **(A)** Longitudinal view shows hypoechoic nodule in the proximal nail bed (*between markers*) impinging on the bone margin of the distal phalanx (*arrows*). **(B)** Color Doppler longitudinal view shows hypervascularity inside the nodule (*).

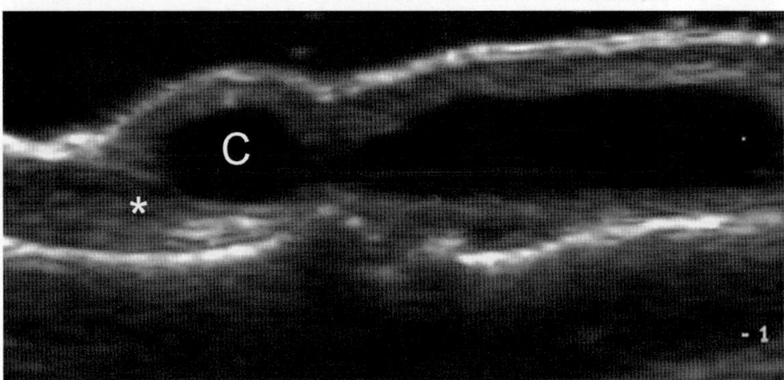

Fig. 9.32 Synovial cyst compressing the matrix of the nail. Longitudinal view shows anechoic cystic structure (C) compressing the surface of the nail matrix (*).

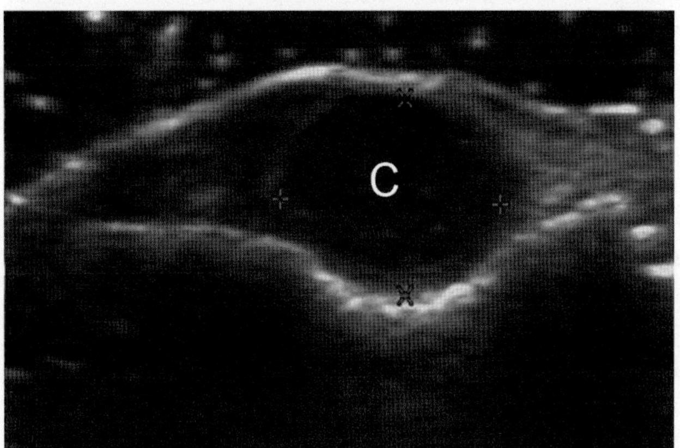

Fig. 9.33 Mucous cyst. Longitudinal view shows a round anechoic cyst (C) in the nail bed impinging on surrounding tissues that includes the nail matrix area and the bone margin of the distal phalanx. No connecting tract to the distal interphalangeal joint is detected.

communicating a synovial cyst to the distal interphalangeal joint (**Figs. 9.32** and **9.33**).

Subungual Exostosis

This refers to bony growths of the distal phalanx that commonly affect the feet; they are sometimes covered by a fibrocartilaginous cap that protrudes into the nail bed, eliciting periungual swelling and deformation of the nail plates. Sonography of subungual exostoses shows a hyperechoic bony extrusion on the surface of the distal phalanx pushing the ungual plates upward (**Fig. 9.34**). Sometimes, exostoses may be covered with hypoechoic chondroid tissue. Again, ultrasound is extremely useful for the differential diagnoses between exostosis and tumoral lesions inside the nail bed because of the limited accessibility of the nail bed to other imaging techniques.

Anatomic Variants

Persistence of a Large-Caliber Artery of the Lip

This is a developmental anomaly caused by the persistence of a large-caliber inferior alveolar artery. Beside a larger size,

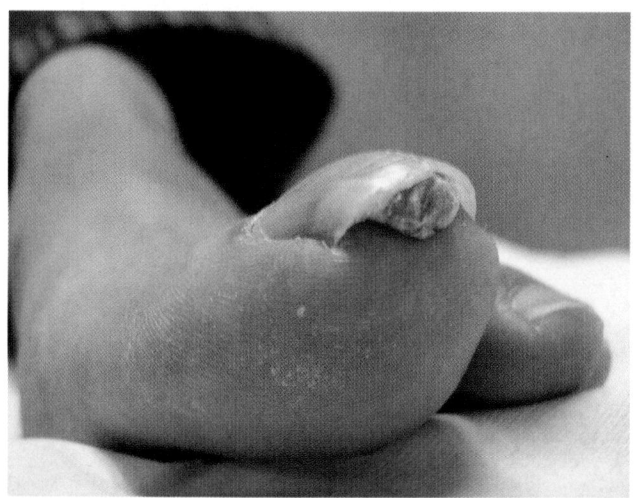

A

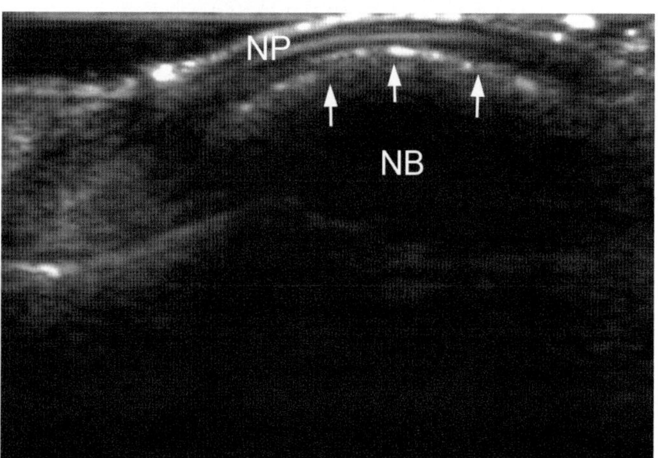

B

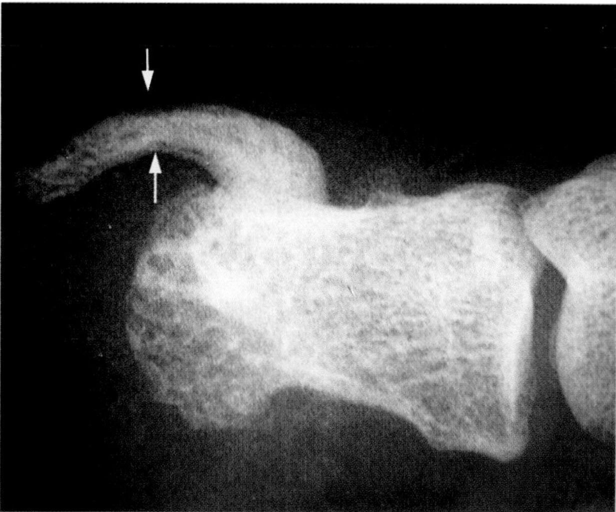

C

Fig. 9.34 Subungual exostosis. **(A)** Clinical picture of a proliferation in the subungual region. **(B)** Longitudinal shows hyperechoic band (*arrows*) below the nail plates (NP) that connects to the bony margin and produces posterior acoustic shadowing artifact. NB, nail bed. **(C)** X-ray (lateral projection) confirmed the diagnosis (*arrows*).

the artery may show thickened walls as it traverses the orbicularis oris muscle in the lower lip to supply the mucosa of the lips. The artery becomes superficial close to the midline and palpable a few millimeters below the vermillion border. Because of the nodular appearance of the large-caliber artery, it may be mislabeled as basal cell carcinoma or a vascular tumor. Nevertheless, color Doppler ultrasound clearly shows the thick artery passing through the lip layers and coming closer to the mucosa.

Accessory Muscles

These are congenital variations in the muscular system that present as localized swellings; on ultrasound accessory muscles exhibit well-defined hypoechoic structure and tendinous insertions similar to the normal muscle, as well as dynamic contractile properties (**Fig. 9.35**). They are more common in the wrist, hand, and ankle regions, but can be located in other body areas. Most are asymptomatic, but

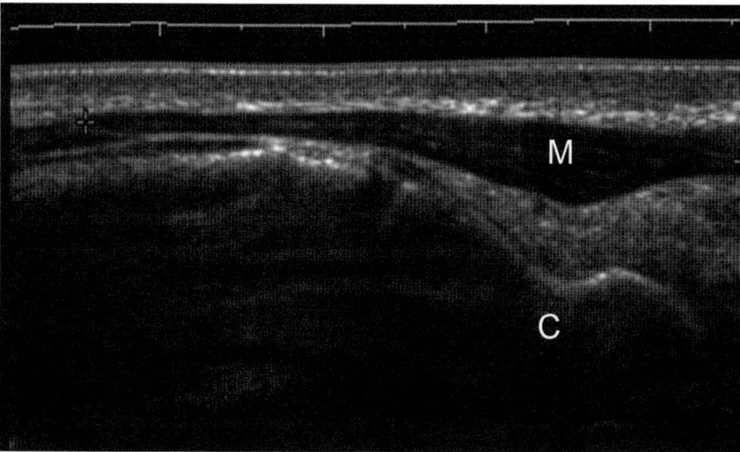

Fig. 9.35 Accessory muscle in the dorsum of the hand. Longitudinal panoramic view shows hypoechoic structure (M) with muscular pattern in the dorsum of the hand (*between markers*). C, capitate.

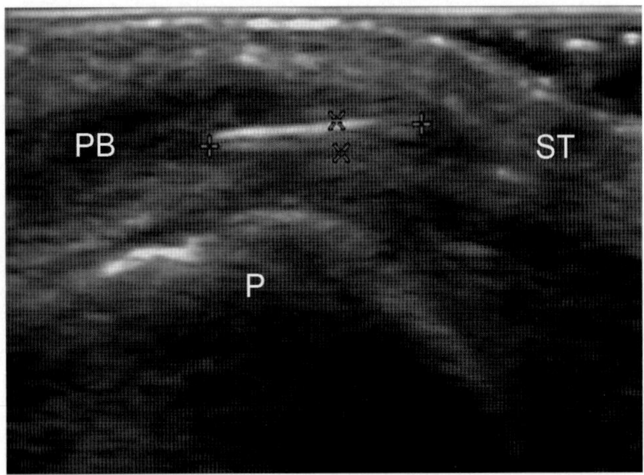

Fig. 9.36 Foreign body. Longitudinal view of the anterior aspect of the knee shows hyperechoic bilaminar structure (*between markers*) in the subcutaneous tissue (ST) and prepatellar bursa (PB) that corresponded with a splinter. P, patella.

they can also cause symptoms from entrapment of normal structures. Another clinical presentation is just as a cosmetic alteration from unexplained swelling simulating a space-occupying lesion such as a lipoma or cyst.

Foreign Bodies

On ultrasound, intruding objects have a variable, composition-dependant echogenicity. The examination also allows for the localization and guided extraction of the foreign body. The most common appearance of foreign bodies can be a hyperechoic line or bilaminar hyperechoic structure surrounded by hypoechoic granulomatous tissue (**Fig. 9.36**). Importantly, biologic materials such as pieces of wood or thorns are not associated with posterior artifacts, in contrast with inert materials (metal or glass) that show posterior acoustic reverberation.

Artifacts

- Depending on the density of the fluid material inside a cyst, echogenicity of the lesion may range from totally anechoic to hypoechoic (mimicking a solid lesion). When in doubt, look for the posterior acoustic enhancement artifact associated with the fluid content in the lesion.
- In malignant tumors, necrotic areas may simulate fluid collections, but compression maneuvers may be helpful to identify the higher elasticity and easier compressibility of free fluid. This free fluid sign is often absent in tumors with areas of necrosis.
- Standoff pads may compress vascular lesions, particularly of low flow. However, large amounts of gel over the lesion site act as a cushion, diffusing pressure on the skin, thus facilitating visualization of the lesion.

Proposed Algorithm for Skin Imaging Investigation

1- Color Doppler ultrasound—first imaging examination for skin and nail pathologies

2- Angio-MRI in multiple vascular skin lesions or vascular lesions that will undergo surgery or an invasive procedure (embolization)

Pearls and Pitfalls

- Do not compress too hard with the probe because it will stop the flow through low-flow vessels
- Use copious amounts of gel to adjust focusing to the upper skin layers
- Use intermittent compression maneuvers to detect venous vascular malformations. Veins are easily compressible, except when they are thrombosed, which generally occurs in parts of the malformation and rarely in the whole vascular malformation.
- Hyperechoic lines inside a hypoechoic oval or round cutaneous structure are suggestive of fragments of hair, therefore a skin cyst should be suspected.
- Registration of the spectral curve in hemangiomas allows comparison of the blood flow velocity among different examinations over time. Generally, blood flow becomes lower when hemangiomas start the regression phase or after treatment. It is important to choose an anatomic landmark for the measurement and to make all the spectral curve analyses in the same point and axis.

Suggested Readings

Bobadilla F, Wortsman X, Muñoz C, Segovia L, Espinoza M, Jemec GBE. Pre-surgical high resolution ultrasound of facial basal cell carcinoma: correlation with histology. Cancer Imaging 2008;8:163–172

Lassau N, Spatz A, Avril MF, et al. Value of high-frequency US for preoperative assessment of skin tumors. Radiographics 1997;17(6):1559–1565

Matsunaga A, Ochiai T, Abel, et al. Subungual glomus tumour: evaluation of ultrasound imaging in preoperative assessment. Eur J Dermatol 2007;17(1):67–69

Mulliken JB, Glowacki J. Hemangiomas and vascular malformations in infants and children: a classification based on endothelial characteristics. Plast Reconstr Surg 1982;69(3):412–422

Wortsman XC, Holm EA, Wulf HC, Jemec GB. Real-time spatial compound ultrasound imaging of skin. Skin Res Technol 2004;10(1):23–31

Wortsman X, Jemec GB. Ultrasound imaging of nails. Dermatol Clin 2006;24(3):323–328

Wortsman X, Jemec GBE. Imaging hidradenitis suppurativa. In: Jemec GBE, Revuz J, Leyden JJ, eds. Hidradenitis Suppurativa. 1st ed. Heidelberg: Springer; 2006: 34–37

10 Peripheral Nerve Imaging

Siegfried Peer and Werner Judmaier

Peripheral nerves are small structures, with a complex course along the extremities. They are often covered by thick layers of muscle and fatty tissue, which obscures them from direct access thus making them difficult to image. In addition, the most common pathologies—such as compression neuropathy at the carpal tunnel, for example—are clinically clearly defined and readily diagnosed entities. There is increasing demand for imaging and especially sonography of peripheral nerves. One of the reasons for this is that clinically similar neurologic findings may be caused by completely different pathologies structurally. For example, carpal tunnel syndrome, which may be idiopathic in nature, may also be caused by a space-occupying lesion in the carpal tunnel, such as ganglia, accessory muscle tissue, or vascular malformations, which may impinge on the median nerve. Various causes of carpal tunnel syndrome may cause quite similar neurologic symptoms and electrophysiologic studies may not reveal the underlying pathology. Imaging provides structural information of a nerve and its surroundings; this is important not only for diagnosis, but also for treatment planning. This is especially true for traumatic nerve lesions, where the definition of the exact site and extent of nerve involvement is crucial for the planning of surgical interventions; this directly affects the patient's postoperative outcome. Another important reason for the revival of nerve imaging lies in the substantial improvement of imaging technology, especially in sonography and magnetic resonance imaging (MRI). This improvement—particularly in resolution—enables imaging of very small structures such that even tiny nerves in the finger may be visualized with sonography. This improved technology opens the field for the detailed study of intraneural structure, neural vasculature, and probably function.

Clinical Indications

Common indications for peripheral nerve imaging may be categorized into three main areas: compression neuropathies, traumatic lesions, and tumors. These are the areas where sufficient expert knowledge based on clinical research in larger patient populations exists. There are attempts to image other nerve pathologies such as inflammatory conditions or systemic peripheral neuropathies, but despite some interesting reports in the literature, reliable data on the value of sonography for imaging of those conditions is currently lacking. Probably the most frequently imaged peripheral nerve pathology is compression neuropathy. The incidence of carpal tunnel syndrome, for example, is as high as 4% in the general population. The value of sonography for the diagnosis of compression neuropathy varies depending on the site of compression and the examination technique used. With high-resolution equipment, sonography can diagnose an idiopathic compression syndrome with high confidence and definitely define an extrinsic lesion with direct compromise of a nerve, such as compression by tumors, ganglia, accessory muscle, or functional impairment by dislocation of a nerve during movement. Another commonly imaged peripheral nerve pathology is trauma; the results of these imaging studies may substantially alter a patient's therapeutic regime. For brachial plexus trauma and peripheral nerve injury in the extremities, ultrasound defines the location, extent, and severity of the lesion (i.e., if a lesion is complete or incomplete). Peripheral nerve tumors may be investigated with ultrasound based on the clinical suspicion of a lesion (i.e., a lesion with a positive Tinel sign or neurologic symptoms), but more often such a lesion is incidentally found during examination of an otherwise unclear soft tissue mass. A musculoskeletal sonographer should therefore be aware of the sonographic appearances of peripheral nerve tumors to have them included in the differential diagnosis.

Technical Guidelines

Equipment

Sonographic imaging relies on contrast and resolution. High-frequency transducers of up to 17 MHz result in an axial resolution of ~250 microns. High-frequency broadband linear arrays therefore are the state of the art for musculoskeletal and nerve imaging. High resolution, however, is not without problems; generally, improved resolution comes with a reduction in penetration. The choice of transducer for imaging of a specific nerve is therefore influenced by its location (**Table 10.1**).

Requirements for ultrasound scanner hard- and software warrant a short comment: while until recently only big and bulky top-notch ultrasound scanners had sufficient hardware power and software to enable imaging of tiny structures, this has recently changed. High-quality portable ultrasound systems, equipped with tissue harmonic

Table 10.1 Choice of Transducer Depending on Type of Nerve Examined and Clinical Question

Transducer	Nerve	Clinical question
3–9 MHz or similar	Sciatic nerve (proximal)	Trauma
5–12 MHz or similar	Sciatic nerve (distal), brachial plexus, femoral nerve, radial/ulnar/median nerve	Trauma, tumor, compression neuropathy (cross sectional measurements), postoperative lesions (scar tissue compression), sonography guided interventions
5–17 MHz or similar	Radial/ulnar/median/peroneal/tibial/ nerve	Compression neuropathy (structural analysis of nerve), trauma, neuritis, small tumors

imaging, image compounding, and various other artifact-reduction software similar to what we are used to apply on high-end scanners are becoming increasingly available. Combined with efficient high-frequency transducers, these small systems result in very high image quality, allow for bedside examination of peripheral nerves, and are now a valuable adjunct to the diagnostic toolbox of neurologists, orthopedists, and specialists in electrophysiology alike.

General Examination Technique

The general examination technique for sonography of peripheral nerves is similar to what we recommend for other musculoskeletal structures: findings are documented in two perpendicular planes and so on, but it differs especially in how a nerve and neural pathology are identified. It is desirable to scan a nerve in a short axis plane along its complete course along an extremity to search for suspected pathology. Sometimes (especially in traumatic lesions), it is more reliable to first identify the nerve at an area with distinct anatomic landmarks, where it may be easily found and then followed proximally or distally to the site of possible impairment. When scars or hematoma obscure direct access to a nerve at the level of impairment, the latter approach is more feasible.

The general appearance of a peripheral nerve on sonography is fairly uniform: on long axis sonograms the nerve is a longitudinal tubular structure with continuous hypoechoic elements (the axon bundles) interspersed and bordered by hyperechoic connective tissue (epi- and perineurium) (**Fig. 10.1A**). On short axis sonograms, a nerve shows a dotted appearance, like a cross-section of an electric cable, with quite regularly sized individual fascicular elements (**Fig. 10.1B**). The number of discernible fascicles and the amount of connective tissue may vary depending on the size of a nerve and its location in the body. Nerves that run along bony surfaces—especially in a curved fashion—or in osteofibrous tunnels, may undergo some normal amount of stretching and pressure and therefore show tighter packed fascicles with less echogenic elements. Nerves are mobile structures and are easily displaced during joint motion or even with light pressure of the transducer. The functional assessment of nerve motion may be an important sonographic technique to investigate impaction of a nerve under some tight ligament or in a postoperative scar.

A
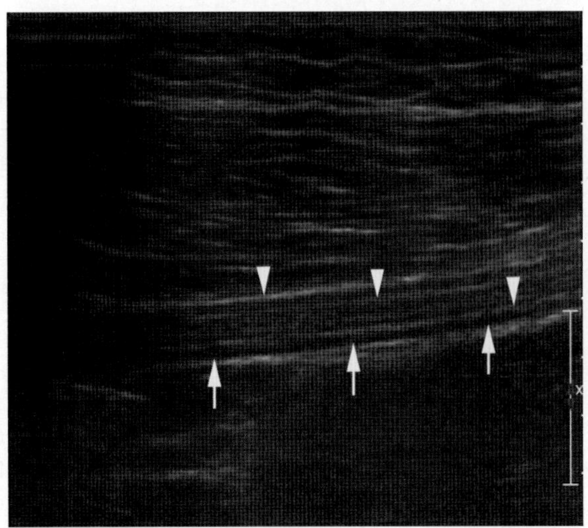
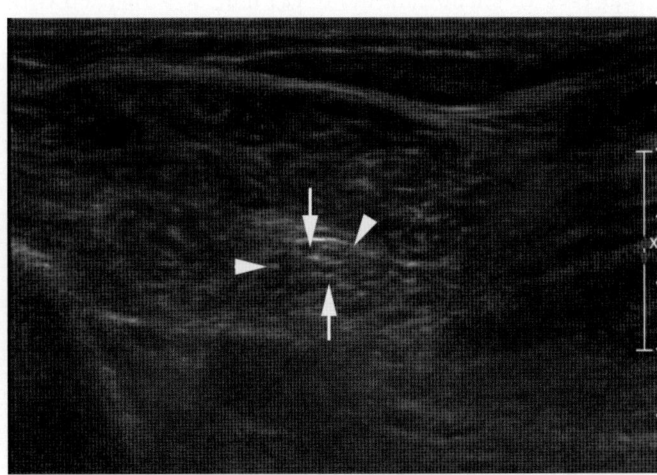
B

Fig. 10.1 **(A)** Long and **(B)** short axis sonogram of sciatic nerve in a volunteer. Continuous hypoechoic fascicular elements (*arrows*) interspersed and bordered by echoic epineurial tissue are seen (*arrowheads*).

In general, nerves accessible for sonography are nerves of the extremities and some of the nerves in the neck region, the latter often only along a limited distance. Although examination of nerves of the extremities may be performed with a high degree of confidence, important neural elements such as the spinal intraforaminal nerve root, the lumbar plexus, or cranial nerves may barely be accessible on sonography. The patient's body habitus such as obesity, muscular atrophy with loss of contrast between degenerated fatty muscle and nerves, as well as concomitant pathology, such as edema, hematoma, or scar tissue, may render the sonographic examination of peripheral nerves difficult, even impossible.

Normal Anatomy

Peripheral nerves are small structures covered and surrounded by various elements of soft tissue (such as fat or muscle). This aspect, together with their peculiar anatomic course, combines to make nerves sometimes difficult to identify with sonography. In the following sections, we will focus on the topographic anatomy of the nerves that are more commonly imaged in routine clinical practice, providing details of their anatomic/sonographic and magnetic resonance imaging (MRI) correlation. Sonographic examination of other less commonly imaged nerves, their detailed anatomy, and description may be found elsewhere (see Suggested Readings); it is beyond the scope of this book, which is directed more toward the general sonographer.

The Cervical/Brachial Plexus

The cervical/brachial plexus is easiest identified in a transverse plane perpendicular and just slightly cranial to the clavicle. In this region, the plexus elements are seen surrounding the subclavian artery (**Fig. 10.2A,B**). If you slide your transducer upward along the plexus, you will easily reach the interscalene gap, where the plexus trunks are lined up one behind the other (**Fig. 10.2C,D**). From here it is easy to follow the individual root to its corresponding neural foramen (**Fig. 10.2E,F**).

For identification of an individual nerve root, the exact level of the neural foramen has to be determined, which can be achieved by two methods: either identify the transverse process of the sixth cervical vertebra searching for the entry of the vertebral artery into its foramen, or search for the transverse process with only a large posterior but no anterior tubercle, which is a distinct feature of the seventh cervical vertebra (**Fig. 10.3**).

The nerve root C5 to C7 is always accessible to sonography; however, the root C8 and TH1 may be obscured from direct access in patients with thick, short necks. The outlet of the neural foramen is best analyzed with oblique scanning in a coronal plane. This scan for example is best suited for the identification of an avulsed nerve root with pseudomeningocele (**Fig. 10.4**). The infraclavicular portion of the plexus may be assessed from an axillary approach with the patient's arm abducted or elevated above the head. In slender individuals we may be able to assess the whole course of the plexus behind the clavicle with supra- and infraclavicular views, but often a short segment lying directly posterior to the clavicle is obscured from direct access.

The Cubital Tunnel

The cubital tunnel is an osteofibrous canal at the medial epicondyle of the humerus. It houses the ulnar nerve in its course to the forearm and is covered by a fibrous band called the cubital tunnel retinaculum also known as the Osborne fascia. The distal extension of this band connects the two heads of the flexor carpi ulnaris muscle and is called the arcuate ligament. Although you may identify the ulnar nerve on short axis views directly behind the tip of the medial epicondyle (**Fig. 10.5**) (the patient is best positioned with the lower arm in forced supination and slight elbow flexion with outward rotation of the upper arm), it is sometimes more feasible to identify it in the upper arm where it runs adjacent to the posterior margin of the biceps muscle. Hereafter, the nerve is continuously scanned distal until it exits the cubital tunnel. Normal diameters and cross-section areas of the nerve are documented in short axis views at the entry, in the middle (tip of the epicondyle), and exit of the tunnel and at any site of a sudden change in caliber. Normal values for cross-section areas range from 4 to 10 mm^2. Note that the ulnar nerve is slightly enlarged in the middle section of the tunnel with a more hypoechoic appearance and less identifiable epineurial tissue in normal subjects. This is most probably due to its close contact with the bony bottom of the tunnel and some normal amount of constant stretching during elbow flexion/extension. Longitudinal scans should always be added, as they allow for easier identification of an abrupt change in nerve caliber (**Fig. 10.6**). Functional scanning with flexion/extension of the elbow is important to diagnose a snapping ulnaris/snapping triceps syndrome, which is a rare, but important cause for ulnar neuropathy at the elbow.

The Carpal Tunnel

The median nerve inside the carpal tunnel is probably the most easily assessed peripheral nerve. Attempts to diagnose carpal tunnel syndrome with sonography date back to the early 1990s. The carpal tunnel holds the flexor tendons and the median nerve and is covered by the flexor retinaculum, sometimes also called the transverse carpal ligament. The retinaculum is readily identified on sonograms and MRIs alike as a small band-like structure traversing from its attachment at the pisiform bone to the scaphoid (**Fig. 10.7**).

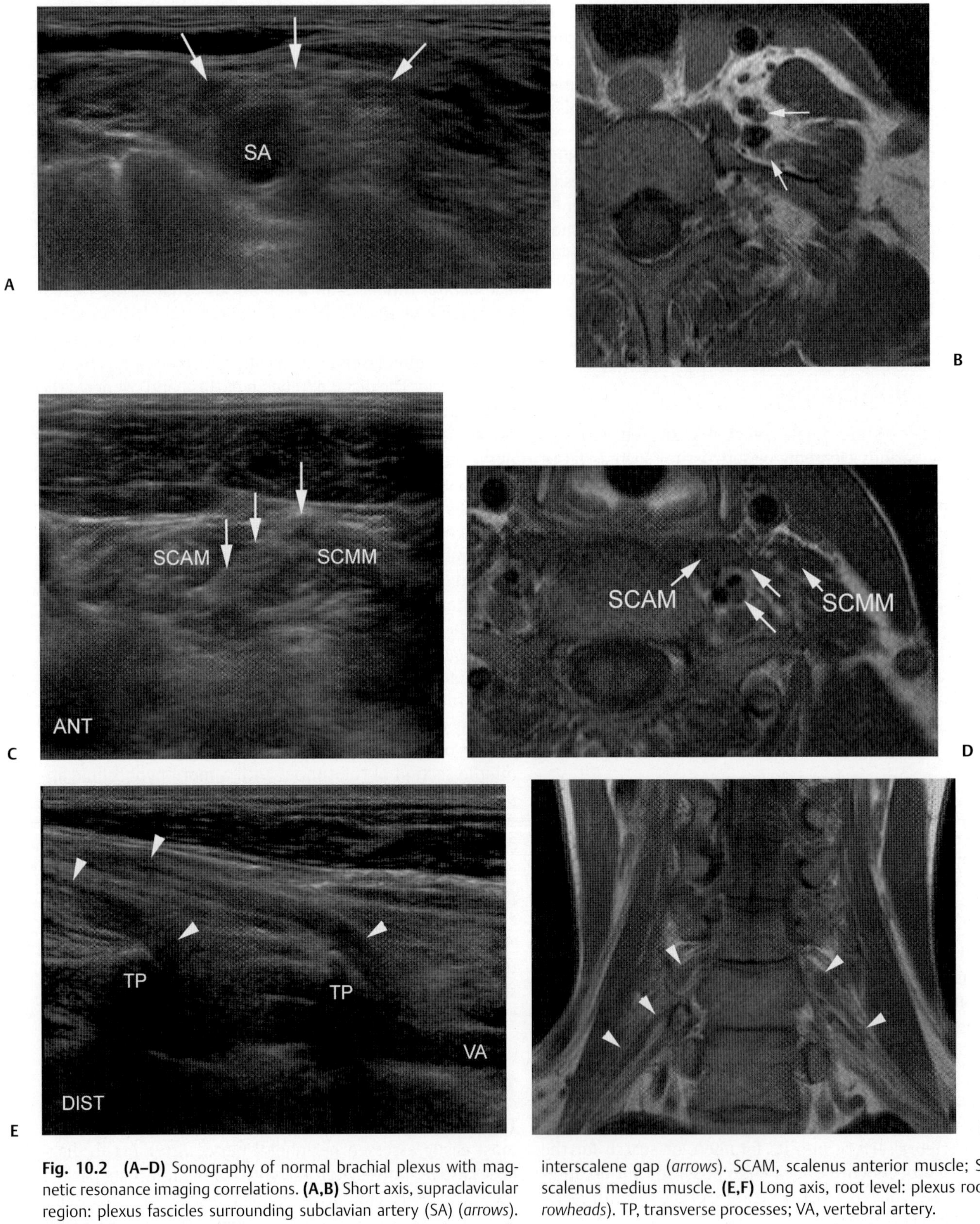

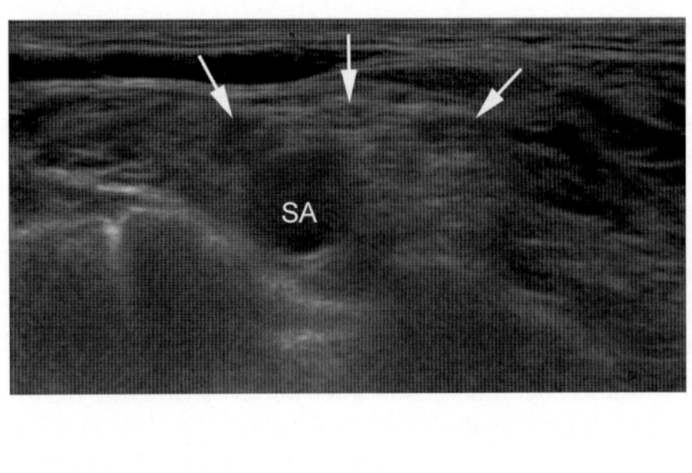

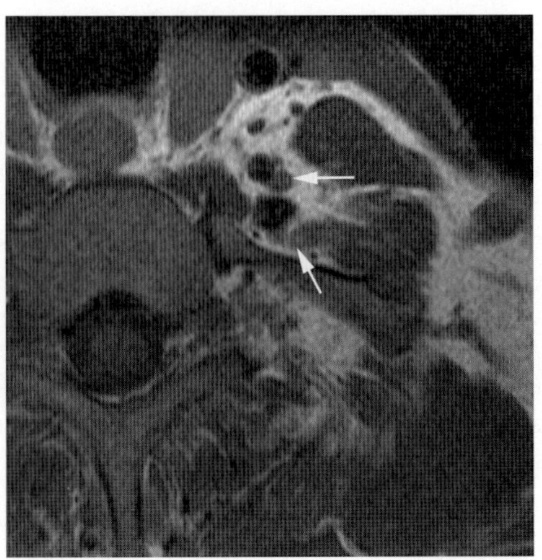

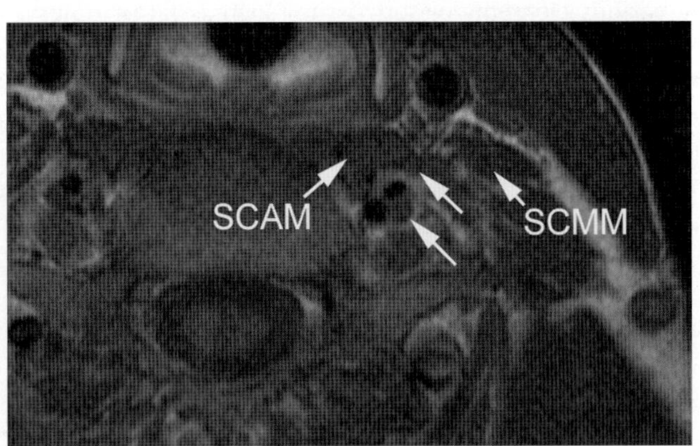

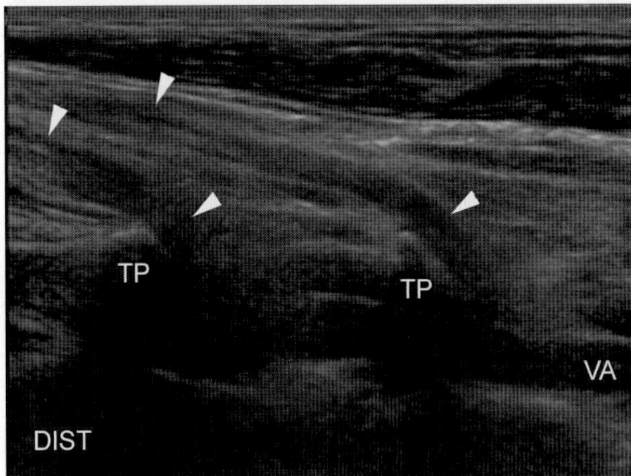

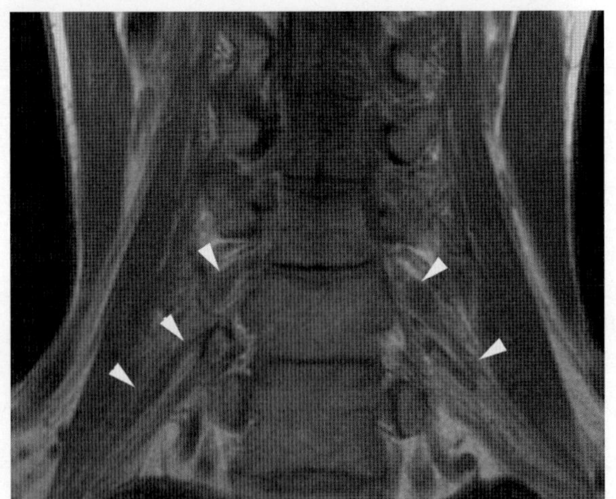

Fig. 10.2 **(A–D)** Sonography of normal brachial plexus with magnetic resonance imaging correlations. **(A,B)** Short axis, supraclavicular region: plexus fascicles surrounding subclavian artery (SA) (*arrows*). **(C,D)** Short axis, interscalene region: plexus trunks lined up inside interscalene gap (*arrows*). SCAM, scalenus anterior muscle; SCMM, scalenus medius muscle. **(E,F)** Long axis, root level: plexus roots (*arrowheads*). TP, transverse processes; VA, vertebral artery.

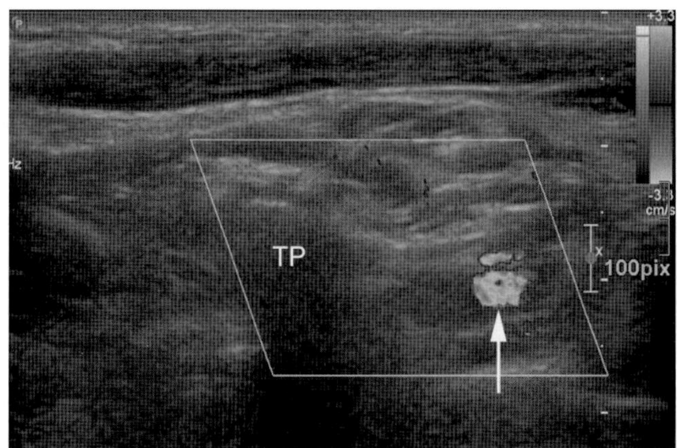

A

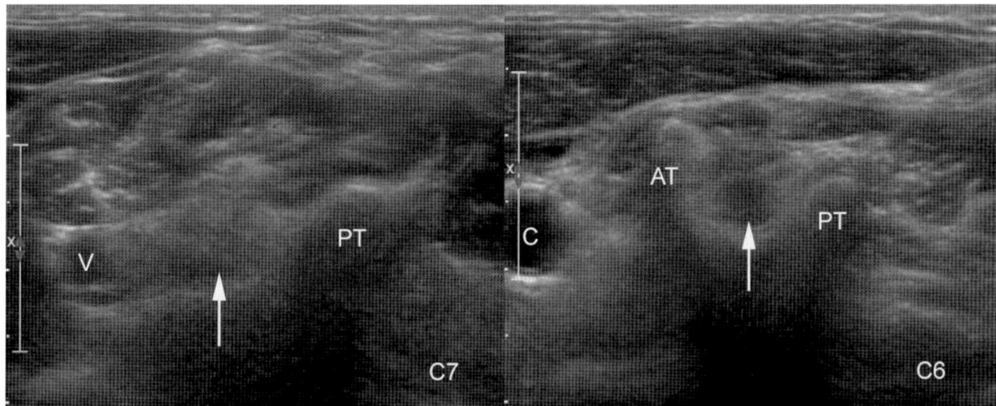

B

Fig. 10.3 Localization of nerve root in plexus sonography. **(A)** Oblique sonogram through transverse process (TP) of 6th cervical vertebra. The vertebral artery can be seen (*arrow*). **(B)** Short axis sonograms through transverse process of 7th and 6th cervical vertebra. Note normal posterior tubercle (PT) in both vertebrae, absence of anterior tubercle (AT) in C7 and prominent anterior (AT) tubercle in C6. V, vertebral artery; C, carotid artery; *arrows*, C6/C7 nerve root.

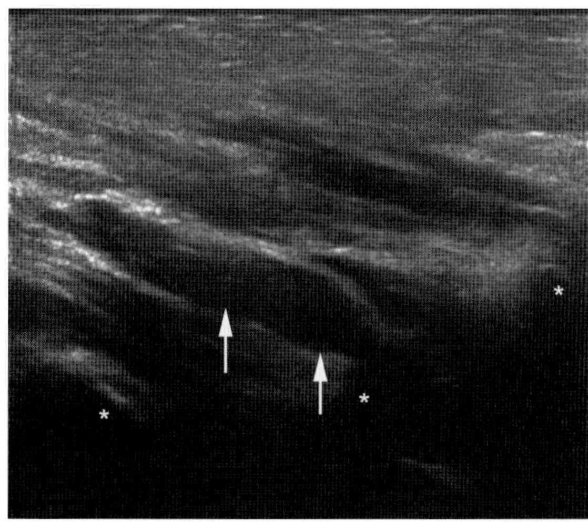

A

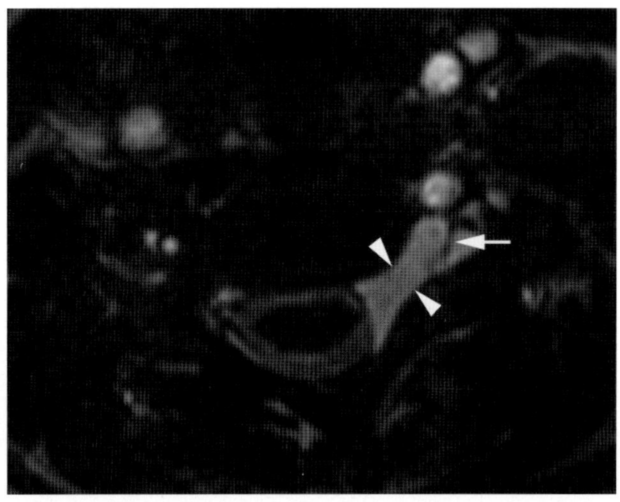

B

Fig. 10.4 **(A)** Long axis sonogram through paravertebral cervical plexus in a patient with root avulsion. Empty extraforaminal root sleeve (*arrows*) is demonstrated and the transverse processes can be seen (*). **(B)** Correlative axial T2-weighted magnetic resonance image confirms fluid-filled pseudomeningocele (*arrowheads*) and avulsed root fragment (*arrow*).

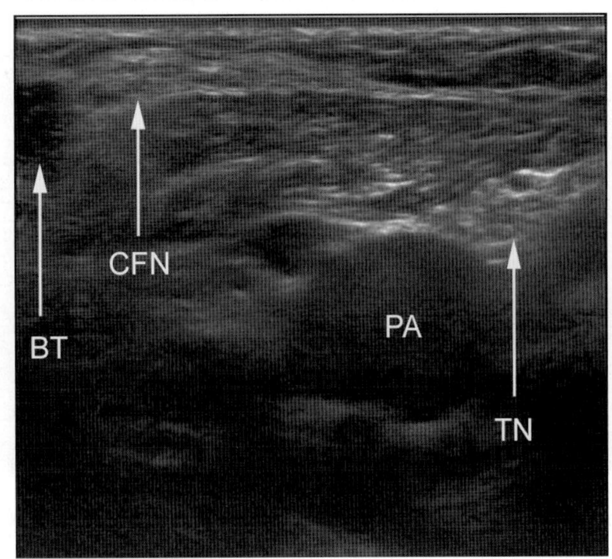

A

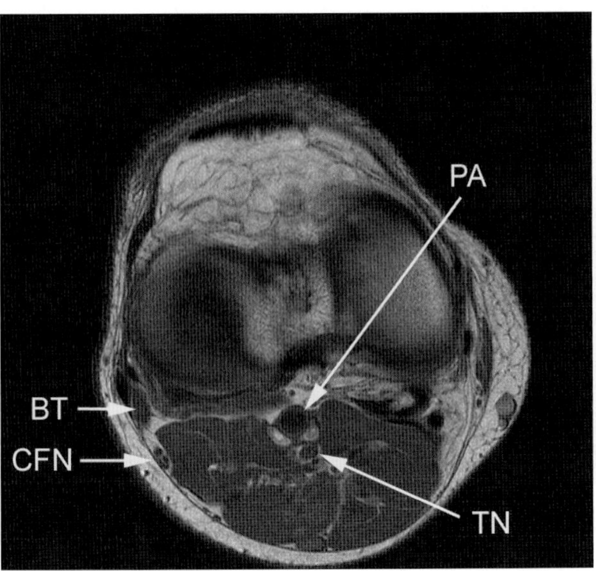

B

Fig. 10.10 **(A)** Transverse sonogram of popliteal fossa. **(B)** Correlative T1-weighted magnetic resonance image. PA, popliteal artery; BT, femoral biceps muscle tendon; TN, tibial nerve; CFN, common fibular nerve.

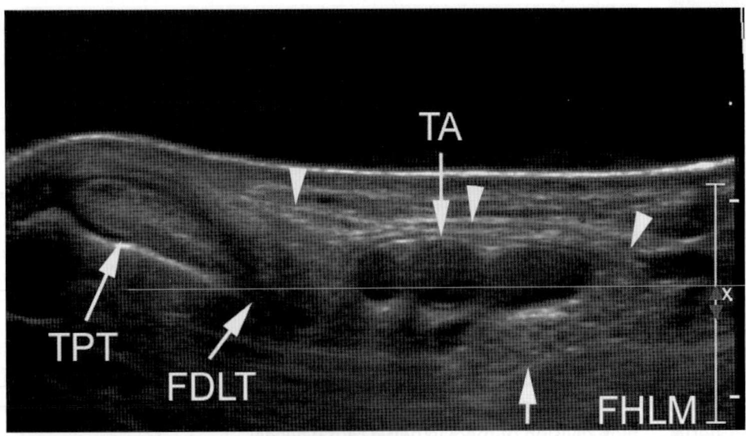

A

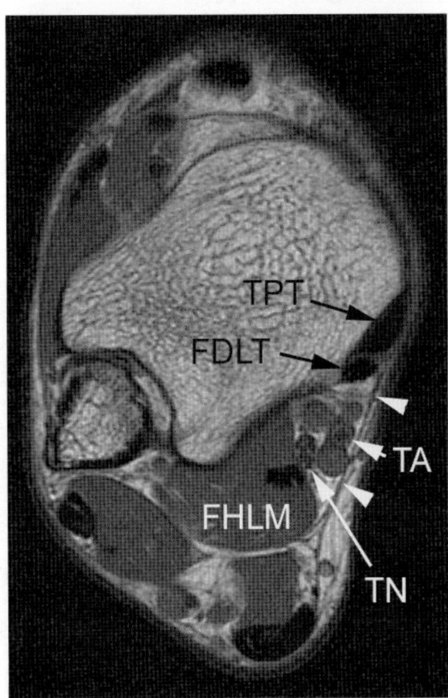

B

Fig. 10.11 **(A)** Transverse sonogram of tarsal tunnel and **(B)** correlative T1-weighted MR image. The flexor retinaculum can be seen in both figures (*arrowheads*). TA, tibial artery; TPT, tibialis posterior tendon; FDLT, flexor digitorum longus tendon; FHLM, flexor hallucis longus muscle; TN, tibial nerve.

directly adjacent to the deep popliteal vein) and followed along its distal course; however, it is easier to localize at its distal portion above the ankle. Although the sciatic nerve division is normally located in the popliteal fossa, a high division at a variable length above knee level may be encountered.

The Tarsal Tunnel

The tibial nerve courses along the medial aspect of the lower leg interposed between the tibialis posterior and flexor hallucis muscle together with the vascular bundle of the posterior tibial artery and veins. The nerve is easily identified at the medial aspect of the lower leg some centimeters above the ankle and is the deepest structure of the neurovascular bundle (**Fig. 10.11**). Proximal to the medial malleolus, it is interposed between the superficial and deep layer of the flexor retinaculum inside the so-called tarsal tunnel. Right at its exit from the tunnel the tibial nerve divides into its two terminal branches, which may be followed for a short length toward the ankle and sole of the foot.

Pathologies

A variety of peripheral nerve pathologies may be imaged with ultrasound; in the next sections, we will focus on the more common ones.

Compression Syndromes

Nerve compression syndrome refers to extrinsic compression of a nerve in special anatomic regions, which according to their regional features—narrow passageways, bony ridges, tight ligaments or retinacula, osteofibrous tunnels—have only limited space for the passage of a nerve and its adjacent structures. Due to chronic tear or compression, a so-called entrapment neuropathy with distinct neurologic signs and symptoms develops. Typical entrapment neuropathies are idiopathic in nature: they are mainly a result of the unfavorable local anatomy often in conjunction with occupational overuse. However, they may also be caused by space-occupying processes—such as ganglia, accessory muscle, tumors, aneurysms—inside an already narrow area; these are secondary compression syndromes.

Quite independent of its location and cause (idiopathic or secondary), a compression neuropathy results in a rather uniform reaction of a peripheral nerve: in general, we may encounter changes in nerve caliber (flattening at the site of compression with enlargement of the proximal portion of the nerve) and structure (loss of inner fascicular discrimination and outer lining because of edema and congestion) (**Fig. 10.12**).

Depending on the site of compression, distinct additional features may be encountered, such as thickening of a retinaculum, which are sonographic hallmarks of the individual syndrome.

A

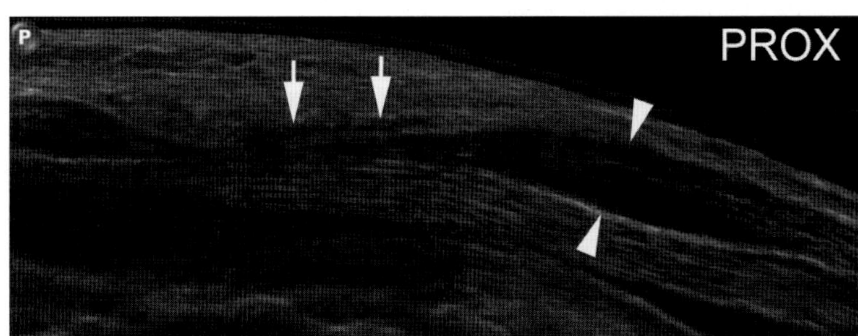

B

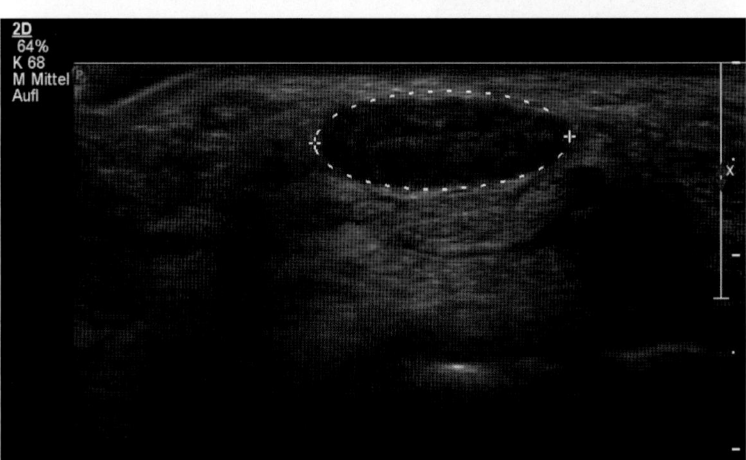

Fig. 10.12 **(A)** Long axis panoramic and **(B)** short axis sonogram of carpal tunnel in a patient with severe long-standing carpal tunnel syndrome. Marked swelling of median nerve proximal to carpal tunnel (*arrowheads* in A) is seen, with a maximum cross section area of 54 mm^2 and loss of inner fascicular discrimination **(B).** In its course underneath the flexor retinaculum [*arrows* in (A)] the median nerve is markedly flattened.

Cubital Tunnel Syndrome

Ulnar neuropathy at the elbow is the second most common form of compression syndrome. Its initial clinical sign is dysesthesia and/or numbness of the fifth and ulnar section of the fourth finger. Local pressure on the nerve at its course along the medial epicondyle may provoke or aggravate the symptoms. Later during the course of neuropathy, ulnar-innervated hand muscles lose function, which results in the typical claw hand and local muscle wasting in the first interosseous space. In the cubital tunnel, the ulnar nerve may be compromised in the epicondylar groove or at the edge of the arcuate ligament. The underlying process leading to ulnar neuropathy may just be abnormal wear and chronic tear in a shallow epicondylar groove. There may be various forms of secondary neuropathies such as a snapping triceps syndrome, accessory muscles like the anconeus epitrochlearis muscle (**Fig. 10.13**), bony abnormalities (osteophytes in arthritis of the elbow, bony prominences or ridges after supracondylar fractures, etc.), or bursal inflammation among others. Therefore, the sonographic assessment of ulnar neuropathy should not focus solely on the ulnar nerve in its course through the epicondylar groove, but also on the surrounding soft tissues. As ulnar neuropathy is a heterogeneous syndrome clinically and electrodiagnosis may frequently show only nonlocalizing findings, it is advisable to scan the ulnar nerve along its complete course from the axilla to the wrist. The latter is especially important, as a second though less common site of ulnar nerve compression is encountered in the Guyon canal at the wrist.

Typical findings of ulnar neuropathy at the elbow are enlargement of the nerve and loss of fascicular discrimination plus surrounding edema (**Fig. 10.14**). In selected cases, the thickened arcuate ligament can even be demonstrated (**Fig. 10.15**).

Measurements of an ulnar nerve cross-section area should be performed above the nerve entrance into the tunnel, along the tunnel (at the level of the epicondyle and 1 to 2 cm above and below that region) and at any region where the nerve shows a sudden change in caliber.

Functional imaging of the ulnar nerve during flexion/extension maneuvers may reveal a snapping triceps/snapping ulnaris syndrome, which is caused by absence of the retinaculum. Ulnar nerve instability is quite frequently encountered in asymptomatic individuals (between 16 to 47%). Ulnar nerve instability is often bilateral clinically and with electrodiagnosis a silent variant. However, it may result in chronic friction of the dislocating nerve, which slides across the epicondyle to the ventral aspect of the forearm during maximum flexion. The snapping sensation may be felt equally by the patient and a careful examiner palpating the nerve during the movement. With sonography, the dislocation of the ulnar nerve alone, or often in conjunction with the medial head of the triceps muscle is nicely demonstrated (**Fig. 10.16**).

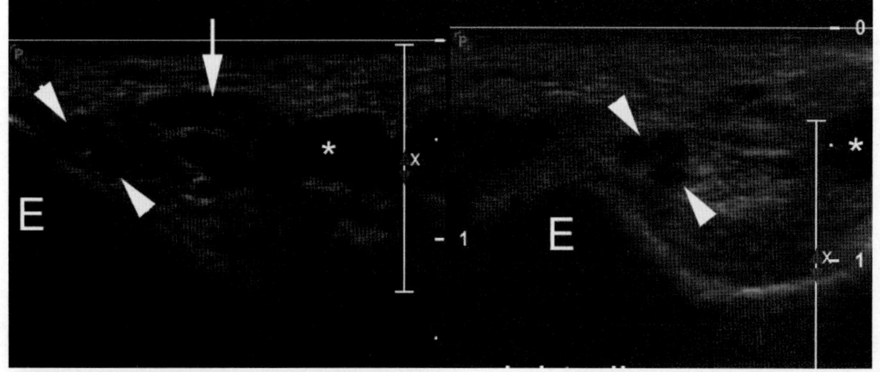

A

B

Fig. 10.13 **(A)** Short axis sonogram of left and right cubital tunnel and **(B)** T1-weighted magnetic resonance image of left cubital tunnel in a patient with ulnar neuropathy at the elbow because of accessory anconeus epitrochlearis muscle [arrow in **(A)** and **(B)**]. The medial head of triceps muscle (*) and the ulnar nerve can be seen (*arrowheads*). Note absence of anconeus epitrochlearis on sonogram of right cubital tunnel. E, medial epicondyle.

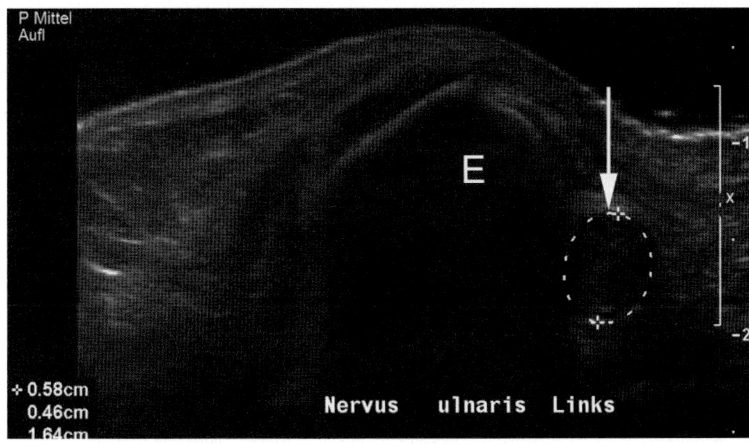

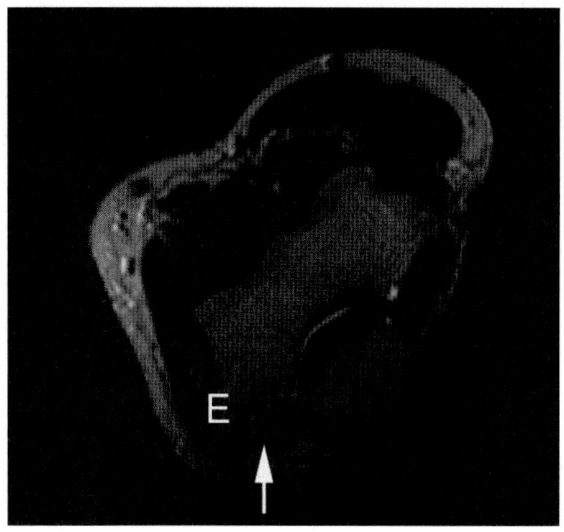

Fig. 10.14 **(A)** Short axis sonogram and **(B)** T2-weighted magnetic resonance image (MRI) of cubital tunnel in a patient with severe ulnar neuropathy at the elbow. The ulnar nerve (*arrow*) is markedly swollen with loss of fascicular texture and a maximum cross-section area of 21 mm^2. In the MRI, the nerve is slightly hyperintense due to edema. E, medical epicondyle.

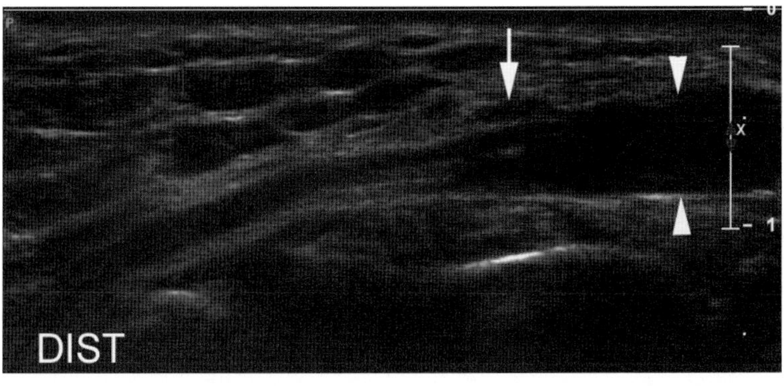

Fig. 10.15 Long axis sonogram along ulnar nerve in a patient with long lasting ulnar neuropathy at the elbow. The ulnar nerve is markedly swollen (*arrowheads*) proximal to the arcuate ligament (*arrow*).

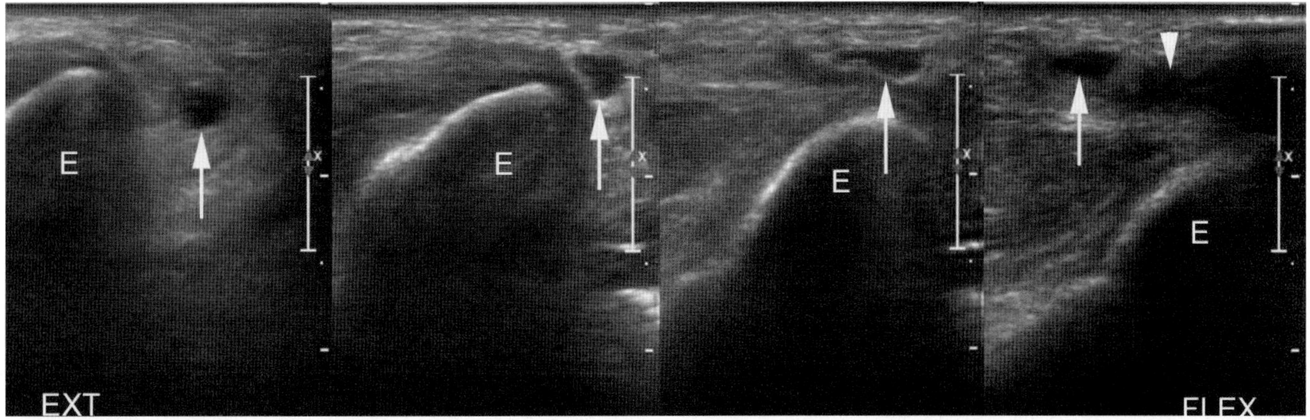

Fig. 10.16 Series of short axis sonograms during extension/flexion of the elbow (from left to right) in an asymptomatic volunteer with snapping ulnaris/snapping triceps. The ulnar nerve (*arrows*) slides across the tip of the epicondyle (E) to the ventral aspect of the forearm during maximum flexion followed by medial head of triceps muscle (*arrowhead*).

Supinator Syndrome

The radial nerve may be compromised in the spiral groove, where it travels close to the bony surface of the humerus; this is encountered with direct pressure in a syndrome commonly referred to as Saturday night nerve palsy (stretching of the nerve during prolonged compression of the arm across a hard support), or in a humeral shaft injury.

Another true idiopathic compression syndrome may be seen with chronic impingement on the deep branch of the radial nerve at the arcade of Frohse, a strong fibrous band at the entry of the nerve into the supinator muscle. A nerve compression at this region, sometimes referred to as the radial tunnel, results in a supinator syndrome with local tenderness and a finger drop instead of the classic wrist drop of a true radial palsy. The syndrome is an important differential in the work-up of patients with a "tennis elbow" and sonography may reliably show the thickened, hypoechoic, edematous nerve proximal to its entry into the supinator arch (**Fig. 10.17**).

Carpal Tunnel Syndrome

Although the median nerve may be compromised in the cubital fossa (pronator syndrome), or its anterior interosseous branch in the forearm (anterior interosseous nerve syndrome) compression at the wrist is most common. The carpal tunnel syndrome (CTS) is the most common entrapment neuropathy with an incidence as high as 3.7% in the general population. In individuals with occupational maneuvers known to result in chronic stretching and compression of the nerve, such as typing, for example, the incidence may even be higher. In almost 50% of cases CTS is bilateral. The clinical presentation of CTS in early stages is that of "brachialgia paresthetica nocturna" with nocturnal pain and/or burning in the thumb, index and middle finger and radial half of the fourth finger, which typically awakens the patient from sleep. Repeated shaking of the hand or massaging of the wrist may result in transient relief. Later during the course of the syndrome, hypesthesia to complete anesthesia develop, with muscular atrophy and function loss being late findings.

Diagnosis is based on clinical examination and electrophysiologic functional testing, which results in reliable detection of CTS in 85 to 90% of patients. While early reports on the application of sonography (and MRI) to the diagnosis of CTS have shown promising results, there is still some debate on the role of sonography in the work-up of CTS. There is a general agreement that sonography is an easily applied, quick, and reliable tool to rule out secondary CTS caused by space-occupying lesions inside the carpal tunnel, but no consensus on its value for diagnosing idiopathic CTS. Recent reports in the literature have shown that sonography alone may have similar diagnostic values compared with electrophysiology and should therefore be applied early in the work-up of CTS. More importantly, it was demonstrated that the combination of electrophysiology and sonography can substantially raise the sensitivity for diagnosing CTS compared with electrophysiology or sonography alone.

The sonographic diagnosis of CTS relies strongly on the demonstration of median nerve enlargement at its entrance into the carpal tunnel (**Fig. 10.18**).

Different cutoff values have been recommended and the choice of threshold results in different sensitivities and specificities. With a cutoff for the cross-section area of 9 mm^2 more mild cases of CTS are detected with a drawback of more false-positive results. A higher cutoff at around 10 to 12 mm^2 may miss some mild cases, but with a higher specificity. Various recommended thresholds are in use based on whether the goal is for detection of mild cases or for cases that warrant treatment. Different threshold values may be caused by differences in measurement sites. The maximum enlargement of the median nerve is not seen in the proxi-

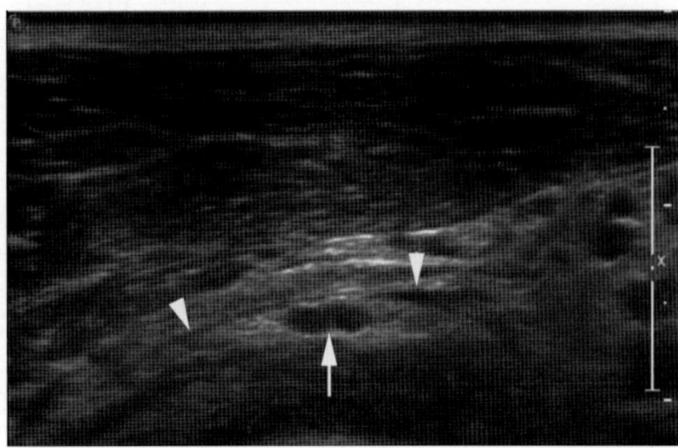

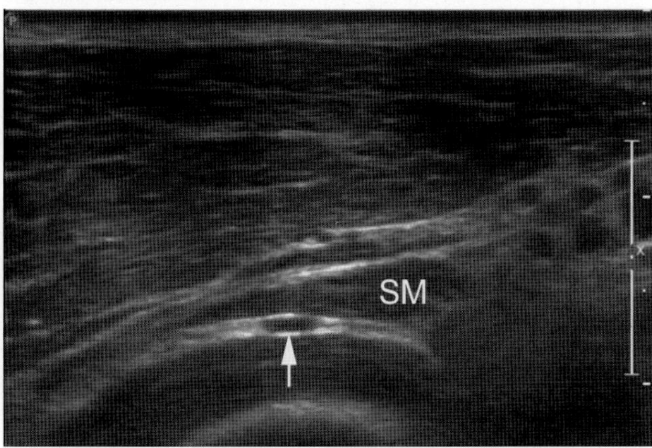

Fig. 10.17 Short axis sonograms at **(A)** proximal and **(B)** more distal entry of deep radial nerve branch (*arrow*) into the supinator muscle (SM) passing underneath the arcade of Frohse (*arrowheads*) in a patient with supinator syndrome. Note swelling and edema of the nerve at its entry underneath the tight ligamentous arc **(A)** with marked flattening in its distal course **(B)**.

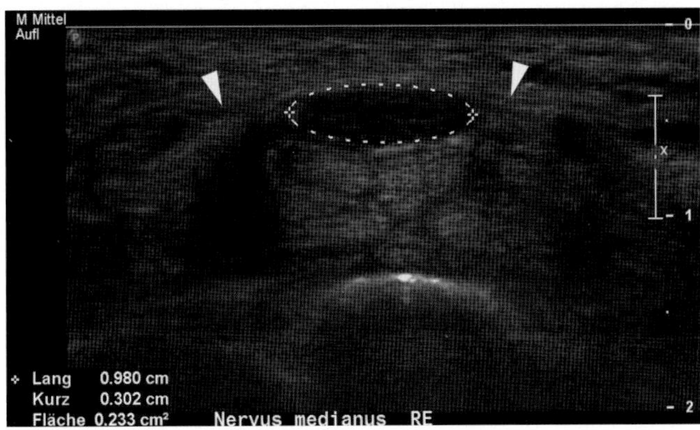

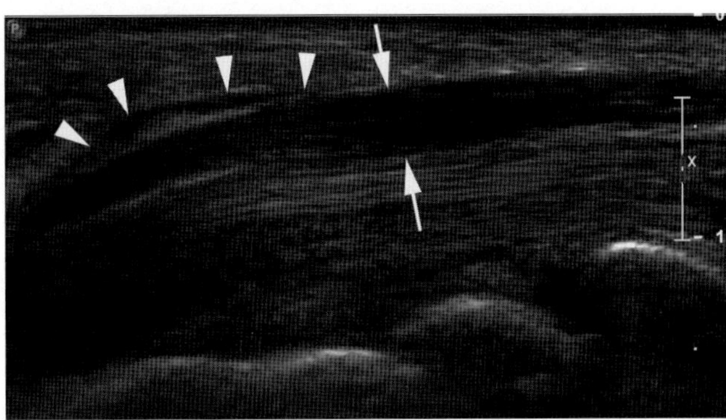

Fig. 10.18 **(A)** Short axis acquired at the proximal edge of the flexor retinaculum (*arrowheads*) and **(B)** long axis sonogram through median nerve in a patient with carpal tunnel syndrome. Note thickening of flexor retinaculum (*arrowheads*) and swelling of median nerve (*arrows*) proximal to the cranial edge of the retinaculum rather than inside proximal carpal tunnel.

mal carpal tunnel, but adjacent to the proximal edge of the flexor retinaculum, hence measuring at this level is more reliable. In the case of a high division of the median nerve, both branches of the nerve must be included in the measurement (**Fig. 10.19**).

Besides changes in caliber and/or shape of the nerve, sonography can also demonstrate structural changes inside the nerve: loss of fascicular discrimination (**Fig. 10.20**) with more or less uniform hypoechoic presentation of the nerve and loss of the nerve's distinct outer epineurial border. These sonographic findings relate to our current pathophysiologic concept of compression neuropathy with edema and vasocongestion constituting a direct consequence of chronic pressure on the nerve. Color Doppler imaging has been proposed by some researchers for identification of hypervascularization inside the longitudinal perineural vascular plexus. State of the art ultrasound equipment can certainly demonstrate tiny intra- and perineural blood vessels, even Duplex spectra may be sampled (**Fig. 10.21**). However, if detection of these vessels reflects a pathologic process—reactive hyperemia and/or inflammation—has to date not been reliably proven in larger controlled trials.

Secondary signs of CTS may be detected with sonography and can help in diagnosing neuropathy: thickening of the flexor retinaculum, bowing of the retinaculum (**Fig. 10.22**), and an enlarged carpal tunnel index (a line is drawn from the hook of the hamate to the trapezium and the maximum distance of the anterior retinaculum to this line at a 90-degree angle is measured; a distance of ≥ 4 mm is considered abnormal).

A variety of space-occupying lesions inside the carpal tunnel can result in secondary CTS: ganglia arising from the palmar wrist capsule are frequently found. Hemangiomas and other tumors are rare causes, whereas chronic tendovaginitis may be seen often. In addition, a CTS-like syndrome may be caused by muscle tissue of a finger flexor, which reaches inside the carpal canal (the carpal canal normally only houses tendons) during extension of the wrist. This muscular impingement syndrome, may be diagnosed with functional dynamic scanning of the wrist, when hy-

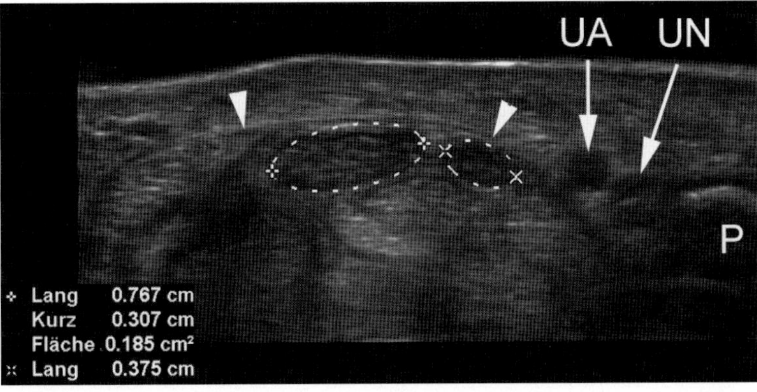

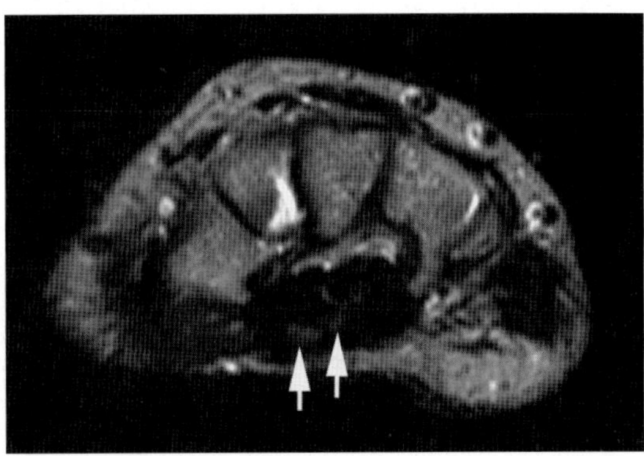

Fig. 10.19 **(A)** Short axis sonogram at proximal edge of flexor retinaculum (*arrowheads*) and **(B)** T2-weighted magnetic resonance image through carpal tunnel in a patient with carpal tunnel syndrome (CTS) and a high division of the median nerve with two differently sized median nerve branches inside carpal canal [*arrows* in **(B)**]. The cross-section area of both median nerve branches is 24 mm^2, which confirms CTS (A). P, pisiform bone; UA, ulnar artery; UN, ulnar nerve.

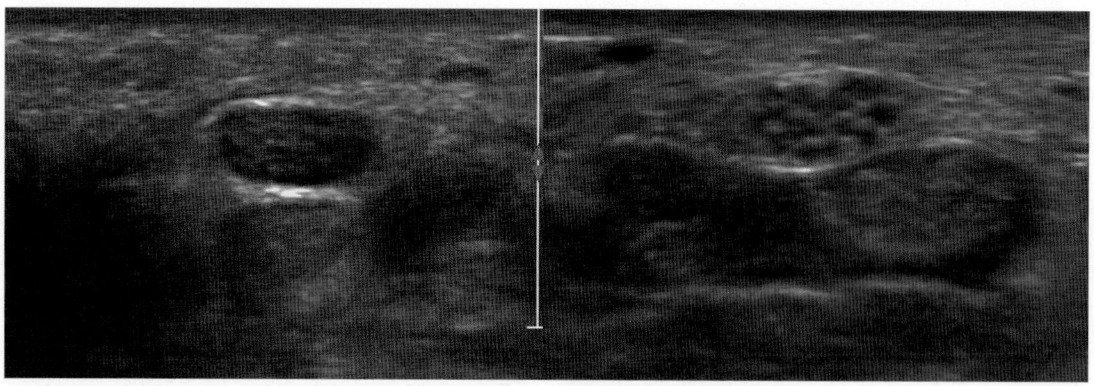

Fig. 10.20 Short axis sonogram of left and right median nerve in a patient with left-sided carpal tunnel syndrome and asymptomatic right wrist. Note loss of fascicular discrimination in left-sided median nerve, compared with normal texture on the right.

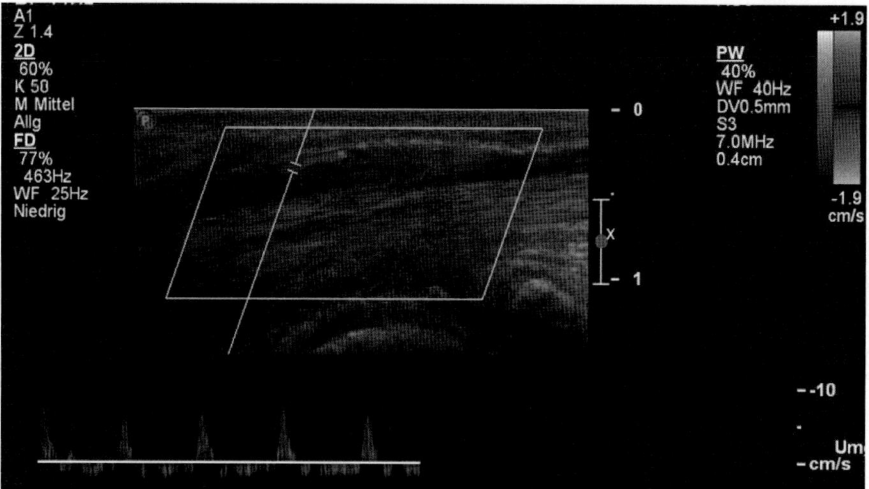

Fig. 10.21 Duplex sonogram of median nerve in a patient with carpal tunnel syndrome demonstrates a thick arterial vessel inside the superficial layer of the nerve, with high resistance waveform.

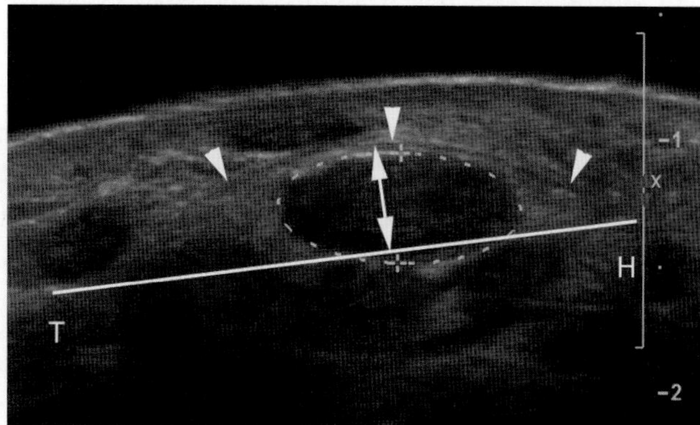

Fig. 10.22 Short axis sonogram through proximal carpal tunnel in a patient with carpal tunnel syndrome. Bowing of the retinaculum (*arrowheads*) and thickened median nerve with loss of fascicular discrimination is seen. The distance between a line from the hook of the hamate (H) to the trapezium (T) and the retinaculum is 4 mm (*double-headed arrow*), which confirms (in this case mild) enlargement of carpal canal.

poechoic muscle tissue—mainly part of the flexor indicis muscle—is seen entering the carpal canal in hyperextension of the wrist (**Fig. 10.23**).

Meralgia Paresthetica

Meralgia paresthetica is a painful condition with compression of the lateral femoral cutaneous nerve at its passage through the inguinal ligament, close to the anterior superior iliac spine. Although this is an uncommon (but not exceedingly rare) syndrome, it may be encountered as a differential in patients with unclear pain in the groin, mostly in obese patients, patients with diabetes, and in patients wearing tight clothes ("hip huggers"). Sonography can reliably demonstrate the enlarged, hypoechoic, edematous nerve in pathologic cases (**Fig. 10.24**); the normal nerve is often hardly visible. Sonography can also be used for the guidance of local corticoid injections (**Fig. 10.25**): this is especially helpful, keeping in mind that the nerve's location alongside the inguinal ligament is quite variable.

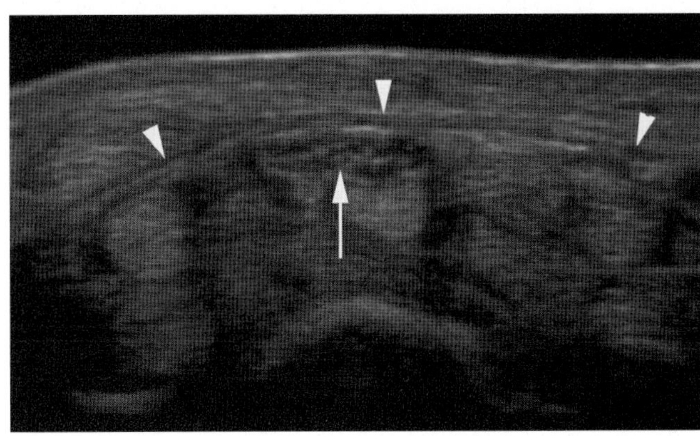

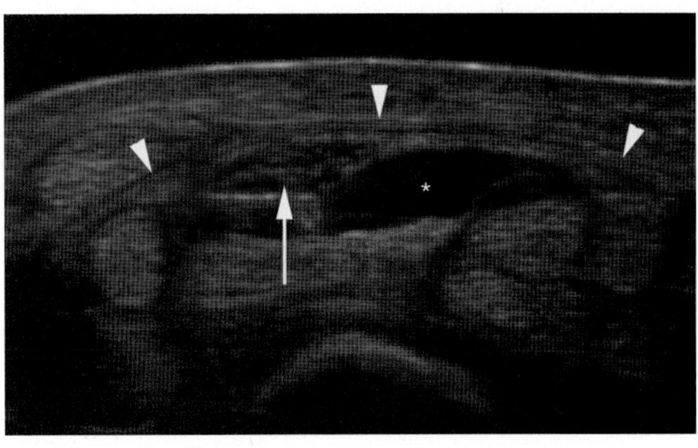

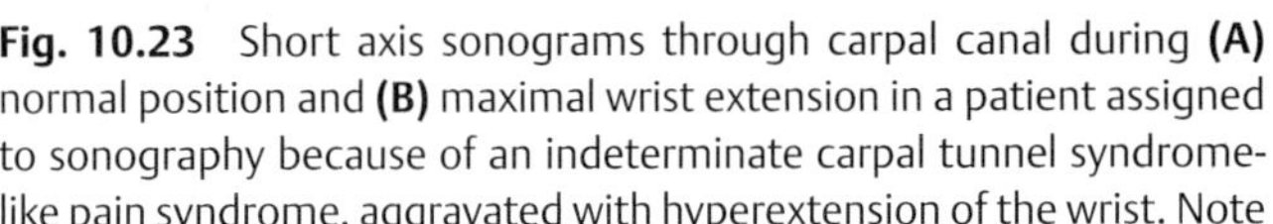

Fig. 10.23 Short axis sonograms through carpal canal during **(A)** normal position and **(B)** maximal wrist extension in a patient assigned to sonography because of an indeterminate carpal tunnel syndrome-like pain syndrome, aggravated with hyperextension of the wrist. Note normal fascicular texture of median nerve (*arrow*), but displacement by muscle belly (*) reaching under the flexor retinaculum (*arrowheads*).

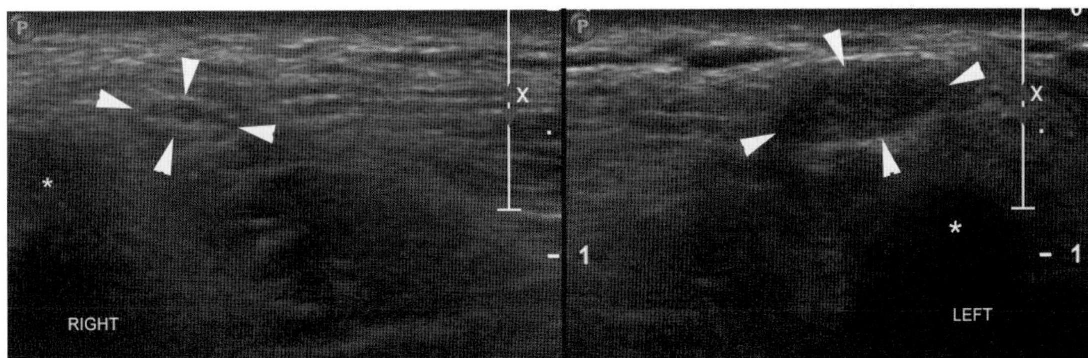

Fig. 10.24 Short axis sonogram of lateral femoral cutaneous nerve in a patient with left-sided meralgia paresthetica nocturna. Note marked enlargement of nerve (*arrowheads*) on the affected side, with edema and loss of fascicular texture (compare with normal nerve on the right). The anterior superior iliac spine is also shown (*).

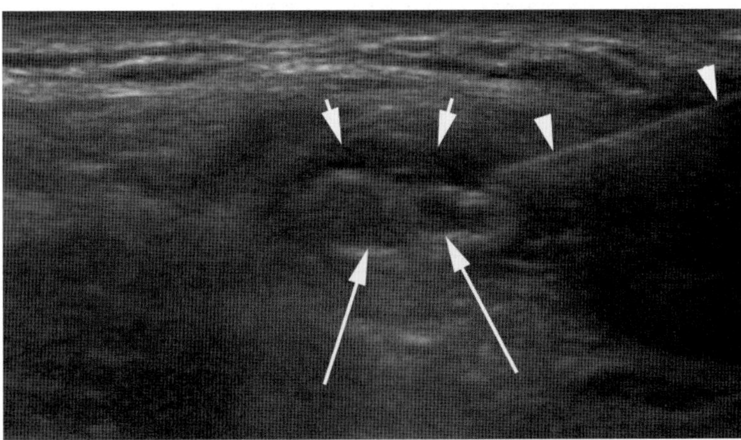

Fig. 10.25 Injection of corticoid around the lateral femoral cutaneous nerve under sonographic guidance (same patient as in **Fig. 10.24**). The needle (*arrowheads*) is placed adjacent to the nerve (*long arrows*), avoiding direct puncture. Hypoechoic fluid (corticoid; *short arrows*) spills around the outer hyperechoic nerve sheath.

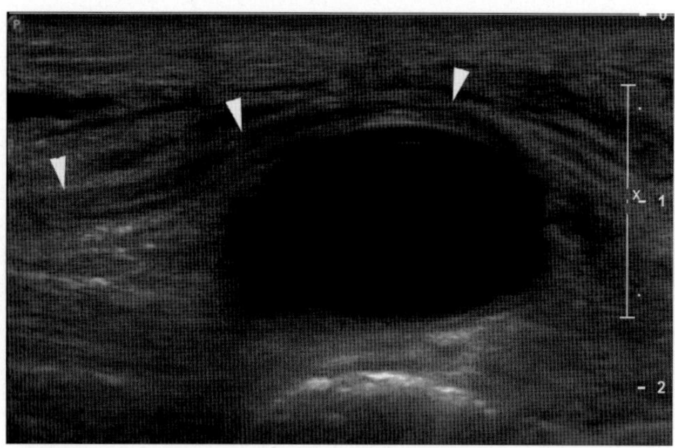

Fig. 10.26 Long axis sonogram of tibial nerve (*arrowheads*) compressed and dislocated by a large fluid-filled ganglion cyst in a patient with tarsal tunnel syndrome.

Tarsal Tunnel Syndrome

The true idiopathic tarsal tunnel syndrome is less frequent than the other compression neuropathies, but indirect compromise of the nerve due to fractures, ganglia, or postoperative scars may be encountered more often. The clinical onset of tibial neuropathy may be subtle; in the case of a pure pain syndrome, it may be demanding to reach a correct differential diagnosis. Sonography is helpful demonstrating an enlargement of the nerve at the proximal level of the tarsal tunnel in a true idiopathic syndrome or the underlying cause in case of external compression (**Fig. 10.26**).

Imaging after Surgery for Compression Neuropathy

Patients with poor outcome or recurring neurologic symptoms after decompression of a neural tunnel warrant imaging to rule out incomplete transection of a retinaculum, direct damage of the nerve during surgery, and/or scar tissue formation with secondary nerve compression. In the first two situations, the patient will never achieve sufficient resolution of symptoms after surgery. In the third situation, the patient's symptoms may improve for a short period, with worsening during ongoing scar tissue compression. Although scar formation is easily seen with sonography, a judgment—whether a scar is the reason for a patient's complaints—is to be based on the demonstration of direct ingrowth of the scar into the outer epineurium (**Fig. 10.27**) and/or flattening of the nerve with loss of mobility.

Peripheral Nerve Trauma

Contrary to general belief, trauma to peripheral nerves is quite common. According to the literature, plexus and peripheral nerve trauma may be found in ~5% of patients admitted to level I trauma centers. The importance of sonography and MRI in imaging nerve trauma lies mainly in the definition of lesion location, extension, and severity. Imaging is especially helpful in the posttraumatic setting, as it sets the path for rehabilitative treatment and surgical intervention. For the latter it is important information, if a nerve is completely or only incompletely transected, where the stumps are located, if a transection is complicated by interpositioning of hematoma or scar tissue. Although direct trauma to a nerve may be readily encountered in the initial clinical setting, late-onset palsy after fracture repair (radial palsy after humeral shaft fracture, for example) or after surgical procedures not directly addressing a nerve (true iatrogenic injuries), as well as nerve lesions caused by anesthesiologic procedures are often more difficult to diagnose.

Cervical/Brachial Plexus Trauma

A variety of traumatic events, ranging from direct head and neck trauma to traction injuries of the upper extremity can

A

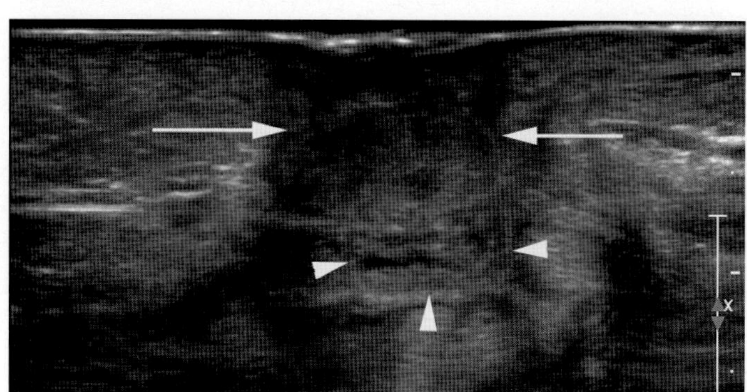

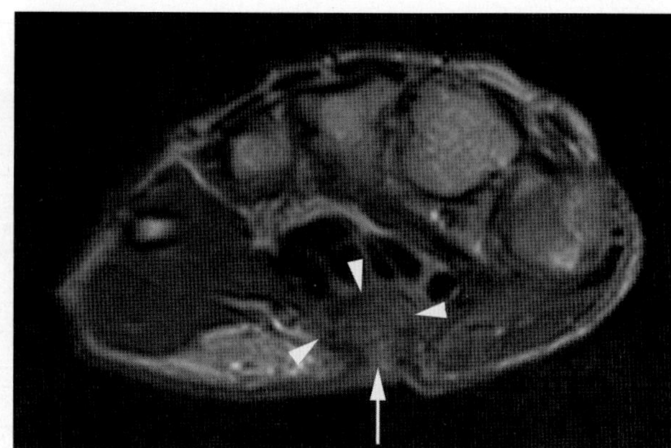

B

Fig. 10.27 **(A)** Short axis sonogram and **(B)** correlative T2-weighted magnetic resonance image in a patient after carpal tunnel release with postoperative worsening symptoms. Median nerve (*arrowheads*) is markedly deformed and compressed by overlying hypertrophic scar tissue (*arrows*).

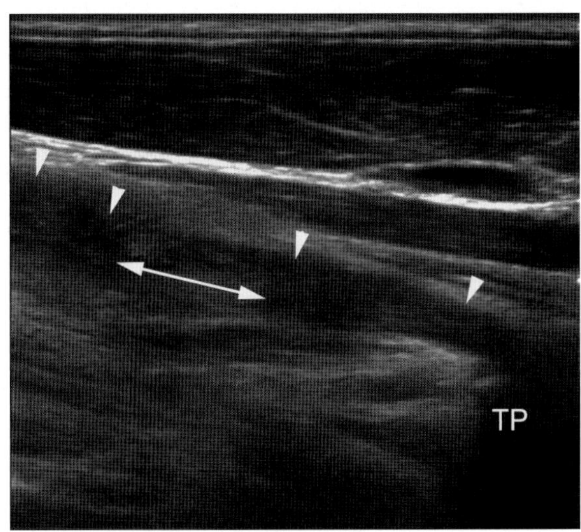

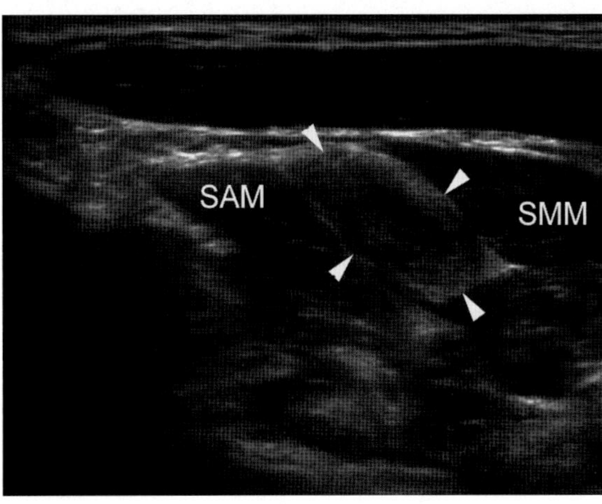

Fig. 10.28 **(A)** Long and **(B)** short axis sonogram through sixth cervical plexus root in a 15-year-old patient with incomplete plexus palsy since birth. **(A)** Two nerve stumps (*arrowheads*) and a gap (*double-headed arrow*) filled with organized hematoma and scar tissue are seen. **(B)** A grossly enlarged mass of scar tissue and hematoma (*arrowheads*) is seen inside the interscalene gap. SAM, scalenus anterior muscle; SMM, scalenus medius muscle.

result in traumatic plexus palsy. Sonographic imaging—generally with a 7 to 12 or 3 to 9 MHz transducer—should aim at definition of the plexus elements involved, the level of injury (root, trunk, or fascicular level), and the severity (complete disruption, traction injury). Due to the complex nature of plexus injuries, MRI and sonography yield complementary information and are therefore always combined in the work-up of plexus injuries at our institution. A complete rupture of a plexus root (**Fig. 10.28**) may be easily diagnosed with longitudinal scanning (we always ask for the demonstration of two distinct nerve stumps with a gap between the neural elements; which may be filled with fluid, hematoma, and/or other interpositioned soft tissue elements); however, so-called traction neuromas are more often encountered. A traction neuroma is an incomplete nerve lesion caused by overt stretching of fascicular elements inside a nerve and may not only be found in plexus lesions, but also with trauma of peripheral nerves in the extremities. Although the outer nerve sheath is normal, the inner structure of a variable segment of the nerve is abnormal. Sonography reveals a segment of indistinct inner structure with hypoechoic and often inhomogeneous loss of texture due to edema and internal hematoma (**Fig. 10.29**). Sometimes, these lesions may appear as several discontinuous sections of a nerve with interposed segments of normal structure in the form of a so-called chain lesion. Side-by-side comparison of the compromised and normal plexus may be needed to detect subtle lesions. Root avulsion may sometimes be detected with sonography if the root is retracted peripherally and an empty foraminal outlet can be demonstrated, but the diagnosis of root avulsion and pseudomeningocele is definitely a domain of MRI (**Fig. 10.4**).

Peripheral Nerve Trauma in the Extremities

Direct sharp transections or traumatic disruption of a peripheral nerve are easily diagnosed with sonography by demonstration of the individual nerve stumps (**Fig. 10.30**).

A lesion known as traction neuroma, also known as neuroma in continuity, warrants further discussion. It may be seen especially in the peroneal nerve after knee joint dislocation. Though the outer nerve sheath stays intact, the fascicular elements are ruptured—often at several levels—and retracted at a variable length (**Fig. 10.31**). For the surgeon,

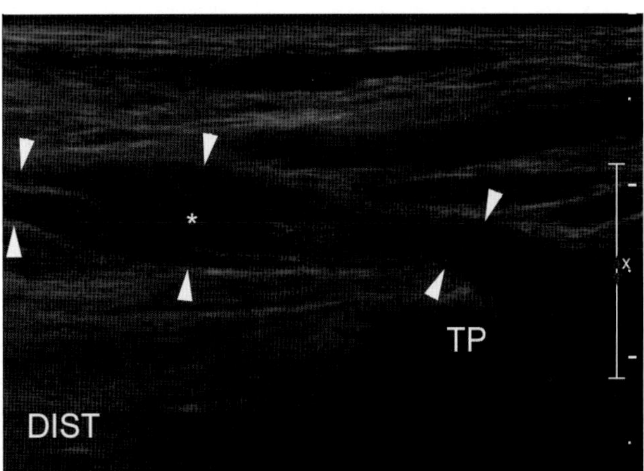

Fig. 10.29 Long axis sonogram through sixth cervical plexus root in a female patient with traction injury of brachial plexus during a motor vehicle accident. Note swelling with hypoechoic inhomogeneous texture of nerve root (*arrowheads*) at the section where it enters the interscalene gap (*). TP, transverse process.

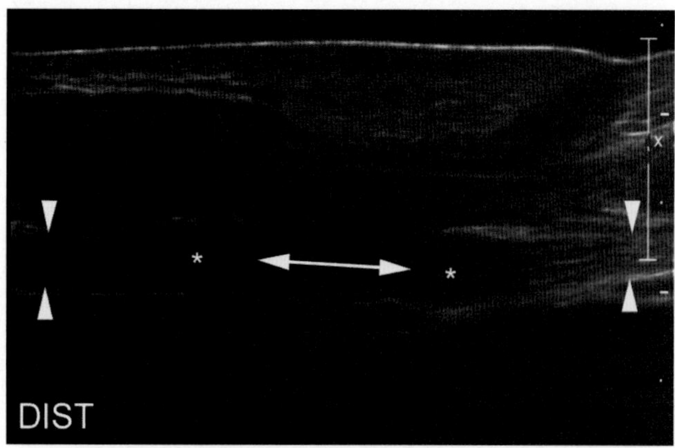

Fig. 10.30 Long axis sonogram through ulnar nerve (*arrowheads*) at the forearm in a patient with sharp transection of the nerve and overlying soft tissues. Note gap (*double-headed arrow*) between the two nerve stumps (*) and damaged overlying muscle.

aiming at reconstruction of the nerve, it is important to know how much of a nerve is internally deranged because normally only a limited access to the nerve is chosen and the extent of damage may be quite difficult to realize with inspection. Exploration of a nerve along a long distance is to be avoided as it may be harmful to the nerve and its surroundings.

The most frequent nerve lesions together with bone and joint trauma occur in humeral shaft fractures (radial nerve palsy in up to 18% of patients) and in shoulder and knee dislocations (axillary and peroneal nerve palsies). Although direct traumatic nerve lesions—which range from traction edema (**Fig. 10.32**) to interposition inside the fracture gap and piercing of a nerve by bony fragments (**Fig. 10.33**)—may be readily diagnosed with sonography, postoperative lesions of a nerve are sometimes more difficult to diagnose.

Postoperative lesions may occur because of the natural process of fracture healing with compression of a nerve by

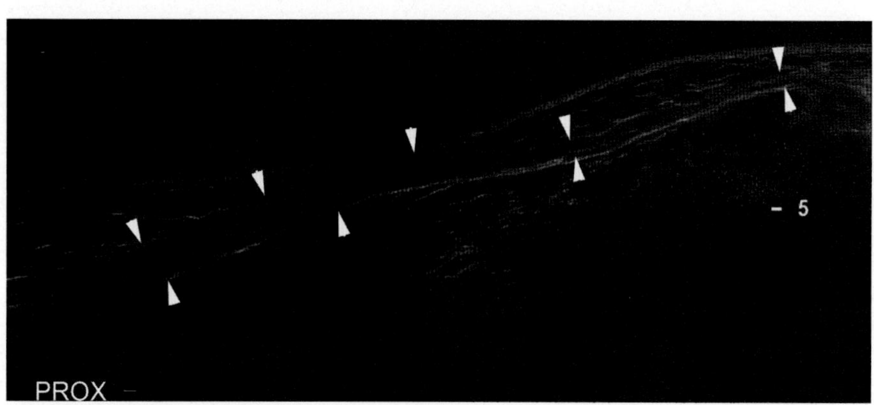

Fig. 10.31 Long axis panoramic sonogram along peroneal nerve (*arrowheads*) in a patient with peroneal nerve palsy after knee dislocation. Preserved outer nerve sheath (*arrowheads*), but inhomogeneous internal structure with swelling of the nerve consistent with internal fascicular rupture and hematoma—traction neuroma is demonstrated.

A

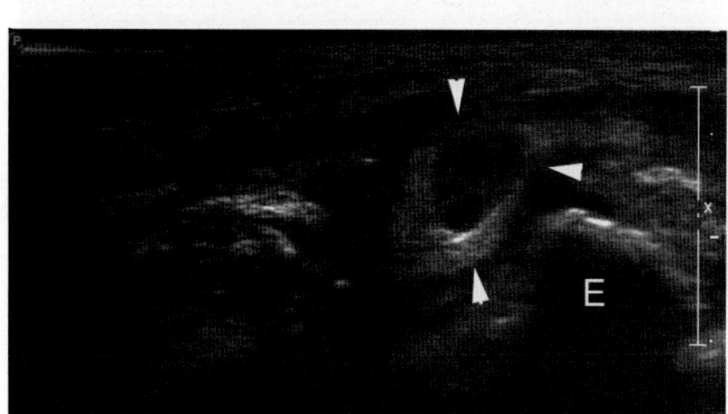

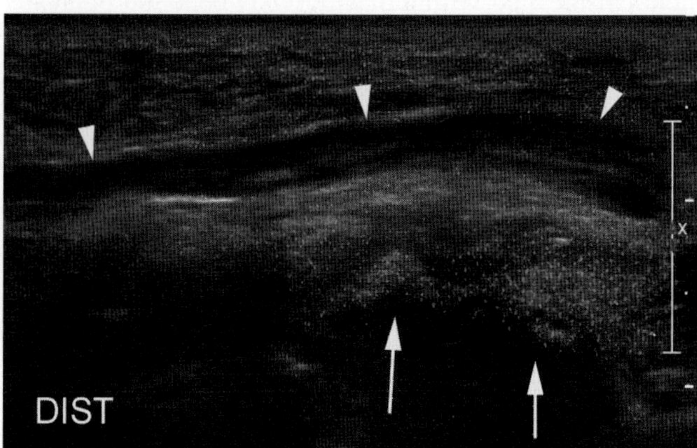

B

Fig. 10.32 **(A)** Short and **(B)** long axis sonogram through ulnar nerve in a patient after fracture dislocation of the elbow and ulnar nerve palsy. The ulnar nerve is markedly swollen and inhomogeneous with hyperechoic perineural edema [*arrowheads* in **(A)**]. A fracture callus can be seen (*arrows*). E, medial epicondyle.

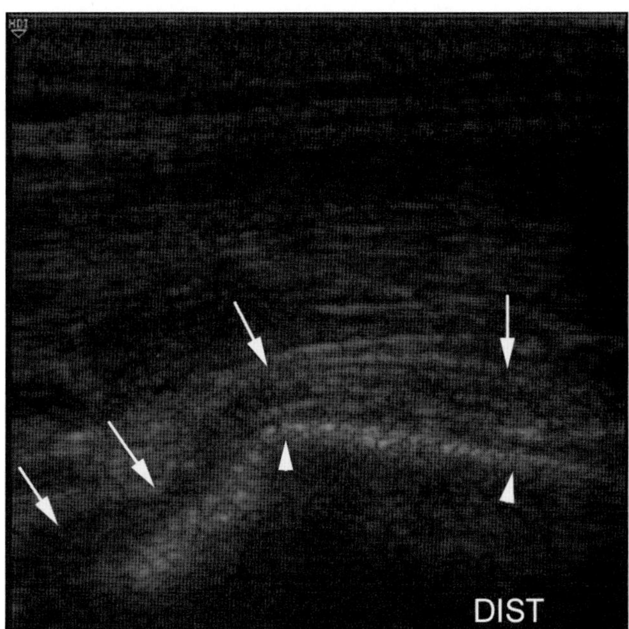

Fig. 10.33 Long axis sonogram of radial nerve (*arrows*) in a patient with radial palsy after humeral shaft fracture. Displaced bony fragment (*arrowheads*) abuts the nerve. Note edema with hypoechoic nerve texture proximal to the fracture.

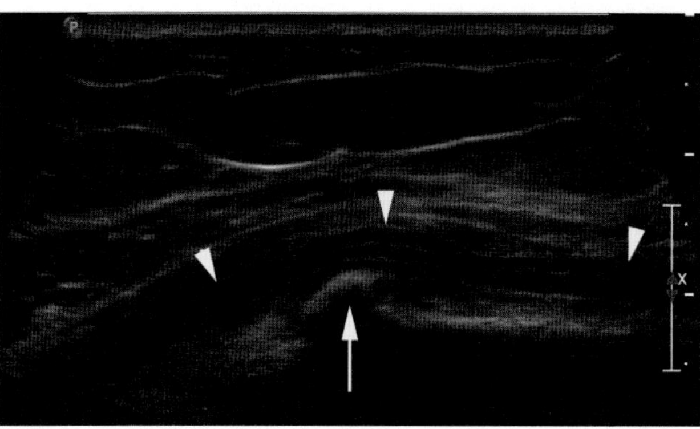

Fig. 10.34 Long axis sonogram of ulnar nerve (*arrowheads*) in a patient with ulnar palsy after supracondylar fracture. The nerve is displaced by abutting bony callus (*arrow*).

scar tissue or bony callus (**Fig. 10.34**), but may also be caused by compression of a nerve by surgical material (**Fig. 10.35**).

With appropriate expertise, sonography can play an important role in the follow-up of nerve surgery. The rehabilitation process after fascicular repair or nerve grafting can be tedious and may be disturbed by well-known processes like neuroma formation, loosening of sutures, and scarring. In this setting, the sonographer should strive at definition of nerve continuity, which may be difficult. Although outer continuity of a nerve is often readily demonstrated (**Fig. 10.36**) by definition of a continuous outer nerve sheath at the level of the suture (note that even the tiny sutures used in nerve repair can be seen with sonography), continuity of fascicular elements is often difficult to define. Suture sites may look grossly enlarged and swollen in the early postoperative period despite favorable functional rehabilitation. Therefore, the aim should be the detection of truly discontinuous elements and neuroma, which is a definite sign of impaired healing (**Fig. 10.37**).

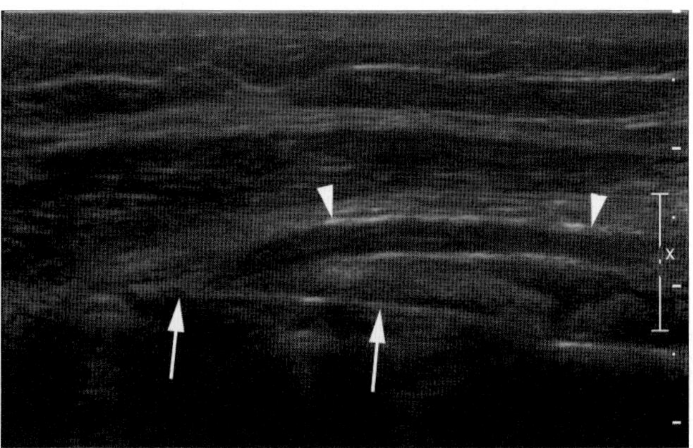

Fig. 10.35 Long axis sonogram of radial nerve (*arrowheads*) in a patient after humeral shaft fracture. Radial nerve palsy developed after fracture repair. Sonogram shows compression of nerve at edge of surgical plate (*arrows*).

Tumors of the Peripheral Nervous System

Peripheral nerve tumors are uncommon, with schwannomas, neurofibromas, and nerve sheath ganglia being most frequent. The musculoskeletal sonographer may incidentally find these lesions during the work-up of a soft tissue mass. Whenever a soft tissue mass can be shown in direct continuity with a nerve, a nerve tumor is probable. While schwannoma has an eccentric location, and is seen as a roundish lesion positioned along the surface of a nerve (**Fig. 10.38**), neurofibroma grows inside a nerve and has a more spindle-shaped appearance (**Fig. 10.39**). Additional sonographic features of schwannoma include inhomogeneous hypoechoic texture, regressive, internal cystic changes (**Fig. 10.40**), and high vascularity (**Fig. 10.41**).

Nerve sheath ganglia are rare but interesting lesions, hardly known by the general sonographer and clinician alike. This is regrettable, as many patients with this type of benign nonneoplastic neural tumor suffer long-lasting painful symptoms without a definite diagnosis. Nerve sheath ganglia consist of small tubular cyst-like structures inside the nerve—either singular or multiple—and often along a substantial distance. They are caused by leakage of joint fluid into the sheath of a close-lying peripheral nerve through a small capsular gap. Because of this pathophysiologic mechanism the peroneal nerve close to the proximal

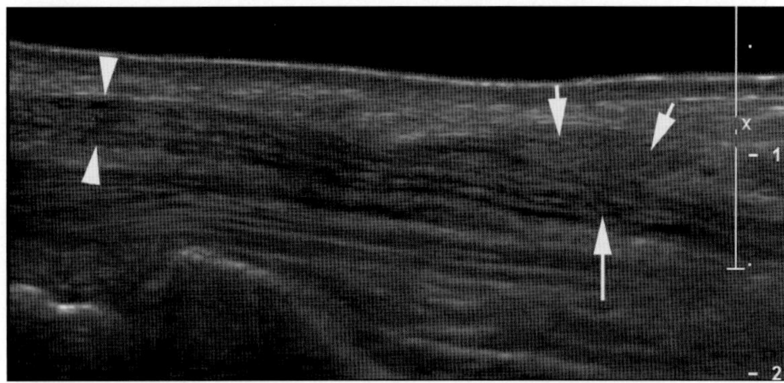

Fig. 10.36 Long axis sonogram through ulnar nerve (*arrowheads*) in a patient after sharp transection of nerve and primary suture. Outer continuity of nerve is readily established at the suture site, which is identified by small suture artifacts (*long arrow*). Close to the nerve surface, a small scar is demonstrated (*short arrows*).

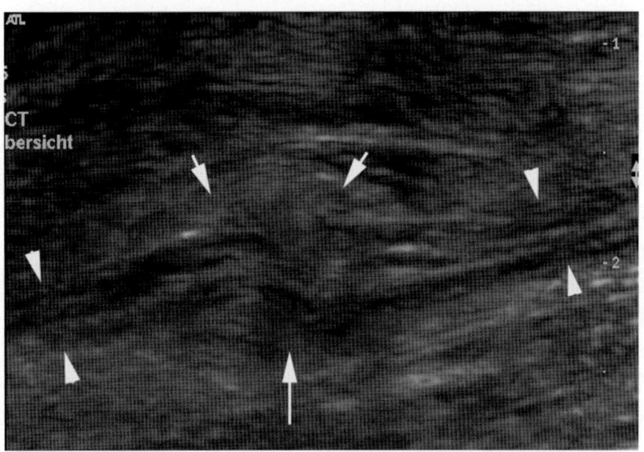

Fig. 10.37 Long axis sonogram through median nerve (*arrowheads*) in a patient after nerve suture. Postoperative rehabilitation was dismal with lasting neural deficit. A gap (*long arrow*) filled with scar tissue and an eccentric anastomotic neuroma (*short arrows*) is seen.

tibiofibular joint, the tibial nerve close to the popliteal recess of the knee capsule (**Fig. 10.42**), or the ulnar nerve close to the wrist/pisotriquetral joint are most often involved. Again, sonographic definition of the extent of the ganglia inside the nerve and if possible the connection to the joint is crucial.

Miscellaneous

Because of its high versatility in terms of choice of imaging planes and patient positioning, sonography is the number one tool for the guidance of injections to peripheral nerves. This is equally true for therapeutic instillation with various types of medications (cortisone, alcohol, phenol injections) and for the guidance of regional anesthesia.

At our institution, we generally prefer a freehand technique with an in-plane needle approach (**Fig. 10.43**). This technique combines optimum visualization of the needle along its course toward the nerve; it is therefore a secure

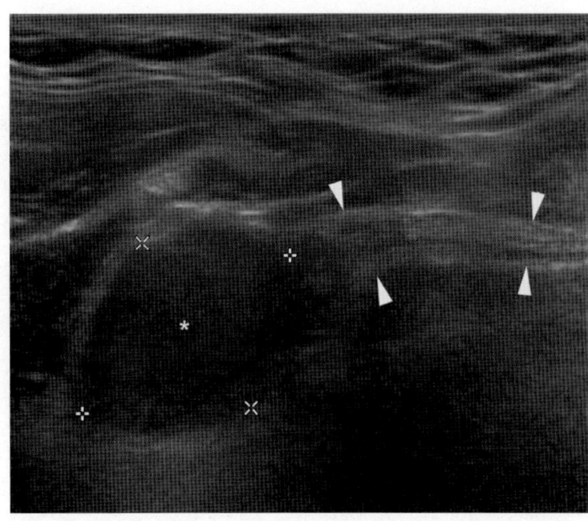

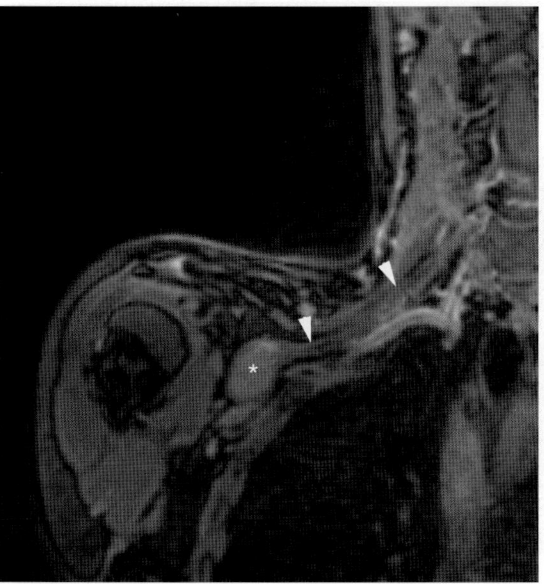

Fig. 10.38 **(A)** Long axis sonogram and **(B)** corresponding magnetic resonance image (MRI) of anterior plexus fascicle (*arrowheads*) in the axillary region. A roundish lesion (*), located eccentrically to the nerve, with hypoechoic echotexture and hyperintense signal in MRI is demonstrated consistent with a schwannoma.

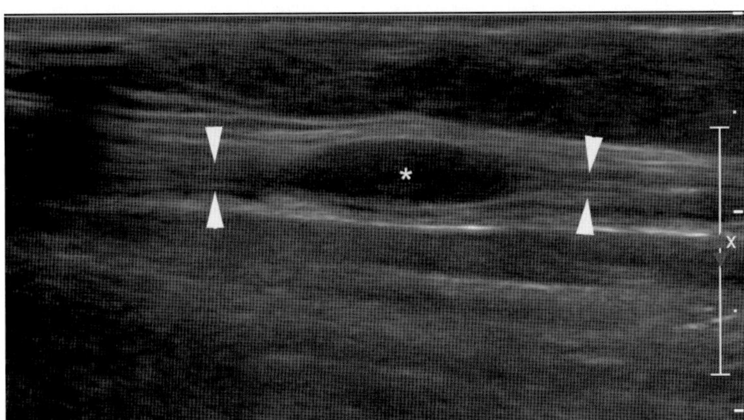

Fig. 10.39 Long axis sonogram through ulnar nerve (*arrowheads*) at forearm level of a patient with neurofibromatosis type I. A small spindle-shaped hypoechoic neurofibroma (*) located concentrically inside the nerve is demonstrated.

Fig. 10.40 **(A)** Long axis sonogram and **(B)** T1-weighted magnetic resonance image (MRI) after application of gadolinium contrast in a patient with tibial nerve schwannoma. Note eccentrically located nerve (*arrowheads*) and internal regressive, cystic changes in the sonogram (*arrow*). Inhomogeneous, but marked contrast uptake is seen in the MRI.

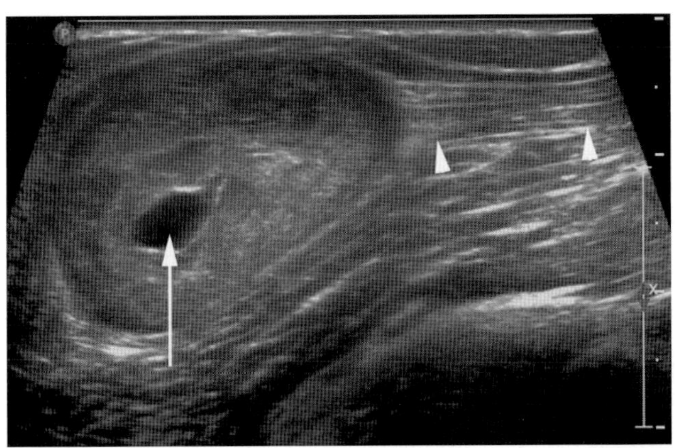

A

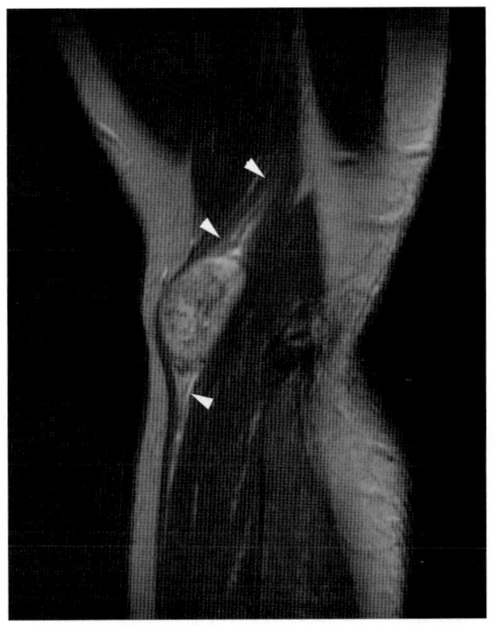

B

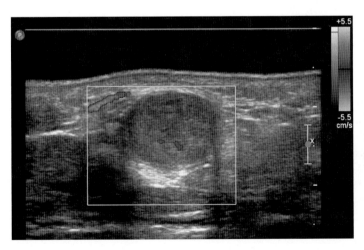

A

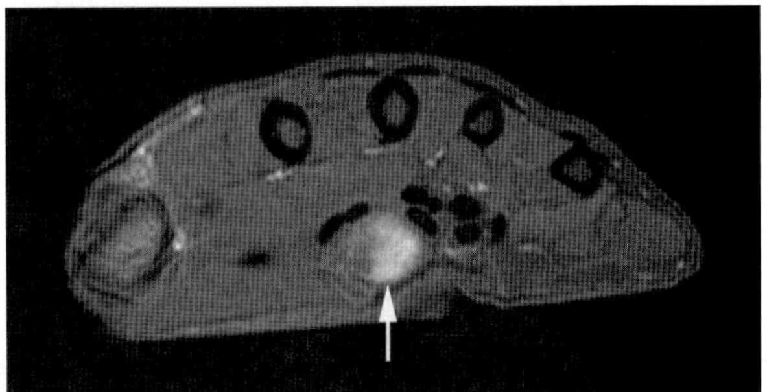

B

Fig. 10.41 **(A)** Short axis color Doppler sonogram and **(B)** T1-weighted fat-saturated magnetic resonance image (MRI) after a gadolinium contrast in a patient with a median nerve schwannoma at the wrist. Note multiple internal vessels in color Doppler image and inhomogeneous, high-contrast uptake [*arrow* in **(B)**] in the MRI.

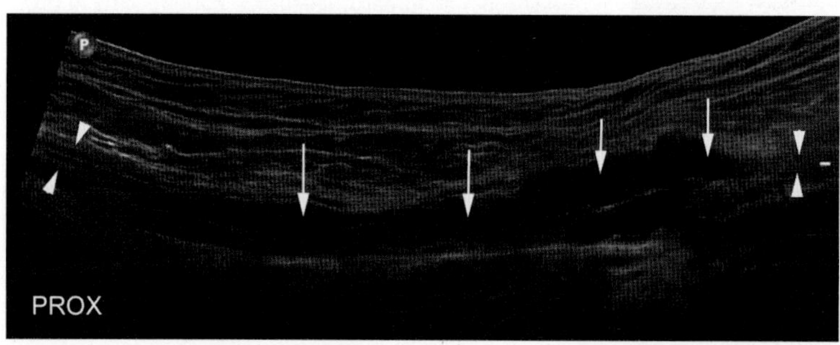

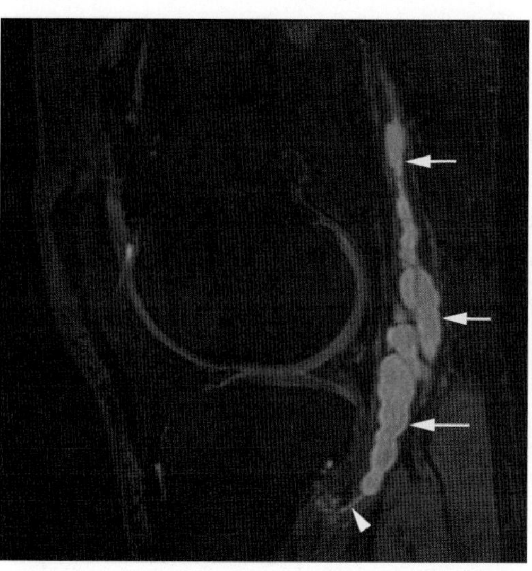

Fig. 10.42 **(A)** Long axis sonogram and **(B)** corresponding magnetic resonance image (MRI) of tibial nerve at knee level in a patient assigned for sonography because of tibial nerve impairment. A tubular fluid-filled intraneural structure (*arrows*) inside the tibial nerve [*arrowheads* in **(A)**] is demonstrated. Note tiny connection of intraneural ganglion toward the capsular recess in the MRI [*arrowhead* in **(B)**].

technique with only a very low risk of nerve damage. It also allows access to a nerve via a wide range of angulations, depending on the anatomic situation. Vast experience exists with almost every known type of anesthetic block, injections to peripheral nerves, and radicular as well as facet joint injections in the cervical and lumbar spine.

In this context, the problem of a stump neuroma in patients with chronic pain syndromes after amputation of a limb will be discussed briefly. Most commonly occurring in patients after lower leg amputation because of peripheral arterial occlusive disease or severe trauma, phantom limb pain significantly reduces a patient's quality of life. Many of these patients are on chronic drug therapy, most of them on morphines; even so, they do not experience sufficient pain control. Phantom limb pain is a rather complex condition with various physiologic and psychologic aspects. Neverthe-

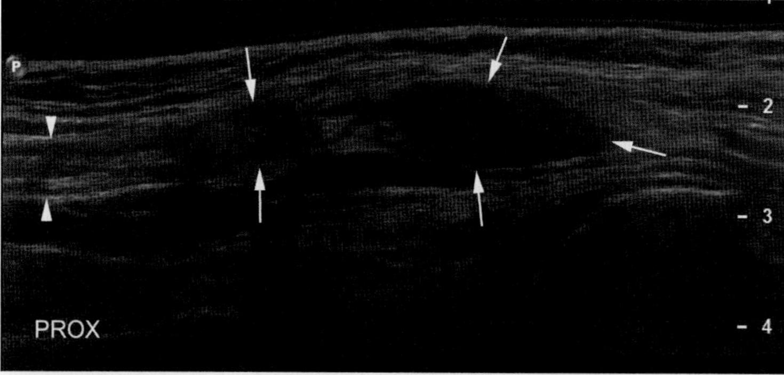

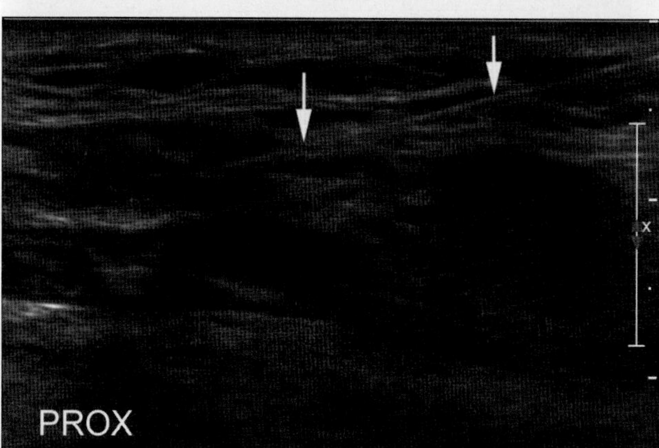

Fig. 10.43 **(A)** Long axis sonogram through tibial nerve (*arrowheads*) in a patient with long-lasting phantom limb pain after lower leg amputation and a large terminal type stump neuroma and a smaller, more proximally located neuroma, a "chain lesion" (*arrows*). **(B)** Application of phenol with sonographic guidance of needle (*arrows*) by in-plane needle approach.

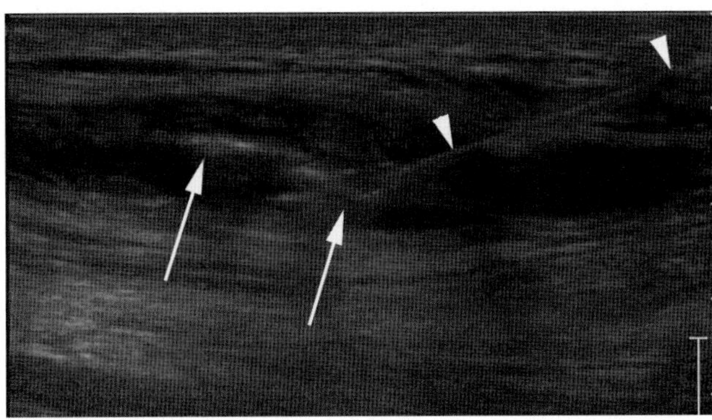

Fig. 10.44 Neurosclerosis with phenol under sonographic guidance in another patient with phantom limb pain and stump neuroma. After placement of the needle (*arrowheads*) into the parent nerve of the neuroma, true intraneural application of phenol (*arrows*) is easily monitored under sonographic control.

less, we do know that terminal-type neuroma at the stump of a severed nerve plays an important role in pain generation. Local instillation of phenol into the neck of the neuroma under sonographic guidance has proved to be helpful in a substantial percentage of patients with phantom limb pain. A low risk of adverse effects (soft tissue inflammation or necrosis due to spilling of phenol) is achieved with careful sonographic application of up to 1 milliliter of phenol into the parent nerve in regional anesthesia (**Fig. 10.44**). Phenol must be placed as close to the neck of the neuroma as possible, to spare functioning neural branches proximal to the neuroma from necrosis, which may result in deterioration of limb function. Additional care has to be taken to flush the needle with saline during withdrawal, to avoid spilling phenol into the soft tissues. Although one injection may quickly result in substantial improvement in some patients, two or more injections within some weeks or months may be needed in others. Only a few patients remain pain-free for a long time; however, pain is reduced in most and phenol treatment substantially reduces the need for oral analgesics.

Artifacts

In general, nerve sonography is free of typical artifacts. Important to mention, however, is the different reaction of nerves and tendons to scanning at different angles. Although varying the scan angle results in the well-known change from a hyper- to a hypoechoic representation of tendons and muscle due to their anisotropic tissue components, this behavior is not seen with peripheral nerves. Therefore, dynamic scanning can help in differentiating a nerve from close lying tendon and muscle.

Proposed Algorithm for Peripheral Nerve Investigation

1- High-resolution sonography for superficial nerves.
2- MRI for deep lying neural structures such as lumbar plexus
3- Additional functional sonography and/or color Doppler/duplex sonography when appropriate
4- Always use additional MRI for lesions of brachial plexus

Pearls and Pitfalls

- Due to its unrivaled resolution, sonography is the modality of choice for imaging of peripheral nerve ultrastructure.
- The number of fascicles discernible with sonography varies in individual nerves. Nerves with a normal amount of constant stretching (such as the ulnar nerve at the elbow) may even be completely hypoechoic.
- Sonographic findings such as edema with loss of fascicular discrimination, indistinct hypoechoic outer nerve sheath, and hypervascularization of a nerve reflect the underlying pathophysiological process of compression neuropathy and thus are reliable diagnostic signs of disease.
- Although secondary neuropathy is quite uncommon in other regions, ulnar neuropathy due to the accessory anconeus epitrochlearis muscle or snapping ulnaris/triceps syndrome may be encountered in the cubital tunnel.
- Sonography with an in-plane needle approach is an elegant method for the guidance of local injection into nerves.

Suggested Readings

There exists abounding literature on sonography of peripheral nerves, especially on sonography of compression neuropathy and trauma; the following list represents a subjective choice of the most important sources.

Chiou HJ, Chou YH, Chiou SY, Liu JB, Chang CY. Peripheral nerve lesions: role of high-resolution US. Radiographics 2003;23(6):e15. Epub 2003 Aug 25

Gruber H, Glodny B, Bendix N, Tzankov A, Peer S. High-resolution ultrasound of peripheral neurogenic tumors. Eur Radiol 2007;17(11):2880–2888

Jacobson JA. Musculoskeletal ultrasound and MRI: which do I choose? Semin Musculoskelet Radiol 2005;9(2):135–149

Peer S, Bodner G, eds. High resolution sonography of the peripheral nervous system. 2nd ed. New York: Springer; 2008

Walker FO. Imaging nerve and muscle with ultrasound. Suppl Clin Neurophysiol 2004;57:243–254

11 Ultrasound for Rheumatoid Arthritis

Robert R. Lopez-Ben

Rheumatoid arthritis (RA) is a severe multisystem autoimmune disease with an overall prevalence of ~1% worldwide—thus affecting tens of millions of people, with approximately a 3:1 female-to-male incidence ratio. The course of the disease is unpredictable and highly variable from patient to patient, but chronic joint inflammation can lead to fixed joint deformities. This can lead to significant disabilities and loss of function or ability to care for oneself.

It has now been shown that early treatment with anti-inflammatory and disease-modifying antirheumatic drugs (DMARDS) will decrease the extent of joint damage and in some cases achieve a remission of the disease. By intervening early in the disease course, functional outcomes in these patients will improve. Some of the newer therapeutic agents used in the treatment of inflammatory arthritis like tumor-necrosis factor α inhibitors, and other agents targeting different components of the inflammatory response like rituximab and abatacept, can be very effective. However, they are expensive and can be associated with significant side effects. Establishing the diagnosis accurately early in the disease course, as well as assessing disease activity frequently, is of critical clinical significance.

The classic clinical presentation of bilaterally symmetrical polyarticular pain and swelling in a rheumatoid-type distribution in the hands and feet, along with the presence of morning stiffness, usually suggests the diagnosis of RA in most cases. The presence of serologic markers of chronic inflammation like rheumatoid factor, and typical radiographic findings including joint space narrowing and marginal erosions, will then usually establish the diagnosis in clinical practice. Radiographs of the hands and feet have been the traditional imaging method to assess disease diagnosis and progression in RA patients.

However, determining active synovial inflammation on physical exam may be difficult, especially in obese patients, patients with an asymmetrical involved joints distribution, or patients with long-standing diseases who may have fibrotic pannus. Serologic markers of inflammation are nonspecific. More specific radiographic markers of active synovial inflammation like marginal bone erosions may not be detected early in the disease course, with up to 70% of patients reported to have normal radiographs at clinical presentation. Because radiography cannot directly visualize the synovium and cartilage, radiographic assessment of synovitis depends on secondary findings like joint space narrowing and periarticular osteopenia. These have significant interobserver variability. Bone erosions are only diagnosed with confidence when the radiographic beam has profiled them in tangent.

Identifying these early RA patients from patients with a self-limiting undifferentiated arthritis clinical syndrome or other conditions like seronegative spondyloarthropathies, and even noninflammatory conditions like fibromyalgia or knucklepads, can be at times difficult for the clinician and lead to diagnostic uncertainty (**Fig. 11.1**).

Cross-sectional imaging techniques like computed tomography (CT), magnetic resonance imaging (MRI), and ultrasound have traditionally been used in this patient population to evaluate for complications of chronic inflammation of RA like tendon tears, entrapment neuropathies, or secondary joint infections (**Figs. 11.2, 11.3, 11.4**).

Based on more aggressive treatment planning in early disease and the high false-negative rate of radiographs in early RA, cross-sectional imaging is now used to directly evaluate the synovium, as well as assess the bone, marrow, and cartilage for evidence of inflammation and joint damage.

Cross-sectional imaging is more sensitive to bone erosion detection when compared with radiographs. MRI and ultrasound have been shown to be more sensitive than clinical exam in determining extent of synovitis and erosions. They

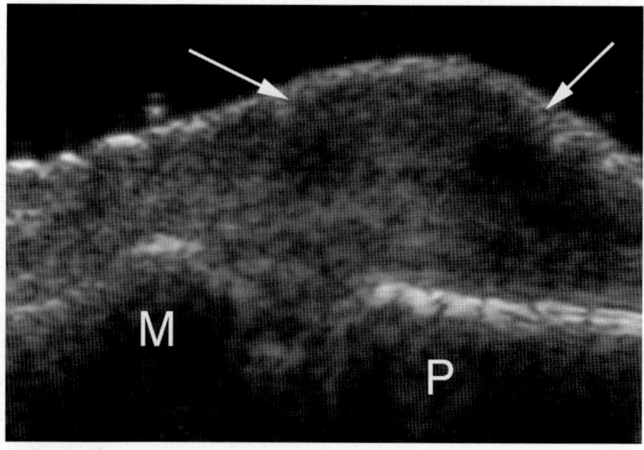

Fig. 11.1 Knucklepads. This patient presented with periarticular soft tissue swelling and presumed rheumatoid arthritis. Longitudinal ultrasound image of the dorsal soft tissue fullness shows a subcutaneous hypoechoic soft tissue mass (*arrows*) with a normal underlying proximal interphalangeal joint. P, distal aspect of the proximal phalanx; MP, base middle phalanx ring finger.

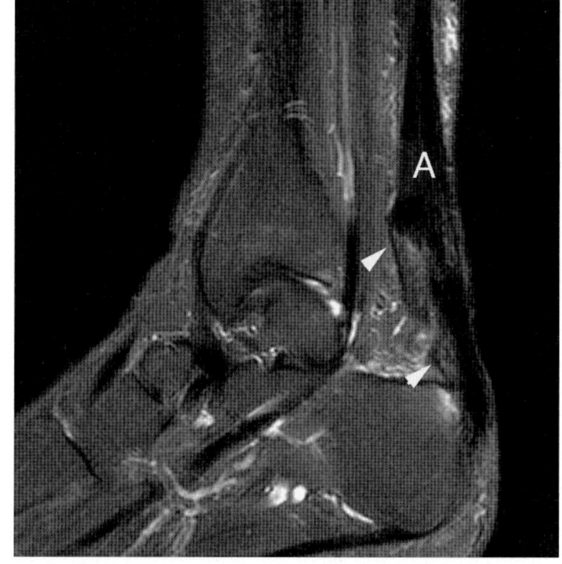

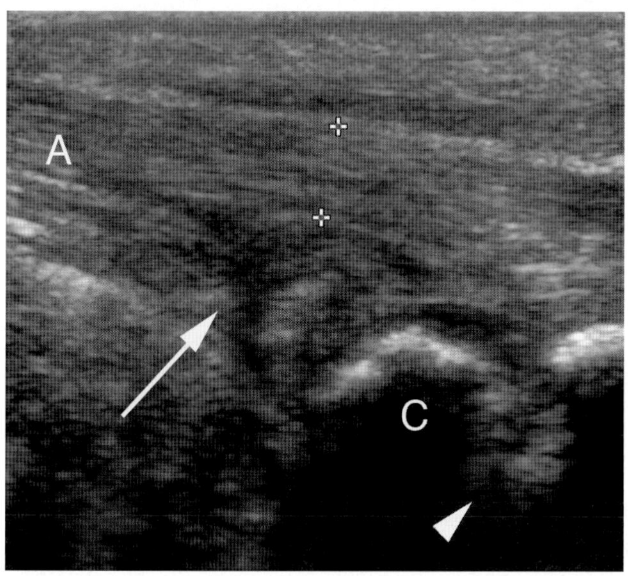

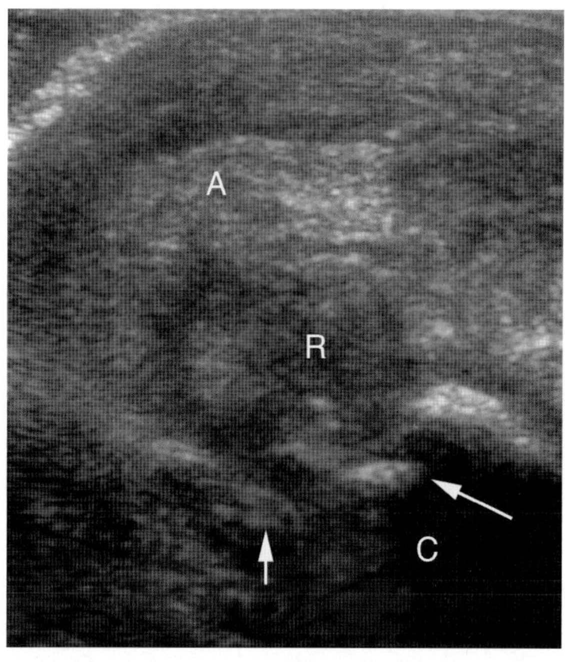

Fig. 11.2 Achilles tendon tears in patients with longstanding rheumatoid arthritis (RA). **(A)** Sagittal T2-weighted magnetic resonance image of the ankle shows a partial thickness tear of the anterior fibers of the distal Achilles tendon (A) (*arrowheads* denote tear extent). Note the focal high signal in the marrow of the calcaneus at the insertion of the tendon. These focal areas of subcortical marrow edema can progress to frank marginal erosions. **(B)** Longitudinal ultrasound image of a different patient. There is disruption of the anterior fibers of the Achilles tendon by a partial tear (*arrow*). *Calipers* bracket the intact posterior fibers. There is an erosion (*arrowhead*) at the calcaneal (C) insertion site of the tendon. **(C)** Transverse ultrasound image of the same patient at the level of the Achilles insertion. The posterior intact Achilles fibers (A) remain hyperechoic. There is disruption of the Achilles anteriorly and distension of the retrocalcaneal bursa (R), adjacent to the calcaneal (C) erosion (*arrows*).

can be utilized earlier in the disease course to determine, as well as to follow, more objective parameters of joint inflammation like effusions, synovial proliferation, and small marginal erosions that can be radiographically occult. These techniques can better gauge the severity of the inflammation and monitor objective parameters to possible response to therapeutic agents.

MRI has been touted as the new gold standard in RA clinical trials for assessment of synovial and tenosynovial inflammation (**Fig. 11.5**). When compared with ultrasound, MRI is unique in that it can depict early marrow "edema"—a marker for abnormal overlying cartilage and possible future erosion development (**Fig. 11.6**). MRI may also quantitate overall synovial volumes and rate of enhancement better,

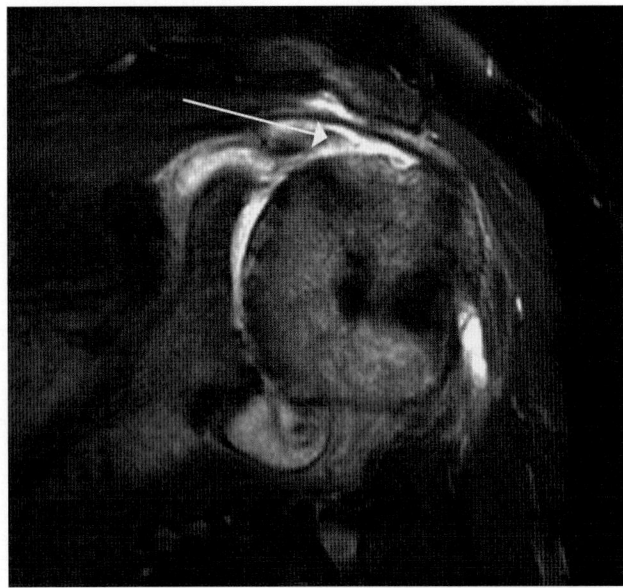

Fig. 11.3 Rotator cuff tears in the setting of long-standing rheumatoid arthritis. Coronal T2-weighted fat-suppressed magnetic resonance image of the left shoulder. There is a high-grade, partially retracted and delaminating tear of the articular surface of the distal supraspinatus tendon (*arrow*). There is marked joint effusion and synovitis as well as pancartilage loss in the glenohumeral joint.

which may be a quantitative measure to assess drug response. However, in clinical practice, utilizing MRI for the assessment of disease activity in RA patients has definite shortcomings. It remains relatively expensive and not as readily accessible to patients in most rheumatology clinics when compared with radiography and even ultrasound. To maximize detail of intraarticular anatomy in small joints, a limited field of view with high spatial resolution is often necessary. This limited field of view can make overall assessment of multiple joints time consuming. Small erosions in very small joints like the proximal interphalangeal (PIP) joints can be difficult to resolve from underlying edema or due to partial volume averaging.

Ultrasound is a safe, portable, more readily available, and less-expensive alternative imaging modality to evaluate synovitis and joint erosions in multiple joints with immediate diagnostic information. Ultrasound is also effective for interventional guidance for joint and tendon sheath aspirations or injections. The limitations of ultrasound include the dependence on operator technique, and the limited sonographic window for visualization of certain portions of joints with complex bony anatomy like the wrist.

Although scanning protocols and techniques can be variable and not standardized among different practitioners,

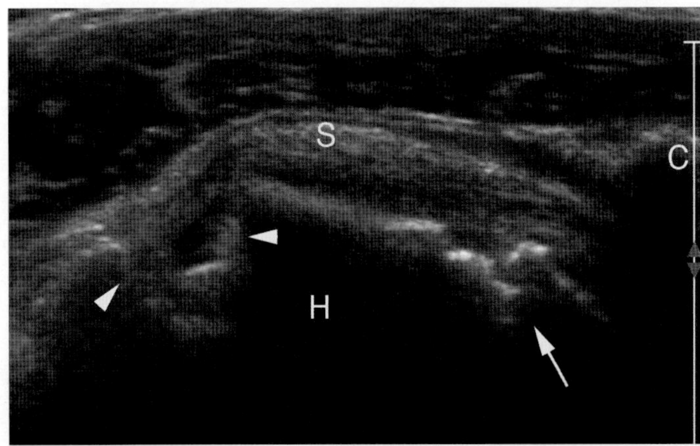

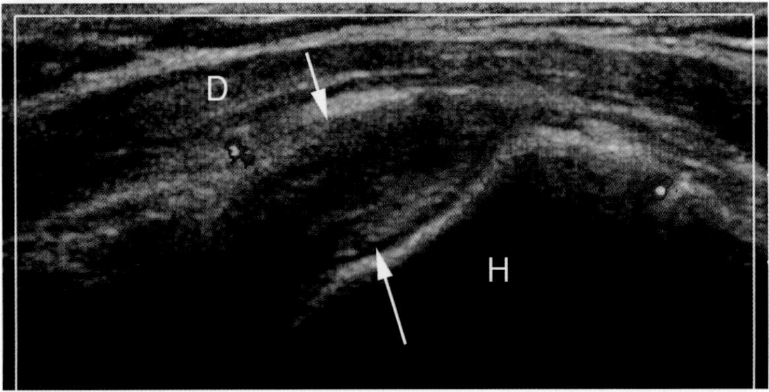

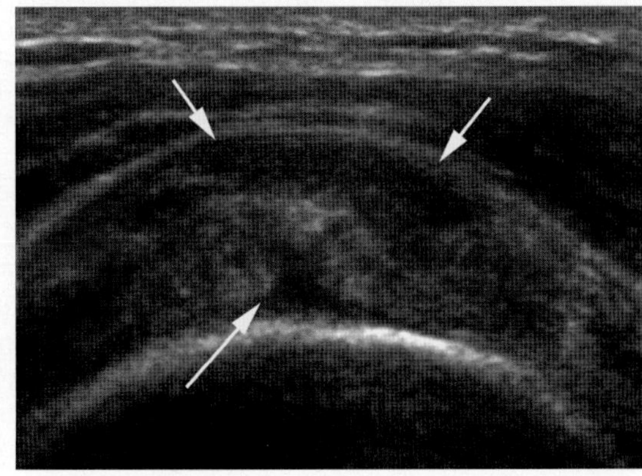

Fig. 11.4 Rheumatoid arthritis patient complaining of shoulder pain. **(A)** Transverse ultrasound image of the right shoulder at the level of the bicipital groove (*arrowheads*). The subscapularis tendon (S) shows normal echogenicity. Its course can be seen from the coracoid (C) to its lesser tuberosity insertion at the humeral head (H). A marginal erosion is seen (*arrow*) in the anterior humeral head and erosive changes of the bicipital groove (*arrowheads*) are present as well as a partial tear of the long head of the biceps tendon at this location. **(B)** Longitudinal ultrasound image at the level of the greater tuberosity of the humerus (H) anteriorly. There is marked hypoechogenicity and loss of the normal fibrillar structure of the distal supraspinatus tendon (*arrows*), with increased power Doppler signal in the distal tendon tear. The overlying deltoid muscle (D) is noted. **(C)** Transverse ultrasound image at the level of the greater tuberosity anteriorly. There is marked swelling and hypoechogenicity extending from articular to bursal surface consistent with a complete tear of the distal supraspinatus tendon (*arrows*).

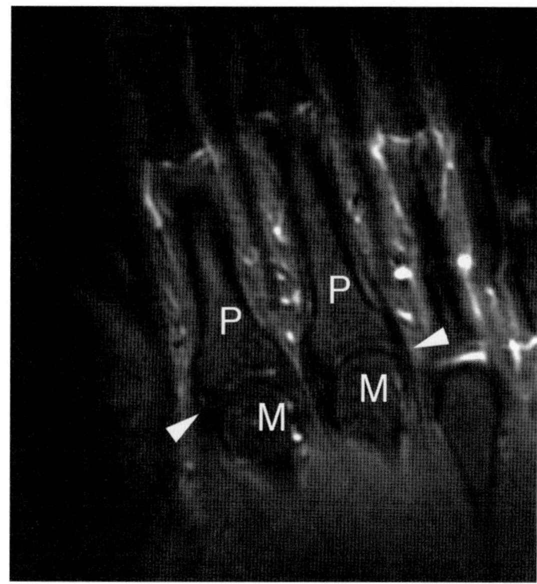

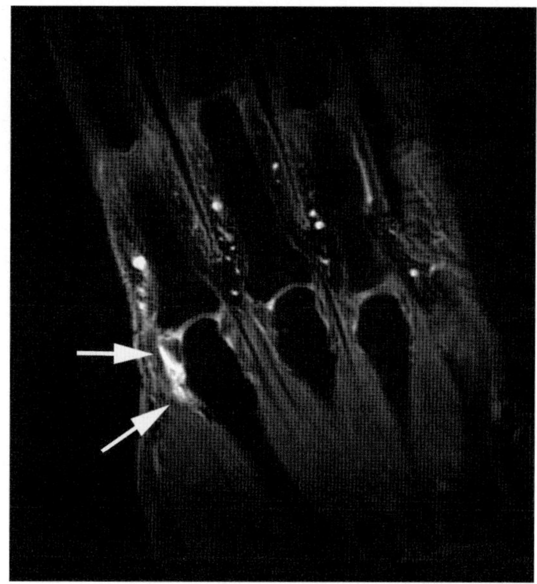

Fig. 11.5 Magnetic resonance imaging (MRI) assessment of metacarpophalangeal (MCP) joints. Coronal T1-weighted fat suppressed gradient recall MRIs after contrast enhancement with gadolinium contrast. **(A)** Normal appearance of the metacarpal head (M) and proximal phalanx (P) of the index and long finger marrow and cartilage. The collateral ligaments and tightly apposed joint capsule are denoted by the *arrowheads*. **(B)** Patient with early rheumatoid arthritis on a new therapeutic agent. *Arrows* show nodular synovial enhancement and thickening of the index finger MCP joint. The exam is centered on the MCP joints, and the proximal interphalangeal joints are included in the field of view, but the wrists are not completely included.

there is increasing validation for the use of ultrasound in the early diagnosis and monitoring of therapy response in RA patients. Given the typical involvement of the hands and feet early in the disease course, we routinely evaluate with ultrasound the metacarpophalangeal (MCP) and PIP joints of the hands, the wrists, and the metatarsophalangeal (MTP) joints of the feet in these patients.

Fig. 11.6 Axial T2-weighted fat suppressed magnetic resonance image of the knee in a patient with known rheumatoid arthritis. There is marked joint effusion and synovitis. *Arrowhead* denotes focal area of subchondral marrow edema in the posterior medial femoral condyle at an area of overlying cartilage loss. *Arrow* shows marginal erosion and surrounding marrow edema in the lateral condyle posteriorly.

Sonographic Intraarticular Anatomy

Unfortunately, there are few validated studies in the literature detailing the sonographic appearance of normal intraarticular structures in the joints of the hands and feet. The sonographic anatomy of the MCP joints has been best described of these small joints. The MCP joints consistently show a hyperechoic structure between the metacarpal head and the base of the proximal phalanx under the deep surface of the extensor and flexor tendons. This represents vascularized connective tissue lined by synovium. On the dorsal side of the MCP joints, this structure forms a triangle (**Fig. 11.7**). A similar finding is also seen in the MTP joints of the toes. Scant power Doppler activity may be found in the joints of healthy volunteers, most commonly in the wrist, but rarely in the MCP joints, and hardly ever in the PIP joints. The MCP joint has a palmar and a dorsal joint recess that is best seen when there is a joint effusion or synovitis (**Fig. 11.8**). A slight depression on the dorsal aspect of the distal metacarpal can be seen in ~33% of the index, long, and ring finger MCP joints (**Fig. 11.9**). The cartilage of the metacarpal head is usually well seen on either the dorsal side or the palmar side as a thin hypoechoic layer. The radial collateral ligament of the second MCP joint and

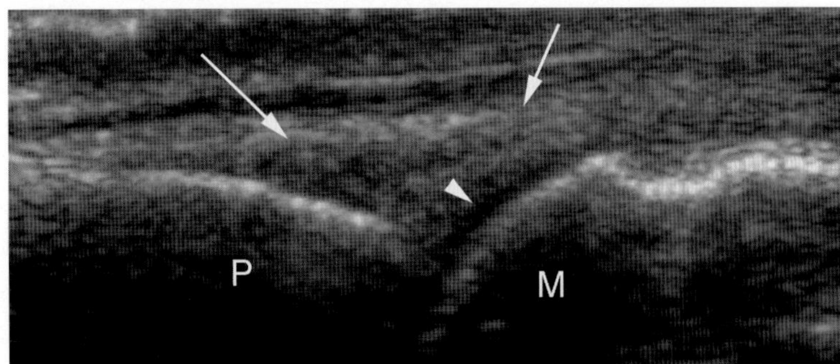

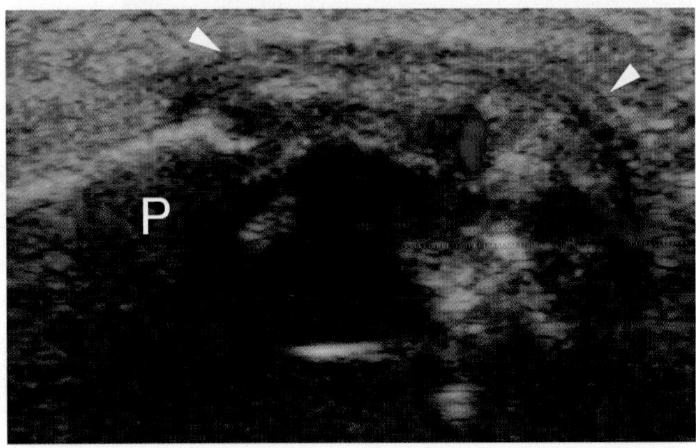

Fig. 11.7 Longitudinal ultrasound image of the metacarpophalangeal (MCP) and metatarsophalangeal (MTP) joints, dorsal view. Note smooth echogenic cortex of the metacarpal or metatarsal heads (M) and proximal phalanx (P). **(A)** Normal index finger MCP joint. *Arrows* show echogenic triangular connective tissue lined by synovium as described in text within the joint capsule. *Arrowhead* shows normal hypoechoic articular cartilage of the metacarpal head. **(B)** Normal fourth toe MTP joint. The normal fibrillar structure of the overlying common extensor tendon sheath is denoted by *arrows*. The echogenic intraarticular triangular connective tissue can also be seen (T). *Arrowheads* show normal hypoechoic articular cartilage of the metatarsal head.

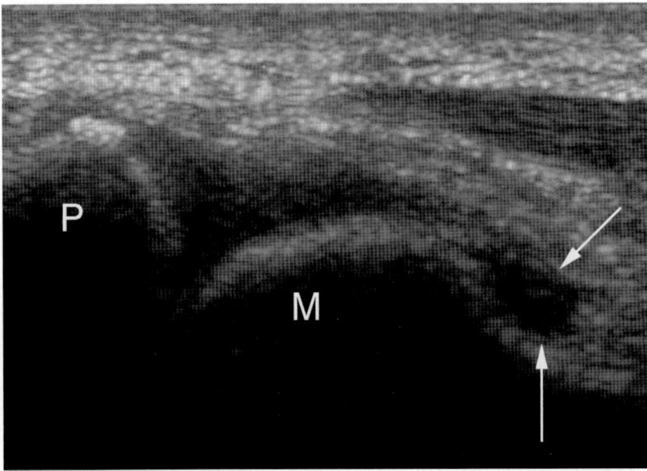

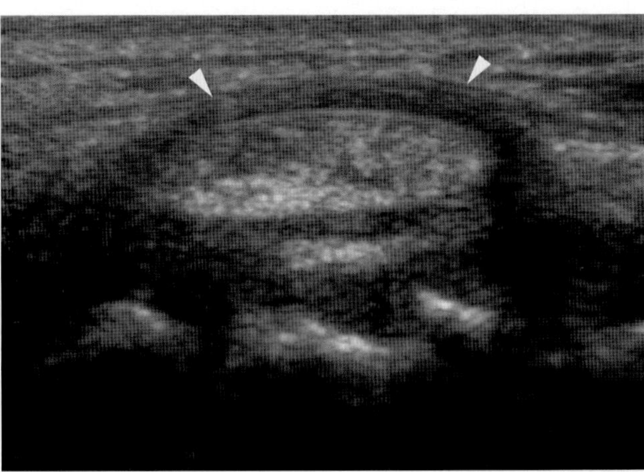

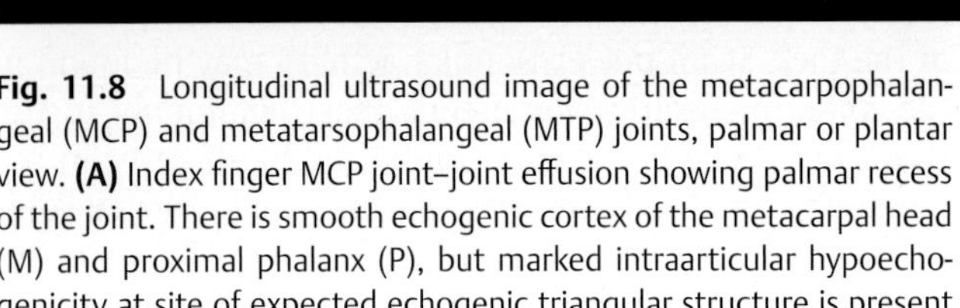

Fig. 11.8 Longitudinal ultrasound image of the metacarpophalangeal (MCP) and metatarsophalangeal (MTP) joints, palmar or plantar view. **(A)** Index finger MCP joint–joint effusion showing palmar recess of the joint. There is smooth echogenic cortex of the metacarpal head (M) and proximal phalanx (P), but marked intraarticular hypoechogenicity at site of expected echogenic triangular structure is present in this patient with a joint effusion. *Arrows* denote palmar recess of joint capsule overlying distal metacarpal cortex. **(B)** Normal little toe MTP joint, plantar view. The normal fibrillar structure of the overlying flexor tendon sheath is denoted by *arrows*. The echogenic intraarticular triangular connective tissue can be seen (T). *Arrowheads* shows normal hypoechoic articular cartilage of the metatarsal head (M).

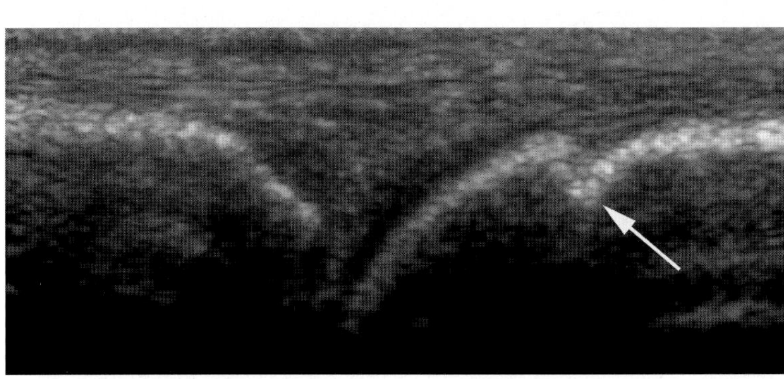

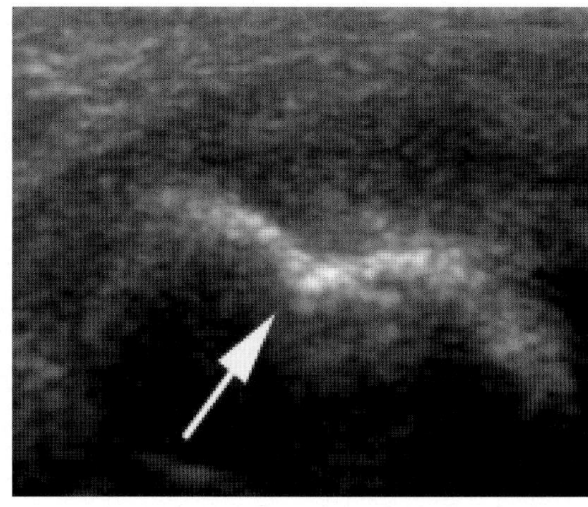

Fig. 11.9 Dorsal depression of the cortex of the distal metacarpal. **(A)** Longitudinal ultrasound image of the index finger metacarpophalangeal joint showing typical location and appearance of dorsal depression (*arrow*). Note the well-defined echogenic floor of the depression in contrast to a marginal erosion. **(B)** Transverse ultrasound image of the same area shows smooth cortical outline (*arrow*) proving it is not an erosion.

the ulnar collateral ligament of the fifth MCP joint can be visualized as fibrillar hyperechoic structures between the attachments at the metacarpal head and base of the proximal phalanx. Similar findings are present in the MTP joints when evaluating the lateral or medial aspects of the first and fifth toe MTP joints (**Fig. 11.10**). The extensor and flexor tendon sheaths are seen overlying the joints of the hands and feet when examining them dorsal or palmar/plantar. At the PIP joints, similar overlying structures are routinely identified (**Fig. 11.11**).

The wrist joint is examined both volar and dorsal to evaluate the normal cortical outlines and synovium, with attention to the overlying extensor tendon compartments dorsally and the flexor tendons volarly for the presence of tenosynovitis or tendon tears, as well as ganglion cysts, which occur with higher prevalence in patients with RA. Dorsally, the scapholunate and lunotriquetral intrinsic ligaments of the proximal radiocarpal row can be best identified as hyperechoic structures.

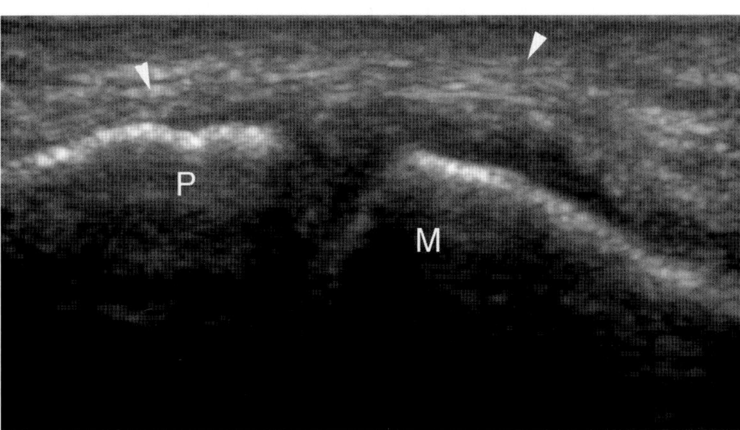

Fig. 11.10 Longitudinal ultrasound image of the first toe metatarsophalangeal joint, medial view. *Arrowheads* show normal echogenic fibrillar structure of the overlying collateral ligament. There is smooth echogenic cortex of the metatarsal head (M) and proximal phalanx (P).

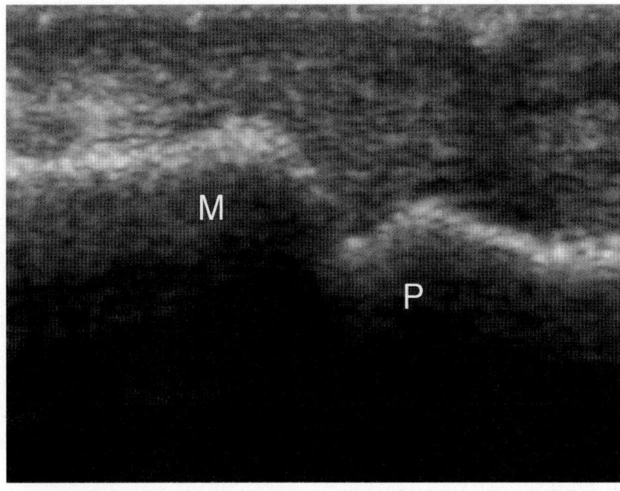

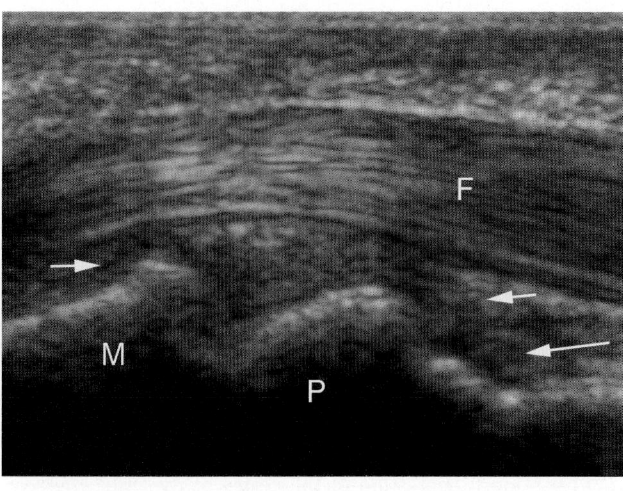

Fig. 11.11 Proximal interphalangeal (PIP) joint—normal appearance. **(A)** Dorsal longitudinal ultrasound image of the ring finger PIP joint. Note the difference from the MCP in the more rectangular cortical outlines of the distal proximal phalanx (P) and proximal middle phalanx (M). **(B)** Palmar longitudinal ultrasound image of the ring finger PIP joint. The flexor tendons (F) overlying the normal joint (joint capsule extent denoted by the *short arrows*—the *long arrow* is showing the palmar recess of the joint). The juxtaarticular distal aspect of the proximal phalanx (P) and proximal aspect of the middle phalanx (M) show normal cortical echogenic outline.

Technique of Sonography

Ultrasound exams of the hand and wrist joints are best performed with high-frequency (10 MHz or greater) linear transducers with small footprints. The palmar and dorsal aspects of the MCP and PIP joints of both hands are imaged as well as the wrists in longitudinal and transverse planes. The lateral aspects of the index and little finger MCP joints as well as the wrists are also imaged. The MTP joints of the feet are also imaged in a similar fashion in patients with foot complaints. To expedite the exam, some investigators select the 2nd and 5th MCP and wrists as well as the 5th MTP as target joints to image given their high likelihood of involvement in RA as well as increased visualization of a greater portion of the joint to the transducer.

Power Doppler interrogation is used to assess synovial vascularity. Power Doppler is more sensitive than color Doppler in assessing blood flow within small vessels. It is sensitive in measuring synovitis, with accuracy comparable to dynamic contrast-enhanced MRI. The Doppler gain setting should be set just above the level of noise to increase sensitivity, but there should be no signal arising within normal cortical bone.

Pathology

Synovitis

A commonly used definition of synovitis on ultrasound is that of thickened, hypoechoic intraarticular tissue poorly compressible on gray-scale B-mode imaging that can demonstrate increased Doppler signals with color or power Doppler interrogation. Utilizing this definition can be helpful in distinguishing synovial proliferation from joint effusion (**Fig. 11.12**). Effusions are sensitive, but obviously not specific for RA activity. The joints affected with RA will have increased synovial vascularity as well as increased synovial volume correlating with disease activity (**Fig. 11.13**). Power Doppler can also be used to ascertain treatment response. Tenosynovitis can be similarly assessed for power Doppler when present in the flexor or extensor tendons (**Fig. 11.14**).

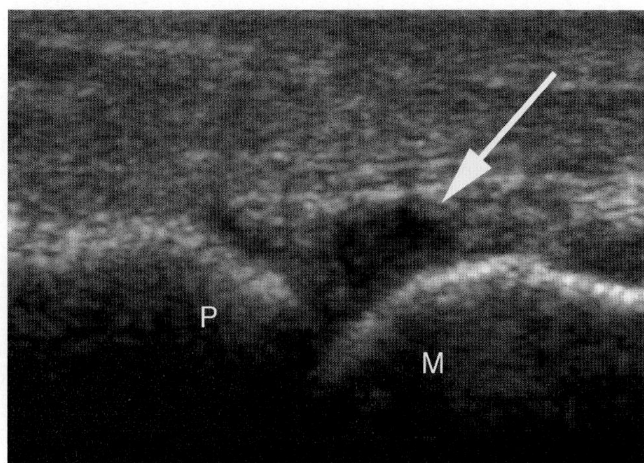

Fig. 11.12 Joint effusion. Longitudinal ultrasound image of the dorsal great toe metatarsophalangeal joint shows hypoechoic area slightly distending the joint capsule (*arrow*). This area was compressible and showed no Doppler signal. P, proximal phalanx; M, middle phalanx.

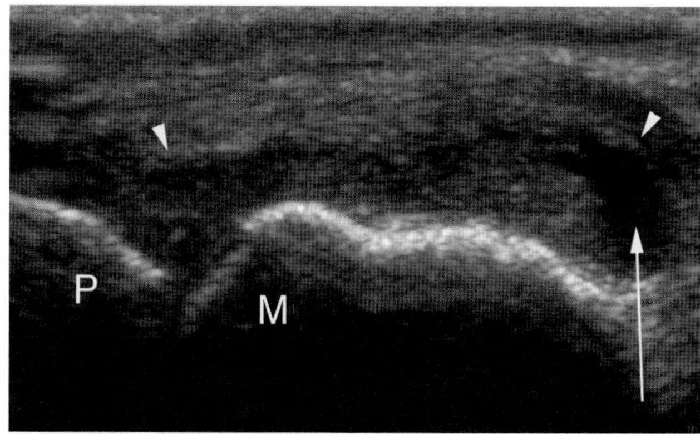

A

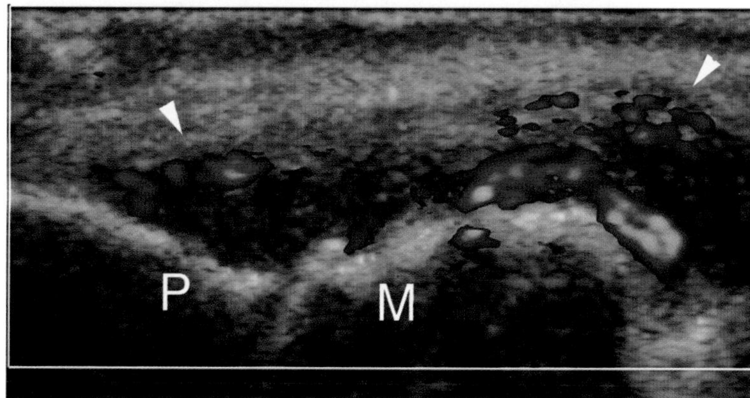

B

Fig. 11.13 Synovitis and effusion—using power Doppler to help distinguish. **(A)** Longitudinal ultrasound image of the dorsal little finger metacarpophalangeal (MCP) joint in a patient with early rheumatoid arthritis (RA). There is marked distension of the joint capsule (*arrowheads*) by synovitis, which appears more echogenic than the small effusion component that is noted in the dorsal recess of the joint (*arrow*). **(B)** Longitudinal ultrasound image of the dorsal little finger MCP joint in a patient with early RA—interrogation with power Doppler. There is marked grade 3 Doppler activity (*arrowheads*) by the synovial pannus.

A semiquantitative grading of synovial power Doppler signal is commonly used to assess extent of synovitis. A commonly used grading system is as follows: 1 = single vessel demonstrated, 2 = confluent vessels, and 3 = greater than 50% of the imaged synovial tissue has visualized vessels (**Fig. 11.15**). Others add a grade 0 when there is no intraarticular power Doppler signal, but increased hypoechoic synovium is present.

Fig. 11.14 Tenosynovitis in a patient with new-onset rheumatoid arthritis. Longitudinal ultrasound image of the ulnar styloid (u). There is diffuse hypoechoic thickening surrounding the extensor carpi ulnaris tendon (ECU) with marked power Doppler signal within the tendon sheath consistent with tenosynovitis (*arrows*).

Erosions

Marginal erosions (located at the periphery of a synovial joint) seen early in RA are predictive of an aggressive disease course. Erosions can be diagnosed on ultrasound when a discontinuity of the smooth echogenic bone surface or cortex is visualized in two perpendicular planes (**Fig. 11.16**). They will have an irregular floor and increased through transmission if there is infiltrating hypoechoic pannus within it. Sometimes, interrogation with power Doppler will show increased signal within this pannus (**Fig. 11.16**). In some studies, greater than 2 mm in depth as a minimal size cutoff in cortical disruption is used to confidently diagnose bone erosions by ultrasound. In contrast, the previously described metacarpal head depressions that can be encountered in the dorsal cortex have regular margins, no discontinuity of the cortex, and a maximum depth of 2.0 mm.

When compared with MRI, ultrasound is at least as sensitive, and some feel superior to MRI, in diagnosing bone erosions of the MCP and MTP joints. However, as with synovitis assessment, the variability between ultrasound machines in diagnosis of erosions has not been explored.

One of the roles of ultrasound in future clinical practice will lie in the monitoring of disease and treatment response

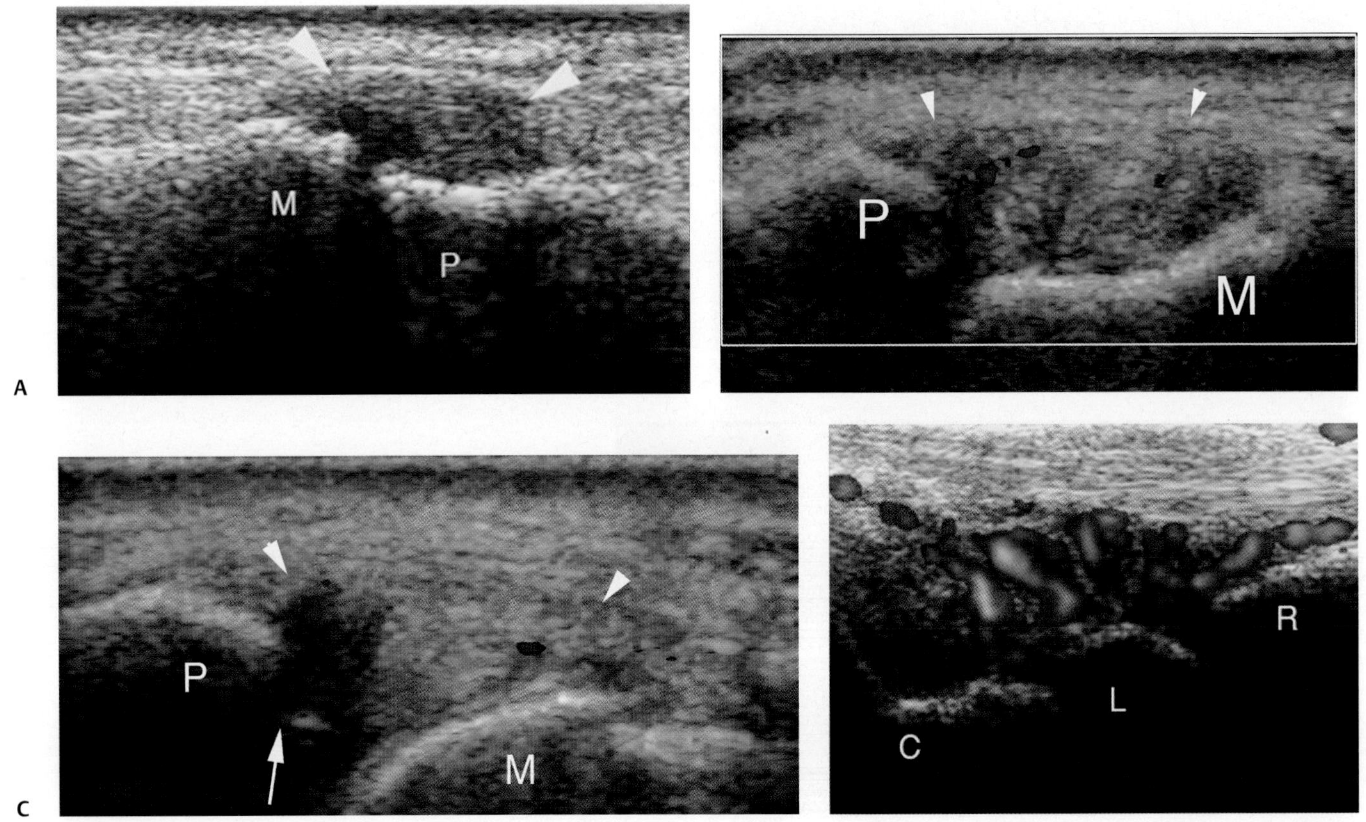

Fig. 11.15 Doppler signal semiquantitative grading. **(A)** Longitudinal ultrasound image lateral aspect of the right index finger proximal interphalangeal joint (M, middle phalanx; P, proximal phalanx) shows a distended joint capsule (*arrowheads*) with grade 1 of 3 intraarticular synovial signal. **(B)** Longitudinal ultrasound image dorsal aspect of the left index finger metacarpophalangeal (MCP) joint (M, metacarpal head; P, proximal phalanx) shows a distended joint capsule (*arrowheads*) with grade 2 of 3 intraarticular synovial signal. **(C)** Longitudinal ultrasound image dorsal aspect of the index finger MCP joint of a different patient (M, metacarpal head; P, proximal phalanx) with a similarly distended joint capsule (*arrowheads*) with confluent vessels consistent with grade 2 of 3 intraarticular synovial signal. Note the erosion in the proximal phalanx (*arrow*) adjacent to the hypoechoic synovium. **(D)** Longitudinal ultrasound image dorsal right wrist (C, capitate; L, lunate; R, radius dorsal cortical outline) shows marked power Doppler intraarticular signals consistent with grade 3+ synovial hyperemia in a distended proximal carpal joint recess.

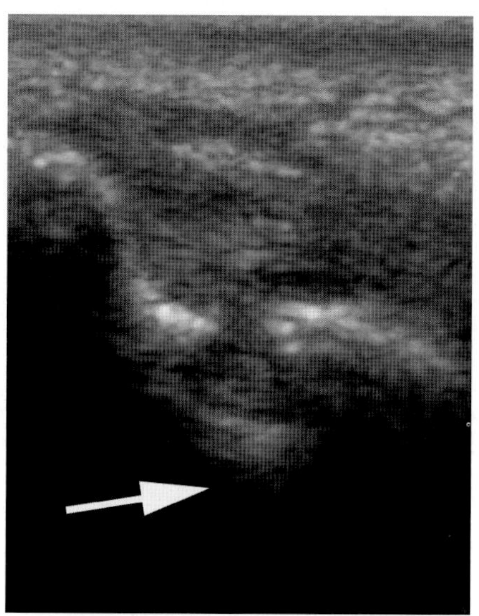

Fig. 11.16 Marginal erosions—ultrasound image. **(A)** Transverse ultrasound image of the index finger metacarpal head radial aspect. There is a well-defined discontinuity of the cortex and increased through transmission adjacent to the erosion floor (*arrow*). **(B)** Longitudinal ultrasound image of the distal lateral ulna with a large and deep marginal erosion (*arrowheads*) and increased through transmission artifact at the floor of the erosion. **(C)** Transverse ultrasound image of the index finger metacarpal head radial aspect [same image as **(A)**]. Power Doppler is now utilized and shows increased Doppler signal within infiltrating synovium in the previously identified erosion (*arrow*). **(D)** A more subtle erosion is identified (*arrow*) in the dorsal aspect of the long finger metacarpal head in a different patient with rheumatoid arthritis. Note the Doppler signal at the periphery of the joint synovitis as well as within the erosion. **(E)** Longitudinal ultrasound image of the dorsal proximal interphalangeal joint ring finger. Small erosion (*arrow*) is present within the proximal phalanx (P). Note distension of joint capsule by synovitis and effusion (*arrowheads*). M, middle phalanx.

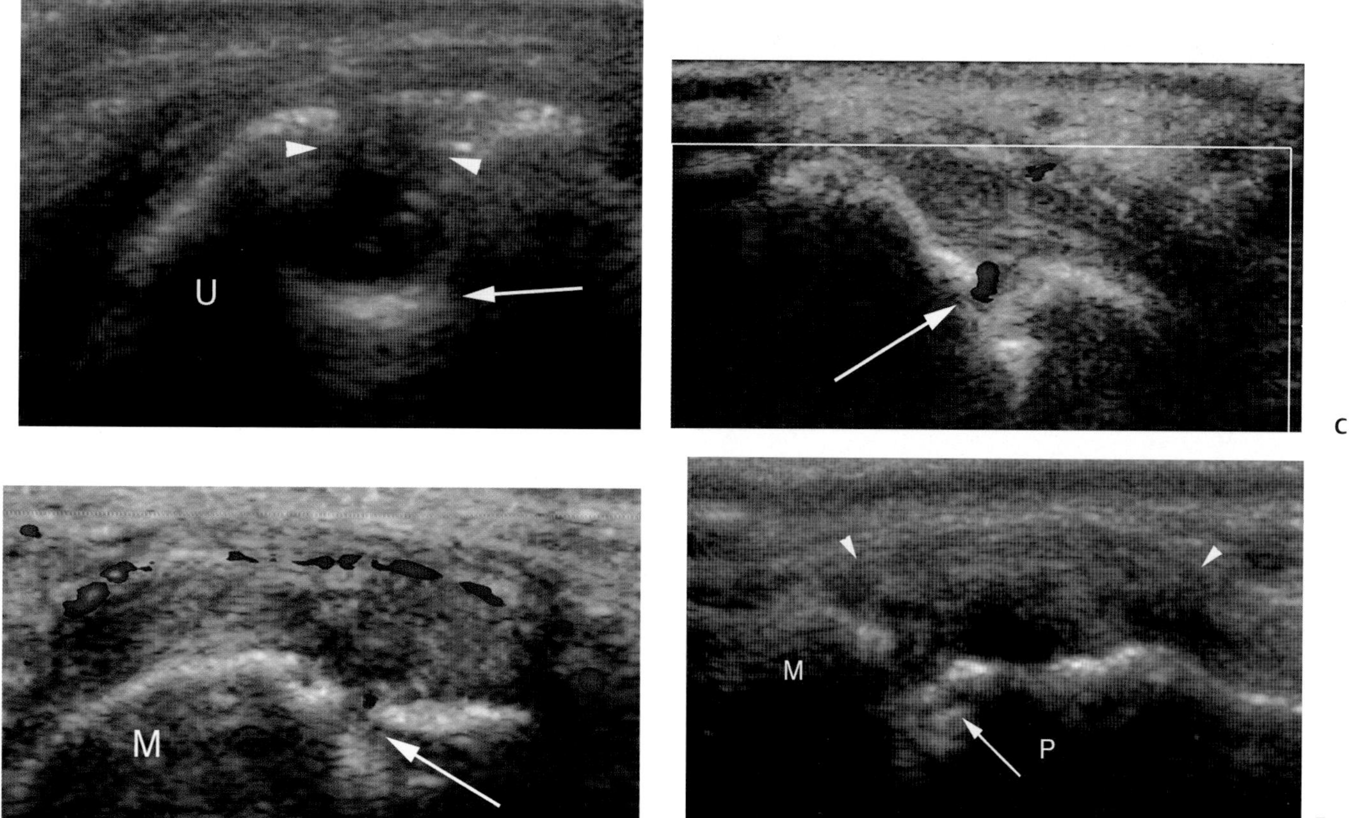

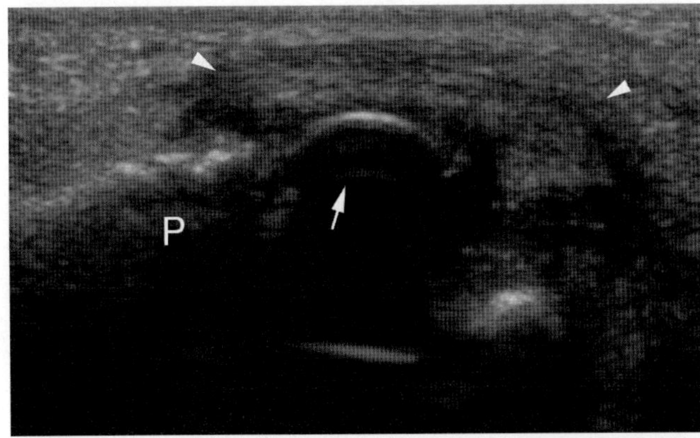

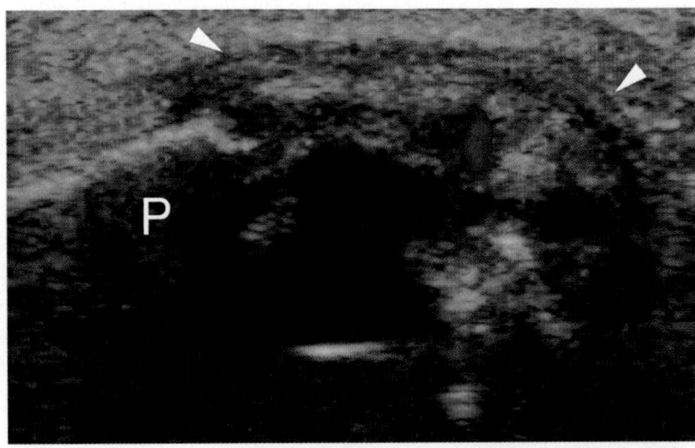

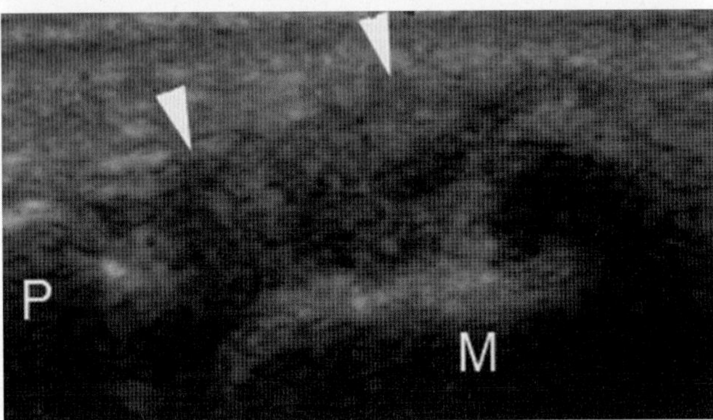

Fig. 11.17 Assessing for active synovial inflammation during treatment. **(A)** Longitudinal ultrasound image of the dorsal metacarpophalangeal (MCP) joint index finger. The patient has had a prior arthroplasty [arrow notes reverberation artifact inferior to the markedly echogenic surface of the metacarpal head prosthesis adjacent to the base of the proximal phalanx (P)]. The referring rheumatologist was unsure if this patient with long-standing rheumatoid arthritis (RA) had persistent joint inflammation. There is distension of joint capsule by possible persistent synovitis (*arrowheads*). **(B)** Same patient as in **(A)** with MCP arthroplasty. Longitudinal ultrasound power Doppler image of the dorsal MCP joint index finger. There is increased intraarticular Doppler signal (grade 1) consistent with active synovitis within the distended joint capsule (*arrowheads*). The results of this ultrasound exam led to a change in medication and better control of her inflammation. **(C)** Different patient with RA now with side effects from longstanding methotrexate usage. Ultrasound was requested to evaluate for possible synovial inflammation as clinical exam was suspicious for persistent synovitis. Longitudinal ultrasound power Doppler image of the dorsal MCP long index finger (M, metacarpal head; P, proximal phalanx). There is no intraarticular Doppler signal detected within the distended joint capsule (*arrowheads*) with likely fibrotic "burned-out" synovial pannus. The patient was taken off the antiinflammatory medications without complication.

in patients with RA (**Fig. 11.17**). In a recent prospective study of patients with early RA, ultrasound showed the number of erosions doubled within a 6-month follow-up period. Identification of patients with faster progression may help in selecting appropriate DMARD therapy to prevent further joint deterioration.

Artifacts

Certain artifacts like motion/flash and edge artifact are common with power Doppler and should not be confused with true increased synovial blood flow.

Artifacts like increased through transmission can help in identifying bone erosions.

Anisotropy can make the extensor retinaculum appear hypoechoic, especially when imaging the fourth extensor compartment (**Fig. 11.18**) at the dorsal wrist and can potentially be confused as tenosynovitis. Careful attention to a perpendicular insonation angle will reveal the hyperechoic fibrillar structures. In addition, as opposed to tenosynovitis, the hypoechogenicity will only be dorsal to the tendons and not surround them.

Proposed Algorithm for Ultrasound in Rheumatoid Arthritis

A. For initial diagnosis of suspected RA:
   1- Radiographs of the hands and feet
   If radiographs are negative for RA, then:
   2- Ultrasound of the hands (PIP, MCP joints and wrists)
   3- Ultrasound of the feet (MTP joints)
B. For evaluation of active synovial inflammation:
   1- Physical examination
   2- Ultrasound of the hands (PIP, MCP joints and wrists)
   3- Ultrasound of the feet (MTP joints)

A 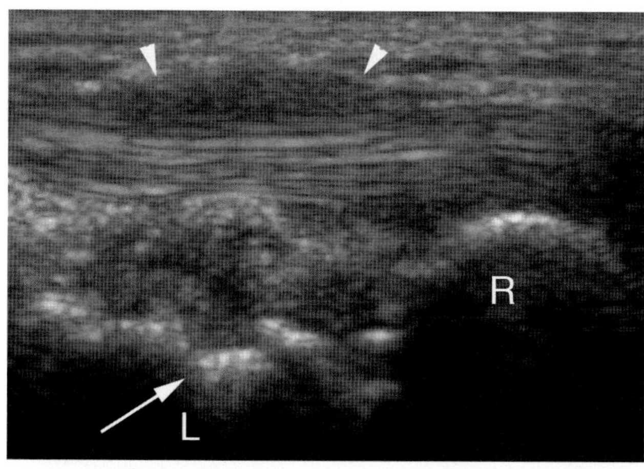

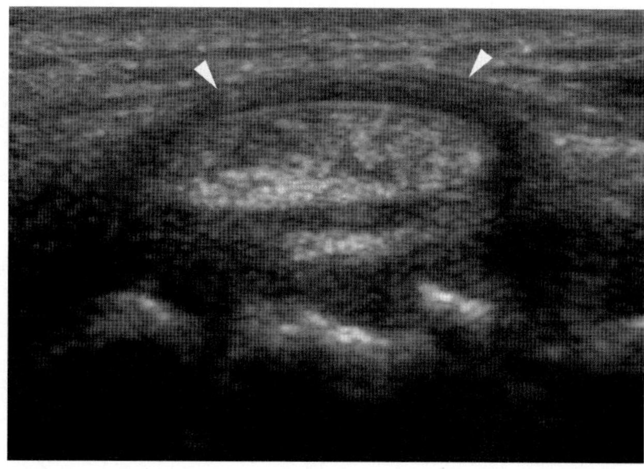 B

C 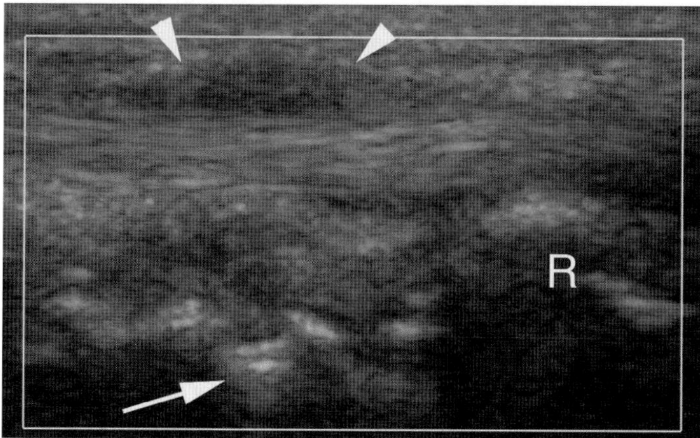

Fig. 11.18 Potential pitfall for tenosynovitis—extensor retinaculum. **(A)** Longitudinal ultrasound image of the dorsal wrist in a patient with rheumatoid arthritis [note erosion (*arrow*) on the dorsal cortical outline of the lunate (L) adjacent to radius (R)]. *Arrowhead* shows focal hypoechogenicity over the dorsal extensor tendon that could be mistaken for focal tenosynovial thickening. **(B)** Transverse ultrasound image at the same location as above. *Arrowhead* shows the increased echogenicity and fibrillar structure of the extensor retinaculum at its expected location over the fourth extensor compartment of the wrist best as the transducer is now at a more perpendicular insonation angle. **(C)** Power Doppler of **(A)**. The erosion (*arrow*) on the dorsal cortical outline of the lunate (L) adjacent to radius (R) is again seen in this longitudinal ultrasound image of the dorsal wrist. *Arrowhead* shows the absence of any Doppler signal within the extensor retinaculum.

C. For monitoring of therapeutic response:
   1- Radiographs
   2- Ultrasound
   3- MRI with gadolinium
D. For complications of disease or therapy like tendon rupture or infection
   1- Radiographs
   2- Ultrasound
   If joint effusion in setting if possible superimposed infection, then ultrasound-guided aspiration.
   3- MRI (especially if osteomyelitis is a clinical concern)

Pearls and Pitfalls

- When examining the patient, ask which joints have been involved longest or more severely as the prevalence of finding erosive change or synovial proliferation in these will be the highest. Similarly, if the patient complains of foot pain, examine the MTP joints as 10 to 15% of patients at clinical presentation will have erosions detected on the feet, but not the hands.
- Synovitis will be identified earliest in the dorsal synovial recess on the MCP joints and the palmar synovial recess on the PIP joints (**Figs. 11.8** and **11.13**).
- When utilizing power Doppler it is important to minimize transducer pressure on the joint as the signal from the small synovial vessels can be obliterated if one is not careful in this regard (**Fig. 11.19**).
- It is important to distinguish erosions from normal findings like dorsal metacarpal head depressions (**Fig. 11.9**). These are usually less than 2 mm in depth and will have a smooth floor. Conversely, almost all erosions that measure at least 2 mm at baseline can be detected on 6-month follow-up at the same site whereas smaller bone irregularities are less constant on follow-up.
- Erosions should be documented as cortical disruptions on two planes to increase specificity.
- The ulnar styloid may show surface bone resorptive-erosive changes early in the disease secondary to inflammation of the overlying extensor carpi ulnaris tendon. Always evaluate this cortical outline carefully.

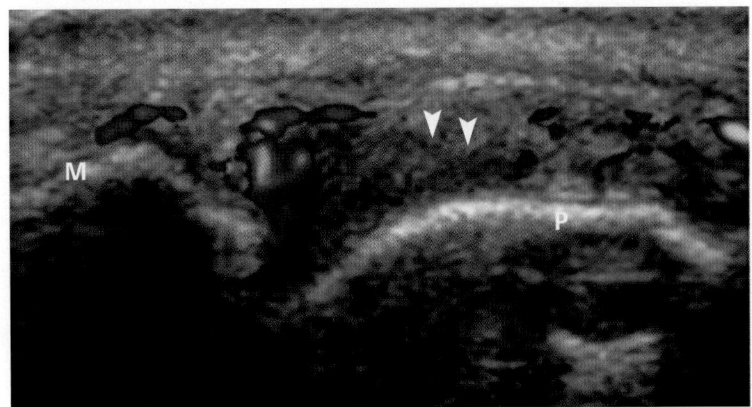

A

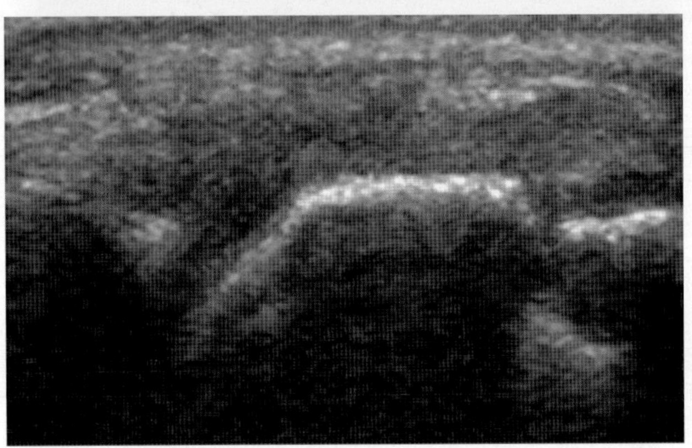

B

Fig. 11.19 Potential pitfall—transducer pressure and power Doppler imaging of synovitis. **(A)** Longitudinal ultrasound image with power Doppler of the right index finger metacarpophalangeal joint (P, proximal phalanx; M, metacarpal head) with grade 3 synovitis (*arrowheads*). **(B)** By increasing transducer pressure, there is compression of the intraarticular vessels and now near complete absence of Doppler signal.

Suggested Readings

Boutry N, Morel M, Flipo R-M, Demondion X, Cotten A. Early rheumatoid arthritis: a review of MRI and sonographic findings. AJR Am J Roentgenol 2007;189(6):1502–1509

Farrant JM, O'Connor PJ, Grainger AJ. Advanced imaging in rheumatoid arthritis. Part 1: synovitis. Skeletal Radiol 2007;36(4):269–279

Farrant JM, Grainger AJ, O'Connor PJ. Advanced imaging in rheumatoid arthritis: part 2: erosions. Skeletal Radiol 2007;36(5):381–389

Keen HI, Brown AK, Wakefield RJ, Conaghan PG. MRI and musculoskeletal ultrasonography as diagnostic tools in early arthritis. Rheum Dis Clin North Am 2005;31(4):699–714

Tehranzadeh J, Ashikyan O, Dascalos J. Advanced imaging of early rheumatoid arthritis. Radiol Clin North Am 2004;42(1):89–107

Wakefield RJ, Balint PV, Szkudlarek M, et al; OMERACT 7 Special Interest Group. Musculoskeletal ultrasound including definitions for ultrasonographic pathology. J Rheumatol 2005;32(12):2485–2487

Wakefield RJ, Gibbon WW, Conaghan PG, et al. The value of sonography in the detection of bone erosions in patients with rheumatoid arthritis: a comparison with conventional radiography. Arthritis Rheum 2000;43(12):2762–2770

12 Imaging of Muscle, Soft Tissue, and Foreign Bodies

Michael A. Bruno, Ashok Kumar Nath, A. U. Sethu, and Khamis Al Muzahmi

Ultrasound is unusually well suited for the detection of foreign bodies within soft tissue. It has been shown to have greater sensitivity and specificity in the detection of a wider variety of foreign bodies than any other imaging modality, including computed tomography (CT), which is the second most-versatile method. Ultrasound has a significant advantage in that real-time imaging may also be utilized for retrieval of soft tissue foreign bodies, especially those that are not readily visualized by other methods. Nonradiopaque foreign bodies generally are quite conspicuous on ultrasound due to the striking difference between their acoustic impedance and that of the surrounding soft tissues (**Figs. 12.1, 12.2, 12.3, 12.4**). In addition, soft tissue foreign bodies generally are located in a superficial position, amenable to sonography.

One of the first reports of the use of ultrasound for this purpose was by Fornage et al in 1986. This succinct report led to a clinical paradigm shift in the management of soft tissue foreign bodies and their conclusions were verified and extended by many other workers, notably by Little et al in 1986 and Jacobsen et al in 1998. Wood fragments, glass, plastic, and other nonradiopaque materials were shown to be easily identified on ultrasound. Currently, the preference

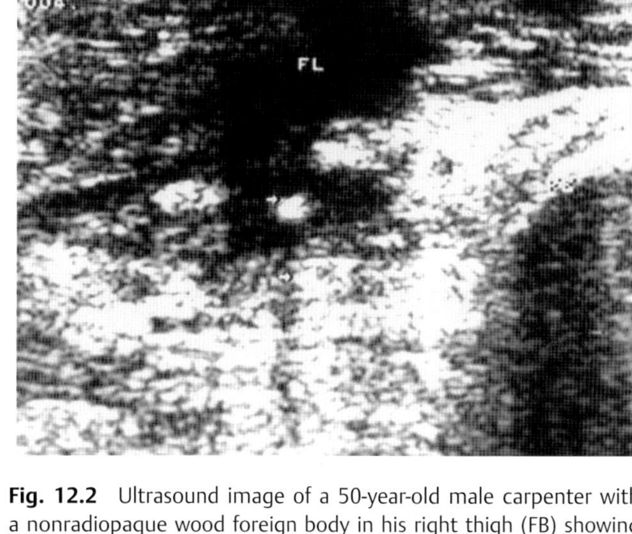

Fig. 12.2 Ultrasound image of a 50-year-old male carpenter with a nonradiopaque wood foreign body in his right thigh (FB) showing as an echogenic lesion with acoustic shadowing (AC) in thigh with a draining sinus (FL) formation leading up to skin surface seen as echolucent tract.

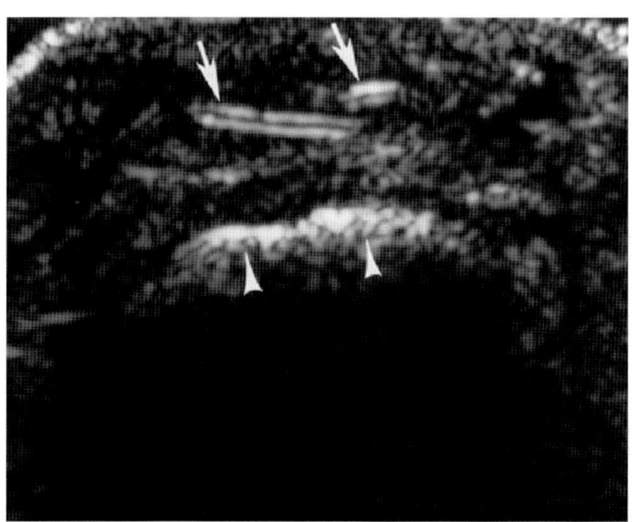

Fig. 12.1 A cactus thorn (*long arrows*) in the superficial soft tissues. This small foreign body would probably not be detectable by any other imaging modality. The bone cortical margin is also seen (*arrowheads*). (Image courtesy of Dr. M. Taljanovic, University of Arizona).

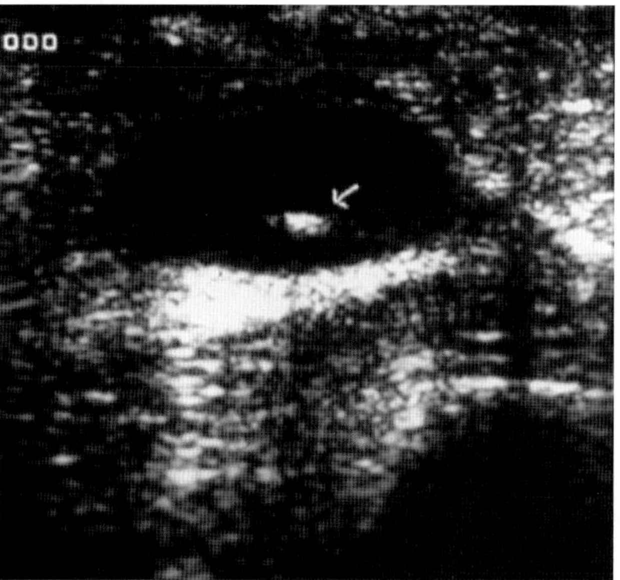

Fig. 12.3 Ultrasound of an 18-year-old village boy with history of a thorn prick and swollen calf and fever. Sonography shows an echogenic foreign body (*arrow*) within an echolucent abscess; the case was proven surgically.

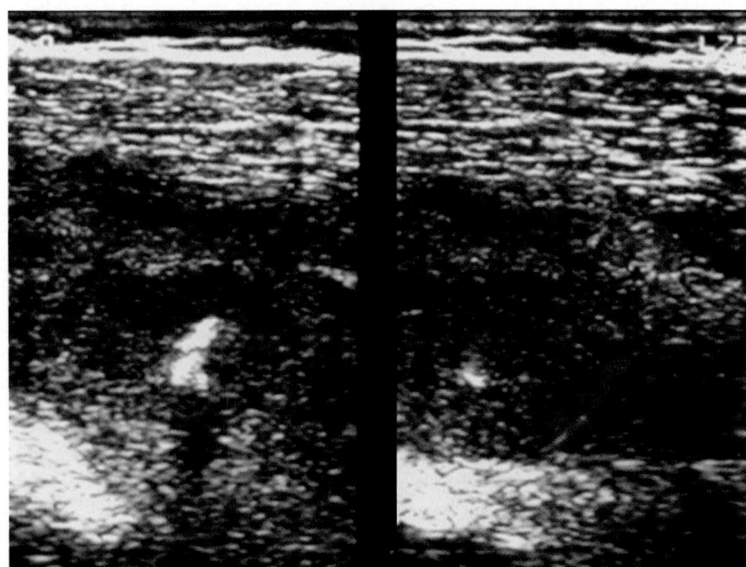

Fig. 12.4 (A) Ultrasound image of 16-year-old boy with a history of a date thorn prick in the anterior thigh showing an echogenic foreign body (FB). **(B)** Image shows surrounding pyomyositis with increased color flow on power Doppler. The case was proven surgically.

for ultrasound for detection, identification, and localization of nonradiopaque foreign bodies is well established. In addition, the use of real-time ultrasound to guide removal of foreign bodies of all types has been well described for over a decade and indeed has become the standard of care in most major centers throughout the world (see, for example, Chapter 13).

In this chapter, we will illustrate the use of ultrasound in the diagnosis and management of soft tissue foreign bodies in the extremities, as well as the identification and management of their complications.

Ultrasound also has proven utility in evaluating diseases and injuries of muscles and surrounding soft tissues; in this application there is overlap with magnetic resonance imaging (MRI), which should be considered the primary modality for the evaluation of muscle disease. We will illustrate cases where the application of ultrasound is clinically useful and decisive.

Muscle, like tendons, are arranged in linear, orderly bundles called fascicles, with linear echogenic echoes oriented in parallel in the midmuscle belly, but characteristically are convergent in the distal muscle as viewed closer to the terminus tendon or aponeurosis (**Fig. 12.5A**). They show some degree of anisotropy to the ultrasound beam, as do tendons (see Chapters 1, 4, and 11). The most common muscle pathologies encountered in imaging are myotendinous tears and strains, contusions, and lacerations (**Figs. 12.5B, 12.6, 12.7**), neurogenic atrophy, infection (including abscess and pyomyositis), and inflammation (**Figs. 12.8, 12.9, 12.10, 12.11, 12.12, 12.13**), diabetic infarction, and necrosis. Discrete lesions such as intramuscular ganglia (cysts) are also sometimes encountered, as are occasional intramuscular

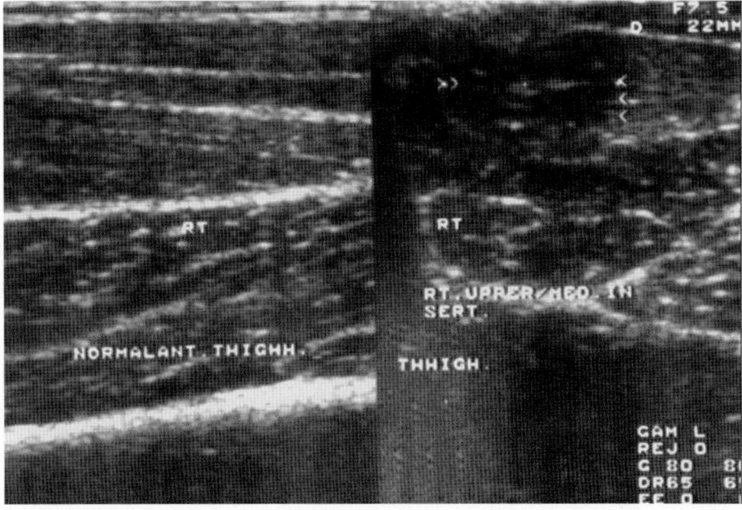

Fig. 12.5 (A) Ultrasound image of normal muscle showing typical herringbone pattern of echogenic septae. **(B)** Evidence of hypoechoic partial muscle tear in 20-year-old male soccer player during the game.

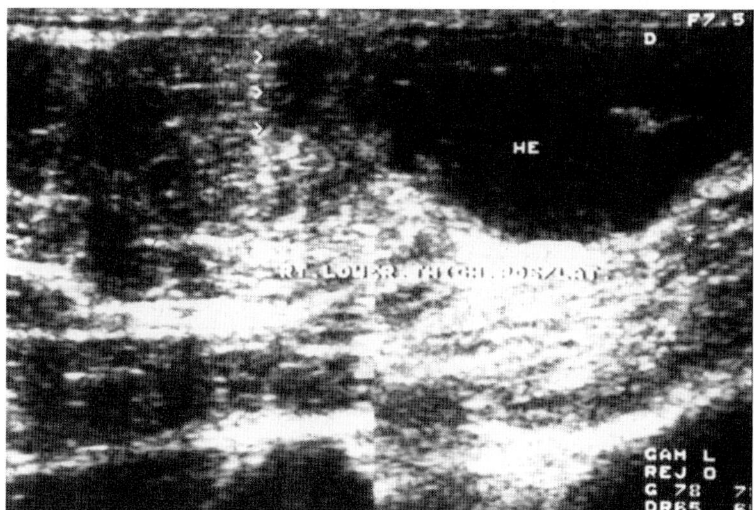

Fig. 12.6 Ultrasound image of a 20-year-male football player with complete muscle tear (CMT) (*arrowheads*) in anterior right thigh muscle with an echolucent hematoma (HE).

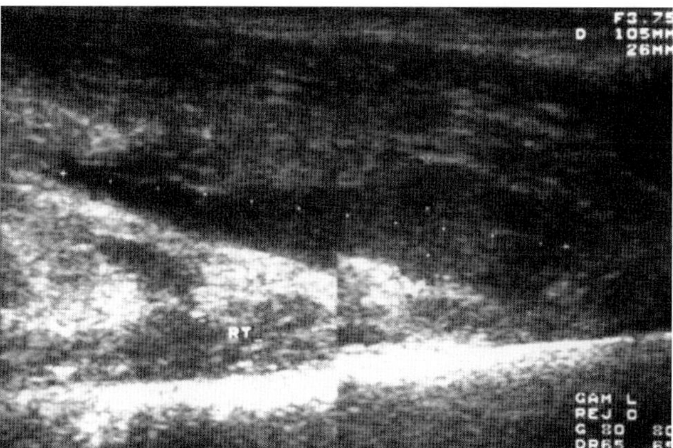

Fig. 12.7 Ultrasound of a 20-year-old soccer player showing large intramuscular hematoma with interrupted muscle fibers (MF) floating within the echolucent blood.

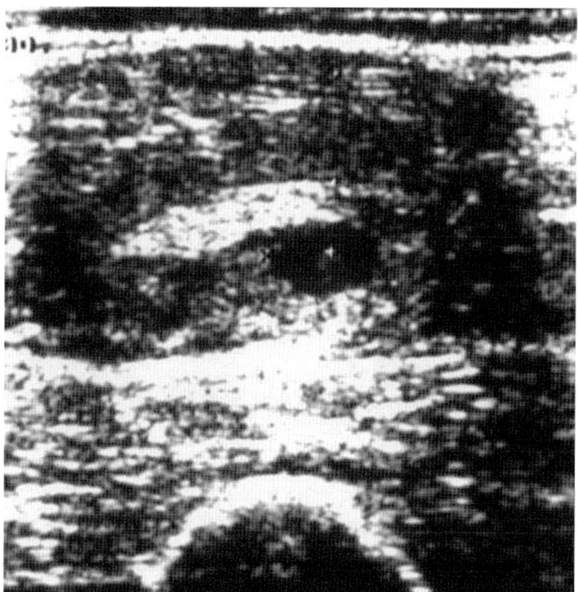

Fig. 12.8 Ultrasound image of a 25-year-old man with hot swollen right thigh with fever and evidence of fluid (FL) in the muscle septae. Pyomyositis (PY) and abscess formation (AB) can be seen with no fluid in contact with the bone (B) ruling out osteomyelitis.

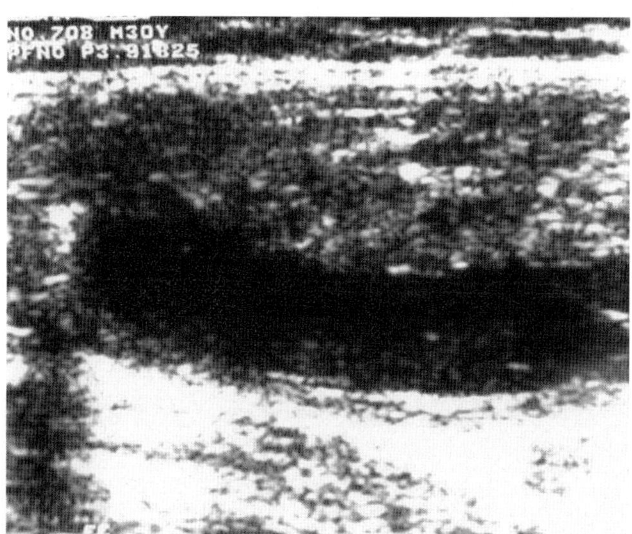

Fig. 12.9 Ultrasound image of a 60-year-diabetic man with fever and a swollen thigh. Ultrasound demonstrates a big sausage-shaped muscle abscess in the thigh with surrounding pyomyositis.

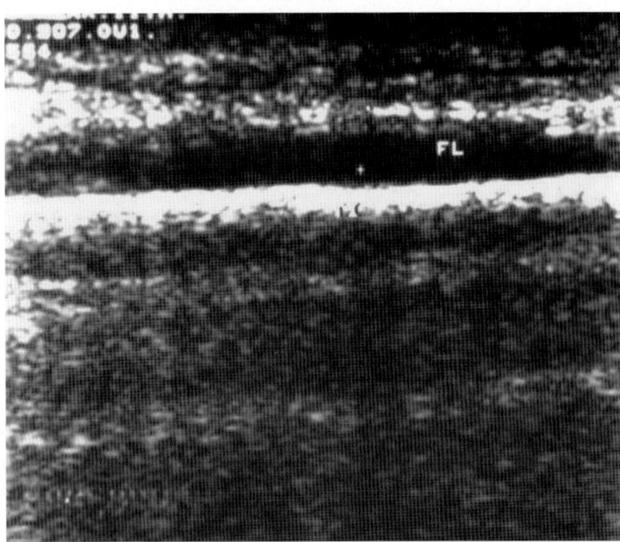

Fig. 12.10 Osteomyelitis. Ultrasound image of a 16-year-old boy with a hot swollen thigh showing fluid (FL) in contact with the bony cortex, with cortical erosion and no soft tissue intervening between the bone and fluid. The fluid was confirmed to represent frank pus at surgery.

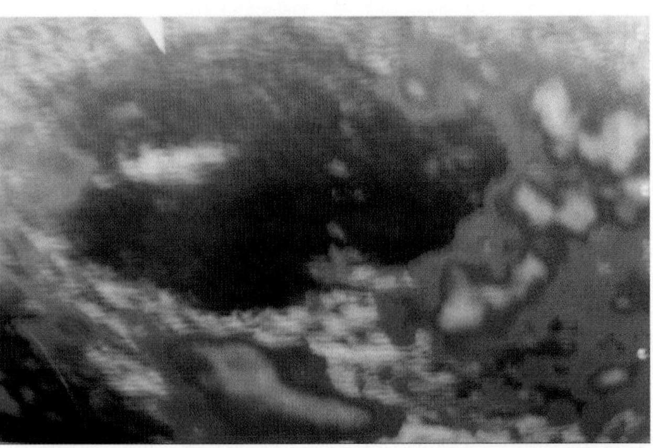

Fig. 12.12 Muscle abscess. Ultrasound image of a 14-year-old boy with a hot swollen thigh with fever and evidence of an echolucent muscle abscess (ABS) with grossly increased color flow on color Doppler.

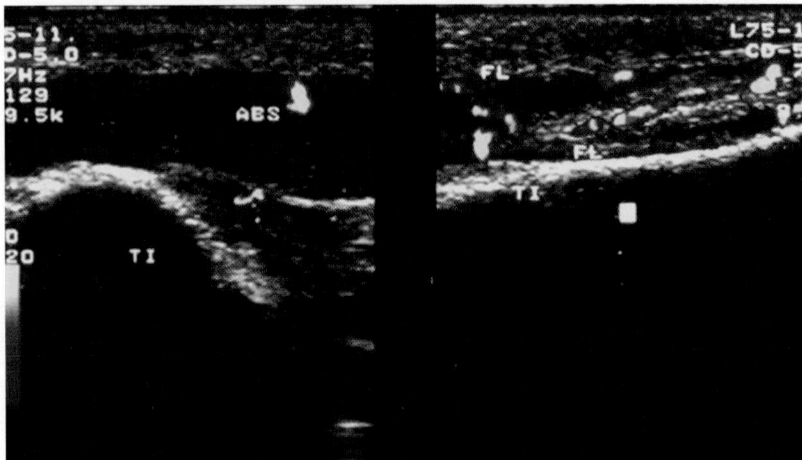

Fig. 12.11 Muscle abscess with pyomyositis. Ultrasound image of a 15-year-old boy with fever and a swollen leg, demonstrating an intramuscular abscess (ABS) medial to the tibia (TI) with evidence of fluid in the muscle planes and increased color flow on power Doppler. Infection was confirmed on aspiration.

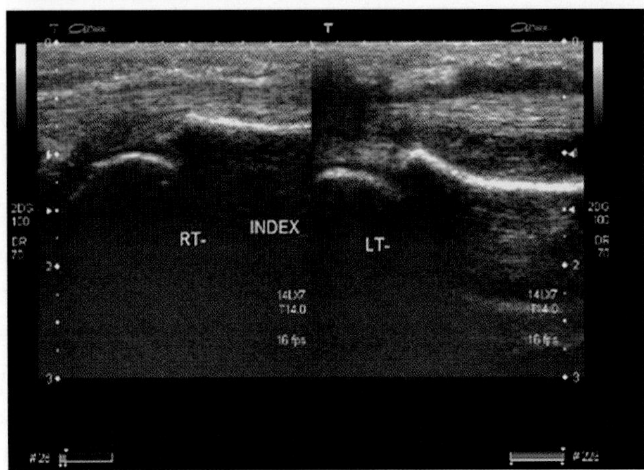

A

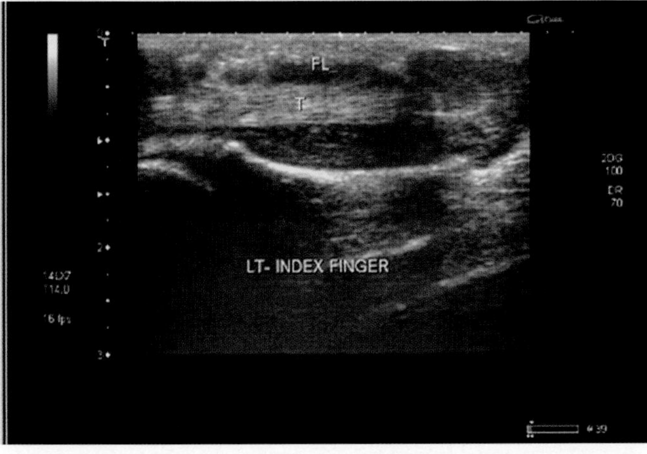

B

Fig. 12.13 Tenosynovitis. Ultrasound image of a 27-year-old woman with a history of fever with swollen left index finger. Hypoechoic fluid (FL) surrounding the flexor tendon can be seen in the scan.

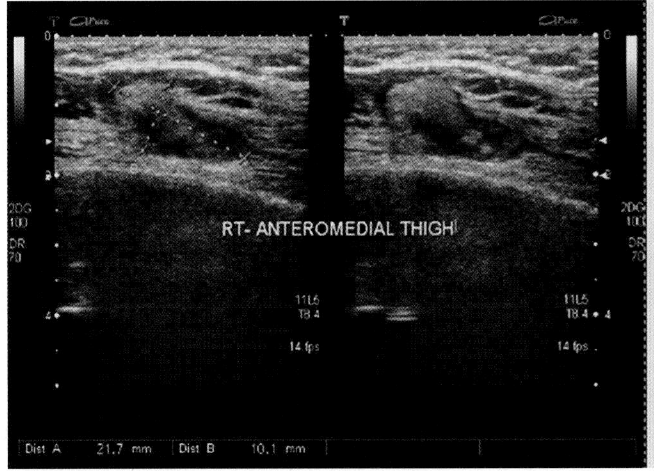

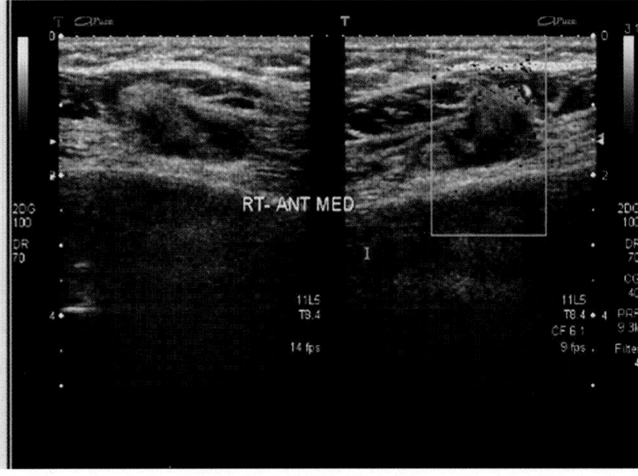

Fig. 12.14 Muscle tumor. Ultrasound image of a 41-year-old woman with history of pain and swelling of one year's duration. Ultrasound shows a muscular mass lesion with evidence of local invasion. The mass demonstrates mixed echogenicity and increased color flow signal internally.

lipomas and hemangiomas (**Figs. 12.14, 12.15, 12.16**). Malignant tumors, such as rhabdomyosarcomas, liposarcomas, and metastases are less common (**Figs. 12.17, 12.18, 12.19**). Although some, like myotendinous tears and intramuscular ganglia, have a characteristic sonographic appearance, most other muscular lesions present a spectrum of overlapping appearances. No single appearance is pathognomonic on ultrasound. Although either modality performs well in the setting of injury or infection, MRI is generally preferred for muscular tumor imaging; ultrasound is generally preferred for biopsy/procedural guidance.

Technical Guidelines

For these applications, technical considerations and equipment do not differ from other types of musculoskeletal ultrasound discussed in the foregoing chapters. In general, all modern (i.e., manufactured within the last 5 or 6 years) ultrasound equipment will allow excellent visualization of nonopaque foreign bodies. Generally, a high-frequency (7–15 MHz) small footprint linear-array probe with good nearfield focus is chosen for this application. Such transducers are typically offered as optional equipment for dedicated

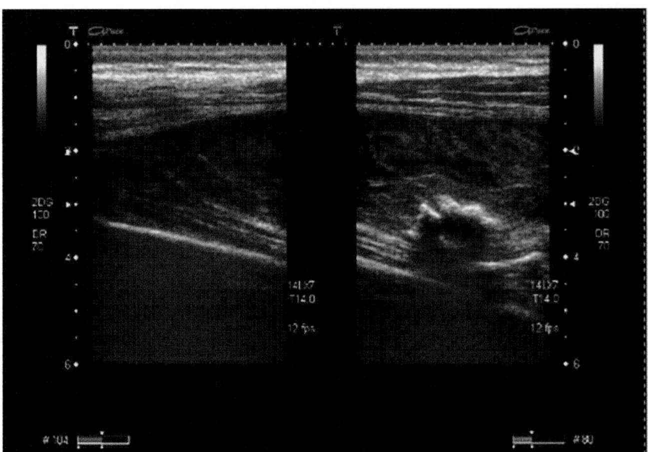

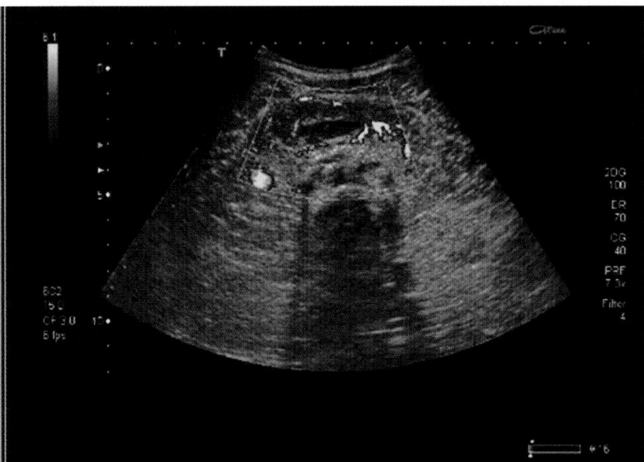

Fig. 12.15 Calcified muscle mass. Ultrasound demonstrates 1.2 × 2.5 cm calcified mass arising from the muscle with increased flow signal on power Doppler. This may represent myositis ossificans or possibly a calcified intramuscular hematoma.

Fig. 12.16 (A-H) Intramuscular hemangioma. A 42-year-old man with swelling over the thenar eminence over one year. **(A)** Plain film showing phleboliths within the lesion. **(B)** Ultrasound heterogeneous mass with calcifications, but no significant signal on Doppler. **(C-F)** Magnetic resonance images (MRI) of same lesion showing isointense signal on T1-weighted **(C)**, brighter signal on T2-weighted **(D)**, and short T1 inversion recovery (STIR) **(E)**, and enhancement in **(F)** and **(G,H)**.

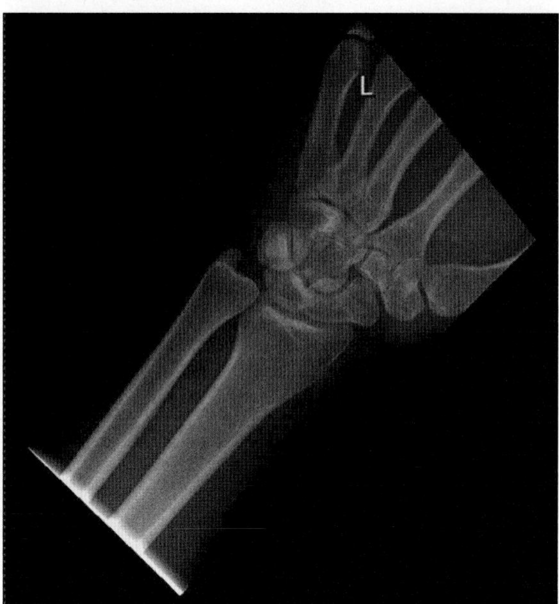

A

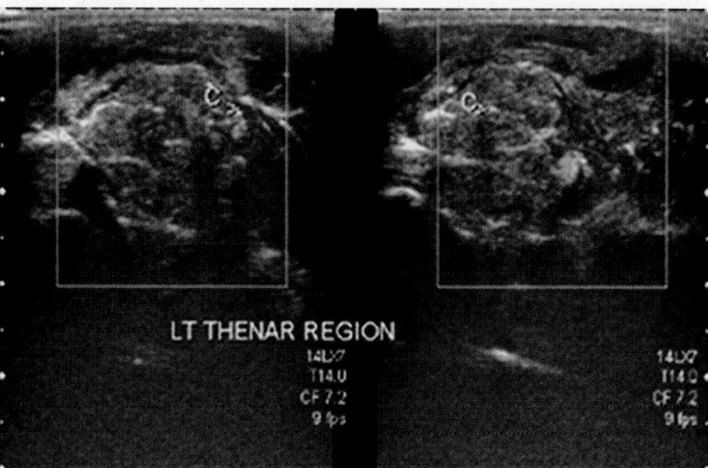

B

C

D

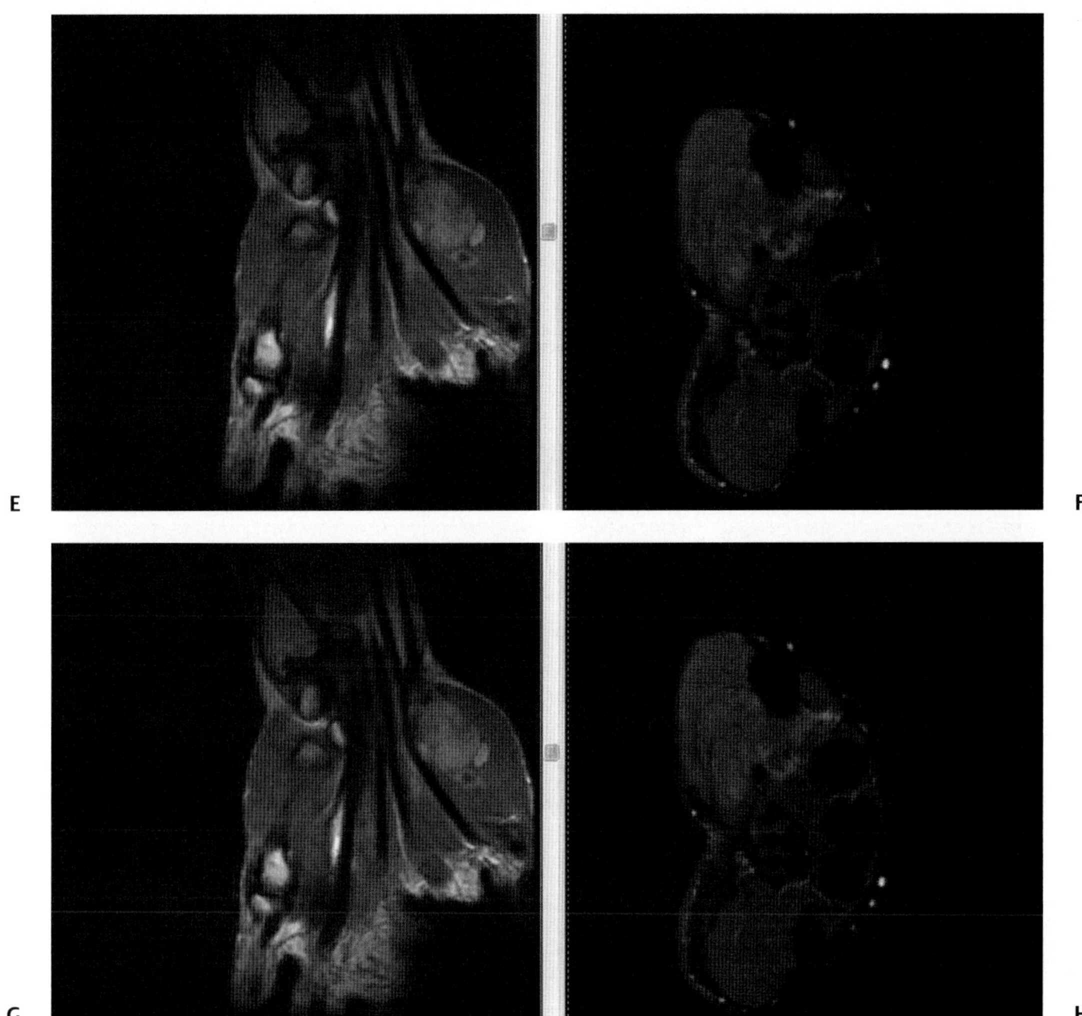
E
F
G
H

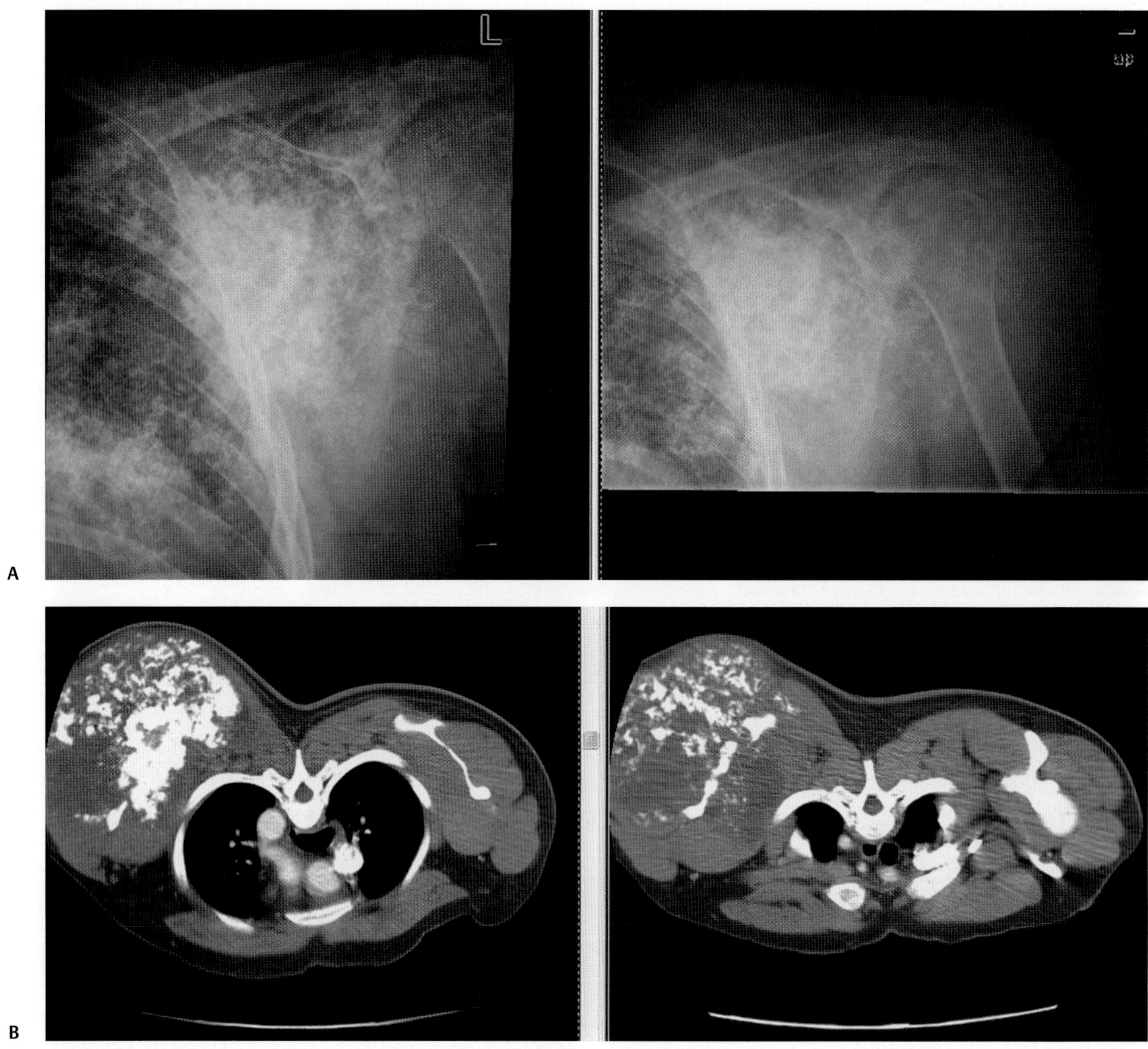

Fig. 12.17 (A-D) Chondrosarcoma. A 30-year-old man with a slowly growing mass over his left shoulder for over 3 years. **(A)** Plain x-ray shows heavily calcified mass, without gross bony involvement. **(B)** Same lesion on computed tomography (CT). Involvement of the scapula is noted on CT.

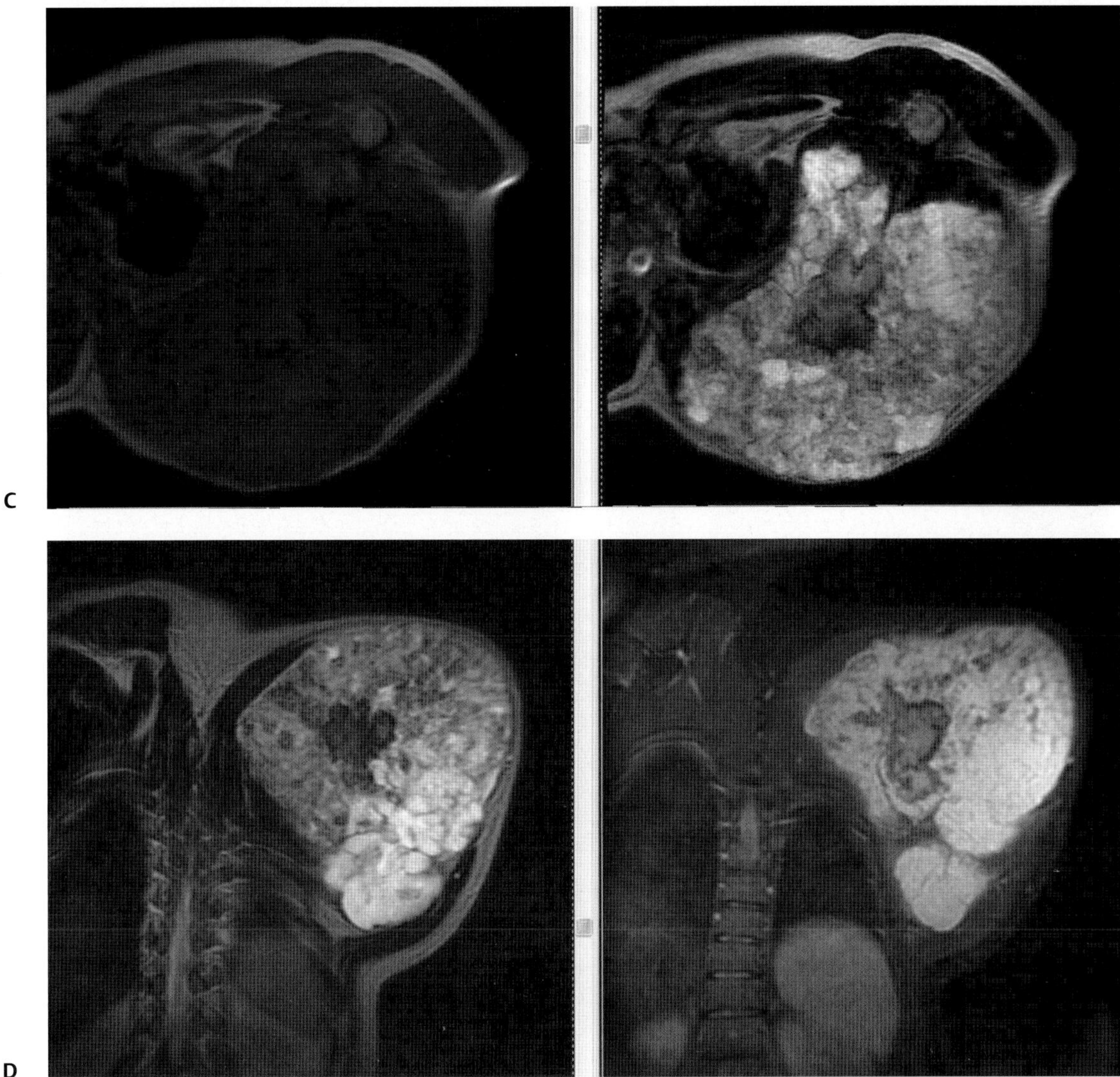

Fig. 12.17 (*Continued*) **(C,D)** Magnetic resonance images (MRI) of same lesion. **(C)** T1-weighted MRI (left) and T1-weighted MRI (right). **(D)** Short T1 inversion recovery (STIR) sequences.

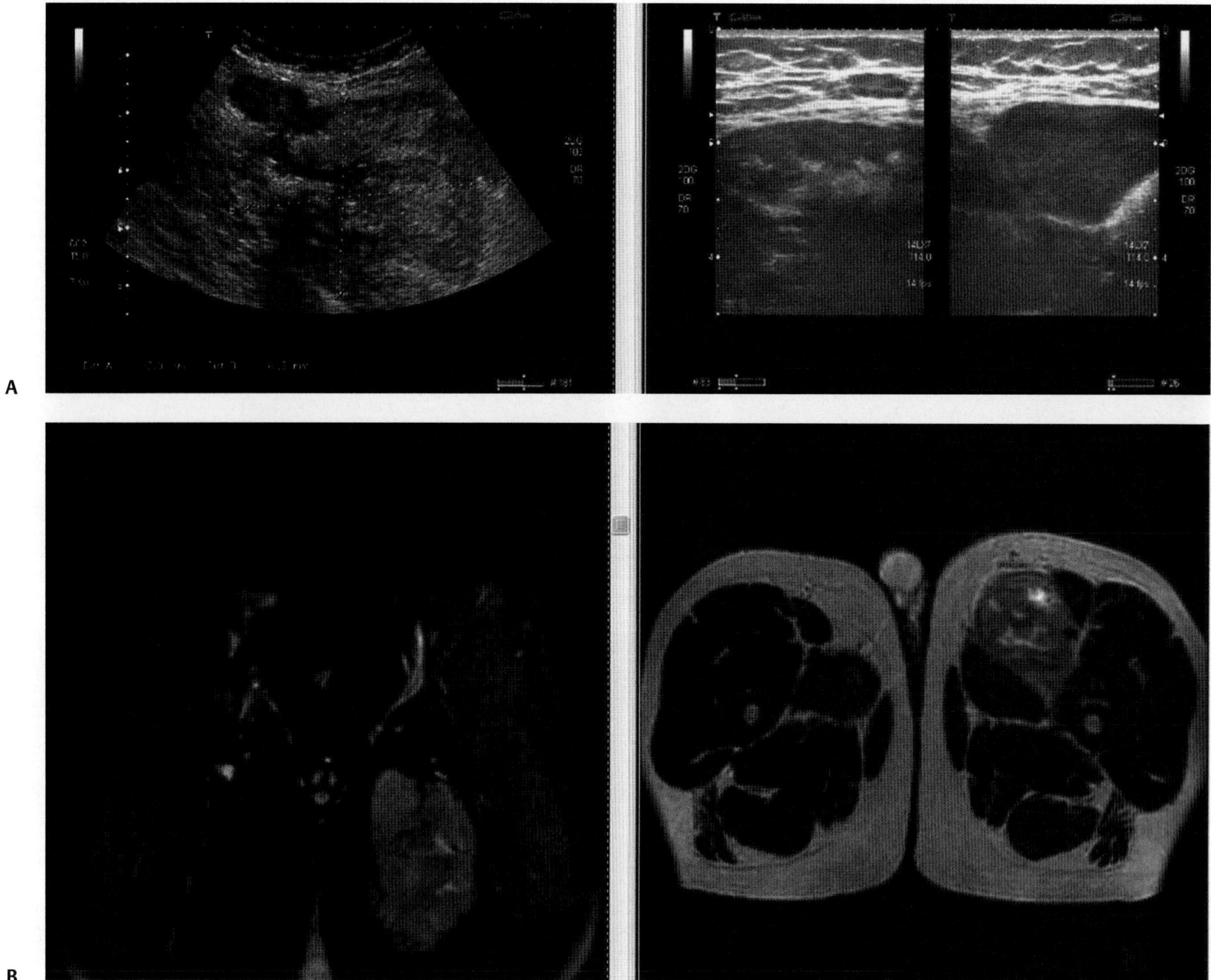

Fig. 12.18 (A-D) Synovial cell sarcoma. A 22-year-old man presented with a slowly growing, painful swelling in his proximal left thigh and on physical examination revealed a firm lump arising from the adductor longus muscle, having mixed echogenicity on ultrasound **(A)**, and high signal on T2-weighted magnetic resonance imaging (MRI) images **(B)** and **(C)**. Mass shows mild contrast enhancement on computed tomography **(D)**.

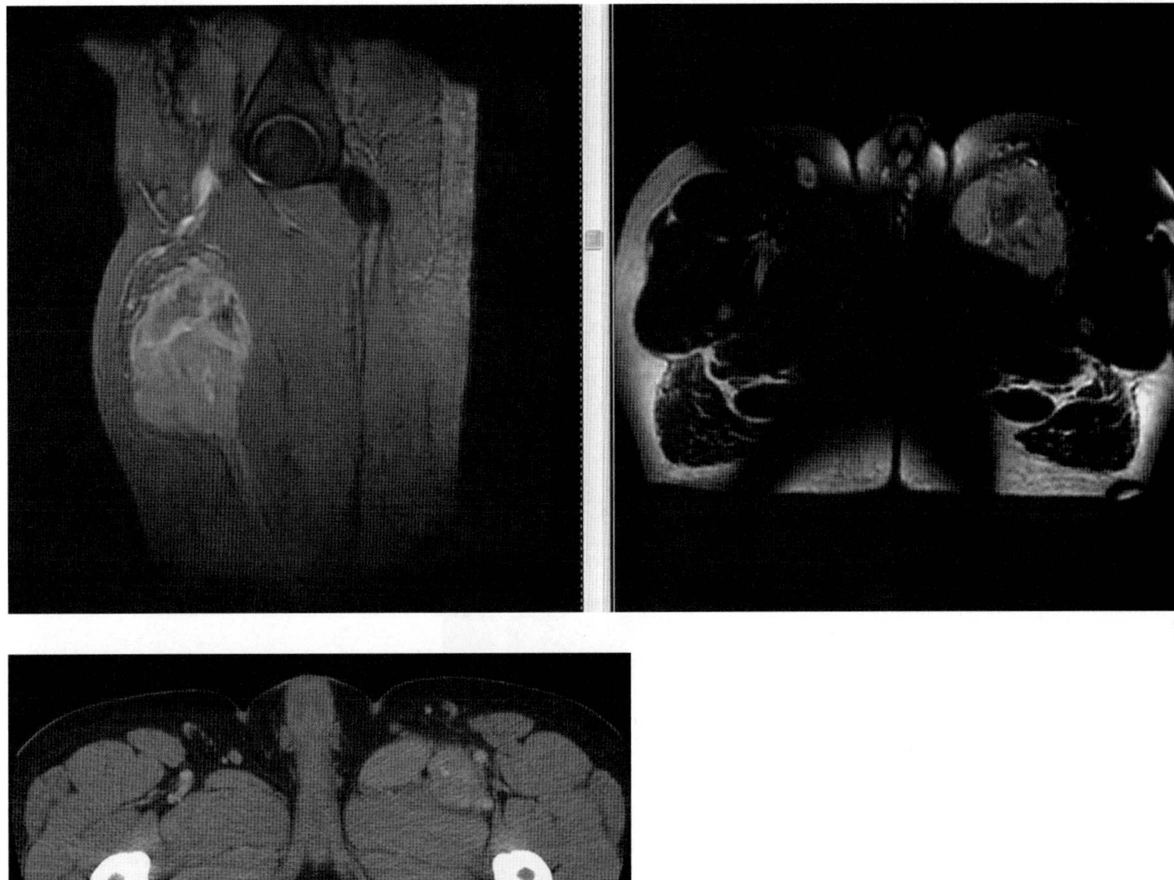

C

D

Fig. 12.18 (*Continued*)

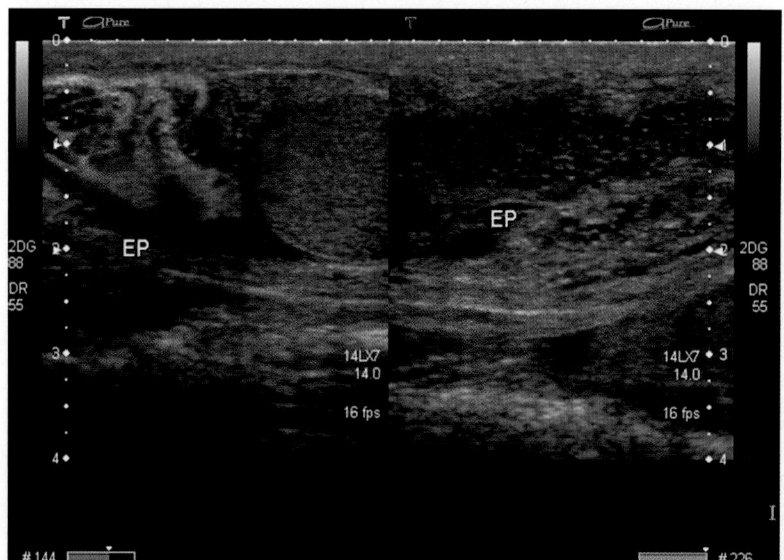

Fig. 12.19 (A-F) Liposarcoma with mixed spindle cell and pleomorphic sarcoma. A 39-year-old man with a swelling over his left thigh region extending over his left scrotum. **(A)** Ultrasound image of lesion (left) shows mixed echogenicity mass attached to the deep surface of the fascia and adductor longus muscle, extending to the medial end of the inguinal ligament and occupying the left hemiscrotum **(A)**, and encroaching on the epididymis **(B).** In **(C)** this same mass is shown to be separate from the testicle and in **(D)** to have increased flow on color Doppler. In **(E)** the mass is shown on unenhanced computed tomography to have both low- and high-attenuation areas. It is shown to enter the left inguinal canal. In **(F)** the lesion is shown to enhance heterogeneously. (Courtesy of Dr. KVS Parsad, General Surgery, Khoula Hospital, Muscat, Oman.)

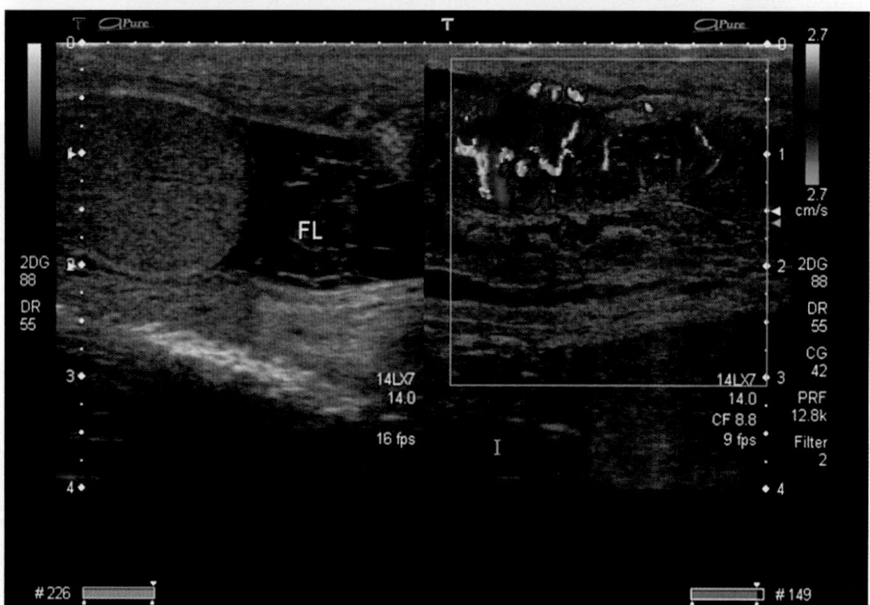

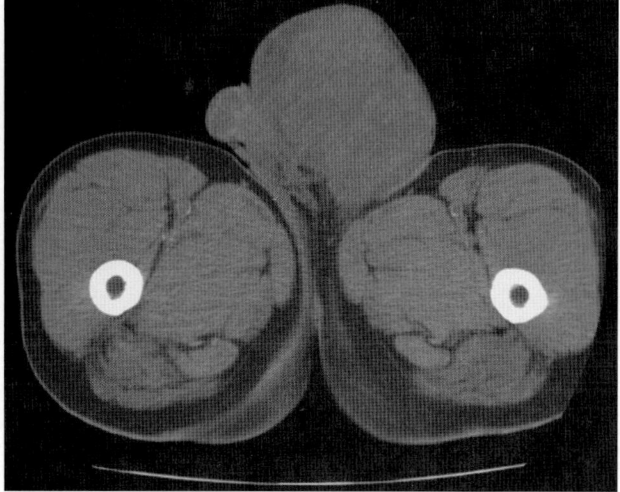

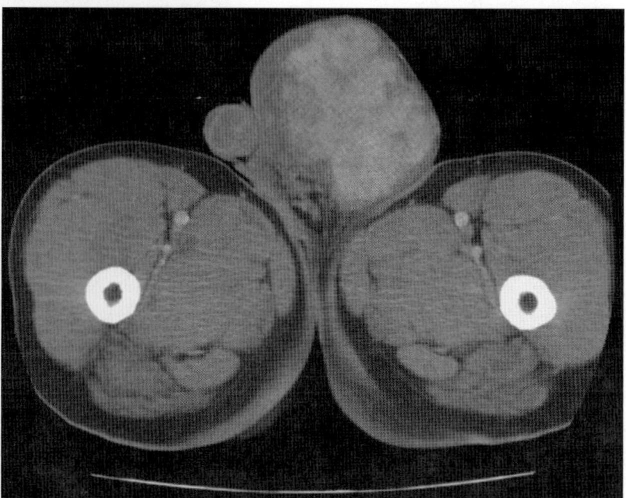

evaluation of small parts and musculoskeletal applications. Doppler, especially power Doppler, is helpful for the identification of secondary inflammation and hyperemia, which often surrounds a retained foreign body (**Fig. 12.4B**).

Pearls and Pitfalls

- Small nonradiopaque foreign bodies, such as cactus thorns and small shards of glass or slivers of wood, may be detectable only by ultrasound, and not by physical examination (even with dissection) nor by any other imaging modality (**Figs. 12.1, 12.2, 12.3, 12.4**).
- Retained soft tissue foreign bodies are often surrounded by a rim of hematoma or purulent material, which can aid in their detection. Power Doppler may aid detection by revealing hyperemic blood flow.
- Ultrasound is extremely well suited to guide the removal of such objects in real time.

Acknowledgment

We thank Mr. Arjun Nath, Mr. Hamed Al Busaidy, and Mr. Rajesh George for their assistance.

Suggested Readings

The following two textbooks, published more than a decade apart, provide extensive background on the application of musculoskeletal ultrasound.

Bianchi S, Martinoli C. Ultrasound of the Musculoskeletal System. In Baert AL, Knauth M, Sartor K, Eds. Heidelberg/New York: Springer; 2007

Fornage B. Musculoskeletal Ultrasound, Clinics in Diagnostic Ultrasound. Vol. 30. New York: Churchill Livingstone; 1995

Additional Readings

Fornage BD, Schernberg FL. Sonographic diagnosis of foreign bodies of the distal extremities. AJR Am J Roentgenol 1986;147(3):567–569

Jacobson JA, Powell A, Craig JG, Bouffard JA, van Holsbeeck MT. Wooden foreign bodies in soft tissue: detection at US. Radiology 1998;206(1):45–48

Kransdorf MJ, Jelinek JS, Moser RP Jr. Imaging of soft tissue tumors. Radiol Clin North Am 1993;31(2):359–372

Kransdorf MJ, Murphey MD. Imaging of Soft-Tissue Tumors. Philadelphia: Lippincott Williams & Wilkins; 2006

Küllmer K, Sievers KW, Reimers CD, et al. Changes of sonographic, magnetic resonance tomographic, electromyographic, and histopathologic findings within a 2-month period of examinations after experimental muscle denervation. Arch Orthop Trauma Surg 1998;117(4-5):228–234

Little CM, Parker MG, Callowich MC, Sartori JC. The ultrasonic detection of soft tissue foreign bodies. Invest Radiol 1986;21(3):275–277

Oikarinen KS, Nieminen TM, Mäkäräinen H, Pyhtinen J. Visibility of foreign bodies in soft tissue in plain radiographs, computed tomography, magnetic resonance imaging, and ultrasound. An in vitro study. Int J Oral Maxillofac Surg 1993;22(2):119–124

Soudack M, Nachtigal A, Gaitini D. Clinically unsuspected foreign bodies: the importance of sonography. J Ultrasound Med 2003;22(12):1381–1385

Trusen A, Beissert M, Schultz G, Chittka B, Darge K. Ultrasound and MRI features of pyomyositis in children. Eur Radiol 2003;13(5):1050–1055

Turner J, Wilde CH, Hughes KC, Meilstrup JW, Manders EK. Ultrasound-guided retrieval of small foreign objects in subcutaneous tissue. Ann Emerg Med 1997;29(6):731–734

13 Ultrasound-Guided Procedures

Cesare Romagnoli, Tobias De Zordo, Andrea S. Klauser, and Rethy Chhem

The importance of ultrasound-guided musculoskeletal interventions has been increasingly recognized over the last decade, largely due to the development of high-frequency probes (10–20 MHz), which provide better spatial resolution in superficial structures. This increased spatial resolution has enhanced the feasibility of ultrasound diagnosis of musculoskeletal pathologies and the use of ultrasound as guidance for diagnostic and therapeutic procedures. The most common ultrasound-guided interventions are aspiration of fluid; injections of joints, tendons, and nerves; biopsy of soft tissue masses; aspiration and lavage of calcifications; and removal of foreign bodies, all of which will be discussed in more detail in this chapter.

Ultrasound is a readily available, nonionizing, lower-cost imaging modality for assessing musculoskeletal disorders. Although clinically guided techniques, using palpation as guidance are mainly used, the reliability of correct needle localization is low. However, ultrasound is an excellent tool for guiding minimally invasive interventional procedures in the musculoskeletal system when lesions are visible in the ultrasound images.

It is important to distinguish between diagnostic procedures and therapeutic procedures. When fluid from joints or tendons is aspirated to differentiate inflammatory from infective synovitis, or when biopsy of synovium or soft tissue masses is performed, or when local anesthetics are injected to confirm a clinical diagnosis, these are diagnostic interventions. Therapeutic interventions include aspiration of cysts; foreign body extraction; lavage of calcifications; and injections of drugs into joints, tendon sheaths, bursae, and around ligaments or nerves. Under ultrasound guidance, direct visualization of the underlying pathology is possible and needle insertion can be seen in real-time. The surrounding vessels and tendons and also nerves and articular cartilage can be displayed and therefore avoided during needle insertion, which leads to a more painless procedure for the patient and results in minimization of adverse effects. Ultrasound guidance has been shown to improve intraarticular placement in various regions, but is particularly useful in obese patients, poorly accessible joints (e.g., hip), or when only small joint effusions are present. In localizing the lesion and guiding the procedure, ultrasound can be used to control the efficacy of the intervention and for follow-up imaging.

General Considerations

After informed consent, a thorough ultrasound examination of the patient's area of complaint is mandatory before beginning any procedure to better delineate the clinically suspected pathology and to localize it precisely with respect to adjacent structures. This allows planning of the entry site and the orientation of needle placement. The patient should be positioned appropriately to ensure the most comfortable procedure for both the physician and patient. Surrounding structures of the target should be kept in a relaxed position to decrease resistance during needle insertion.

Although the risk of complications (e.g., septic arthritis) is low, disinfection of the patient's skin and the instruments is performed. The surrounding area should be covered with a sterile drape and only the field of interest should remain uncovered to minimize the risk of contamination. Other critical issues in musculoskeletal interventions are existing coagulative disorders and anticoagulant treatment. However, bleeding diathesis represents no absolute contraindication in most cases where needles are used for the procedure. If large needles have to be used, coagulation tests including prothrombin time, international normalized ratio (INR), and a platelet count should be performed at least 24 hours before the intervention.

The ultrasound scanner should be fitted with high-frequency probes (10–15 MHz or higher) for superficial regions (hands, feet, elbow, shoulder) and with lower frequencies for deeper structures such as the knee, hip, and sacroiliac joint (5–12 MHz). A small footprint probe may allow better access to small superficial structures and an easier handling of the probe and the syringe. Normally, no needle-guidance kit is required because a freehand technique allows for a faster and more flexible (no fixed angle) intervention. The shortest needle path should be selected, avoiding vessels, nerves, and tendons, and the entry point may be marked on the skin with an indelible ink marker. After entering with the needle under the skin, sterile ultrasound gel should be used for better real-time visualization of the needle.

Biopsy

Biopsies of soft tissue masses are required when imaging does not allow for a definite characterization of the lesion.

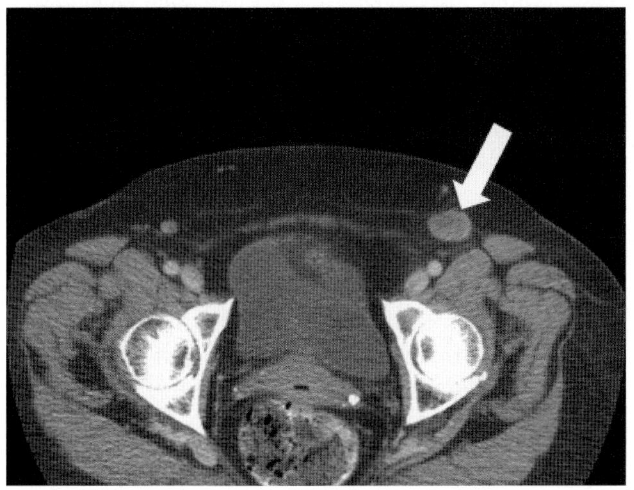

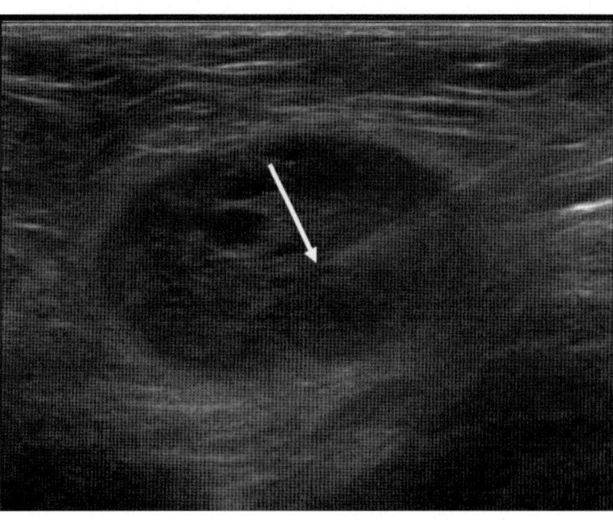

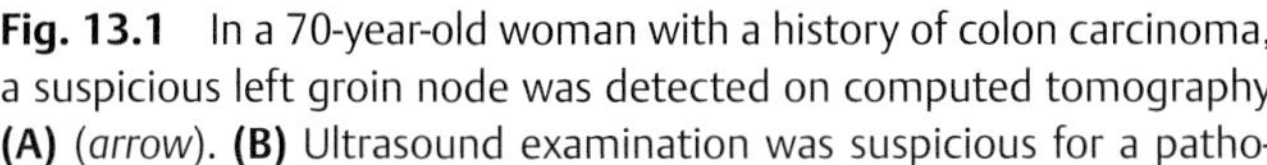

Fig. 13.1 In a 70-year-old woman with a history of colon carcinoma, a suspicious left groin node was detected on computed tomography **(A)** (*arrow*). **(B)** Ultrasound examination was suspicious for a pathologic lymph node and fine needle aspiration confirmed metastatic colon carcinoma (*arrow*).

Lipoma, sarcoma, desmoid, nodular fasciitis, metastatic lesions (**Fig. 13.1**), lymphoma, and epidermal cysts (**Fig. 13.2**) are some common examples where biopsy might be necessary for a better differentiation, and ultrasound-guided biopsy of masses in the musculoskeletal system can be acquired quickly, accurately, and safely. The most common complications of surgical biopsies, including wound infection, local pain, hematoma, seroma, keloids, and problems related to general anesthesia, are almost nonexistent in image-guided percutaneous biopsies. The reported complication rate of image-guided percutaneous biopsies is between 0 and 0.5%. However, malignant masses can spread along the needle track (e.g., sarcoma); therefore, an appropriate needle pathway should be discussed with the surgeons before the intervention. Considering compartment anatomy is critical in tumor biopsies to avoid seeding into ulterior compartments, which also might be resected after histologic confirmation. Fine needle aspiration, moving end-cutting 20- or 22-gauge spinal or Chiba needles up and down inside the mass, is used for cytologic examination and might be sufficient for diagnosis. However, most solid masses require larger needle biopsies to provide samples for histologic assessment.

For local anesthesia, a solution of lidocaine at a concentration of 1 to 2% can be used, and bicarbonate can be added to prevent a burning sensation on the skin. Using the freehand technique with a long axis view of the needle, a 14- to 18-gauge automatic core biopsy needle may be used to gather multiple core samples (3–6) for each biopsy, which are then

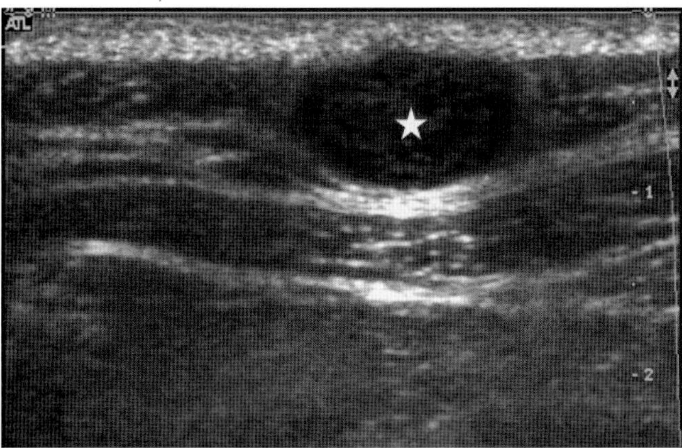

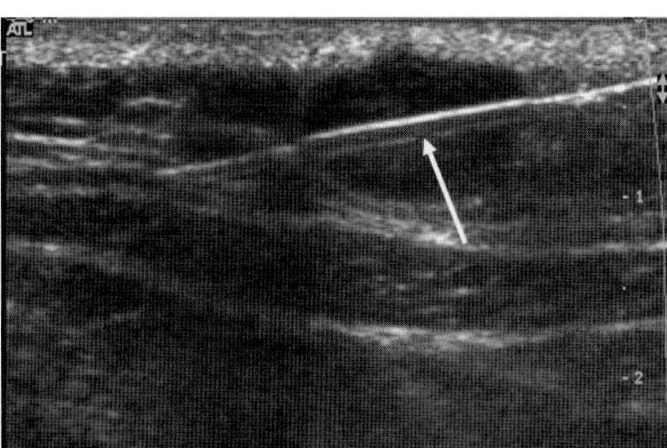

Fig. 13.2 A 49-year-old man with a soft tissue mass at the right side of the posterior neck. **(A)** Ultrasound showed a subcutaneous oval nodule with clear margins and inhomogeneously hypoechoic echotexture (*). **(B)** The underlying muscle fascia was compressed, but not infiltrated. To rule out malignancy, a biopsy was performed under ultrasound guidance using an 18-gauge core biopsy needle (*arrow*). Histologic analysis of the sample was diagnostic for an epidermal cyst.

placed in formaldehyde solution. After reaching the lesion with the tip of the needle, it should be remembered that after activation the needle will advance an additional 18 to 19 mm into the lesion, and care should be taken to preserve soft tissue structures that are located dorsally to the lesion. Therefore, surrounding tissue has to be assessed routinely before the procedure, and color Doppler ultrasound allows visualization of viable tissue and adjacent vessels.

An ambulatory setting is normally sufficient except for severely ill patients and patients requiring sedation. Outpatients should be observed for at least 1 hour after biopsy. They should be discharged with stable blood pressure and no evidence of active bleeding.

Ultrasound may also be used to identify selected muscle involvement in neuromuscular disorders such as Duchenne or Becker muscular dystrophies and to guide muscle biopsy in these cases.

Analysis of synovial tissue can provide relevant information about the pathophysiologic mechanism, the degree of inflammation, and prognosis. Ultrasound-guided biopsy can be used to obtain synovial samples, but it is mainly performed for research purposes.

In summary, ultrasound-guided biopsy is a reliable technique to characterize soft tissue lesions in most cases. However, if histologic diagnosis is equivocal or negative for malignancy, but a high clinical or radiologic suspicion for malignancy still exists, open biopsy should be performed.

Foreign Body Extraction

Identification of soft tissue foreign bodies is routinely performed by using radiographs. However, ultrasound is able to detect and assess a variety of foreign bodies of different shapes and material compositions, with the added advantage of being able to detect nonradiopaque foreign bodies such as wood, plastic, and often glass. Foreign bodies appear mainly as a hyperechoic structure surrounded by hypoechoic granulation tissue. Ultrasound can be used for preoperative localization of the foreign body, and also to guide the extraction process and avoid surgery.

Ultrasound-guided removal of superficial foreign bodies can be performed more easily when the compositions of the fragments are metallic splinters (**Fig. 13.3**) or gravel, but removal of pieces of glass (**Fig. 13.4**) and wood (**Figs. 13.5** and **13.6**) require more patience and meticulous technique. Besides adequate local anesthesia, a set of sterilized surgical instruments, including Mosquito, Kelly, Kocher, and Splinter forceps is needed. After marking the position of the best extractable side of the foreign body, a skin incision is usually necessary to allow the instrument to enter the soft tissue and to proceed toward the foreign body. When an open wound is present, it may be possible to extract the foreign body through the same path that it entered. If an incision is necessary, care should be taken to ensure an adequate incision width to allow extraction of the foreign body without significant injury to adjacent soft tissues. Real-time ultrasound guidance allows for a simpler extraction procedure, as it is easier to estimate the location and angle at which the foreign body is lying.

Calcification Puncture and Lavage

Calcific tendinitis is caused by calcium hydroxyapatite deposition, which can theoretically affect all tendons, but it is found most commonly in the rotator cuff tendons of the shoulder. Predominantly, the supraspinatus tendon is involved either unilaterally or bilaterally in 30- to 60-year-old patients, with a higher incidence range in women (57–76.7%). Although calcific tendinitis is a self-limited process in which the calcifications tend to be reabsorbed, in 50% of patients these deposits become symptomatic, causing acute or chronic pain. The disease is divided into two stages: the formative phase in which calcium hydroxyapatite is deposited into the tendon and the resorptive phase where these deposits resolve. Systemic antiinflammatory drugs, iontophoresis, physiotherapy, and subacromial injections of corticosteroids often provide only temporary relief and these patients may benefit from removing the calcium. Surgery and high-intensity shock waves are two more invasive and relatively expensive procedures, but a simpler and more inexpensive method to remove the calcium crystals is ultrasound-guided needle puncture of the calcification followed by lavage.

Ultrasound scanning helps to localize the calcification, which appears as a hyperechoic structure with or without posterior shadowing. After local freezing, the calcification is repeatedly punctured with a 16- to 22-gauge needle under ultrasound guidance in an attempt to fragment the calcific deposit. Different methods are described for the second part of the procedure, where after injections of small amounts of 1% lidocaine or 0.9% saline using a 10- to 20-mL syringe, aspiration of the calcium is performed. Although some authors are using a single needle for puncture, injection, and aspiration, we prefer using a two-needle technique. One is inserted for injection of saline and the second one is used for aspiration; in our experience, there is less frequent occlusion of the needle using this technique. Aspiration is easier in tuff-like or semiliquid calcifications representing reabsorptive states (**Fig. 13.7**), but more difficult when a solid calcification is present (**Fig. 13.8**). In both cases, aspiration of a cloudy, milky fluid or a solid gritty substance is performed until the aspirated fluid becomes clear. Generally, only a part of the calcification can be aspirated, but this does not represent a failure of the treatment as the residual calcium tends to undergo spontaneous resorption over the weeks following the procedure (**Fig. 13.9**). Before extracting the needle, intrabursal injection of corticosteroids and long-acting anesthetics is performed to decrease crystal-in-

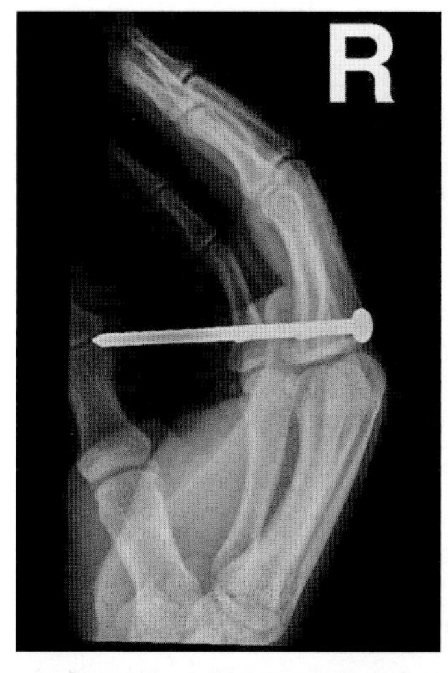

A

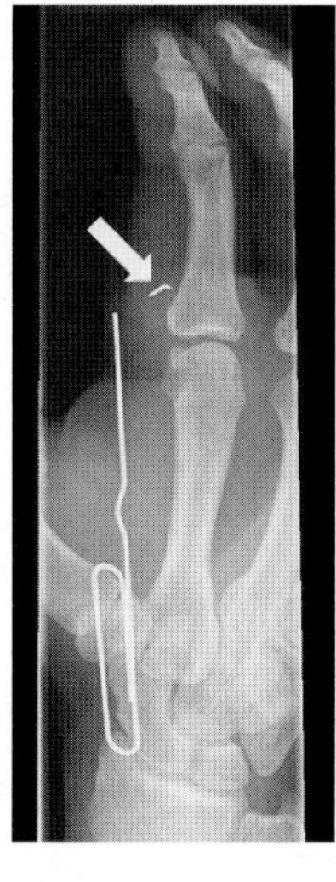

B

Fig. 13.3 Radiograph shows right hand of a 17-year-old man with a screw penetrating his second finger at the level of the proximal phalanx, but not penetrating the bone **(A)**. **(B-D)** After extraction of the screw in the emergency department, a 7 mm foreign body piece was still detectable and ultrasound scanning detected the intravascular location of the foreign body (*arrows*). **(C)** Note the reverberation artifact, consistent with the presence of metal. **(E)** Photograph shows the extracted metallic foreign body. **(F)** Plain film radiograph confirmed complete extraction of the foreign body with some residual soft tissue swelling.

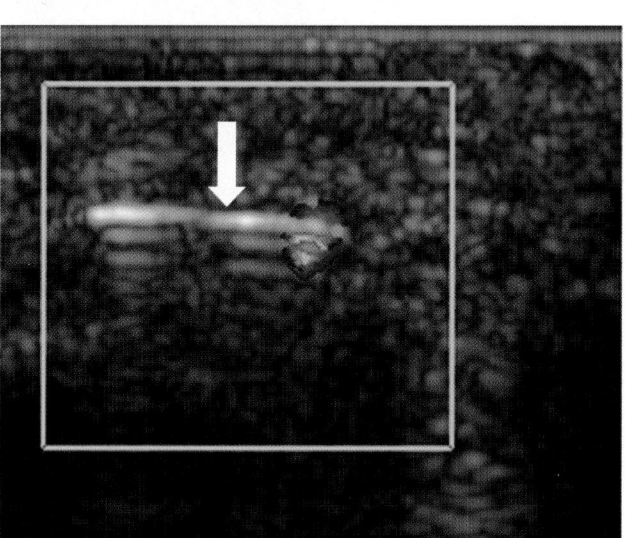

C

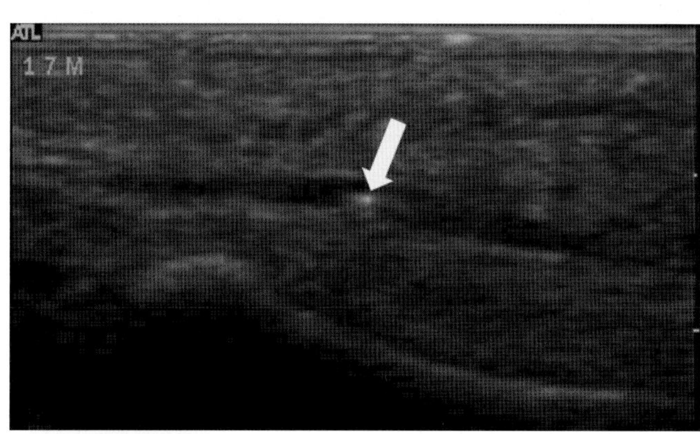

D

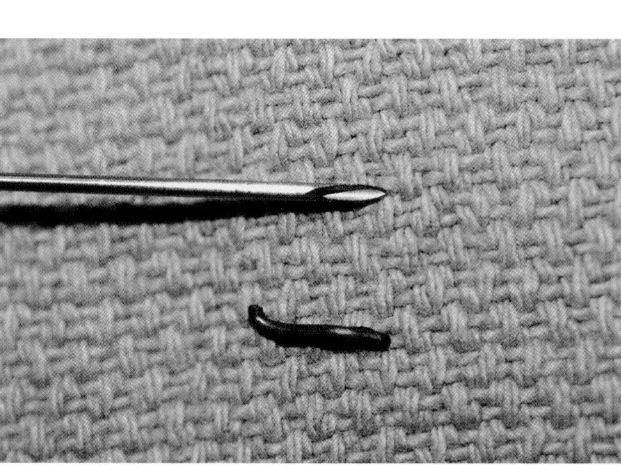

E

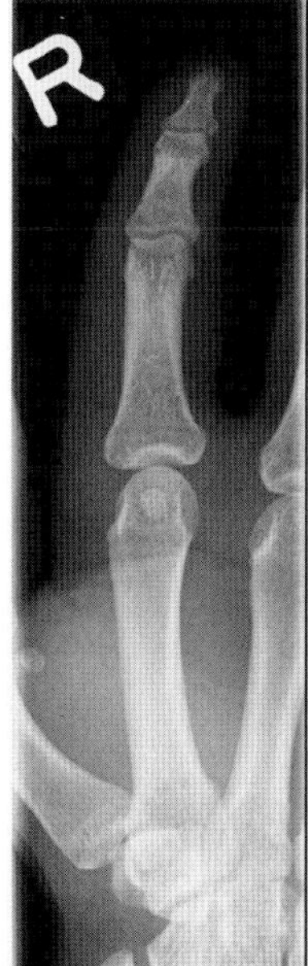

F

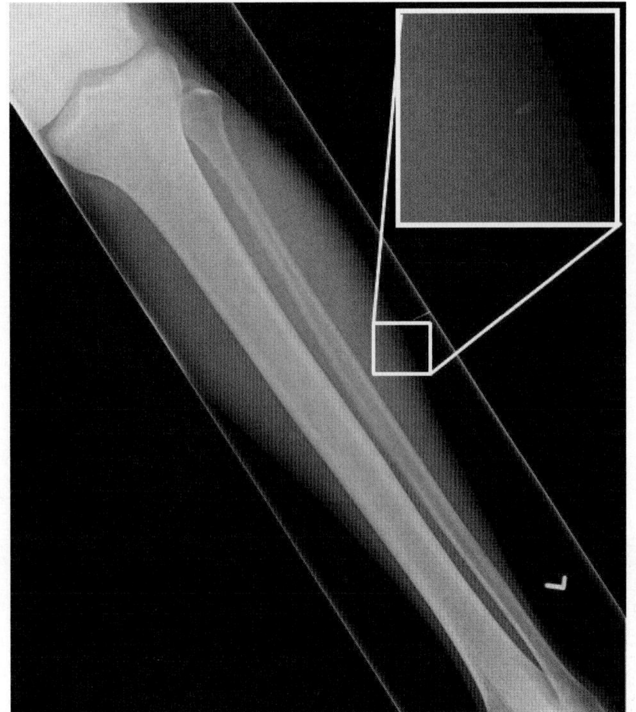

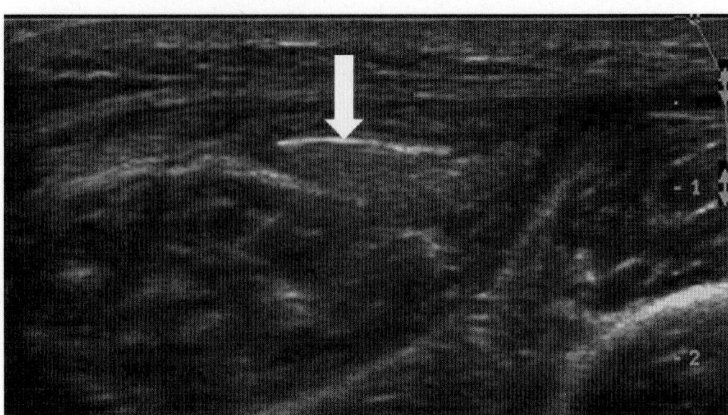

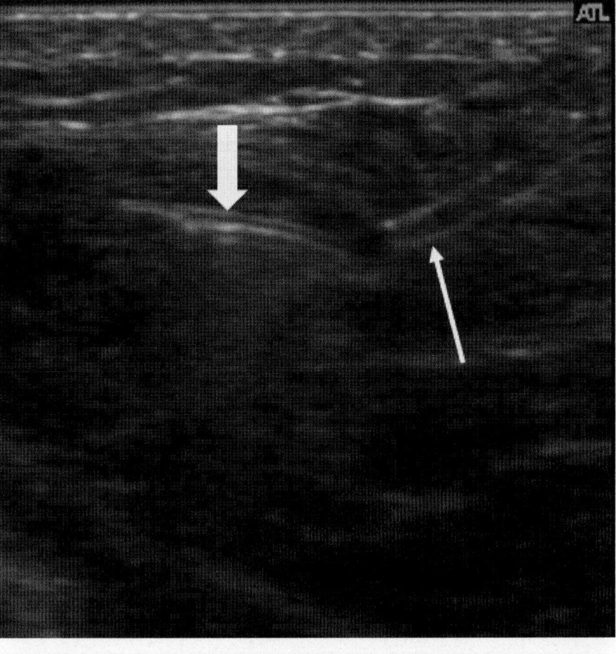

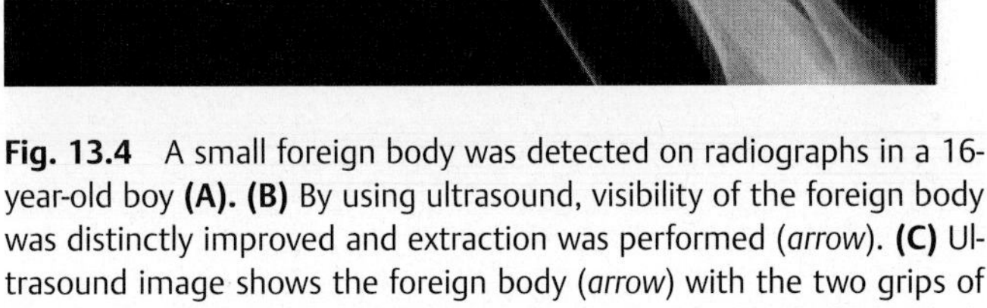

Fig. 13.4 A small foreign body was detected on radiographs in a 16-year-old boy **(A). (B)** By using ultrasound, visibility of the foreign body was distinctly improved and extraction was performed (*arrow*). **(C)** Ultrasound image shows the foreign body (*arrow*) with the two grips of the forceps (*thin arrow*). The foreign body was made of glass, which explained the poor visibility on plain films.

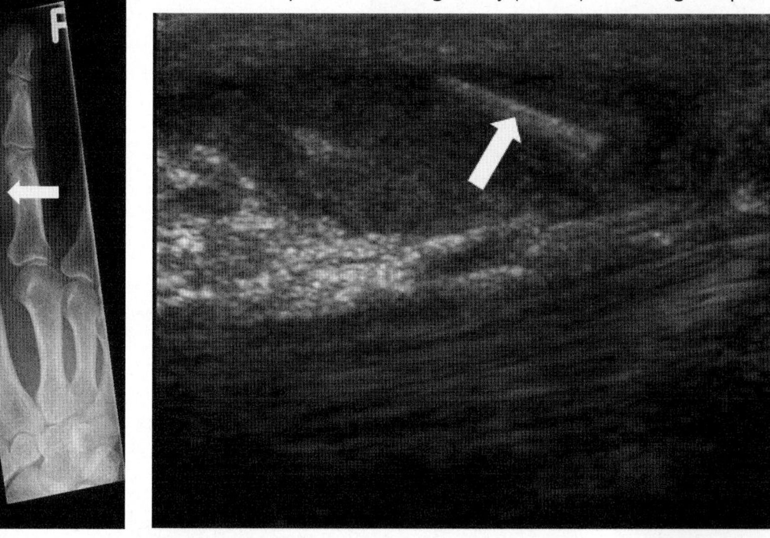

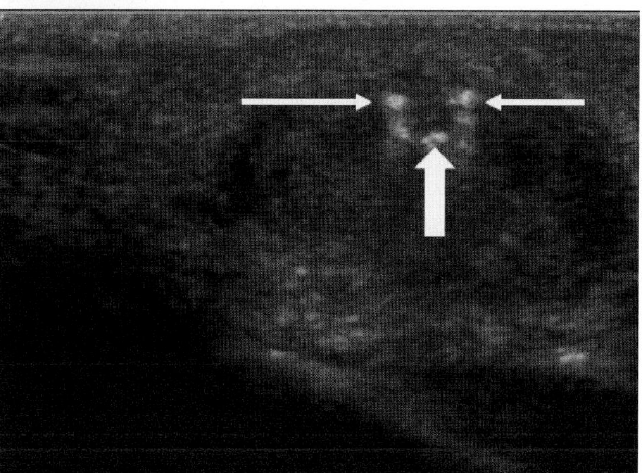

Fig. 13.5 A 53-year-old patient with a painful third right finger for 3 months after gardening. On plain films only soft tissue swelling was detectable **(A)** (*arrow*). **(B)** Ultrasound showed a foreign body surrounded by granulomatous tissue (*arrow*). Ultrasound-guided foreign body removal was performed and a thorn was extracted. **(C,D)** Ultrasound images show the forceps and the foreign body (*arrows*) on orthogonal planes.

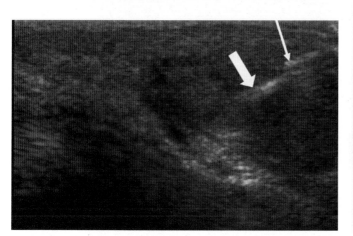

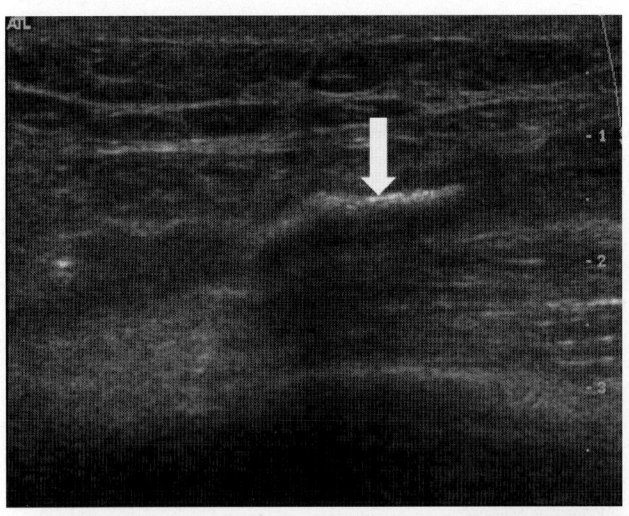

A

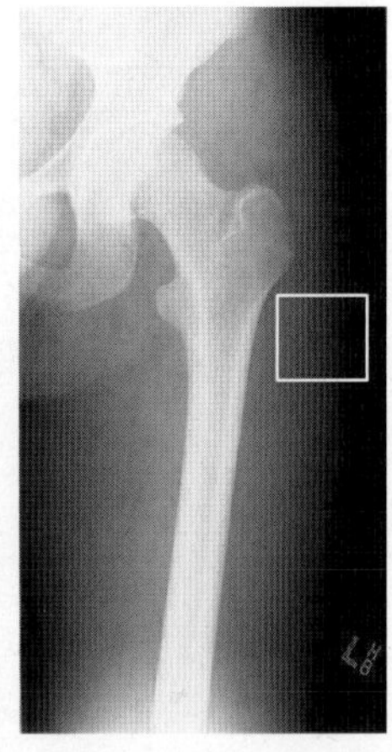

B

Fig. 13.6 After three episodes of local infection in an 18-year-old male patient, a foreign body was detected in the posterolateral thigh on ultrasound **(A). (B,C)** On radiographs, the same lesion was barely seen (*arrow*). (**D)** After ultrasound-guided removal, fluoroscopy of the specimen was performed showing a calcified splinter (*arrow*).

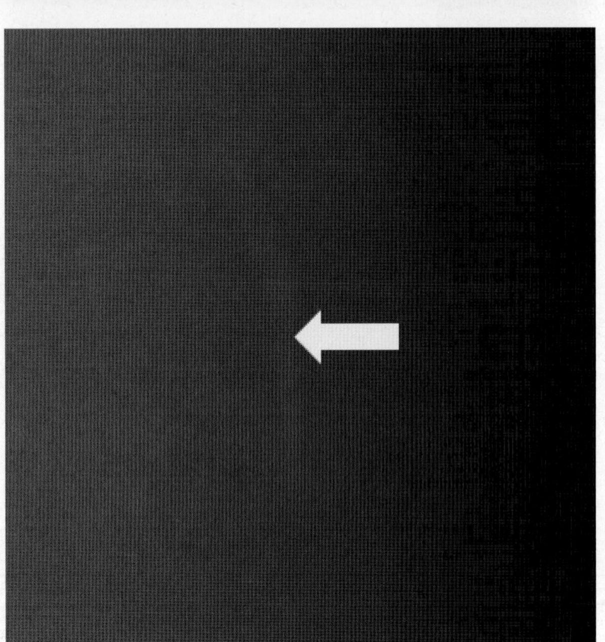

C

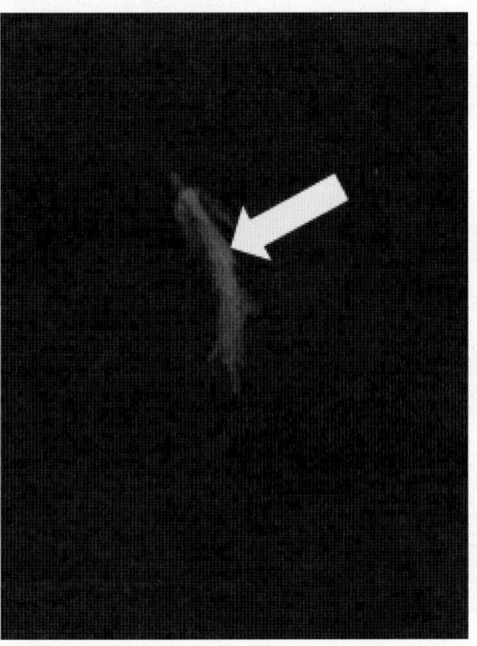

D

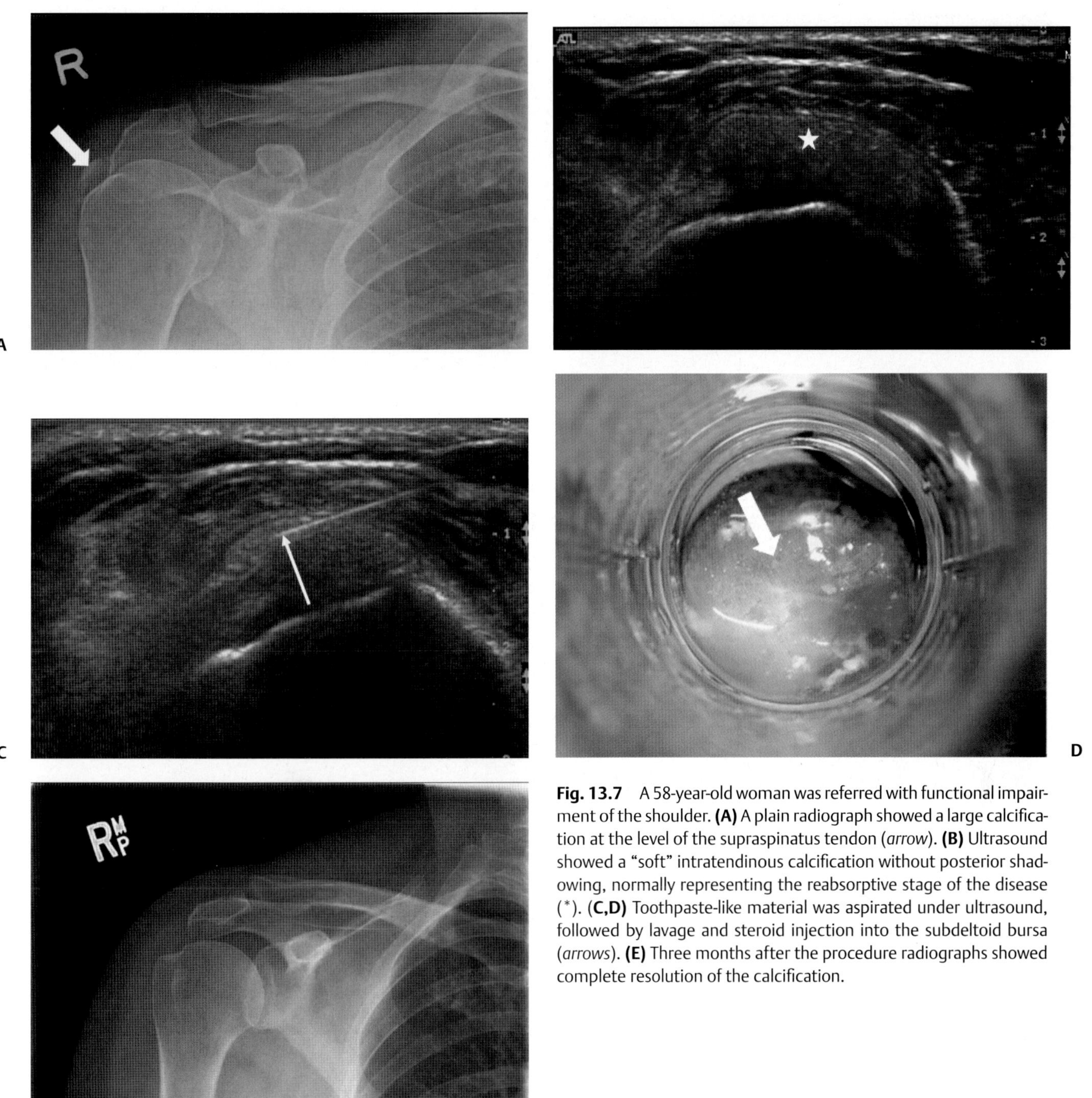

Fig. 13.7 A 58-year-old woman was referred with functional impairment of the shoulder. **(A)** A plain radiograph showed a large calcification at the level of the supraspinatus tendon (*arrow*). **(B)** Ultrasound showed a "soft" intratendinous calcification without posterior shadowing, normally representing the reabsorptive stage of the disease (*). **(C,D)** Toothpaste-like material was aspirated under ultrasound, followed by lavage and steroid injection into the subdeltoid bursa (*arrows*). **(E)** Three months after the procedure radiographs showed complete resolution of the calcification.

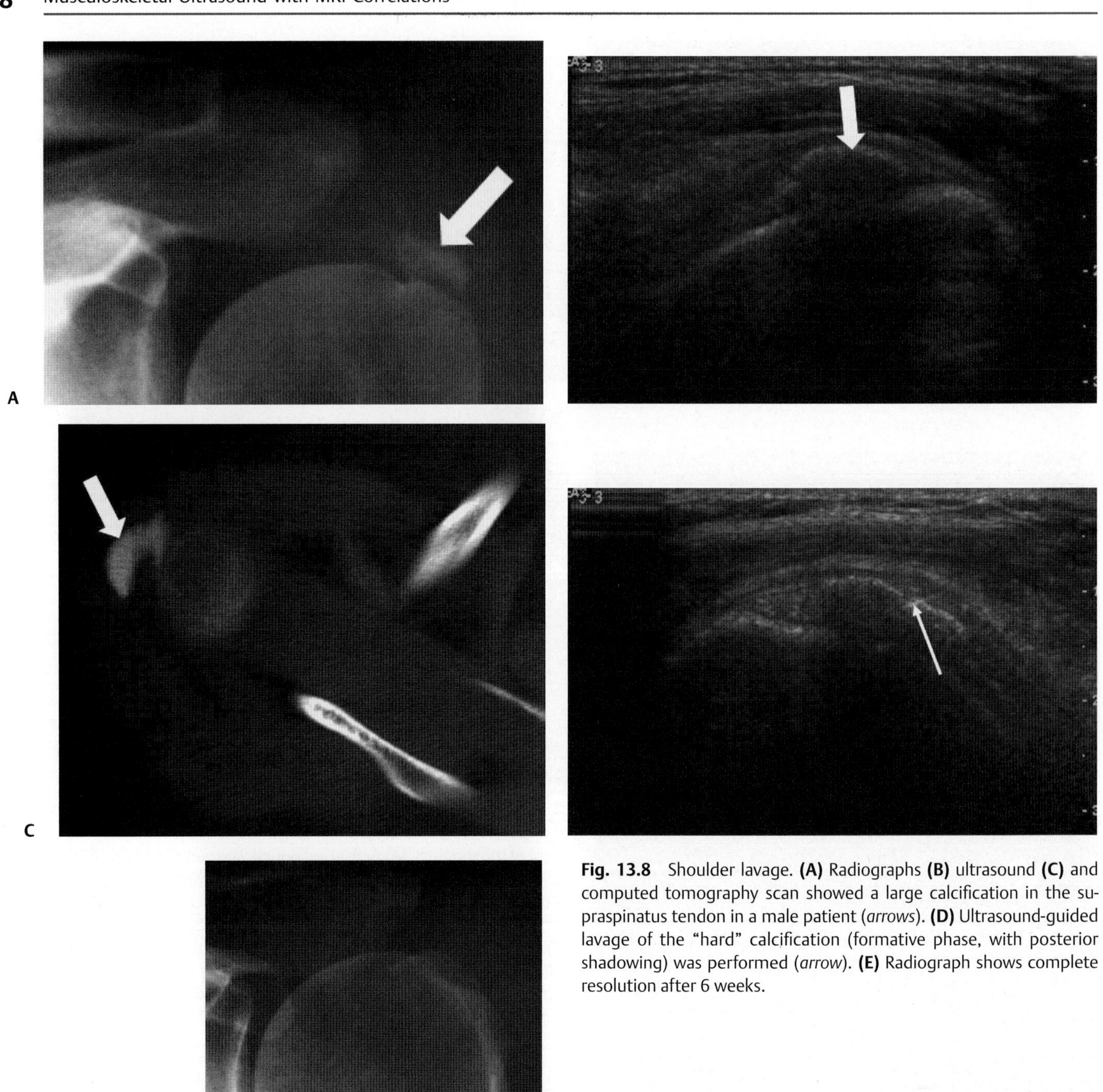

Fig. 13.8 Shoulder lavage. **(A)** Radiographs **(B)** ultrasound **(C)** and computed tomography scan showed a large calcification in the supraspinatus tendon in a male patient (*arrows*). **(D)** Ultrasound-guided lavage of the "hard" calcification (formative phase, with posterior shadowing) was performed (*arrow*). **(E)** Radiograph shows complete resolution after 6 weeks.

Fig. 13.9 A 53-year-old woman complaining of lateral elbow pain, clinically diagnosed as golfer's elbow. **(A)** A radiograph shows a large calcification at the common flexor tendon insertion (*arrow*). **(B,C)** Ultrasound shows the "soft" calcification (*) and the close relationship to the ulnar nerve (N) (*arrow*). **(C)** Ultrasound-guided lavage was performed, carefully avoiding damaging the ulnar nerve. **(D)** Milky fluid was aspirated and the **(E)** computed tomography performed right after the procedure shows significant reduction of the calcification (*arrow*). (F) One month after the procedure, the patient reported significant pain reduction and only tiny residual calcifications were seen on radiographs (*arrow*).

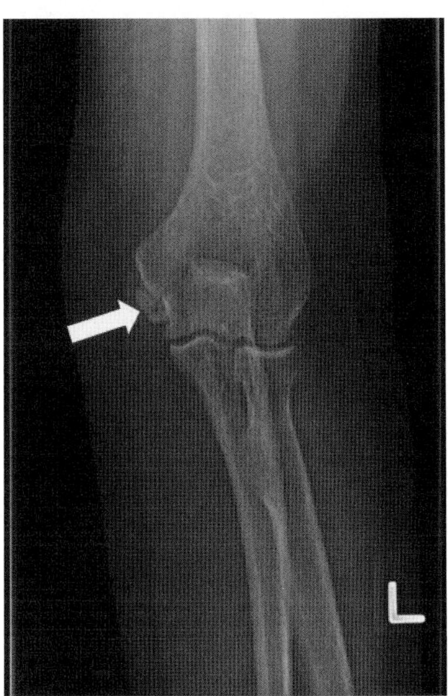

A

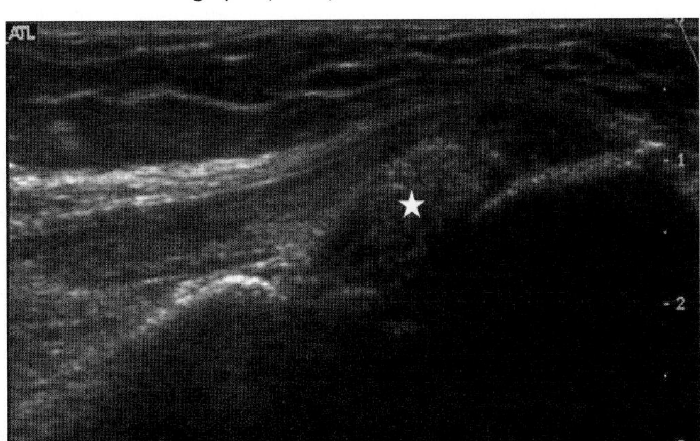

B

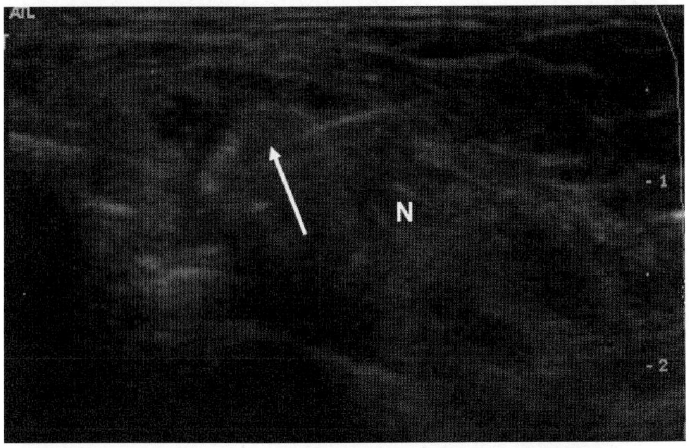

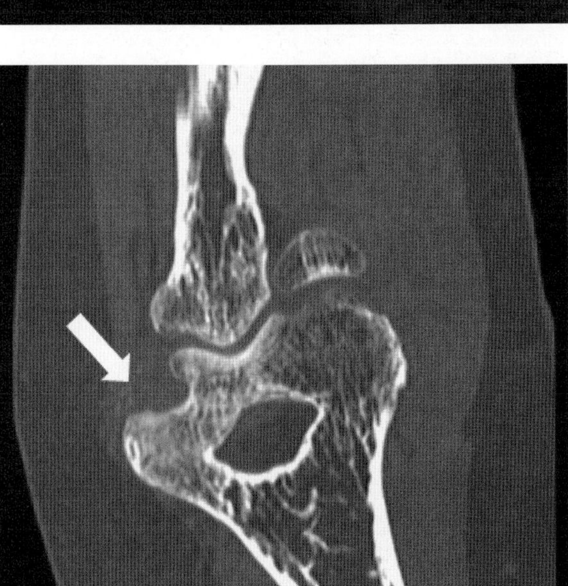

C

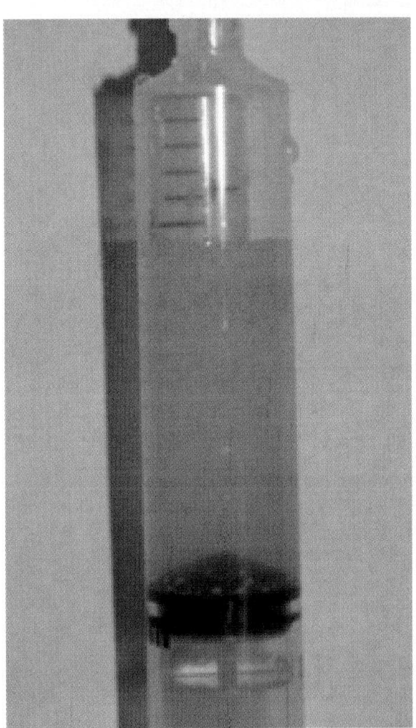

D

E

duced inflammation caused by local diffusion of the calcific material.

Clinical improvement during the first weeks is reported in up to 91% of procedures, but in our experience a few patients, mostly those with large calcifications, experience recurrent pain after 2 to 3 weeks. A further subdeltoid bursa injection with steroids is usually effective in these cases, we consider this as an ongoing crystal-induced bursitis when drug effectiveness decreases. On radiographs, calcifications disappear or at least reduce in size and density over the first month after lavage. However, once ruptured, calcifications almost invariably evolve toward resorption, and pain and disability improve in most cases. If calcifications are still present, repeated lavage should be performed after 6 to 8 weeks. In cases of unsuccessful lavage, pain of other origin should be considered (**Fig. 13.10**).

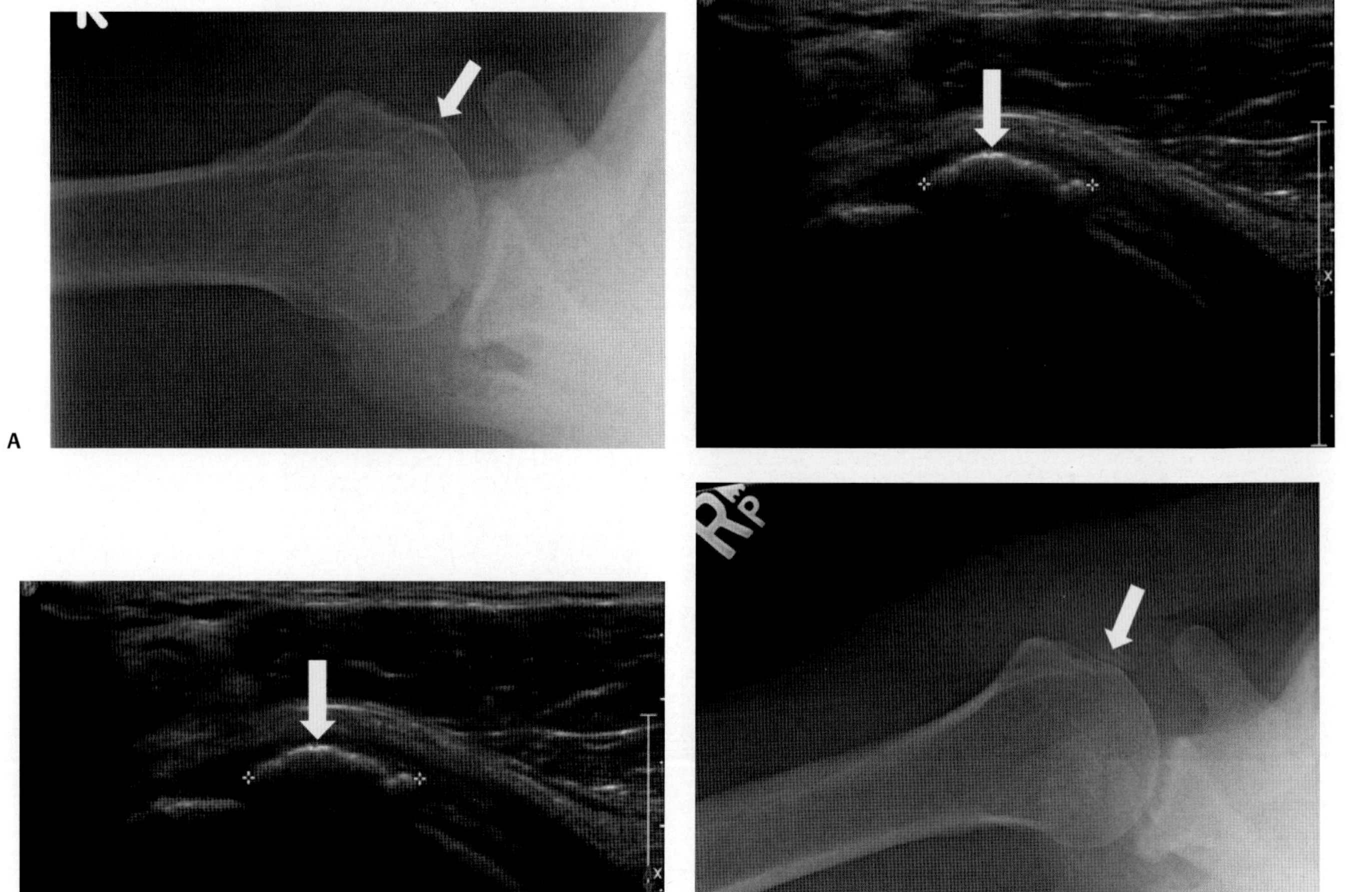

Fig. 13.10 **(A)** A 44-year-old male patient with a calcification at the level of the subscapularis tendon on radiographs was sent for ultrasound-guided aspiration and lavage of the calcification. **(B)** Although a solid calcification was noted on ultrasound (*arrow*), **(C)** lavage of the calcification was not successful (*arrow*). **(D)** Radiographs were repeated and they showed the calcification was actually a bone fragment, most likely from previous avulsion (*arrow*). Therefore, correct diagnosis is crucial for a successful treatment.

Fluid Drainage

Ultrasound is the method of choice for imaging fluid-containing lesions of the musculoskeletal system. Using ultrasound guidance, aspiration of cysts, abscesses, hematomas, and joint effusions can be easily and accurately performed. The purpose of fluid aspiration is twofold: laboratory analysis of aspirated fluid allows for better diagnosis and leads to local decompression, which reduces the patient's pain. Ultrasound also can be used to monitor the efficacy of the intervention.

Cysts

Ganglion cysts (**Figs. 13.11** and **13.12**), meniscal cysts, labral cysts (**Fig. 13.13**), and synovial cysts are other indications for percutaneous needle aspiration when they become symptomatic. The most frequent cysts are ganglion cysts at the wrist and Baker cysts in the popliteal fossa, appearing as anechoic or hypoechoic lesions with posterior acoustic enhancement and delimited by fibrous walls. Rarely, cysts present with heterogeneous or hyperechoic patterns, but septation of cysts is a common finding and should be considered during intervention.

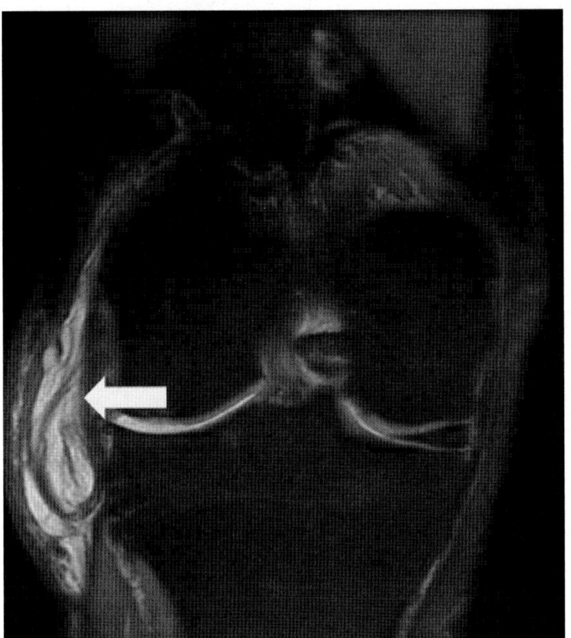

A

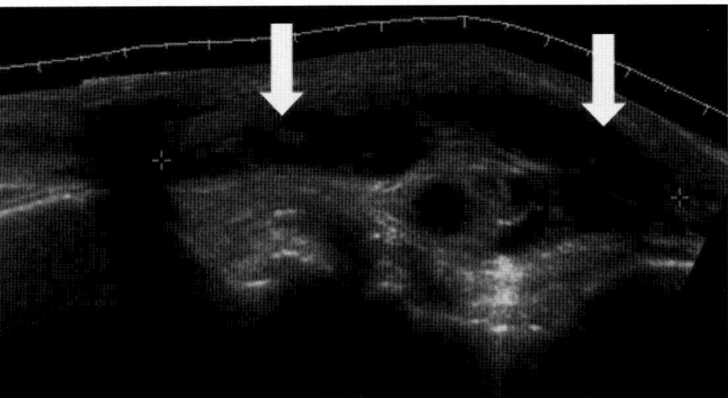

B

C

Fig. 13.11 Right knee pain in a 65-year-old man with known osteoarthritis. **(A)** A multilobulated ganglion cyst adjacent to the posterior aspect of the iliotibial band was present in a coronal fat-saturated fast spin echo proton density magnetic resonance image (*arrow*) and **(B)** on ultrasound (*arrows*). **(C)** Ultrasound-guided aspiration and injection was performed (*arrow*), but the cyst recurred in a few months and knee arthroplasty was necessary.

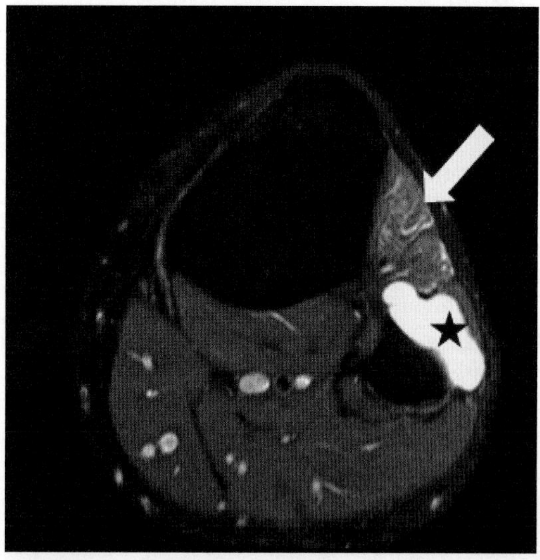
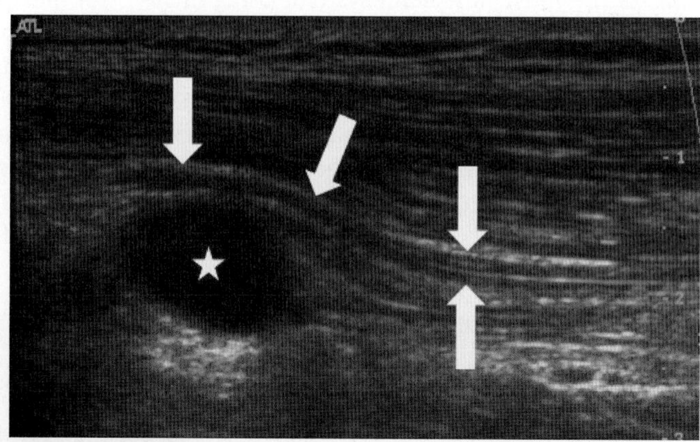
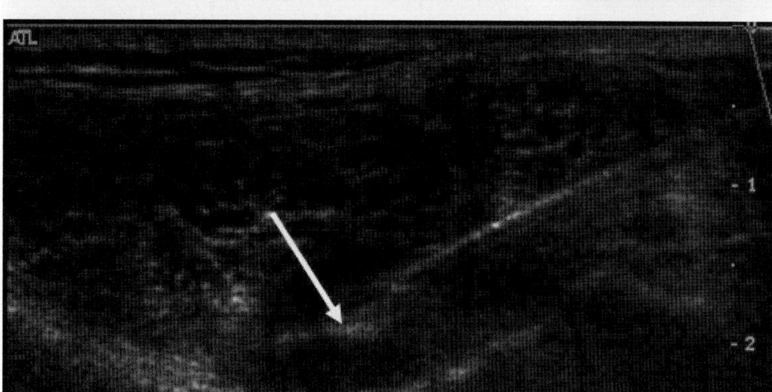

A B C

Fig. 13.12 An intraneural mass was suspected in this 17-year-old man. **(A)** An axial fat-saturated proton density magnetic resonance image (MRI) demonstrated a lobulated cystic mass (*) arising from the proximal tibiofibular joint. **(B)** On ultrasound, compression of the common peroneal nerve (*arrows*) by the ganglion cyst (*) was noted, which would explain the high signal in the peroneus muscles on MRI representing muscle denervation. **(C)** Ultrasound-guided aspiration and injection of corticosteroids and anesthetics was performed (*arrow*).

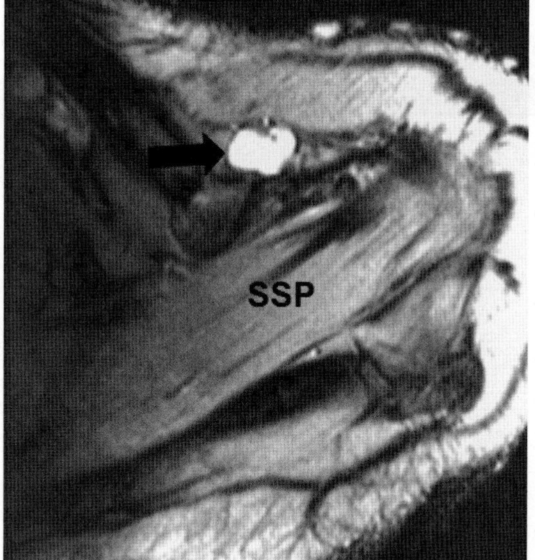

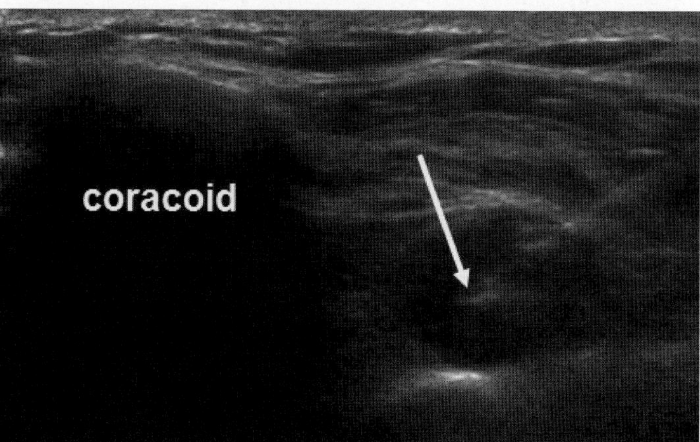

A B

Fig. 13.13 **(A)** Axial multiplanar gradient recalled acquisition in the steady state (MPGR) magnetic resonance image sequence at the level of the supraspinatus tendon (SSP) of a 50-year-old man with clinically suspected frozen shoulder syndrome. **(B)** A ganglion cyst (*arrow*) located between the coracoid and subscapularis tendon with a connection to the glenohumeral joint was present. Aspiration and injection of corticosteroids was performed using ultrasound guidance, resulting in an immediate decrease of pain and increased functionality.

Color Doppler is useful for differentiation of vascular alterations, such as aneurysm and pseudoaneurysm. Dynamic compression under ultrasound may reveal the fluctuant nature of cysts, although some cysts are solid and noncompressible. All cysts may become symptomatic due to increased internal pressure, compression of surrounding structures as nerves and vessels, rupture, or chronic inflammation. Besides surgery, ultrasound-guided percutaneous needle aspiration also should be considered as a treatment option. The content of the cysts, especially ganglion cysts, can be extremely gelatinous and dense; therefore, larger needles of 14- to 20-gauge should be used for aspiration. For complete drainage of the collection, a wash-out of the cyst with saline solution can be helpful, but whether they should undergo further injection with corticosteroids is controversial. Short-term results of this procedure are very good, although a recurrence rate of 21 to 60% is described in the literature. Therefore, it cannot be considered as the definitive treatment, but it is nevertheless a minimally invasive technique to manage the ganglia. In case of symptomatic recurrence, repeating ultrasound-guided aspiration or surgery (recurrence rate of 1–34%) can be considered.

Abscesses

Abscesses of the soft tissue can be caused by trauma, surgery, foreign bodies, osteomyelitis, and as a result of the extension of nearby or distant infectious processes under predisposing conditions, such as diabetes, renal insufficiency, and immunosuppression. Instead of surgical removal, abscesses can be aspirated or drained under ultrasound guidance, which allows the assessment of the best pathway toward the accumulation and the accurate placement of the needle or drainage catheter. For aspiration, a large, 18- to 20-gauge needle is recommended for suction of the viscous pus (**Fig. 13.14**). Because the diagnosis of an abscess is not always clear by imaging alone, bacteriologic culture of the aspirated fluid can confirm an abscess and the best antibiotic treatment can be assessed by an antibiogram. Aspiration in combination with an appropriate antibiotic regimen can be sufficient to cure the infection. Drainage catheters may be required for larger abscesses, which can be installed by using the Seldinger technique or the trocar system. The Seldinger technique uses a needle to puncture the accumulation and a guide wire is placed inside the abscess through this needle (**Fig. 13.15**). After serial dilatation of the track over the wire, a drainage catheter is finally placed in the cavity and allowed to curl inside. For large, superficial abscesses the trocar system is used as it requires less time and less manipulation. It consists of an 8- to 10-F catheter mounted on a hollow rigid metallic guide, through which a mobile needle can puncture through the soft tissue and then be pulled out after the catheter is inserted. The catheter is connected to a collector, and is maintained until the patient is afebrile, has normal blood tests, and the drain is producing

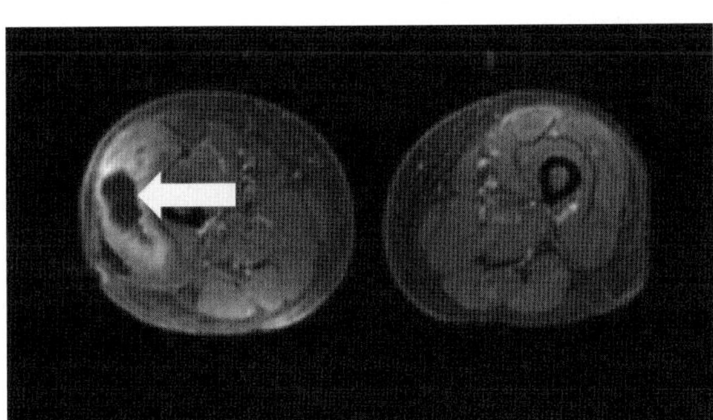
A

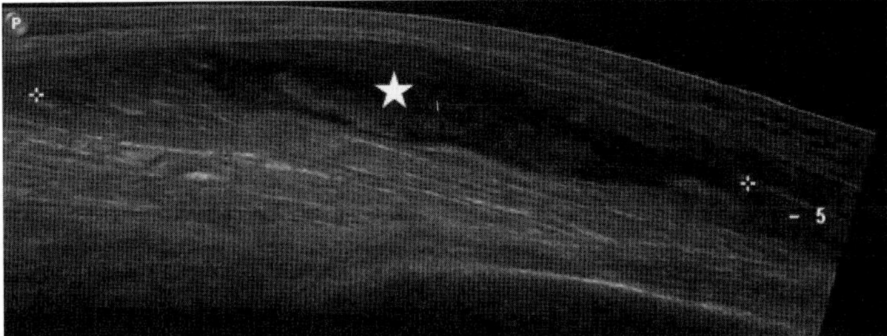
B

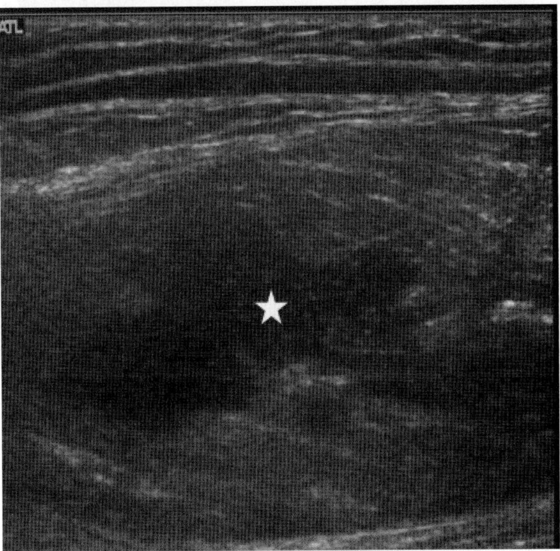
C

Fig. 13.14 Clinically suspected thigh abscess in a 60-year-old patient. **(A)** Axial T1 fat-saturated gadolinium enhanced magnetic resonance image showing peripheral enhancing lesion (*arrow*) in the vastus medialis muscle. **(B,C)** Ultrasound scanning demonstrated a large echogenic fluid collection (*), suggestive of infection. Fluid aspirated under ultrasound guidance appeared to be pus mixed with hemorrhage and microbiology revealed *Staphylococcus aureus* infection.

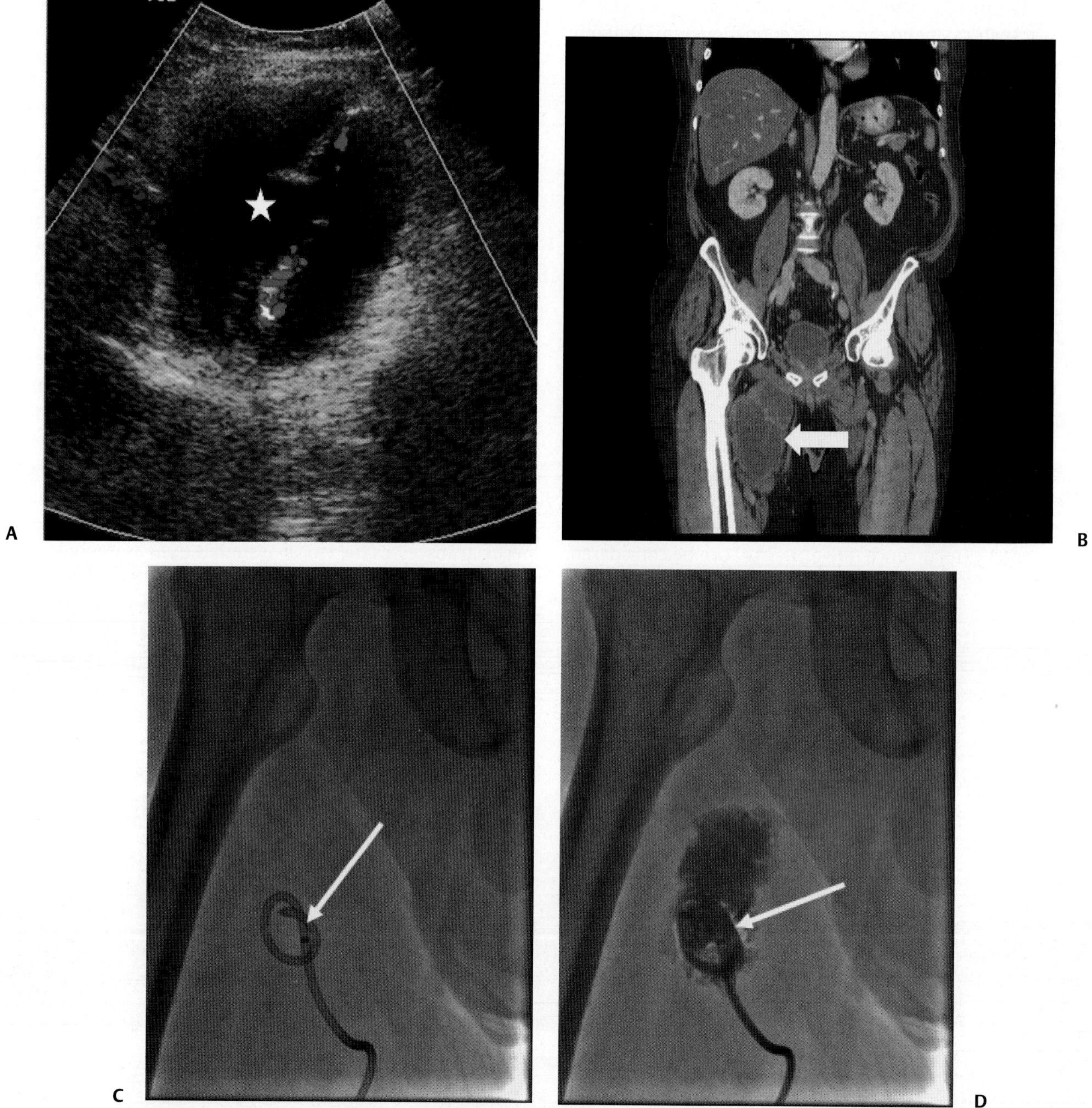

Fig. 13.15 After radical prostatectomy, an urinoma was detected in the right adductor compartment on ultrasound **(A)** **(*)** and computed tomography (CT) (*arrow*) **(B)** in a 60-year-old patient. Ultrasound detected hyperemia and septation inside the lesion that was suspicious for infection. Aspiration under ultrasound confirmed the presence of pus; a drainage catheter was placed using the Seldinger technique. Culture of the aspirated fluid revealed a *Candida* infection and antifungal treatment was initialized. **(C)** Fluoroscopy before contrast injection (*arrow*). **(D)** Fluoroscopy after contrast injection (*arrow*).

less than 10 mL/day for three consecutive days. Obstruction of the catheter occurs very commonly due to clots or viscous pus, so frequent flushing with saline should be performed. In the literature, healing of the abscess using this method is reported in ~80% of cases. In the cases in which it is unsuccessful, drainage can help to control infection and reduce the size of the abscess to make surgery easier.

Hematomas

Hematomas of the musculoskeletal system have generally a traumatic origin and appear as more or less well-defined hypoechoic lesions with internal echoes on ultrasound. They also may have fluid–fluid levels and will become hyperechoic when healing is followed by fibrous encasement, calcifications, or ossification of the hematoma. The usefulness of evacuating hematomas is still debated. Some physicians believe they should be aspirated to obtain prompt recovery and reduce the risk of fibrous adhesions; others consider these lesions to be a self-healing condition and believe that aspiration is an unnecessary procedure with an increased risk of secondary infections. Small asymptomatic hematomas may require only conservative treatment because they are spontaneously reabsorbed. Larger hematomas can produce pain, mass effects, and may cause a compartment syndrome. In all these cases, evacuation by ultrasound-guided aspiration should be performed (**Fig. 13.16**). For some pa-

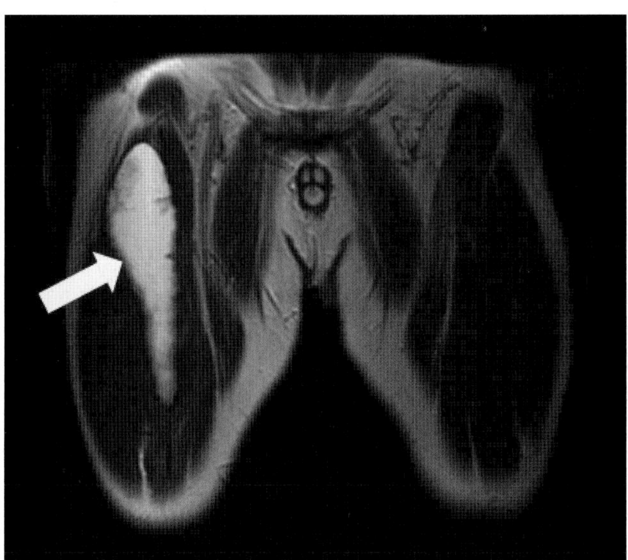

A

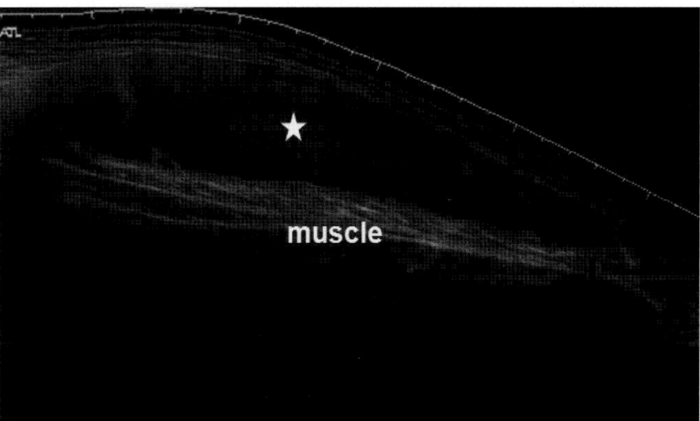

B

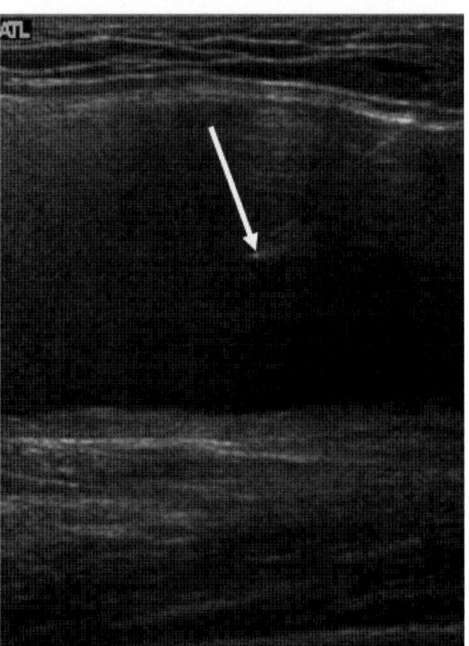

C

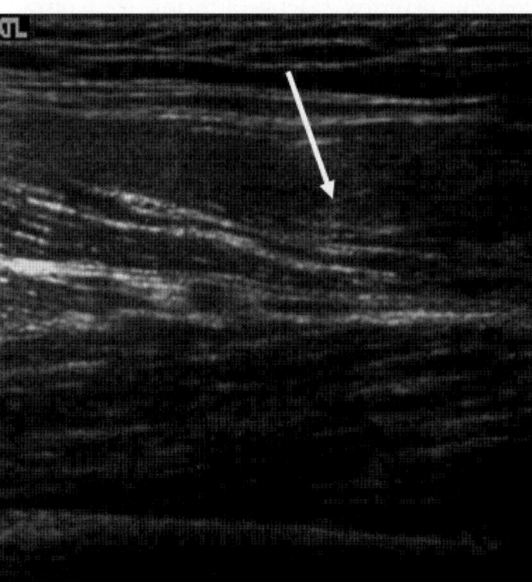

D

Fig. 13.16 After trauma in a 41-year-old man, a large hematoma (*arrow*) was detected in the rectus femoris muscle of the right thigh on coronal T2-weighted fast spin echo magnetic resonance image **(A)**. After 5 months, the lesion (*) was still present on ultrasound **(B)**, and an ultrasound-guided procedure was performed with aspiration of 200 cc of fluid (*arrow*) **(C)** and complete collapse (*arrow*) of the collection **(D)**.

tients, drainage catheters as described for abscesses are necessary and fibrinolytic substances may be used to resolve the hematoma. In muscular strains, particularly in athletes, hematoma aspiration with 18- to 20-gauge needles can be used to accelerate the healing process by reapproximating muscle fibers. Clinical improvement with total or partial resolution is usually achieved in all patients. If symptoms are still present in cases of partial resolution, repeating the procedure and/or installing a drainage catheter may be a treatment option.

Joints

Fluid aspiration of joints may be required in various conditions, such as infection, inflammatory disease, osteoarthritis, and crystal arthropathies, and less commonly in amyloidosis. Although aspiration can be performed by a clinician in acute cases, ultrasound guidance provides real-time visibility of the needle during the procedure, confirms the intraarticular placement of the needle, and shows immediately if the intervention was successful or if residual fluid remains. Furthermore, ultrasound allows for detecting small fluid accumulations where saline may be first injected within the joint and reaspirated for further analysis. Aspiration not only acquires fluid for laboratory analysis, but also relieves pain and disability. Aspiration and injections of joints usually are performed at the same time, except when infection is suspected. A more-detailed description of the procedure in different joints will be given later.

■ Injection

In rheumatoid arthritis, osteoarthritis, or other forms of systemic disease with joint or tendon involvement (e.g., juvenile idiopathic arthritis, reactive arthritis, etc.), ultrasound-guided intraarticular steroid injection is a relatively simple and cost-effective treatment option. If bursae, tendon, or tendon sheath involvement is more dominant (e.g., psoriasis, overuse), injections of these structures can be performed. Corticosteroids are widely considered as the drug of choice for injection, but newer studies address other substances in different diseases (e.g., hyaluronic acid in osteoarthritis). The goal of injections in all pathologies is the reduction of inflammation, what can be easily monitored by ultrasound, although infection of the region of interest should be excluded prior to ultrasound-guided injection.

In general, the injection within joints, bursae, and tendon sheaths (**Fig. 13.17**) consists of corticosteroids alone or a mixture of corticosteroid and local anesthetic. We use a mixture of corticosteroids (e.g., Betaject, Bayer Healthcare, LLC, Shawnee Mission, KS, and Celestone, Schering-Plough, Kenilworth, NJ) and a long-acting anesthetic. Marcaine 0.5% was commonly used for intra- and extraarticular injection, but there has been a recent warning about possible cartilage damage caused by this particular anesthetic. Therefore, our institution presently uses ropivacaine for intraarticular injections. The dose and volume of the injected steroid should be adjusted for the individual size of the cavity and the size of the joint. It is possible to use less in interphalangeal joints (2.5 mg/0.5 mL) compared with larger regions, where injection of 40 mg/2 mL is possible. However, an injection should be stopped when a "sensation of ballooning" is reported by the patient because this is a sign prior to disruption. Efficacy of local therapy depends not only on the amount and type of the injected drugs, but also on the appropriate space or structure into which the solution is injected. A small dose of steroids instilled within an inflamed bursa is far more effective than a larger dose injected in the adjacent tissues and has fewer side effects, which highlights the usefulness of ultrasound guidance.

The most common indication for aspirations and injections is osteoarthritis, but it is also used in rheumatoid arthritis and spondyloarthritis, or in other systemic diseases involving joints and tendons.

Shoulder

In glenohumeral joint arthritis, fluid tends to accumulate in the posterior aspect of the joint; therefore, a posterior approach through the infraspinatus muscle with the patient sitting or in a semiprone position is mostly used. The needle pathway should be directed to the joint space immediately deep to the free margin of the glenoid labrum and tangential to the curvature of the humeral head.

For acromioclavicular joint injection, a cranial approach with the patient supine or sitting is suggested. Only small amounts of a drug should be injected in this joint because of the risk of capsule or ligament rupture.

The subdeltoid-subacromial bursa is another frequently injected area of the shoulder, where blind injection failure was reported in 13 to 71% of cases. Therefore, ultrasound-guided injections should be considered seriously, particularly in patients with no or insufficient response to previous blind injection. An anterior or lateral approach with the patient sitting or supine is recommended, with real-time visualization of the needle in a parallel position.

Ultrasound-guided injection is also useful for the treatment of inflammation of the long head of the biceps tendon, a common finding in overuse injuries. A longitudinal view of the tendon with the patient sitting or supine allows for best visualization of the intervention.

Elbow

When a large amount of fluid is present, the cubital joint can be punctured from a posterior approach to allow access to the olecranon recess. As an alternative, an anterolateral approach through the radiocapitellar joint or anteromedial toward the humeroulnar joint is feasible.

Enthesopathy at the lateral (tennis elbow) or medial epicondyles (golfer's elbow) are other common causes of elbow

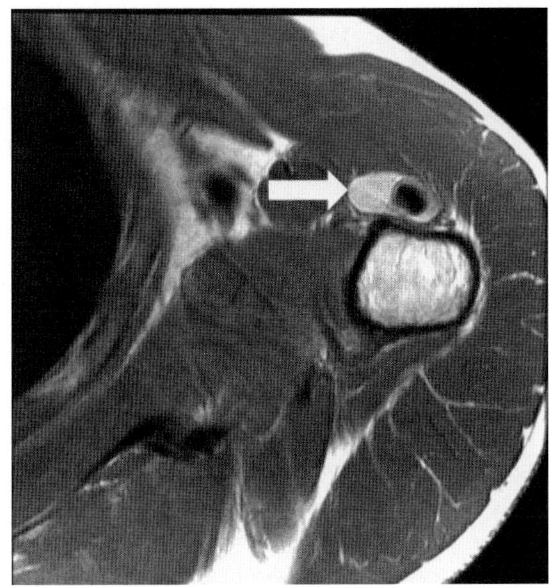

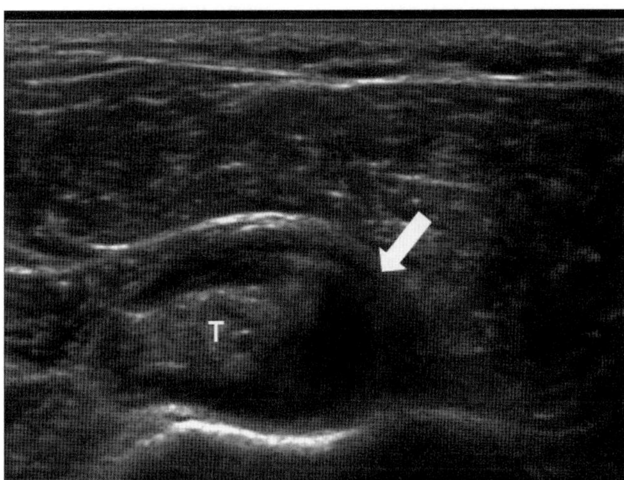

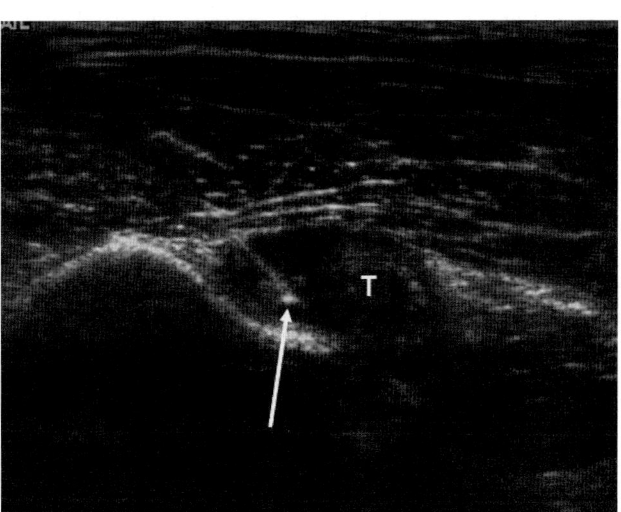

Fig. 13.17 **(A)** Axial proton density magnetic resonance image at the level of the left proximal humerus showed high signal intensity around the long head of the biceps tendon with thickening of the tendon (*arrow*). **(B)** Corresponding axial ultrasound image demonstrated distinct tenovaginitis and tendinopathy (*arrow*) in a 46-year-old patient with chronic alterations and no response to conservative measures. **(C)** Steroid injection was performed using a 25-gauge needle with good response. T, tendon.

pain. Ultrasound guidance can be useful for peritendinous injection to avoid intratendinous placement of corticosteroids. Puncture is performed parallel to the tendon and drugs can be injected immediately superficial to the tendon origin. Another option in these enthesopathies is tenotomy (or dry needling), where repeated puncture (needling) of the areas of mucoid degeneration is performed under local anesthesia. Peritendinous polidocanol injections or intratendinous autologous blood injections also have been described in the literature.

Wrist

The radiocarpal joint can be injected easily under ultrasound guidance using a dorsal approach. Comfortable positioning with the patient supine, and their arm placed at the side of the body with the dorsal aspect of the wrist facing upward should be attempted. The puncture point is localized ~1 to 2 cm distal to the Lister tubercle, between the second and third, or third and fourth extensor tendon compartments. Using ultrasound guidance, needle placement through the tendons, tendon sheaths, or small vessels can be avoided. In some cases, separate injections of the distal radioulnar joint may be necessary.

Tenosynovitis is a frequent finding in rheumatoid arthritis and spondyloarthropathies, but it may also result from overuse injury. Because intratendinous injections may result in tendon rupture, care has to be taken to guarantee peritendinous placement of the drugs (**Fig. 13.18**). Detailed assessment regarding the degree of tendinopathy (partial tears, full-thickness tears) that could bear a higher risk of tendon damage is necessary, and should be discussed with the patient. Generally, injection into the tendon sheath is a safe procedure with very few complications. The affected tendon is best approached first longitudinally; then after the needle

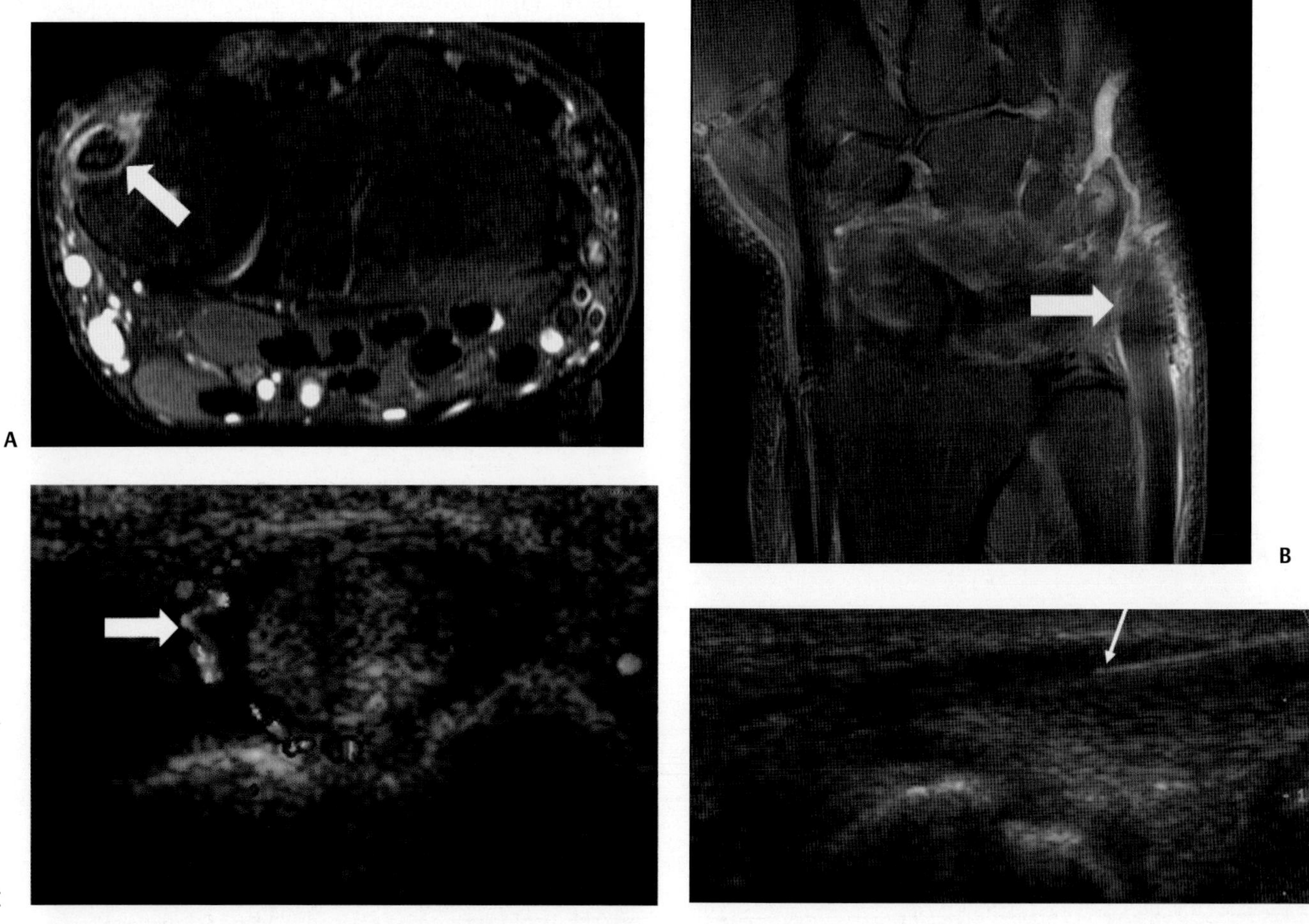

Fig. 13.18 **(A)** Axial inversion recovery magnetic resonance image (MRI) at the level of the distal radius shows high signal around the extensor carpi ulnaris (ECU) tendon (*arrow*) in a 45-year-old man with a history of injury. **(B)** Coronal proton density turbo spin echo T2-weighted MRI demonstrates tenovaginitis and tendinopathy at the insertion of the ECU tendon (*arrow*). **(C)** Axial ultrasound scan confirmed MRI findings and showed increased vascular flow on Doppler signal in the tendon sheath (*arrow*). **(D)** Longitudinal ultrasound image shows peritendinous placement of 25-gauge needle (*arrow*). Care must be taken to avoid intratendinous steroid injections due to the risk of further tendon damage.

tip is placed inside the tendon sheath, an axial plane image should verify correct needle placement. During injection, both planes should be used to ascertain peritendinous placement of the drug because intratendinous injection may result in local damage and increased risk of rupture. A 27-gauge needle can be used in most cases for tendon injection, and injection should result in distension of the tendon sheath; however, this can be compromised by tendon sheath adhesions, resulting in local accumulation of the administrated drug and consequently repeated injections may be necessary.

Small Joints

For intercarpal, intertarsal, metacarpophalangeal, metatarsophalangeal, proximal, and distal interphalangeal joints, a dorsal oblique approach, laterally or medially to the extensor tendon using a hockey stick probe is an easy and safe pathway for aspiration and/or injection. Fluid accumulations are normally very small in these joints; therefore, injection by real-time ultrasound guidance seems to be the best way to access these small joints (**Fig. 13.19**).

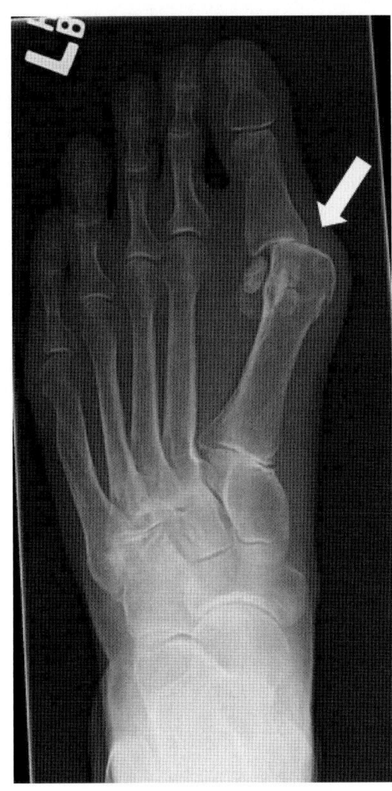

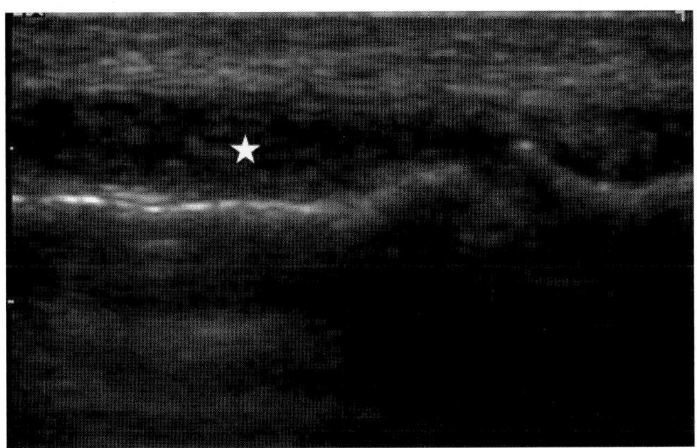

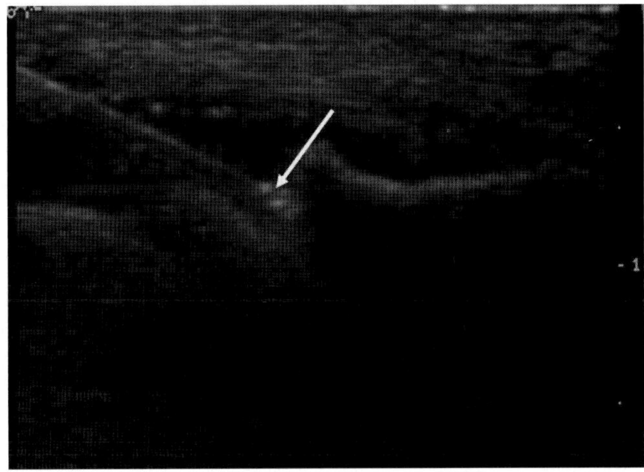

Fig. 13.19 **(A)** Hallux valgus in a 58-year-old woman showing deformity of the first left metatarsophalangeal joint (*arrow*) on plain film. **(B)** On ultrasound, an intraarticular fluid collection (*) was seen due to the osteoarthritic alterations. Fluoroscopy-guided injection was requested, but because the joint space was very small, ultrasound guidance was preferred by the radiologist. **(C)** Ultrasound image shows intraarticular needle placement and joint capsule enlarging after injection (*arrow*).

Hip

With the patient in supine position, an anterolateral access under the inguinal ligament toward the anterior synovial recess at the junction of the femoral head and neck should be chosen. As the needle passes the iliofemoral ligament, a slight increase in resistance can be encountered. With further advance, the needle can be felt to "pop" through the ligament and enter the hip joint. Caution has to be taken to avoid large vessels and nerves at this region, and direct injection into the ligament should be avoided due to the risk of rupture.

Knee

Knee joint injection without image guidance can be readily performed with a high degree of accuracy; however, a more accurate needle placement can be obtained using ultrasound guidance. Image guidance is especially useful in obese patients, patients with swollen legs, and when only a small amount of fluid is present. With the patient lying in supine position and the knee angulated at 20 to 30 degrees, the needle is inserted from the lateral aspect of the joint at the superior margin of the patella toward the suprapatellar recess, where in pathologic conditions fluid is detectable. If the recess is not discernible on ultrasound, the needle can be placed in the joint cavity, but using this traditional approach the needle is covered by bone and intraarticular placement cannot be demonstrated. Some authors have proposed injecting air inside the joint cavity, which will move to the suprapatellar recess, thus making it visible. However, air is not sterile and we prefer not to use this method. Symptomatic Baker cysts are accessed from a dorsal approach (**Fig. 13.20**), and ultrasound-guided aspiration and injection can be especially helpful when septation or a multilobulated Baker cyst is present.

Ankle

For injection or aspiration of the ankle, an anterior approach is recommended after localizing the anterior tibial artery. Avoiding artery and extensor tendons, the needle can be directly inserted toward the joint where fluid or synovial proliferation can be detected in most pathologic conditions. Tendons such as the Achilles tendon, plantar fascia, flexor hallucis longus, peroneus (**Fig. 13.21**), and tibialis tendons are commonly involved in systemic diseases and sports injuries, and are often referred for corticosteroid injection. No general technique can be implemented in these cases, but an intratendinous placement of drugs should be avoided because of the risk of tendon rupture. After assessing the needle's position in relation to the neurovascular bundles and other tendons, a longitudinal scan perpendicular to the needle should be attempted, as it affords better visualiza-

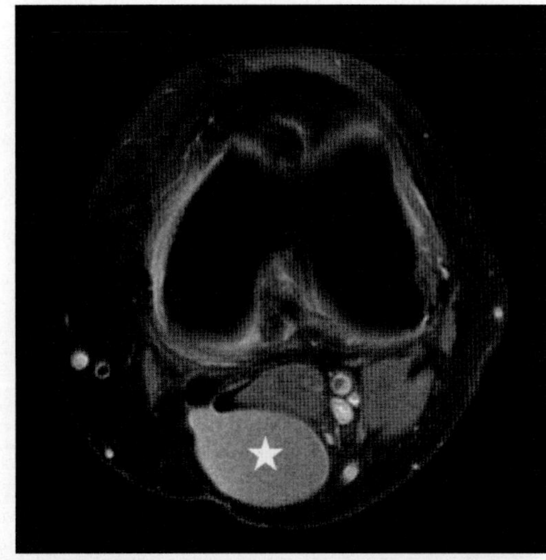

Fig. 13.20 Symptomatic Baker cyst in the left knee in a 57-year-old woman. **(A)** Axial fat-saturated fast spin echo proton density magnetic resonance image and **(B)** longitudinal ultrasound scan showed a large fluid accumulation in the popliteal fossa (*). **(C)** Aspiration was performed under ultrasound guidance (axial view) and 20 cc of clear viscous fluid were obtained (*arrow*), with complete collapse of the Baker cyst.

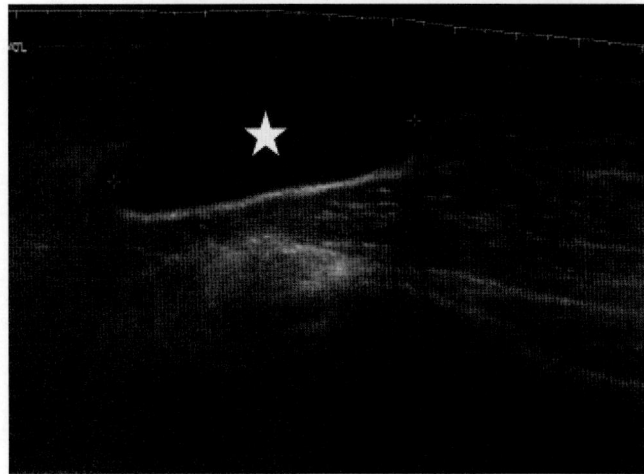

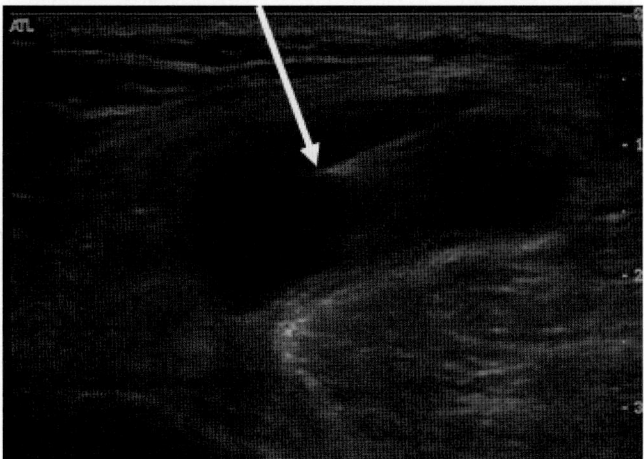

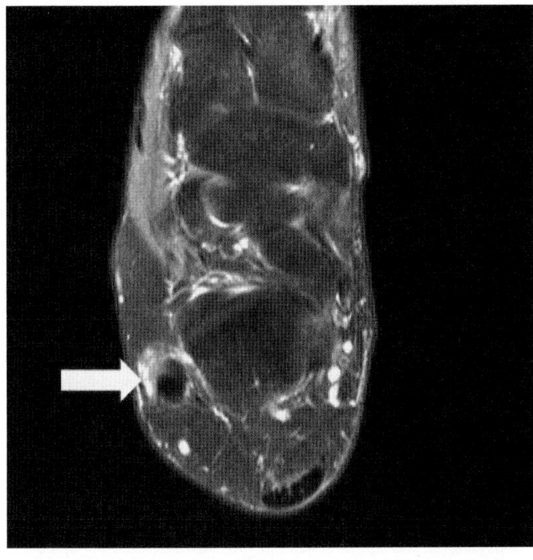

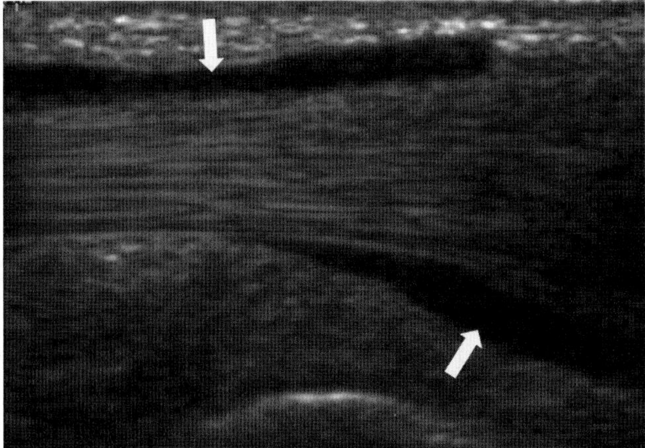

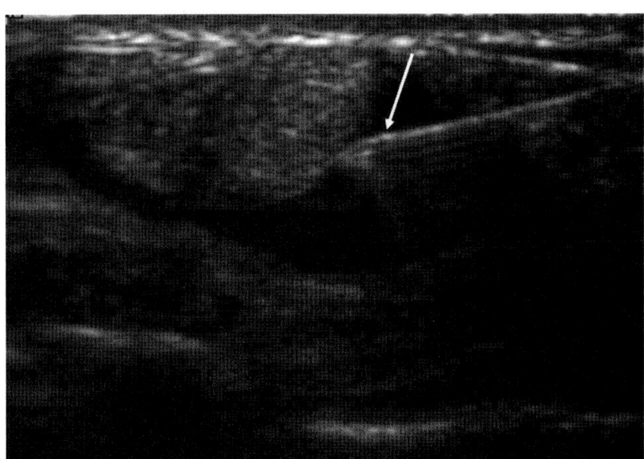

Fig. 13.21 **(A)** Axial fat-saturated T2-weighted magnetic resonance image shows high signal around the peroneus tendons representing tenovaginitis in a 58-year-old woman. A longitudinal tear of the peroneus brevis tendon (*arrow*) was present. Conservative treatment showed no improvement and ultrasound-guided injection was suggested. **(B)** Longitudinal ultrasound scan shows a hypoechoic fluid collection around the peroneus longus tendon (*arrows*). **(C)** Ultrasound-guided (axial view) injection of corticosteroids and anesthetics (*arrow*) was performed twice, resulting in a significant improvement of symptoms.

tion of the needle tip. During injection, fluid distension of the sheath results in a tenosonographic effect, which also enables improved visualization of the tendon margins.

Artifacts and Drawbacks

In ultrasound-guided interventions, the needle appears as a bright echoic line in the longitudinal view, whereas in the transverse view only a bright dot can be seen. Reverberation artifacts of the needle may be seen behind the needle when it is ~90 degrees to the ultrasound beam, which helps to highlight the needle. For accurate guidance, the tip of the needle must be visualized during the whole procedure and confirmation of the end position of the needle tip in two planes is recommended. However, it is sometimes difficult to visualize smaller caliber needles and gentle shaking of the needle can facilitate visualization, particularly when calcifications (e.g., gout) or "solid masses" (e.g., chronic synovitis) hamper clear differentiation between tissue and needle. Although some authors suggest injecting a small quantity of saline, anesthetics, or air, in our experience this can cause artifacts that decrease the visibility of the underlying structures.

Complications

Different drugs can be used for injections in the musculoskeletal system, but the most common is a mixture of anesthetic (lidocaine, bupivacaine, etc.) and corticosteroids (Betaject, triamcinolone acetonide, methylprednisolone, etc.). Although this combination is widely used, both drugs have chondrotoxic effects; therefore, each injection should be evaluated carefully. For a single joint, a maximal injection rate of 4 times is advised, with a period of 6 weeks between injections. The other side effects of steroids must also be noted, such as skin atrophy, fat necrosis, and skin depigmentation. In up to one-third of patients, local corticosteroids also may cause a local flare-up of symptoms a few days following the procedure, which may be caused by a sterile synovitis. Special care must be taken in tendon procedures to avoid intratendinous steroid placement, which has been reported to cause tendon rupture.

Ultrasound-guided interventions are operator dependent and require detailed knowledge of the relevant anatomy and a good understanding of the pathology in question, but accurate needle placement is possible after appropriate training. Ultrasound-guided procedures have also been shown to be feasible in nerve entrapment (**Fig. 13.22**), peripheral neuromas, or for local/regional anesthesia. Ultrasound is not the best imaging modality for visualizing deep lesions, lesions encased by bone, and those with overlying air-containing structures, but these cases are very rare and alternative image guidance such as CT or MRI can be used in such circumstances.

Conclusion

Ultrasound-guided interventions of the musculoskeletal system are a well-established technique for aspiration, injection, and biopsy. The advantages of ultrasound include real-time imaging, multiplanar visualization, lack of ionizing radiation exposure, and more flexible positioning of the patient. Nearby neurovascular structures can be identified and thus avoided during the procedures. Ultrasound is relatively inexpensive, widely available, and permits comparison with the asymptomatic side of the patient. All these advantages highlight the utility of this technique, but interdisciplinary discussion of each procedure is necessary to guarantee best patient care.

Proposed Algorithm for Ultrasound Guided Interventions

A. For soft tissue mass:
  1- Radiographs
  2- Ultrasound
    If cystic: aspiration
    If solid: needle biopsy after discussion with orthopedic surgeon
    If malignant: MRI for staging
B. For joint disease:
  1- Radiographs
  2- Ultrasound
    If effusion: aspiration
    If requested by rheumatologist: therapeutic injection
C. For calcific tendinitis:
  1- Radiographs
  2- Ultrasound
  3- Ultrasound-guided puncture and aspiration
  4- Ultrasound or radiographs for follow-up
D. Tendon sheath injection:
  1- Ultrasound
    If fluid in tendon sheath or thickening of tendon sheath: aspiration with or without therapeutic injection
E. Foreign body extraction:
  1- Radiographs
  2- Ultrasound
  3- Ultrasound-guided extraction if possible

A

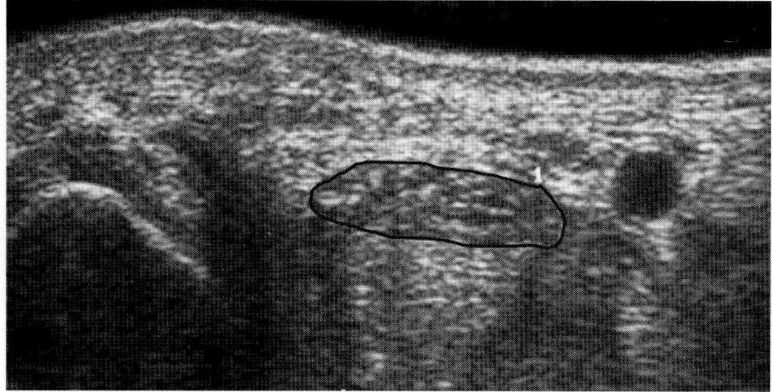

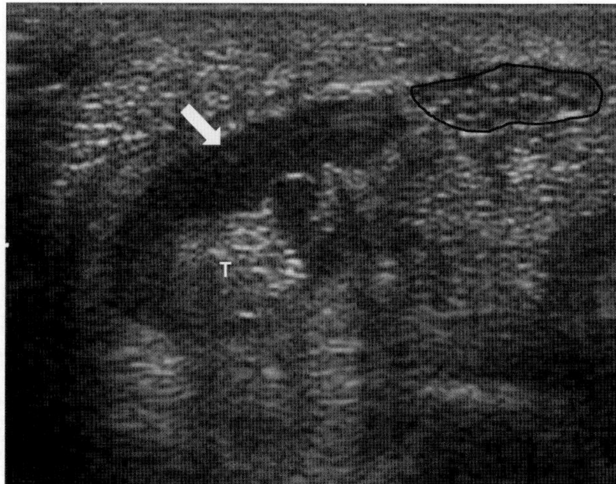

B

Fig. 13.22 Perineural injections in carpal tunnel syndrome. **(A)** Ultrasound image shows a thickened median nerve measuring 33 mm^2 in a patient complaining of typical symptoms of carpal tunnel syndrome. A 27-gauge needle was placed between the median nerve and the flexor pollicis longus tendon and a mixture of 40 mg triamcinolone acetonide and 2 mL of 0.5% Marcaine was injected adjacent to the median nerve. **(B)** After injection, widening of the radial flexor tendon sheaths (*arrow*) can be observed. Care should be taken to avoid intraneural injection as this may lead to dysesthesia and nerve damage.

Pearls and Pitfalls

- Ultrasound is a widely and readily available, nonionizing, low-cost imaging modality for guiding musculoskeletal interventions.
- Real-time ultrasound guidance allows for a highly accurate needle/instrument placement in a variety of musculoskeletal procedures, such as aspiration, injection, biopsies, foreign body extraction, and calcification puncture and lavage.
- Ultrasound provides a good anatomic overview of musculoskeletal lesions, allowing the establishment of the best pathway for the needle/instrument, but good anatomic and pathophysiologic knowledge is essential to perform accurate ultrasound-guided procedures.
- Although ultrasound-guided techniques can be learned quite quickly, initial training on a phantom model and supervision by an experienced physician is essential.
- For soft tissue tumors, careful biopsy planning is necessary to avoid seeding in adjacent compartments, which could jeopardize limb salvage surgery.
- Calcific tendinosis is generally a self-limited disease, and so risks and benefits should be carefully discussed with the patient.
- Accurate aseptic procedure is mandatory to avoid infection during all interventions, particularly during joint aspiration and injection.

Acknowledgment

The authors gratefully thank Jackie Williams for her help in editing this manuscript.

Suggested Readings

Bianchi S, Martinoli C. Ultrasound of the Musculoskeletal System. Berlin: Springer; 2007

del Cura JL, Torre I, Zabala R, Legórburu A. Sonographically guided percutaneous needle lavage in calcific tendinitis of the shoulder: short- and long-term results. AJR Am J Roentgenol 2007;189(3):W128–34

Jacobsen JA. Fundamentals of Musculoskeletal Ultrasound. Philadelphia: Saunders; 2007

McNally EG. Practical Musculoskeletal Ultrasound. Oxford: Churchill Livingstone; 2004

Van Holsbeeck MT, Introcaso JH. Musculoskeletal Ultrasound. Philadelphia: Mosby Publishing;2001

Index

Note: Page numbers followed by *f* and *t* indicate figures and tables, respectively.

A

Abductor digiti minimi muscle, 64, 77*f*, 78
Abductor pollicis brevis muscle, 77–78, 77*f*
Abductor pollicis longus tendon, 47, 47*f*, 76, 77*f*
Abscess
  aspiration, ultrasound-guided, 233, 233*f*, 234*f*
  drainage catheter installation
    Seldinger technique, 233, 234*f*
    trocar system, 233–235
  muscle, ultrasound appearance, 209*f*, 210*f*
  skin, 161
Accessory muscle(s)
  and cubital tunnel syndrome, 180, 180*f*
  in foot and ankle, 169
  in hand and fingers, 169, 169*f*
  and skin, 169–170, 169*f*
  in wrist, 46, 64–66, 66*f*–68*f*, 169
Achilles tendon, 108, 110*f*
  repair, postoperative infection, 111, 112*f*
  tear, 111*f*
    in rheumatoid arthritis, 195*f*
ACL. *See* Anterior cruciate ligament
Acoustic impedance *(Z)*
  equation for, 132
  tissue-specific, 132
Acromioclavicular joint
  inflammation, ultrasound, 14*f*
  subluxation, 135, 137*f*
  ultrasound, transverse image, 6–7, 7*f*
  ultrasound-guided injection in, 236
  widened by hematoma, ultrasound, 14*f*
Acromioplasty, postoperative ultrasound, 11–13, 14*f*
Adductor pollicis muscle, 77–78, 77*f*
ADM. *See* Abductor digiti minimi muscle
Anconeus epitrochlearis muscle, 180
Ankle. *See* Foot and ankle
Anterior cruciate ligament, tears, 102
Anterior talofibular ligament, 106, 107*f*
  anatomy, 116
  injury, 111, 113*f*
  normal anatomy, 113*f*
Anterior talotibial ligament, 108
AP. *See* Adductor pollicis muscle
APB. *See* Abductor pollicis brevis muscle
APL. *See* Abductor pollicis longus tendon
Arcade of Frohse, 182, 182*f*
Arcuate ligament, 173
Arteriovenous fistula, 59
Arthritis. *See also* Rheumatoid arthritis (RA)
  of carpometacarpal joint of thumb, 81, 81*f*
  crystal-related, wrist involvement in, 46, 52
  cubital, 24*f*, 27*f*, 30*f*, 33*f*, 40, 40*f*–41*f*
  in foot and ankle, 110
  psoriatic
    periostitis in, 139, 142*f*
    and tenosynovitis in hand and fingers, 82, 84*f*

B

Baker cyst, 94*f*, 100–101, 100*f*–101*f*
  ultrasound-guided aspiration/injection, 240, 240*f*
Basal cell carcinoma, 150–151, 153*f*
BCC. *See* Basal cell carcinoma
Biceps femoris tendon, 93, 178*f*
  tendinopathy, 103
Biceps tendon
  dislocation, 19, 19*f*
  distal, rupture, 26*f*, 39, 39*f*
  long head
    dislocation, 19, 19*f*
    ultrasound
      longitudinal image, 1, 2*f*
      transverse image, 1, 2*f*
    ultrasound-guided injection in, 236
  tear, 19, 19*f*
  tenosynovitis, 18*f*, 19
Biceps tendon sheath, fluid in, 18*f*, 19, 19*f*
Bicipital groove
  congenital narrow or shallow, 19
  erosion, in rheumatoid arthritis, 196*f*
  ultrasound
    longitudinal image, 1, 2*f*
    transverse image, 1, 2*f*
Biopsy, ultrasound-guided, 220–222
  of bone tumors, 142, 144*f*, 145*f*, 146*f*
Blood vessel(s). *See also specific vessel*
  in hand and fingers, 78–79, 79*f*
  large, thrombosis, skin changes with, 156, 160*f*
Bone. *See also specific bone*
  computed tomography, 146
  Doppler ultrasound, 146
  erosions, 135, 137*f*
  fractures
    healing, and peripheral nerve compression, 188–189, 189*f*

Bone (*continued*)
    linear, 132, 133*f*
    occult, 135, 135*f*, 136*f*
    and peripheral nerve injury, 188–189, 188*f*, 189*f*
    surgery for, and peripheral nerve compression, 188–189, 189*f*
    ultrasound, 132–135, 133*f*–136*f*
  imaging, algorithm for, 146
  magnetic resonance imaging, 146
  pathology, 132–144
    imaging, 144
  radiography, 146
  scintigraphy, 146
  tumors
    biopsy, ultrasound-guided, 142, 144*f*, 145*f*, 146*f*
    computed tomography, 142, 144*f*, 146*f*
    Doppler ultrasound, 142, 143*f*, 145*f*
    magnetic resonance imaging, 142, 144*f*, 145*f*
    ultrasound, 142, 143*f*, 144*f*, 145*f*, 146*f*
  ultrasound, 146
    equipment for, 132
    normal anatomy on, 132
    patient positioning for, 132
    pearls and pitfalls, 146
    physics, 132
    technical guidelines for, 132
    transducer for, 132
Brachialgia paresthetica nocturna, 182
Brachial plexus. *See* Cervical/brachial plexus
Bursitis olecrani. *See* Olecranon bursitis

C

Calcaneofibular ligament, 106, 107*f*
  injury, 111
Calcaneotibial ligament, 108
Calcaneum, 107*f*, 110*f*
  spur, 112*f*
Calcaneus, tumor in, 143*f*–144*f*
Calcification
  differential diagnosis, 230, 230*f*
  puncture and lavage, ultrasound-guided, 222–230, 227*f*–230*f*
Calcifying Malherbe epitheliomas. *See* Pilomatrixomas
Calcium pyrophosphate dihydrate (CPPD) deposition, 52
Capitate, fractures, 57
Carpal bones, fractures, 55, 56*f*–58*f*
Carpal boss, 49–50, 51*f*
Carpal tunnel
  anatomy, 46–47, 173–176
  content, changes, in carpal tunnel syndrome, 62
  muscular impingement syndrome, 183–184, 185*f*
  space-occupying lesions in, 183–184
Carpal tunnel index, 183
Carpal tunnel syndrome, 46, 60–62, 179*f*
  causes, 60, 171, 182
  diagnosis, 182
  epidemiology, 60–61, 171, 182
  symptoms, 61, 171, 182
  ultrasound diagnostic criteria, 61–62, 61*f*–62*f*
  ultrasound in, 171, 182–184, 182*f*–185*f*
Carpometacarpal boss, 49–50, 51*f*
Carpometacarpal joint(s)
  fingers, 79
  thumb, 79, 79*f*
    degeneration, 81, 81*f*
    osteoarthritis, 81, 81*f*
    osteophytes, 81, 81*f*
    range of motion, 81
Cellulitis, in foot, 111, 112*f*
Cervical/brachial plexus
  normal anatomy, 173, 174*f*, 175*f*
  palsy, 186–187, 187*f*
  trauma, 186–187, 187*f*
Chondritis
  of nose, 164
  of pinna, 164, 165*f*
Chondromatosis, elbow, 26*f*, 29*f*, 32*f*, 34, 36*f*
Chondrosarcoma, 214*f*–215*f*
Clergyman's knee, 99
Common fibular nerve, 176, 178*f*
Common peroneal nerve, 93
  anatomy, 103
  ganglion cyst of proximal tibiofibular joint and, 103, 104*f*
Common tibial nerve, 176–179
Compression neuropathy(ies), 171, 179–186. *See also* Carpal tunnel syndrome
  idiopathic, 179
  postoperative imaging, 186, 186*f*
  secondary, 179
  sonographic findings in, 179, 179*f*
  ultrasound-guided injection for, 242, 242*f*
Corticosteroid(s)
  adverse effects and side effects, 241–242
  chondrotoxic effects, 241
  ultrasound-guided injection, 236, 237*f*
Crossover syndrome. *See* Distal intersection syndrome
CTS. *See* Carpal tunnel syndrome
Cubital arthritis, 24*f*, 27*f*, 30*f*, 33*f*, 40, 40*f*–41*f*
Cubital tunnel
  contents, 173
  normal anatomy, 173, 176*f*
Cubital tunnel retinaculum, 173
Cubital tunnel syndrome, 176*f*, 180, 180*f*, 181*f*
Cuneiform bone, 111*f*
Cyst(s)
  aspiration, ultrasound-guided, 231–233, 231*f*, 232*f*
  Baker. *See* Baker cyst
  epidermal, 149, 149*f*, 150*f*

biopsy, ultrasound-guided, 221, 221*f*
ganglion. *See* Ganglion (pl., ganglia) cyst
meniscal, 102*f*, 103, 103*f*
nail bed, 167–168, 168*f*
pilonidal, 149, 151*f*
sebaceous. *See* Cyst(s), epidermal
trichilemmal, 149, 150*f*

D
DDH. *See* Hip, developmental dysplasia
Deep infrapatellar bursitis, 99
Deep palmar arch, 79
Deep palmar artery, 78
Deep vein thrombosis, differential diagnosis, 100–101
Deltoid ligament, 108, 108*f*
injury, 111
De Quervain tenosynovitis, in wrist, 46, 47–48, 48*f*
postoperative complication, 48, 49*f*
Dermatomyositis-calcinosis, 161–162, 164*f*
Dermis, ultrasound appearance, 148, 148*f*
Desmoid tumor, biopsy, ultrasound-guided, 221
Developmental dysplasia of hip. *See* Hip, developmental dysplasia
DIP. *See* Distal interphalangeal (DIP) joint
Distal interphalangeal (DIP) joint, ultrasound-guided injection in, 238
Distal intersection syndrome, 46, 48–49, 49*f*
Doppler ultrasound. *See also* Power Doppler imaging
in rheumatoid arthritis, 200, 201, 201*f*, 202*f*
Dorsalis pedis artery, 108
Double contour sign, 52, 53*f*
Drug(s), chondrotoxic effects, 241
DVT. *See* Deep vein thrombosis

E
Ear cartilage, chondritis, 164, 165*f*
ECU. *See* Extensor carpi ulnaris tendon
ED. *See* Extensor digitorum tendon (ankle)
EHL. *See* Extensor hallucis longus tendon
Elbow
avascular osteonecrosis, 34
bony changes in, 22*t*
bursae, changes in, 22*t*
bursitis olecrani. *See* Elbow, olecranon bursitis
calcification puncture and lavage, ultrasound-guided, 229*f*
chondromatosis, 26*f*, 29*f*, 32*f*, 34, 36*f*
cubital arthritis, 24*f*, 27*f*, 30*f*, 33*f*, 40, 40*f*–41*f*
dorsal region, ultrasound
longitudinal image, 28, 30–31, 31*f*
pathology on, differential diagnosis, 28, 29*f*–31*f*, 31, 32*f*–34*f*, 36*f*, 38*f*, 39*f*, 40*f*, 41*f*, 42*f*, 44*f*
transverse image, 28, 29*f*
pathology on, differential diagnosis, 28, 29*f*–31*f*, 36*f*, 38*f*, 41*f*, 42*f*, 44*f*
fracture, peripheral nerve injury in, 188*f*
fracture of coronoid process, 28*f*, 37, 37*f*
free joint body, 23*f*, 26*f*, 27*f*, 34, 35*f*
gouty tophus, 30*f*, 34*f*, 41, 41*f*
intraarticular hemorrhage, 37, 37*f*–38*f*
joint cavity, changes in, 22*t*
ligaments, changes in, 22*t*
metastatic disease in, 42, 44*f*
olecranon bursitis, 29*f*, 32*f*, 38, 38*f*–39*f*
osteochondroses, 34
osteochondrosis dissecans, 34, 35*f*
pathology, 22*t*, 34–42, 35*f*–44*f*
differential diagnosis, 28, 29*f*–31*f*, 31, 32*f*–34*f*
radial head fracture, 24*f*, 33*f*, 37, 37*f*–38*f*
radiography
anteroposterior projection, 38*f*
pathology on, differential diagnosis, 35*f*, 38*f*, 40*f*, 44*f*
regional lymphadenitis, 24*f*, 28*f*, 42, 42*f*
rheumatic node, 30*f*, 34*f*, 42, 42*f*
rheumatoid arthritis in, soft-tissue changes with, 33*f*
tendons, changes in, 22*t*
tumor, 24*f*, 28*f*, 31*f*, 34*f*, 42, 43*f*, 44*f*
ultrasound, 22
examination technique, 22–34
indications for, 22*t*
pearls and pitfalls, 45
ultrasound-guided injection in, 236–237
ventral region
osteochondritis dissecans, 25*f*
radiography, pathology on, differential diagnosis, 35*f*
ventral region, ultrasound
humeroradial longitudinal image, 22–23, 25*f*
pathology on, differential diagnosis, 23, 25*f*–27*f*, 35*f*, 36*f*, 39*f*, 40*f*
humeroradial transverse image, 22, 23*f*
pathology on, differential diagnosis, 22, 23*f*, 24*f*, 40*f*
humeroulnar longitudinal image, 26, 27*f*
pathology on, differential diagnosis, 26, 27*f*, 28*f*, 35*f*, 37*f*, 43*f*
Enthesitis, 139, 139*f*
Entrapment neuropathy, 179
Eosinophilic granuloma, 145*f*
EPB. *See* Extensor pollicis brevis tendon
Epidermal cyst, 149, 149*f*, 150*f*
biopsy, ultrasound-guided, 221, 221*f*
Epidermis, ultrasound appearance, 148, 148*f*
EPL. *See* Extensor pollicis longus tendon
Ewing sarcoma, 143*f*–144*f*
Exostoses, 137, 138*f*
subungual, 168, 169*f*
Extensor carpi radialis brevis tendon, 47*f*
Extensor carpi radialis longus tendon, 47*f*
Extensor carpi radialis tendon, 47

Extensor carpi ulnaris tendon, 47, 47*f*
- recurrent dislocation, 55
- tenosynovitis, 50, 51*f*

Extensor digiti minimi tendon, 47, 47*f*
Extensor digitorum brevis manus muscle, 64–66, 66*f*–67*f*
Extensor digitorum longus tendon, 47, 47*f*
Extensor digitorum tendon (ankle), 108, 109*f*
Extensor hallucis longus tendon, 109*f*
Extensor hallucis tendon, 108
Extensor indicis proprius tendon, 47, 47*f*
Extensor pollicis brevis tendon, 47, 47*f*, 76, 77*f*
- rupture, 54

Extensor pollicis longus tendon, 47, 47*f*, 76, 77*f*
- rupture, 54, 54*f*

Extensor radialis brevis tendon, 47
Extensor radialis longus tendon, 47
Extensor retinaculum, 47
- in rheumatoid arthritis, 204, 205*f*

External jugular vein, thrombosis, 160*f*

F

Fat necrosis, 160–161, 163*f*
FCR. *See* Flexor carpi radialis tendon
FCU. *See* Flexor carpi ulnaris tendon
FDL. *See* Flexor digitorum tendon (ankle)
FDMB. *See* Flexor digiti minimi brevis muscle
FDP. *See* Flexor digitorum profundus tendon
FDS. *See* Flexor digitorum superficialis tendon
Femoral head, 118*f*
- ossification center, 118, 127
- ultrasound appearance, in newborn, 118

Femoral neck, proximal, ultrasound appearance, in newborn, 118
Femur
- distal, exostosis, 138*f*
- proximal
  - diaphysis, occult fracture, 136*f*
  - focal deficiency, 117, 131

FHL. *See* Flexor hallucis longus tendon
Fibrolipomatous hamartoma, in hand, 90, 90*f*
Fibroma(s), in hand, 90, 91*f*
Fibular nerve, 176
Fingers. *See* Hand and fingers
Fistula(s)
- odontogenic, 157, 162*f*
- in skin, 157–160, 162*f*

Flexor carpi radialis tendon, 46*f*, 47
- tendinitis, 52

Flexor carpi ulnaris tendon, 47
- tendinitis, 52

Flexor digiti minimi brevis muscle, 77*f*, 78
Flexor digitorum longus tendon, 178*f*
Flexor digitorum muscle, anomalous bellies, 66
Flexor digitorum profundus tendon, 46, 46*f*, 73–74, 73*f*–74*f*, 75
Flexor digitorum superficialis tendon, 46, 46*f*, 73–74, 73*f*–74*f*
Flexor digitorum tendon (ankle), 108, 109*f*
Flexor hallucis longus muscle, 178*f*
Flexor hallucis longus tendon, 108, 109*f*
Flexor pollicis brevis muscle, 77–78, 77*f*
Flexor pollicis longus tendon, 46, 46*f*, 75, 76*f*
Flexor retinaculum (ankle), 178*f*
Flexor retinaculum (wrist), 46–47, 46*f*, 173, 177*f*
- in carpal tunnel syndrome, 183, 183*f*, 184*f*
- changes, in carpal tunnel syndrome, 62

Fluid drainage, ultrasound-guided, 231
Foot and ankle
- accessory muscles in, 169
- ankle injuries, Lauge-Hansen classification, 111, 113*t*
- anterior ankle structures, normal anatomy, 108, 109*f*
- cellulitis, 111, 112*f*
- degenerative changes, 110–111, 111*f*
- forefoot structures, normal anatomy, 110
- foreign bodies in, 106, 113, 114*f*
- fractures, 113, 114*f*
- ganglion cyst, 115, 115*f*
- infection, 106, 111, 112*f*
- inflammatory disorders, 111, 112*f*
- lateral-sided ankle structures, normal anatomy, 106, 107*f*–108*f*
- ligaments
  - anatomy, 116
  - injury, 111, 113*f*
- magnetic resonance imaging, normal anatomy, 107*f*, 108*f*, 109*f*, 110*f*
- masses, 106, 115
- medial-sided ankle structures, normal anatomy, 108, 108*f*–109*f*
- normal anatomy, 106–110, 107*f*–110*f*
- osteoarthritis, 110
- osteophytes in, 110, 111*f*
- pathology, 110–115, 111*f*–115*f*
- plantar structures, normal anatomy, 108–110, 110*f*
- posterior ankle structures, normal anatomy, 108, 110*f*
- radiography, indications for, 106
- sonographic intraarticular anatomy, 197–199, 198*f*
- tendons
  - anatomy, 116
  - injury, 111, 114*f*
  - overuse, 111, 111*f*
  - postoperative infection, 111, 112*f*
- trauma, 106, 111–113, 113*f*, 114*f*
- tumors, 115
- ultrasound
  - artifacts, 116
  - indications for, 106
  - normal anatomy, 107*f*, 108*f*, 109*f*, 110*f*

pearls and pitfalls, 116
technical guidelines, 106
ultrasound-guided injection in, 240–241, 241*f*
Foreign body(ies)
in foot and ankle, 106, 113, 114*f*
in hand and fingers
granulation tissue caused by, ultrasound, 87, 87*f*
ultrasound, 71, 86–87, 86*f*, 87*f*
removal
algorithm for, 242
ultrasound-guided, 208, 222, 223*f*–226*f*
in skin, 170, 170*f*
soft-tissue, ultrasound appearance, 207, 207*f*, 208*f*
ultrasound
advantages, 207
pearls and pitfalls, 219
FPB. *See* Flexor pollicis brevis muscle
FPL. *See* Flexor pollicis longus tendon
Fracture(s). *See also* Bone, fractures; *specific bone*
compression, subchondral, 132, 133*f*
osteochondral avulsion, 134, 134*f*

G
Gamekeeper's thumb, 86
Ganglion (pl., ganglia) cyst
aspiration, ultrasound-guided, 231, 231*f*, 232*f*
in carpal tunnel, 183
in cruciate ligaments, 102
foot and ankle, 115, 115*f*
hand, 81, 81*f*
nerve sheath, 189–190, 192*f*
of proximal tibiofibular joint, 103
wrist, 46, 62–63, 63*f*–64*f*
carpal boss and, 50, 51*f*
extensor carpi ulnaris tenosynovitis and, 50
postoperative ultrasound, 63, 65*f*
Gastrocnemius muscle, 93, 94*f*
GCTTS. *See* Giant cell tumor of tendon sheath
Giant cell tumor of tendon sheath, in hand, 89, 89*f*
Glenohumeral joint
effusion, rotator cuff tear and, 9, 12*f*
fluid in
magnetic resonance imaging, 12*f*
ultrasound, 12*f*
in rheumatoid arthritis, 196*f*
synovitis, magnetic resonance imaging, 12*f*
ultrasound, transverse image, 3, 4*f*
ultrasound-guided injection in, 236
Glenoid labrum, ultrasound, transverse image, 3, 4*f*
Glomus tumor, of finger, 88–89, 88*f*, 89*f*, 167, 168*f*
Golfer's elbow, ultrasound-guided injection in, 236–237
Gout, 166, 166*f*
hand/finger involvement in, 82, 84*f*, 166*f*
wrist involvement in, 52, 53*f*
Gouty tophus, 166, 166*f*
in elbow, 30*f*, 34*f*, 41, 41*f*
Greater tuberosity
fractures
magnetic resonance imaging, 13*f*
ultrasound, 11, 13*f*
irregularity, 11
Guyon canal
anatomy, 47
ulnar nerve compression in, 180
Guyon tunnel, normal anatomy, 62, 62*f*
Guyon tunnel syndrome, 46, 62, 63*f*

H
Hageman disease, 34
Hamate
fractures, 55–57
hook of, 47
fractures, 55–57
Hand and fingers. *See also* Nail bed; Nail unit
accessory muscles in, 169, 169*f*
annular pulleys, normal anatomy, 74–75, 75*f*
blood vessels, 78–79, 79*f*
cruciate pulleys, normal anatomy, 74–75
crystal deposition disease, 82, 84*f*
degenerative disorders, 80–81, 81*f*, 82*f*
erosive arthropathy, ultrasound, 71
extensor tendons, 75, 76*f*
flexor tendons, zones, 75
foreign bodies in
granulation tissue caused by, ultrasound, 87, 87*f*
ultrasound, 71, 86–87, 86*f*, 87*f*
gout in, 82, 84*f*, 166*f*
infection in, 83–84, 85*f*
sinus formation caused by, 83, 85*f*
inflammatory disorders, 81–82
injuries, radiography, 71
joints, 79–80, 79*f*, 80*f*
effusions, 71
swelling, 71
ligaments, injuries, 71
muscles, 77–78
anomalies, 90, 91*f*
normal anatomy, 72–80
normal variants, 90, 91*f*
pathology, 80–90
penetrating injuries, 71
in rheumatoid arthritis, ultrasound technique for, 200
soft-tissue edema, ultrasound, 71
sonographic intraarticular anatomy, 197–199, 198*f*
tendons
atypical courses, 90
injuries, 71
normal anatomy, 73–76, 73*f*–77*f*
postoperative scarring, 88, 88*f*
repaired, re-tear, 85

Hand and fingers (*continued*)
rupture, 84–85, 85*f*
tenosynovitis
from overuse, 82, 84*f*
in psoriatic arthropathy, 82, 84*f*
in rheumatoid arthritis, 82, 83*f*
traumatic injuries, 84–88
tumors, 88–90, 88*f*–91*f*
ultrasound
cine-loop display, 72
dynamic assessment, 72
indications for, 71
limitations, 71
pearls and pitfalls, 91
positioning for, 72
technical guidelines for, 71–72, 72*f*, 73*f*
transducer frequency for, 71
transducer shape and configuration for, 71–72, 72*f*
water-bath examination, 72, 73*f*
ultrasound-guided procedures in, 71
uric acid crystals in, 82, 84*f*
Hemangioma(s), 151–155, 156*f*, 157*f*
in carpal tunnel, 183
intramuscular, 211, 212*f*–213*f*
Hematoma
aspiration, ultrasound-guided, 235–236, 235*f*
intramuscular, calcifying, 211*f*
postacromioplasty, ultrasound, 11, 14*f*
ultrasound appearance, 235
Hemorrhage, subperiosteal, and occult fracture, 135, 136*f*
Hidradenitis suppurativa, 160, 163*f*
Hill–Sachs fracture, 11, 13*f*, 132, 133*f*
Hip
acetabulum
anatomy, 118
bony, 118, 118*f*
bony roof, 118*f*
cartilaginous, 118
hyaline cartilage roof, 118, 118*f*
morphology, reporting, 126
a (cartilage roof triangle acetabular inclination) angle, 119, 120*f*, 126, 127
b (cartilage roof) angle, 119, 120*f*, 126, 127
bony rim, 118*f*, 126
bony rim percentage, 122
cartilage roof line, 127, 128*f*
chondroosseous border, 118, 118*f*
developmental dysplasia, 117–128
arthrography, 117
diagnosis, ultrasound for, 117
incidence, 117–118
magnetic resonance imaging, 117
pathophysiology, 117
risk factors for, 127
screening for, ultrasound, 126–127
sonographic signs, reporting, 126
treatment monitoring, ultrasound for, 127
ultrasound, *pearls and pitfalls*, 127, 128*f*
effusion, 128–131
computed tomography, 128
Doppler ultrasound evaluation, 128, 129*f*
magnetic resonance imaging, 128, 129*f*, 130*f*
radiographic evaluation, 128
ultrasound, technical guidelines, 129–131, 130*f*
femoral head coverage, 122
fluid collections
composition, and echogenicity, 131
percutaneous aspiration, ultrasound-guided, 117
ultrasound, 129–131, 130*f*
Graf's classification, 119, 121*f*
greater trochanter, ultrasound appearance, in newborn, 118
inflammatory arthropathy, 129*f*
intraarticular fluid in, 128–131
joint capsule, 118*f*
Morin ratio
in dislocated hip, 126*f*
in normal hip, 126*f*
normal sonographic anatomy, 118, 118*f*
osteomyelitis, 130*f*
pain in, 117
in Pavlik harness, ultrasound
anterior approach, 127
lateral approach, 127
radiography, indications for, 128
septic, 130*f*
toxic synovitis, 128
transient synovitis, 128, 129*f*, 130*f*
triradiate cartilage, 118, 118*f*
type I (Graf's classification), 119, 121*f*, 126
type IIa (Graf's classification), 119, 121*f*, 126
type IIb (Graf's classification), 119, 126
type IIc (Graf's classification), 119, 126
type IId (Graf's classification), 119
type III (Graf's classification), 119
type IIIa (Graf's classification), 119, 121*f*, 126
type IIIb (Graf's classification), 119
type IV (Graf's classification), 119, 121*f*, 126
ultrasound
advantages, 117
artifacts, 128
coronal flexion view, 122, 125*f*
coronal neutral view, 122
dynamic method, 118
dynamic standard minimum examination, 122
findings in, reporting, 126
Graf's static technique, 118–119, 119*f*
standard coronal plane for, 119, 127, 128*f*
Harcke's dynamic method, 118, 122
imaging planes for, 122, 123*f*–125*f*

indications for, 117
Morin and modified Morin (Terjesen) technique, 122, 126*f*
in newborn, 122
pearls and pitfalls, 131
technical guidelines, 118
transverse flexion view, 122, 124*f*
transverse neutral view, 122, 123*f*
ultrasound-guided injection in, 239
Housemaid's knee, 99
Humeral head
compression fractures, 11, 13*f*–14*f*, 132, 133*f*
elevation, rotator cuff tear and, 7*f*, 9
osteomyelitis, 141*f*
Humeral shaft
distal third, ultrasound, transverse image, 23*f*
fracture, peripheral nerve injury in, 188, 189*f*
Humerus
greater tuberosity, occult fracture, 135, 135*f*
proximal, exostosis, 138*f*
Hypodermis, ultrasound appearance, 148, 148*f*
Hypothenar hammer syndrome, 60
Hypothenar muscles, 77–78, 77*f*

I

Iliac wing, 118, 118*f*, 128*f*
Iliotibial band, 93
tendinopathy, 103
Iliotibial band friction syndrome, 103
Ilium, 118
Impingement syndrome, shoulder, 15, 15*f*
Infrapatellar fat, 93
Infraspinatus tendon
large full-thickness tear
magnetic resonance imaging, 8*f*
ultrasound, 8*f*
ultrasound, transverse image, 2–3, 4*f*
Intercarpal joint, ultrasound-guided injection in, 238
Interossei muscles (hand), 78, 78*f*
dorsal, 78, 78*f*
palmar, 78, 78*f*
Interphalangeal joints (foot), 110
in rheumatoid arthritis, 197
Interphalangeal joints (hand), 80
collateral ligaments, injury, 85–86, 86*f*
Interscalene gap, 173, 174*f*
Intertarsal joint, ultrasound-guided injection in, 238
Interventions. *See* Musculoskeletal interventions
Ischium, 118

J

Joint(s). *See also specific joint*
diseases, algorithm for, 242
effusion, 200, 200*f*, 201*f*
rotator cuff tear and, 9, 12*f*, 18*f*
fluid in, aspiration, ultrasound-guided, 236
small, ultrasound-guided injection in, 238, 239*f*
subluxation, 135, 137*f*
Jumper's knee, 96–97, 97*f*

K

Knee
anterior
active pannus, 99
bursitis, 99
fibrous pannus, 99
intraarticular fracture, 98–99, 99*f*
joint effusion, 98–99, 98*f*, 99*f*
lipohemarthrosis, 98–99, 99*f*
muscle hernia, 99–100, 100*f*
normal anatomy, 92, 92*f*
pathology, 94–100, 94*f*–100*f*
synovitis, 99
ultrasound examination, 92
ganglion cyst in, aspiration, ultrasound-guided, 231, 231*f*
imaging examination
algorithm for, 105
pearls and pitfalls, 105
joint effusion, in rheumatoid arthritis, 197*f*
lateral
normal anatomy, 93
pathology, 103, 104*f*
ultrasound examination, 93
magnetic resonance imaging, 104
indications for, 92
medial
normal anatomy, 93, 94*f*
pathology, 102–103, 102*f*, 103*f*
ultrasound examination, 93
normal anatomy, 92–93, 92*f*–94*f*
pathology, 94–104
pearls and pitfalls, 105
posterior
cruciate ligaments
magnetic resonance imaging, 102
ultrasound, 102
normal anatomy, 93, 94*f*
pathology, 100–102, 100*f*–102*f*
ultrasound examination, 93
prosthesis, granulocytic reaction to, 105*f*
in rheumatoid arthritis, 197*f*
soft-tissue masses, 104, 104*f*, 105*f*
synovitis, in rheumatoid arthritis, 197*f*
ultrasound, 104
advantages, 92
indications for, 92
pearls and pitfalls, 105
technical guidelines, 92
ultrasound-guided injection in, 239–240, 240*f*
Knucklepads, 194, 194*f*

L

Lateral collateral ligament, 93
  sprains, 103
Lateral femoral cutaneous nerve, in meralgia paresthetica, 184, 185*f*
Lateral malleolus, 107*f*, 113*f*
LCL. *See* Lateral collateral ligament
Legg–Calve–Perthes disease, 117, 128, 131
Lip, large-caliber artery, persistence of, 168–169
Lipoma(s), 149, 151*f*, 211
  biopsy, ultrasound-guided, 221
Liposarcoma, 211, 218*f*
Lister tubercle, 47, 47*f*
  fracture, 54
Local anesthetic
  chondrotoxic effects, 241
  ultrasound-guided injection, 236
Lumbrical muscles, 78, 78*f*
  anomalies, 91*f*
Lunotriquetral ligament, 199
Lymphadenitis, in elbow region, 24*f*, 28*f*, 42, 42*f*
Lymphedema, 162, 164*f*
Lymphoma(s), biopsy, ultrasound-guided, 221

M

Malleolar fractures, Lauge-Hansen classification, 111, 113*t*
MCL. *See* Medial collateral ligament
McLaughlin fracture, 11, 14*f*, 132, 133*f*
MCP. *See* Metacarpophalangeal joints
Medial collateral ligament, 93, 94*f*
  injuries, 102
Medial malleolus, 108*f*, 109*f*
Median artery, persistent, 66–68, 69*f*, 176, 177*f*
Median nerve, 177*f*
  anatomy, 173–176, 177*f*
  bifid, 66, 69*f*
  in carpal tunnel syndrome, 179*f*, 182–184, 182*f*
  cross-section area, 176
    in carpal tunnel syndrome, 182
  fibrolipomatous hamartoma, in palm, 90*f*
  forearm to wrist ratio, 176
  high bifurcation, 176, 177*f*
  lipomatosis, 66*f*
  neuroma, 65*f*
  schwannoma, 191*f*
  surgery, sonographic follow-up, 190*f*
  at wrist, 46*f*, 47
    changes, in carpal tunnel syndrome, 61, 61*f*–62*f*
    normal anatomy, 61*f*
Melanoma, 151, 155*f*
Meniscus
  cysts, 102*f*, 103, 103*f*
  lateral, tears, 103, 103*f*
  medial, 93, 94*f*
    chondrocalcinosis, 102
    degeneration, 102
    meniscocapsular separation, 102—103
    pathology, 102–103, 102*f*, 103*f*
    tears, 102, 102*f*
Meralgia paresthetica, 184, 185*f*
Metacarpal, distal, dorsal depression, 197, 199*f*
Metacarpophalangeal joints, 79–80, 80*f*
  articular cartilage, 80, 80*f*
  collateral ligaments, injury, 85–86
  dorsal depression, 197, 199*f*
  joint effusion, 197, 198*f*
  in rheumatoid arthritis, 197, 197*f*
    ultrasound technique for, 200
  sonographic intraarticular anatomy, 197–199, 198*f*, 199*f*
  ultrasound-guided injection in, 238
  volar plate at, 80, 80*f*
Metastatic disease
  biopsy, ultrasound-guided, 221, 221*f*
  in elbow, 42, 44*f*
  in muscle, 211
  in sternum, 146*f*
Metatarsal(s), 108*f*
  fracture, 114*f*, 133*f*
  head, articular cartilage, sonographic appearance, 198*f*
  periosteal new bone formation in, 114*f*
Metatarsophalangeal joint(s), 110
  in rheumatoid arthritis, 197
    ultrasound technique for, 200
  sonographic intraarticular anatomy, 197–199, 198*f*, 199*f*
  ultrasound-guided injection in, 238, 239*f*
Middle collateral ligament (knee), tear, 134*f*
Milwaukee shoulder, 17
Mondor disease, 155–156, 159*f*
Morton neuroma, 115, 115*f*
Muscle(s). *See also specific muscle*
  abscess, ultrasound appearance, 209*f*, 210*f*
  calcified mass in, 211*f*
  hematoma, ultrasound appearance, 209*f*
  pathology, 208–211
    magnetic resonance imaging, 208
    ultrasound, 208
  tears, ultrasound appearance, 208, 208*f*, 209*f*
  tumors, 208–211, 211*f*, 214*f*–218*f*
  ultrasound, technical guidelines, 211–219
  ultrasound appearance, 208, 208*f*
Musculoskeletal disorders, and skin lesions, 147
Musculoskeletal interventions, ultrasound-guided
  advantages, 220
  algorithm for, 242
  artifacts, 241
  complications, 241–242
  diagnostic, 220
  equipment for, 220

general considerations in, 220
pearls and pitfalls, 243
technical guidelines, 220
therapeutic, 220
Myositis ossificans, 211*f*

N
Nail bed
cysts, 167–168, 168*f*
germinal matrix injury, 87, 87*f*
lesions, 166–168
Nail unit
glomus tumor, 167, 168*f*
psoriasis in, 166, 166*f*
subungual exostoses, 168, 169*f*
ultrasound appearance, 148, 148*f*
Navicular, 111*f*
Nerve compression syndrome, 179. *See also* Compression neuropathy(ies)
Nerve root(s)
avulsion, in brachial plexus sonography, 173, 175*f*
localization, in brachial plexus sonography, 173, 175*f*
Neurilemmoma(s). *See* Schwannoma(s)
Neurofibroma(s)
sonographic features, 189, 191*f*
wrist, 63–64
Neuroma(s)
postoperative, 189, 190*f*
stump, after amputation, chronic pain with, 192–193, 193*f*
wrist, 63, 65*f*
Neuroma in continuity. *See* Traction neuroma
Nodular fasciitis, biopsy, ultrasound-guided, 221
Nose, chondritis, 164

O
ODM. *See* Opponens digiti minimi muscle
Olecranon bursitis, 29*f*, 32*f*, 38, 38*f*–39*f*
OP. *See* Opponens pollicis muscle
Opponens digiti minimi muscle, 78
Opponens pollicis muscle, 77–78, 77*f*
Osborne fascia, 173
Osgood–Schlatter disease, 97–98
Os ilium, 118, 118*f*
Os styloideum, in carpal boss, 50, 51*f*
Osteoarthritis. *See also* Arthritis
in foot and ankle, 110
Osteochondroma, 137, 138*f*
Osteochondrosis dissecans
clinical features, 34
in elbow, 34, 35*f*
Osteomyelitis, 139, 140*f*, 141*f*, 210*f*
Osteophyte(s)
degenerative, in carpal boss, 50, 51*f*
in foot and ankle, 110, 111*f*

P
Palmaris longus muscle
musculotendinous variant, 67*f*
variants, 66, 67*f*
Palmaris longus tendon (wrist), 46*f*, 47
absent, as normal variant, 47
variants, 47
Panner disease, 34
Paronychia, 83–84, 85*f*
Patella, 92, 92*f*
osteochondral avulsion fracture, 134*f*
proximal pole, avulsion, 95, 95*f*
Patellar sulcus, 93, 93*f*
Patellar tendon, 92, 92*f*, 93*f*
tears, 94–96, 95*f*
tendinosis/tendinopathy, 96–97, 97*f*, 98*f*
Pavlik harness, scanning hip in
anterior approach, 127
lateral approach, 127
PCL. *See* Posterior cruciate ligament
Periostitis, 139, 142*f*
Peripheral nerve(s). *See also* Compression neuropathy(ies)
imaging investigation, algorithm for, 193
injections, ultrasound-guided, 190–192, 192*f*
normal anatomy, 173–179
pathology, 179–190
stump neuroma, after amputation, chronic pain with, 192–193, 193*f*
surgery, sonographic follow-up, 189, 190*f*
transection, 187, 188*f*
traumatic lesions, 171, 186–189
in extremities, 187–189, 188*f*
tumors, 171, 189–190
ultrasound
advantages, 171
artifacts, 193
equipment for, 171–172, 172*t*
factors affecting, 173
general examination technique, 172–173, 172*f*
indications for, 171
pearls and pitfalls, 193
technical guidelines, 171–173
ultrasound-guided injection in, 242, 242*f*
Peripheral nerve sheath tumor(s), in hand, 89, 90*f*
Peroneal nerve, traction neuroma, 188*f*
Peroneal nerve sheath, ganglion, 189–190
Peroneal tendon(s), 106, 107*f*
Peroneus brevis tendon, 106, 107*f*, 108*f*
tendinitis, 111*f*
Peroneus longus tendon, 106, 107*f*
Pes anserinus bursa
anatomy, 103
bursitis, 103
Pes anserinus tendons, 93
Phantom limb pain, 192–193

Phlebitis, 157
Pigmented villonodular synovitis, 89
Pilomatrixomas, 149–150, 152*f*
Pilonidal cyst(s), 149, 151*f*
Pinna, chondritis, 164, 165*f*
PIP. *See* Proximal interphalangeal (PIP) joint
Pisiform bone, 47, 177*f*
  fracture, 56*f*
Plantar aponeurosis, 108–110, 110*f*
Plantar fascia, 108–110, 110*f*
Plantar fasciitis, 111, 112*f*
Plantar fibromatosis, 115, 115*f*
Plantar warts, 164–166, 165*f*
Popliteal artery, 93, 178*f*
Popliteal fossa, 93, 94*f*
  normal anatomy, 176–179, 178*f*
Popliteal neurovascular bundle, 93
Popliteal vein, 93
Popliteus tendon, tendinopathy, 103
Popliteus tendon sheath, fluid in, 103
Posterior cruciate ligament, tears, 102
Posterior talofibular ligament, 106
Posterior talotibial ligament, 108
Posterior tibial artery, 108
Posterior tibial vein, 108
Power Doppler imaging, of synovitis, in rheumatoid arthritis, 200–201, 201*f*
  pearls and pitfalls, 205, 206*f*
Prepatellar bursae, 99, 99*f*
Princeps pollicis artery, 79
Pronator quadratus muscle (wrist), 46*f*, 47, 49, 50*f*
Pronator quadratus muscle syndrome, 49, 50*f*
Proximal interphalangeal (PIP) joint
  in rheumatoid arthritis, ultrasound technique for, 200
  sonographic intraarticular anatomy, 199, 200*f*
  ultrasound-guided injection in, 238
Proximal intersection syndrome, in wrist, 49
Pseudoaneurysm(s), 58, 59*f*, 157, 162*f*
Pseudogout, 52
Pseudomeningocele, 173, 175*f*
Psoriasis
  nail involvement in, 166, 167*f*
  periostitis in, 139, 142*f*
  and tenosynovitis in hand and fingers, 82, 84*f*
Pubis, 118
PVNS. *See* Pigmented villonodular synovitis
Pyoderma gangrenosum, 156–157
Pyomyositis, ultrasound appearance, 208*f*, 209*f*, 210*f*

Q

Quadriceps muscle(s), 92
  tears, 94–96, 95*f*
Quadriceps tendon, 92, 92*f*
  tears, 94–96, 95*f*

R

Radial artery, 46*f*, 47, 78
  anatomy, 59
  injuries, 59, 59*f*
  pseudoaneurysm, 58, 59*f*
  thrombosis, 58, 58*f*
    postoperative, 65*f*
Radial collateral ligament, 79, 80
  injury, 55
Radial head, fracture, 24*f*, 33*f*, 37, 37*f*–38*f*
Radialis indicis artery, 79, 79*f*
Radial nerve
  compression syndrome, 182
  injury, humeral shaft fracture and, 188, 189*f*
Radial tunnel, 182
Radiocarpal joint, ultrasound-guided injection in, 237
Radioulnar joint, subluxation, 135
Radius
  distal, fracture, 55, 55*f*, 56*f*
  at wrist, 46*f*, 47*f*
Rectus femoris muscle, 92
  tear, 95–96, 95*f*, 96*f*
Rectus femoris tendon, 92, 93*f*
  tear, 95–96
Rhabdomyosarcoma, 211
Rheumatic node, in elbow, 30*f*, 34*f*, 42, 42*f*
Rheumatoid arthritis (RA)
  bone erosion in, 201, 203*f*
    imaging, 194–195, 195*f*, 196*f*
  clinical presentation, 194
  complications, imaging, 205
  computed tomography in, 194
  cross-sectional imaging in, 194–195
  differential diagnosis, 194
  elbow involvement in, soft-tissue changes with, 33*f*
  epidemiology, 194
  extensor carpi ulnaris tenosynovitis in, 50
  hand involvement in, 81–82, 82*f*
  imaging in
    algorithm for, 204–205
    pearls and pitfalls, 205
  magnetic resonance imaging in, 194, 195–196, 195*f*, 197*f*, 205
  pathology, 194
  radiography in, 194, 204–205
  serology, 194
  synovitis in, 200–201, 200*f*, 201*f*, 202*f*
  tenosynovitis in, 52, 52*f*, 82, 83*f*, 200, 201*f*
    differential diagnosis, 204, 205*f*
  therapeutic response, monitoring, 201–204, 204*f*, 205
  treatment, 194
  ultrasound in, 194, 195*f*, 196–197, 196*f*
    artifacts, 204, 205*f*
    pearls and pitfalls, 205, 205*f*, 206*f*
    technique for, 200

wrist involvement in, 46, 52, 52*f*, 53*f*, 82, 83*f*
Rheumatoid nodule(s), 166, 166*f*
Rotator cuff
arthropathy, 11–13
compressibility, tears and, 11
impingement, assessment, dynamic maneuvers for, 5–6, 6*f*
repair, postoperative ultrasound, 11–13
ultrasound, 13–15
pitfalls, 13
Rotator cuff tear
acute *versus* chronic, 7*f*, 11, 11*f*, 12*f*
in critical zone, 7, 9*f*
full-thickness
focal (small)
magnetic resonance imaging, 9*f*
ultrasound, 7, 8*f*–9*f*
total (large)
magnetic resonance imaging, 7*f*, 8*f*
ultrasound, 7, 7*f*, 8*f*
intrasubstance, ultrasound, 9, 10*f*
minor criteria for, 7*f*, 9–11, 11*f*, 12*f*
partial-thickness, ultrasound, 7, 10*f*
recurrence, 11–13
in rheumatoid arthritis, 196*f*

S
Sarcoma, biopsy, ultrasound-guided, 221
Saturday night nerve palsy, 182
Scalenus anterior muscle, 174*f*
Scalenus medius muscle, 174*f*
SCAM. *See* Scalenus anterior muscle
Scaphoid bone, 47
fracture, 55, 56*f*–57*f*
Scapholunate ligament, 199
ganglia, 64*f*
SCC. *See* Squamous cell carcinoma
Schwannoma(s)
hand, 89, 90*f*
sonographic features, 189, 190*f*, 191*f*
wrist, 63–64, 65*f*
Sciatic nerve, 176
division
high, 179
in popliteal fossa, 176, 179
ultrasound, 172*f*
SCMM. *See* Scalenus medius muscle
Sebaceous cyst. *See* Epidermal cyst
Semimembranosus tendon, 93, 94*f*
Semitendinosus tendon, 93, 94*f*
Sesamoid bones, 81, 82*f*
Shoulder
arthrography, 20, 20*t*
bursal effusion, 17–19, 18*f*
calcification puncture and lavage, ultrasound-guided, 222–230, 227*f*–230*f*
calcifying bursitis
computed tomography, 17*f*
magnetic resonance imaging, 16*f*, 17*f*
ultrasound, 15–17, 16*f*
calcifying tendonitis
computed tomography, 15*f*
magnetic resonance imaging, 16*f*
ultrasound, 15, 15*f*, 16*f*
computed tomography, 20, 20*t*
indications for, 20
dislocation, 132
imaging investigation, algorithm for, 20
impingement syndrome, 15, 15*f*
joint effusion, 17–19, 18*f*
magnetic resonance imaging, 20, 20*t*
indications for, 20
pathology, ultrasound, 7–19
ultrasound
artifacts, 19–20
comparison to other imaging modalities, 20, 20*t*
equipment for, 1
examination protocol, 1
indications for, 20
normal anatomy on, 1–7
patient positioning for, 1
pearls and pitfalls, 20
transducer for, 1
ultrasound-guided injection in, 236
Skier's thumb, 86
Skin
abscess, 161
accessory muscles and, 169–170, 169*f*
anatomic variants, 168–170
biopsy, 147
cysts, 149, 149*f*–151*f*
fat necrosis in, 160–161, 163*f*
fistulous tracts, 157–160, 162*f*
fluid collections in, 161
foreign bodies in, 170, 170*f*
hematoma in, 161
histology, 147
imaging investigation, algorithm for, 170
infectious disorders, 157–166
inflammatory disorders, 157–166
large vessel thrombosis and, 156, 160*f*
magnetic resonance imaging, limitations, 147
normal anatomy, 148, 148*f*
pathology, 149–168
perforant veins, insufficiency, 156–157, 161*f*
tumors
benign, 149–150, 149*f*–152*f*
malignant, 150–151, 153*f*–155*f*
vascular, 151–155, 156*f*–159*f*
ultrasound
advantages, 147
for ancillary diagnosis, 147

Skin (*continued*)
- artifacts, 170
- indications for, 147–148
- limitations, 148
- *pearls and pitfalls*, 170
- preoperative, 148
- for primary diagnosis, 147
- technical guidelines for, 148
- in therapeutics, 148
- for treatment monitoring, 147

vascular lesions
- nontumoral, 155–157, 159*f*–162*f*
- tumoral, 151–155, 156*f*–159*f*

Skin cancer, 150–151, 153*f*–155*f*
- nonmelanoma, 150

Skin disorders, and musculoskeletal disorders, 147
Skull tumor, 145*f*
Snapping triceps syndrome, 173, 180, 181*f*
Snapping ulnaris syndrome, 173, 180, 181*f*
Soft-tissue mass(es)
- algorithm for, 242
- biopsy, ultrasound-guided, 220–222

Sound reflection *(R)*
- at air-tissue interface, 132
- at bone-tissue interface, 132

Spinoglenoid notch, ultrasound, transverse image, 3, 4*f*
Squamous cell carcinoma, 150, 154*f*
Stener's lesion, 86
Step-off deformity, 132, 133*f*
Sternal metastasis, 146*f*
Steroid injection
- adverse effects and side effects, 241–242
- chondrotoxic effects, 241
- ultrasound-guided, 236, 237*f*

Subacromial bursa
- concave contour, rotator cuff tear and, 9, 11*f*
- effusion, rotator cuff tear and, 9, 11*f*
- ultrasound-guided injection in, 236

Subacromial-subdeltoid bursa
- bursitis, 17–19, 18*f*
  - communicating, 17
  - noncommunicating, 17–19
- effusion, rotator cuff tear and, 11*f*, 17, 18*f*

Subclavian artery, 173, 174*f*
Subcutaneous tissue, ultrasound appearance, 148, 148*f*
Subdeltoid bursa
- calcifying bursitis, 16*f*, 17*f*
- ultrasound-guided injection in, 236

Subscapularis bursa, calcifying bursitis, 16*f*, 17*f*
Subscapularis tendon
- calcification, 230*f*
- partial-thickness tear
  - magnetic resonance imaging, 10*f*
  - ultrasound, 10*f*
- ultrasound
  - longitudinal image, 2, 3*f*
  - transverse image, 1, 3*f*

Subungual exostoses, 168, 169*f*
Superficial palmar arch, 78–79
Superficial palmar artery, 78
Supinator syndrome, 182, 182*f*
Suprapatellar recess, 92, 92*f*
- fluid in, 98–99, 98*f*, 99*f*

Supraspinatus tendon
- calcific tendinitis, calcification puncture and lavage, ultrasound-guided, 222, 227*f*, 228*f*
- calcifying tendonitis, 15, 15*f*–16*f*
- critical zone
  - focal full-thickness tear, 9*f*
  - partial-thickness tear, 10*f*
- focal full-thickness tear
  - magnetic resonance imaging, 9*f*
  - ultrasound, 8*f*, 9*f*
- full-thickness tear, and biceps tendon dislocation, 19
- ganglion cyst, aspiration, ultrasound-guided, 232*f*
- intrasubstance tear, ultrasound, 10*f*
- large full-thickness tear
  - magnetic resonance imaging, 7*f*
  - ultrasound, 7*f*
- partial-thickness tear, ultrasound, 10*f*
- tear, in rheumatoid arthritis, 196*f*
- ultrasound
  - longitudinal image, 5, 5*f*
  - transverse image, 3–5, 5*f*

Symphysis pubis, subluxation, 135
Synovial cell sarcoma, 216*f*–217*f*
Synovitis
- Doppler signal semiquantitative grading, 201, 202*f*
- in rheumatoid arthritis, 200–201, 200*f*, 201*f*, 202*f*

T

TA. *See* Tibialis anterior tendon
Talonavicular ligament, 108
Talus, 107*f*, 108*f*, 109*f*, 111*f*, 113*f*
Tarsal tunnel, contents, 108, 109*f*, 178*f*, 179
Tarsal tunnel syndrome, 186, 186*f*
Telangiectasis, 156
Tendinitis, calcific
- algorithm for, 242
- calcification puncture and lavage, ultrasound-guided, 222–230, 227*f*–230*f*

Tendon(s), anisotropy, on ultrasound, 1, 2*f*, 18*f*, 19, 91, 116
Tendon sheath injection, algorithm for, 242
Tennis elbow, 182
- ultrasound-guided injection in, 236–237

Tennis leg, 101, 101*f*–102*f*